How to access the supplemental web resource

We are pleased to provide access to a web resource that supplements your textbook, *Core Concepts in Athletic Training and Therapy*. This resource provides 41 modules you can use to demonstrate mastery in key competency areas.

Accessing the web resource is easy!
Follow these steps if you purchased a new book:

1. Visit **www.HumanKinetics.com/CoreConceptsInAthleticTrainingAndTherapy**.

2. Click the <u>first edition</u> link next to the book cover.

3. Click the Sign In link on the left or top of the page. If you do not have an account with Human Kinetics, you will be prompted to create one.

4. If the online product you purchased does not appear in the Ancillary Items box on the left of the page, click the Enter Key Code option in that box. Enter the key code that is printed at the right, including all hyphens. Click the Submit button to unlock your online product.

5. After you have entered your key code the first time, you will never have to enter it again to access this product. Once unlocked, a link to your product will permanently appear in the menu on the left. On future visits to the site, all you need to do is sign in to the textbook's website and follow the link!

→ Click the Need Help? button on the textbook's website if you need assistance along the way.

How to access the web resource if you purchased a used book:

You may purchase access to the web resource by visiting the text's website, **www.HumanKinetics.com/CoreConceptsInAthleticTrainingAndTherapy**, or by calling the following:

800-747-4457 . . . . .U.S. customers
800-465-7301 . . . . .Canadian customers
+44 (0) 113 255 5665 . . . . European customers
08 8372 0999 . . . . Australian customers
0800 222 062 . . . . .New Zealand customers
217-351-5076 . . . . .International customers

For technical support, send an e-mail to:
support@hkusa.com . . . . U.S. and international customers
info@hkcanada.com . . . . Canadian customers
academic@hkeurope.com . . . . European customers
keycodesupport@hkaustralia.com . . . . . Australian and New Zealand customers

HUMAN KINETICS
The Information Leader in Physical Activity & Health

11–2011

Product: Core Concepts in Athletic Training and Therapy web resource

Key code: HILLMAN-LYJK8H-OSG

This unique code allows you access to the web resource.

Access is provided if you have purchased a new book. Once submitted, the code may not be entered for any other user.

Core Concepts in Athletic Training and Therapy

ATHLETIC TRAINING EDUCATION SERIES

Core Concepts in Athletic Training and Therapy

ATHLETIC TRAINING EDUCATION SERIES

Susan Kay Hillman, ATC, PT

A.T. Still University

Editor

▼ ▼ ▼

David H. Perrin, PhD, ATC, FNATA

The University of North Carolina at Greensboro

Series Editor

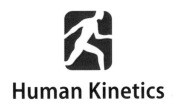

Human Kinetics

Library of Congress Cataloging-in-Publication Data

Core concepts in athletic training and therapy / Susan Kay Hillman, editor.
   p. ; cm. -- (Athletic training education series)
 Includes bibliographical references and index.
 ISBN-13: 978-0-7360-8285-3 (hard cover)
 ISBN-10: 0-7360-8285-9 (hard cover)
 I. Hillman, Susan Kay, 1952- II. Series: Athletic training education series.
 [DNLM: 1. Physical Education and Training. 2. Athletic Injuries--therapy. QT 255]

 617.1'027--dc23

2011032146

ISBN: 978-0-7360-8285-3 (print)

The web addresses cited in this text were current as of July 2011, unless otherwise noted.

Acquisitions Editors: Loarn D. Robertson, PhD, and Melinda Flegel; **Series Developmental Editor:** Amanda S. Ewing; **Developmental Editor:** Amanda S. Ewing; **Assistant Editor:** Kali Cox; **Copyeditor:** Joyce Sexton; **Indexer:** Sharon Duffy; **Permissions Manager:** Dalene Reeder; **Graphic Designer:** Fred Starbird; **Graphic Artist:** Dawn Sills; **Cover Designer:** Keith Blomberg; **Photographer (cover):** Jamie Squire/Getty Images; **Photographs (interior):** © Human Kinetics, unless otherwise noted; **Photo Asset Manager:** Laura Fitch; **Visual Production Assistant:** Joyce Brumfield; **Photo Production Manager:** Jason Allen; **Art Manager:** Kelly Hendren; **Associate Art Manager:** Alan L. Wilborn; **Art Style Development:** Joanne Brummett; **Illustrations:** © Human Kinetics, unless otherwise noted; **Printer:** Walsworth Print

We thank A.T. Still University in Mesa, Arizona, for assistance in providing the location for the photo shoot for this book. We thank Ted Wendel of ImagedByTed, LLC, for taking the photos.

Printed in the United States of America   10 9 8 7 6 5 4 3 2

Human Kinetics
Website: www.HumanKinetics.com

United States: Human Kinetics
P.O. Box 5076
Champaign, IL 61825-5076
800-747-4457
e-mail: humank@hkusa.com

Canada: Human Kinetics
475 Devonshire Road Unit 100
Windsor, ON N8Y 2L5
800-465-7301 (in Canada only)
e-mail: info@hkcanada.com

Europe: Human Kinetics
107 Bradford Road
Stanningley
Leeds LS28 6AT, United Kingdom
+44 (0) 113 255 5665
e-mail: hk@hkeurope.com

Australia: Human Kinetics
57A Price Avenue
Lower Mitcham, South Australia 5062
08 8372 0999
e-mail: info@hkaustralia.com

New Zealand: Human Kinetics
P.O. Box 80
Mitcham Shopping Centre, South Australia 5062
0800 222 062
e-mail: info@hknewzealand.com

E4799

Contents

Introduction to Athletic Training 1

Susan Kay Hillman, ATC, PT

PART I   Prevention and Health Promotion 21

CHAPTER 1   The Preparticipation Physical Examination 23

Susan Kay Hillman, ATC, PT

CHAPTER 2   Fitness Testing and Conditioning 49

Susan Kay Hillman, ATC, PT

Introduction to the Athletic Training Education Series

The six titles of the Athletic Training Education Series—*Core Concepts in Athletic Training and Therapy, Examination of Musculoskeletal Injuries, Therapeutic Exercise for Musculoskeletal Injuries, Therapeutic Modalities for Musculoskeletal Injuries, Management Strategies in Athletic Training,* and *Developing Clinical Proficiency in Athletic Training*—are textbooks for students of athletic training and references for practicing certified athletic trainers. Other allied health care professionals, such as physical therapists, physician's assistants, and occupational therapists, will also find these texts to be invaluable resources in the prevention, examination, treatment, and rehabilitation of injuries to physically active people.

The rapidly evolving profession of athletic training necessitates a continual updating of the educational resources available to educators, students, and practitioners. The authors of the six books in the series have made key improvements and have added information based on the most recent version of the NATA *Athletic Training Educational Competencies* before publication.

- *Core Concepts in Athletic Training and Therapy,* which replaces *Introduction to Athletic Training,* is suitable for introductory athletic training courses. Part I of the text introduces students to the idea of prevention. It also addresses the preparticipation exam (PPE), introduces aspects of fitness testing and conditioning in athletes, looks at the nutrition aspects of health and performance, examines how the environment affects athletic participation, looks at the protective devices used in various sports, and introduces methods of taping and bracing. Part II covers clinical exami-

nation and diagnosis, including injury mechanism and classification; the principles of primary and secondary surveys; injuries and conditions that affect the upper and lower extremities, spine, head, neck, thorax, and abdomen; and general medical conditions. Part III covers acute and emergency care, including planning for emergency situations, immediate care for emergency situations, moving and transporting injured athletes, creating an emergency care plan, and obtaining consent for emergency care. Part IV covers therapeutic interventions, including rehabilitation and healing, therapeutic treatment modalities used in athletics, therapeutic exercise parameters and techniques, and pharmacology in athletic training. Part V introduces topics related to health care administration, including information on management functions and insurance. Part VI covers advanced concepts, such as pathophysiology of tissue injury, psychology of sport injury, and evidence-based practice in athletic training. *Core Concepts in Athletic Training and Therapy* fills the need for a text that covers myriad topics at an introductory level. It sets the stage for the other books in the series, which delve much deeper into specific topics.

- In *Examination of Musculoskeletal Injuries,* new information about sensitivity and specificity strengthens the evidence-based selection of special tests, and an increased emphasis on clinical decision making and problem solving and the integration of skill application in the end-of-chapter activities are now included.

- Two new chapters have been added to *Therapeutic Exercise for Musculoskeletal Injuries*. Chapter 16 focuses on arthroplasty, and chapter 17 contains information regarding various age considerations in rehabilitation. This text also provides more support of evidence-based care resulting from a blend of research results and the author's 40 years of experience as a clinician.

- The new edition of *Developing Clinical Proficiency in Athletic Training* contains 26 new modules, and embedded within it is the NATA *Athletic Training Educational Competencies*. The concepts of progressive clinical skill development, clinical supervision and autonomy, and clinical decision making are introduced and explained. The nature of critical thinking and why it is essential to clinical practice are also discussed.

- The third edition of *Therapeutic Modalities for Musculoskeletal Injuries* continues to provide readers with information on evidence-based practice and includes recent developments in the areas of inflammation and laser therapy.

- The fourth edition of *Management Strategies in Athletic Training* continues to help undergraduate and graduate students master entry-level concepts related to administration in athletic training. Each of the 10 chapters is thoroughly updated, and new material is presented on topics such as evidence-based medicine, professionalism in athletic training, health care financial management, cultural competence, injury surveillance systems, legal updates, and compensation for athletic trainers.

The Athletic Training Education Series offers a coordinated approach to the process of preparing students for the Board of Certification examination. If you are a student of athletic training, you must master the material in each of the content areas delineated in the NATA *Athletic Training Educational Competencies*. The Athletic Training Education Series addresses each of the competencies sequentially and thoroughly. The series covers the content areas developed by the NATA Executive Committee for Education of the National Athletic Trainers' Association for accredited curriculum development. The content areas and the texts that address each content area are as follows:

- Risk management and injury prevention *(Core Concepts* and *Management Strategies)*
- Pathology of injury and illnesses *(Core Concepts, Examination, Therapeutic Exercise,* and *Therapeutic Modalities)*
- Orthopedic assessment and diagnosis *(Examination* and *Therapeutic Exercise)*
- Acute care *(Core Concepts, Examination,* and *Management Strategies)*
- Pharmacology *(Core Concepts* and *Therapeutic Modalities)*
- Conditioning and rehabilitative exercise *(Therapeutic Exercise)*
- Therapeutic modalities *(Core Concepts* and *Therapeutic Modalities)*
- Medical conditions and disabilities *(Core Concepts* and *Examination)*
- Nutrition aspects of injury and illness *(Core Concepts)*
- Psychosocial intervention and referral *(Therapeutic Modalities* and *Therapeutic Exercise)*
- Administration *(Core Concepts* and *Management Strategies)*
- Professional development and responsibilities *(Core Concepts* and *Management Strategies)*

The authors for this series—Craig Denegar, Peggy Houglum, Richard Ray, Jeff Konin, Ethan Saliba, Susan Saliba, Sandra Shultz, Ken Knight, Kirk Brumels, Susan Hillman, and I—are certified athletic trainers with well over a century of collective experience as clinicians, educators, and leaders in the athletic training profession. The clinical experience of the authors spans virtually every setting in which athletic trainers practice: high schools, sports medicine clinics, universities, professional sports, hospitals, and industrial settings. The professional positions of the authors include undergraduate and graduate curriculum director, head athletic trainer, professor, clinic director, and researcher. The authors have chaired or served on the NATA's most prominent committees, including Professional Education Committee, Education Task Force, Education Council, Research Committee of the Research and Education Foundation, Journal Committee, Appropriate Medical Coverage for Intercollegiate Athletics Task Force, and Continuing Education Committee.

This series is the most progressive collection of texts and instructional materials currently available to athletic training students and educators. Several elements are present in most of the books in the series:

- Chapter objectives and summaries are tied to one another so that students will know and achieve their learning goals.
- Chapter-opening scenarios illustrate the relevance of the chapter content.
- Thorough reference lists allow for further reading and research.

To enhance instruction, various ancillaries are included:

- All of the texts (except for *Developing Clinical Proficiency in Athletic Training*) include instructor guides and test banks.
- *Therapeutic Exercise for Musculoskeletal Injuries* includes a presentation package plus image bank.
- *Core Concepts in Athletic Training and Therapy*, *Therapeutic Modalities for Musculoskeletal Injuries*, and *Examination of Musculoskeletal Injuries* all include image banks.

- *Examination of Musculoskeletal Injuries* includes an online student resource.
- *Core Concepts in Athletic Training and Therapy* includes a web resource.

Presentation packages include text slides plus select images from the text. Image banks include most of the figures, tables, and content photos from the book. Instructors can use these images to create their own presentations and to enhance lectures and demonstration sessions. Other features vary from book to book, depending on the subject matter; but all include various aids for assimilation and review of information, extensive illustrations, and material to help students apply the facts in the text to real-world situations.

The order in which the books should be used is determined by the philosophy of each curriculum director. In any case, each book can stand alone so that a curriculum director does not need to revamp an entire curriculum in order to use one or more parts of the series.

When I entered the profession of athletic training over 30 years ago, one text—*Prevention and Care of Athletic Injuries* by Klafs and Arnheim—covered nearly all the subject matter required for passing the Board of Certification examination and practicing as an entry-level athletic trainer. Since that time, we have witnessed an amazing expansion of the information and skills one must master in order to practice athletic training, along with an equally impressive growth of practice settings in which athletic trainers work. You will find these updated editions of the Athletic Training Education Series textbooks to be invaluable resources as you prepare for a career as a certified athletic trainer, and you will find them to be useful references in your professional practice.

__David H. Perrin, PhD, ATC, FNATA__
__Series Editor__

Contributors

Kirk Brumels, PhD, AT, ATC
Director, Athletic Training Program
Associate professor of kinesiology
Athletic trainer
Hope College

Craig R. Denegar, PhD, ATC, PT, FNATA
Professor
University of Connecticut

Frances A. Flint, PhD, CAT(C), ATC
Coordinator of the Athletic Therapy
Certificate
York University

Eric J. Fuchs, DA, ATC, EMT-B
Director, Athletic Training Education
Program
Associate professor
Eastern Kentucky University

Peggy A. Houglum, PhD, ATC, PT
Associate professor
Duquesne University

Laura J. Kenow, MS, ATC
Associate professor and Athletic Training
Education Program director
Linfield College

Tamara C. Valovich McLeod, PhD, ATC, FNATA
John P. Wood, D.O., Endowed Chair for
Sports Medicine
Associate professor, Athletic Training
Program
A.T. Still University

David H. Perrin, PhD, ATC, FNATA
Provost, vice chancellor for academic
affairs
School of Health and Human Performance
Professor
University of North Carolina
at Greensboro

Richard Ray, EdD, ATC
Provost
Hope College

Susan Saliba, PhD, ATC, PT, FNATA
Assistant professor
University of Virginia at Charlottesville

Sandra J. Shultz, PhD, ATC, CSCS, FNATA
Associate professor, director of graduate
study
University of North Carolina
at Greensboro

Diane M. Wiese-Bjornstal, PhD, CC-AASP
Associate professor and director
of graduate studies
University of Minnesota at Minneapolis

Preface

Core Concepts in Athletic Training and Therapy is an excellent textbook for the entry-level athletic training student, the coaching student, and students in other health care fields wishing to further their understanding of the profession of athletic training. The text was written by a unique combination of world-recognized authors who have had years of experience at the professional and collegiate levels and are also highly recognized educators in athletic training. Through the concerted efforts of experts in athletic training and athletic training education, Core Concepts in Athletic Training and Therapy provides a much-needed comprehensive introductory textbook for athletic training courses. It will facilitate the introduction of students to the world and work of the athletic trainer.

Core Concepts in Athletic Training and Therapy provides material sufficient to enable a thorough understanding of athletic training in a course spanning two quarters or one full semester. Using it in chronological order will provide a clear pathway through the field of athletic training, from an introduction to the profession through to evaluation, treatment, and all aspects of sport health care to the more advanced aspects of administration and management. Core Concepts in Athletic Training and Therapy will remain a reference text for curriculum students as they move into the advanced courses. Chapters of Core Concepts in Athletic Training and Therapy will become their quick reference time after time and will certainly be the core text for them to use in reviewing for their certification examination.

Core Concepts in Athletic Training and Therapy is a complete resource for understanding and addressing the National Athletic Trainers' Association (NATA) published competencies. Core Concepts in Athletic Training and Therapy will help students progress to a complete understanding of the athletic trainer's roles and responsibilities, from those involved in the first day of their association with the patient in the preparticipation physical exam through to the more advanced administrative functions of the athletic trainer.

Throughout this text the terms athletic trainer and athletic therapist are to be considered synonymous. Although different, these two terms are the most common international usages and collectively define the scope of the profession. In Canada, for instance, the Canadian Athletic Therapists Association, or CATA (www.athletictherapy. org), maintains a Mutual Recognition Agreement (MRA) with the U.S.-based Board of Certification (BOC) due to the equivalent practice standards and core competencies required of the two organizations. This MRA permits a person who has successfully graduated with a degree from an accredited athletic training or therapy program and holds a current certification with either CATA or BOC to directly challenge the certification exam of the other accrediting organization (CATA or BOC). In reading further, please consider athletic trainer and athletic therapist to be equivalent.

Organization

We begin the book with "Introduction to Athletic Training." This stand-alone chapter familiarizes the reader with the profession of athletic training. It discusses training and education; licensure and certification as an ATC; and the various sports medicine organizations, including NATA. The chapter also covers the history of athletic training, employment opportunities for athletic trainers, and the roles of the members of the sports medicine team.

Part I: Prevention and Health Promotion

This part of the book covers the core area of the athletic trainer's function: prevention. Prevention is not one single function but a multitude of different functions that help to keep the patient healthy and performing on the court or field.

Chapter 1 looks at the athletic trainer's association with the client through the pre-participation physical examination (PPE). The chapter covers the main components of the PPE, methods for setting up an exam for a large group, and various forms that are useful in designing a PPE.

Chapter 2 is devoted to fitness testing procedures and fitness testing parameters, including muscle function, cardiovascular function, agility and speed, flexibility, and body composition. The second half of the chapter focuses on developing an appropriate strength training program and the various types of strength training. Integrating cardiovascular training and flexibility programs is also discussed.

Chapter 3 covers basic nutritional and fluid needs for the physically active patient. The roles of the three major nutrients (carbohydrates, fats, and proteins) and the percentage of daily calories that should come from each are discussed. Nutritional concerns important to patients such as preevent meals, managing weight, and dietary supplements are covered, as are nutritional concerns in injury and illness.

Chapter 4 discusses environmental conditions. Consideration of body cooling mechanisms provides a base for understanding the participant's response to extreme heat and cold. The chapter then presents the symptoms of and treatment for heat illnesses. Information about other environmental conditions will stimulate thought-provoking discussion. These include weather conditions such as storms and lightning as well as facility safety considerations.

Chapter 5 is an eclectic chapter that discusses protective equipment and devices and the standards and regulations surrounding their development. It details the rules and requirements for protective equipment for each sport, as well as legal concerns important to the manufacturer and the athletic trainer. The chapter also introduces basic skills for fitting protective equipment.

Chapter 6 covers techniques for taping and bracing. It focuses on the most common techniques and applications and explains concepts related to supporting athletic injuries with tape.

Part II: Clinical Examination and Diagnosis

This part includes six chapters designed to introduce the student to the problem-solving function inherent to athletic training. Each chapter will give readers an understanding of particular knowledge and skills needed for accurate injury assessment.

Chapter 7 focuses on injury mechanisms and the classification of injuries as an introduction to the clinical exam. Injury mechanisms and the ways in which injuries are classified are discussed. The chapter reviews the anatomical reference position and presents terminology that is important in documentations the athletic trainer must produce. The chapter also discusses acute and chronic conditions and the classification of injuries to soft tissues, bones and joints. and nerve tissue.

Chapter 8, on the components of the athletic injury examination, presents a review of the primary survey and discusses the secondary survey, history taking, and objective measures. These include observation; palpation; and examination of motion, strength, neurological status, and cardiovascular and respiratory status. This chapter also covers the appropriate use of all exam components, depending on the setting (on-site, clinic), and concludes with information on documenting the exam.

Chapters 9, 10, and 11 present region-specific examination strategies. Each chapter focuses on common injuries and emphasizes how to recognize them. Basic objective tests, physical exam strategies, and injury mechanisms are also presented. The chapters in this section cover mechanisms, signs, and symptoms of common injuries occurring in particular anatomical regions:

- The upper body, including the shoulder, arm, elbow, forearm, wrist, and hand (chapter 9)
- The lower body, including the hip and pelvis, thigh, knee, leg, ankle, and foot (chapter 10)
- The spine, head, face, thorax, and abdomen (chapter 11)

These three chapters also cover objective tests and exam strategies appropriate for injuries occurring in these regions.

Chapter 12 deals with medical conditions that an athletic trainer is likely to encounter in physically active individuals. Emphasis is on recognition and referral, based on history and observation, rather than on special diagnostic tests. Conditions are discussed according to body system: the cardiovascular, respiratory, digestive, endocrine, reproductive, urinary, musculoskeletal, nervous, and integumentary systems and EENT (eyes, ears, nose, and throat).

Part III: Acute and Emergency Care

Acute care means two things to the athletic trainer: day-to-day evaluation of athletic illness and injury and the emergency situations that occur from time to time.

Chapter 13 introduces the role of the athletic trainer as both the medical referral point and the first responder in the emergency situation. The chapter begins by discussing the development of an emergency action plan and the role of the athletic trainer as well as others on the emergency medical team. The chapter addresses the acute care of life-threatening as well as non-life-threatening conditions—conditions that frequently call for controlling visible bleeding. The chapter addresses sterile technique in wound care and the use of Universal Precautions to avoid transference of bloodborne pathogens.

Chapter 14 introduces the ABCs of emergency care and begins discussion of cardiopulmonary resuscitation. It also addresses the emergency medical services (EMS) and EMS team. The chapter includes a discussion of the consent forms that should be obtained prior to the first day of participation.

Part IV: Therapeutic Interventions

This part of the book covers topics related to returning the patient to sport participation, from the use and application of therapeutic modalities during healing to the therapeutic exercises that help the individual regain muscle and joint function. The chapter on pharmacology will help students realize the role that pharmaceuticals have in the healing process.

Chapter 15 introduces students to rehabilitation in the athletic training setting. It discusses the basic components of a rehabilitation program and therapeutic exercise, as well as return-to-competition criteria. It also covers the healing process and factors that affect healing.

Chapter 16 provides an overview of the many therapeutic modalities available to the athletic trainer. Beginning with relatively basic heat and cold therapies, the chapter also covers ultrasound, electrotherapy, and massage and manual therapies. For each type of therapy, the physiological basis for its use is discussed, as well as methods of application, indications for use, and contraindications and cautions.

Chapter 17 introduces the athletic training student to the therapeutic exercise techniques that are used in the progression through a rehabilitation program. The first part of the chapter deals with restoring range of motion and flexibility. The discussion then focuses on restoring muscular strength and endurance, reestablishing neuromuscular control and proprioception, and incorporating plyometrics. Functional and sport-specific exercises are the focus of the last part of the chapter.

Chapter 18 introduces the athletic training student to basic concepts of pharmacology, including drug nomenclature and classification, pharmacokinetics, and pharmacodynamics. The bulk of the chapter is devoted to discussion of specific drugs, such as anti-inflammatory agents, analgesics, muscle relaxants, decongestants, bronchodilators, and antibacterial agents.

Part V: Health Care Administration

Part V provides a glimpse into the world of the staff athletic trainer and helps the student understand the vast responsibilities of the ATC. While this material is rarely covered in an introductory athletic training text, it is included here to give students a full picture of the world of athletic training.

Chapter 19 covers the many management strategies that athletic trainers must be aware of. These include program management (strategic planning, developing a policies and procedures manual), human resource management (staff selection, supervision, and evaluation), financial resource management (budgeting, purchasing, inventory management), facility design and planning, and information management (documentation and record keeping).

Chapter 20 discusses how insurance systems function and how to process claims. It briefly covers basic legal principles but places more emphasis on ways to reduce risk of legal liability, such as credentialing, risk management procedures, and awareness of regulations concerning medications.

Part VI: Advanced Athletic Training Concepts

This final part provides the entry-level student with information that is often reserved for the graduate or upper-level student in athletic training. This material is central to a full understanding of the roles and responsibilities of the athletic trainer and is an important addition to an entry-level textbook.

Chapter 21 presents the advanced concepts of the pathophysiology and pathomechanics of sports injury and describes the response of tissue to injury. These are concepts that are often reserved for upper-level students and graduate students but are important to a full understanding of the injury and healing processes.

Chapter 22 explores the patient's psychological response to injury and the ways in which it can affect rehabilitation. The discussion emphasizes maximizing compliance with the rehabilitation protocol and avoiding depression and other barriers to successful recovery.

Chapter 23 presents evidence-based practice as a concept of athletic training. The chapter introduces readers to the process of scrutinizing published research studies to gain a better understanding of the evidence. Application of research to clinical practice is discussed, as are techniques athletic trainers can use to establish their own evidenced-based practice.

Special Features

Several special features throughout the book will help students understand and retain the information presented in each chapter.

- **Chapter objectives.** Each chapter begins with a list of objectives that help set the stage for the discussion and give a glimpse of the topics that will be covered.

- **Key Concepts and Review.** Following study of the chapter, students can compare their thinking on the objectives to those of the author(s) in the Key Concepts and Review section. This section shows how the text addressed each objective.

- **Critical Thinking Questions.** These questions present a scenario and challenge students to apply knowledge that they have gained in the chapter. Instructors can also use these questions to stimulate discussion in class.

- **Case Study.** A number of chapters include case studies to stimulate thought and provide instructors with discussion points. The case studies appear in the more applied chapters of the book, particularly those that have content related to therapy and working with injured patients.

- **Key terms.** Key terms are highlighted throughout the text, giving students a quick reference to terms as they are introduced. Full definitions are provided in the glossary.

- **Web resource.** The web resource provides 41 select clinical competency modules. Each module contains instructions to the student for demonstrating specific knowledge, developing specific skills, practicing the skills on a peer, practicing the skills on a patient, and then demonstrating competence to a peer teacher and to an ACI. Students can access the modules by going to www.HumanKinetics.com/Core ConceptsInAthleticTrainingAndTherapy. Once there, they can either fill out the modules online, or they can print out the modules and fill them out on a hard copy. (See Web Resource Instructions for more detailed information on the web resource.) Students are directed to the web resource at the end of each chapter by this type of wording:

PRACTICE!

For hands-on practice in this area, go to the web resource and complete the following:

Level 3.4, Module O6: Pre-Participation Medical and Physical Examination

In all, *Core Concepts in Athletic Training and Therapy* is a user-friendly text that is sure to become a much-used reference throughout the student's degree curriculum and career.

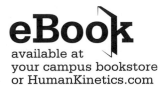

Instructor Resources

Three valuable ancillaries are provided to help instructors teach and test the book's content: the instructor guide, image bank, and test package.

The instructor guide contains several features that will help instructors facilitate the teaching of lecture materials and student activities.

- The chapter objectives listed in the text are repeated, helping you quickly review the main points of the chapter.

- The Chapter at a Glance feature includes the main headings from the chapter, helping you quickly construct lecture slides. The main topics will help you remember the salient points for your individualized lecture. Copy and paste the Chapter at a Glance into Power-Point and add figures and images from the Image Bank, and you have a great start to your chapter lecture.

- Active Learning Suggestions stimulate your thinking on ways to get your students actively involved. Through these helpful questions, you can involve your class in their discovery of information. Students remember better if they experience the learning, so what better way to involve a class in learning? Years of experience contributed to the *Core Concepts in Athletic Training and Therapy* Active Learning Suggestions. The authors' experience with actual situations is sure to bring the chapter material into focus.

- The Critical Thinking Questions are repeated from the chapter, and the authors' answers to the questions are provided. This material can be your lesson for the day, or it may stimulate different questions for your particular class. The excitement of this learning style will quickly make it your favorite. Use the questions in large-group discussions, small-group assignments, home study assignments, or even topics for presentation or reports. Some chapters in the guide include Critical Thinking Questions not presented in the book.

The image bank includes most of the figures, tables, and photos from the book. Instructors can use these images to supplement lecture slides, create handouts, or develop other teaching materials for their class.

The test package provides you with 20 or more multiple-choice, true/false, fill-in-the-blank, and essay-type questions for each chapter. You can use these questions to create quizzes or to supplement quizzes and tests you have created.

In addition to these instructor ancillaries, a web resource is available for students to access. Select clinical competency modules are identified for each chapter; instructors can assign these modules to their students as a way to help demonstrate student proficiency in different areas. Students can either print out these modules from the web resource and complete them on hard copy or can complete them online. (See Web Resource Instructions for more detailed information on the web resource.)

You can access these ancillary items by going to www.HumanKinetics.com/Core ConceptsInAthleticTrainingAndTherapy.

In addition to these ancillary items, instructors can use many of the textbook's features to help facilitate class planning and discussion:

- The Key Concepts and Review section at the end of each chapter gives instructors a review of the chapter objectives;

instructors can quickly compare their thinking with that of the authors.

- The Critical Thinking Questions can be used to foster classroom discussions using the years of experience of 12 seasoned athletic trainers. (Recall that the Instructor Guide provides the authors' answers to these and other Critical Thinking Questions to aid you in formulating discussion points.)

- You will find that slightly fewer than half of the chapters in *Core Concepts in Athletic Training and Therapy* contain case studies. These case studies were carefully selected to work within the more applied chapters of the book, particularly those chapters with content that relates to therapy and working with injured patients. The content of these chapters will be less familiar to students and often comprises more technical information but is presented at an introductory level in athletic training. The case studies present scenarios underscoring principles of rehabilitation and exercise that are appropriate for introductory-level students. The scenarios spotlight important features of the rehabilitation process that athletic trainers are exposed to. Readers will gain clear insights into the application of concepts developed within the chapter. "Think About It" questions that follow each case study require students to work back through the chapter to find appropriate responses or form logical responses to open-ended questions. Instructors can have students work through the case studies individually or in groups; another option is for instructors to elaborate or build on the cases based on their own personal experiences to illustrate other pertinent roles of the athletic trainer.

Web Resource Instructions

The web resource that accompanies this textbook contains 41 modules reproduced from *Developing Clinical Proficiency in Athletic Training: A Modular Approach, Fourth Edition,* by Kenneth L. Knight and Kirk Brumels (Human Kinetics, 2010). Each module contains instructions to the student for demonstrating specific knowledge, developing specific skills, practicing the skills on a peer, practicing the skills on a patient, and then demonstrating competence to a peer teacher and to an ACI. The 41 selected modules allow students to demonstrate mastery in several key competency areas as they relate to the content of *Core Concepts in Athletic Training and Therapy*.

Each module consists of four parts:

1. Objective or purpose of the module
2. NATA educational competencies that are embedded within the module
3. List of competencies, or specific performance skills that students must master to reach the objective
4. Proficiency demonstration and space for signatures of didactic, skills, peer, and clinical teachers when students have demonstrated that they are proficient in performing the competencies

Modules are arranged into three levels (numbered) and subgrouped within those levels (alphabetized and numbered), partly based on the difficulty and complexity of the skills involved. The three main levels are the following:

- Level 1: Introduction to Athletic Training Clinical Education
- Level 2: Individual Athletic Training Skills Development
- Level 3: Integrating and Polishing Skills

Basic skills developed during many level 1 and 2 modules are later integrated into more complex skills required for level 3 modules. Each subject area (block) is designated by a letter:

- A through Q modules develop specific clinical skills.
- X modules involve directed clinical experience.
- T modules are peer-teaching modules.
- O/P modules are oral and practical examinations.

Most of these blocks (A-Q) are located within a specific level; however, blocks X, T, and O/P are found across the three levels.

The skills included in the modules are skills students will use for a lifetime. Therefore, students should not cycle knowledge here (i.e., memorize, pass a test, forget the material, and move on to the next module of material). Students should review the material, work with peer teachers, and then practice, study, and practice. When they can use the material confidently, they demonstrate the competence, first to a peer teacher and then to an ACI.

Most work on the modules (both developing the skills and demonstrating competence) should occur during regular athletic training clinical hours as students study with each other during slack times. Work on modules must not interfere with clinical duties, but there usually is a great deal of time to work on them during team meetings, practices, and so on.

At the end of each chapter, students are directed to the modules that will help reinforce mastery of that chapter's content. Here is an example of the wording students will see at the end of the chapters:

PRACTICE!

For hands-on practice in this area, go to the web resource and complete the following:

Level 3.4, Module 06: Pre-Participation Medical and Physical Examination

Students can access the modules by going to www.HumanKinetics.com/Core

ConceptsInAthleticTrainingAndTherapy. Once there, they can either fill out the modules online, or they can print out the modules and fill them out on a hard copy. Either way, once the module is complete, it can be submitted to the instructor. Instructors can assign these modules as a regular classroom assignment, as a way for students to earn extra credit, or as elective tasks students can complete to gain additional knowledge. Instructors should feel free to integrate these modules into their syllabus to the level they feel will be most useful to their students.

Introduction to Athletic Training

Susan Kay Hillman, ATC, PT

OBJECTIVES

After reading this introduction, the student should be able to do the following:

- Describe the education, training, and licensure and certification of the athletic trainer.
- Provide a general history of the athletic training profession.
- Identify the top three employment settings for athletic trainers in 2009.
- Identify various employment opportunities for athletic trainers.
- Describe five members of the sports medicine team and explain the general duties of each.

"**A**thletic training" has long been thought to be a poor name for the profession. The term often elicits an image of strength training or conditioning rather than the medical service provided. Although agreement has not been reached in the decision to change the name, the profession of athletic training—through the National Athletic Trainers' Association (**NATA**) continues to strive toward greater public recognition. Do you know how the athletic trainer fits into the sports medicine team? Do you know who the other members of the sports medicine team are? This introduction answers these and related questions.

Becoming an NATA Certified Athletic Trainer

Just as students plan their route to becoming a coach, physical therapist, or lawyer, students interested in the athletic training profession should understand what lies ahead. As you progress through this text, you will learn about various aspects of the profession. In addition to your instructor, the athletic trainer at your institution can help guide your learning and skill development. Through your diligent study, your willingness to listen, your ability to learn and practice skills of evaluation and treatment, and your lifelong study and investigation, you can enjoy the exciting and rewarding profession of athletic training. Here we look at the educational and skill training aspects of the profession, the road to certification, and the Code of Ethics for the certified athletic trainer; we also take a look at the governing association, the NATA.

Training and Education

Athletic training requires at least 4 years of college education including at least 2 years of hands-on practice in evaluation, prevention, and management of athletic injuries. If an individual did not attend an athletic training educational program (ATEP)–accredited

school, the NATA would not have proof of completion of both the required course work and the clinical experience needed; thus the person seeking to become certified would not meet the standards set by the NATA. Athletic training educational programs are offered on many college campuses and are housed under programs like medicine, **kinesiology**, physical education, motor learning, **psychology**, human movement, and many others. Each ATEP program leader finds the best program to satisfy his program needs. It is easy to find listings for colleges offering athletic training degrees. Each program may seem a little different from the others, but all meet the same basic requirements of course work and clinical experience.

Colleges and universities offering athletic training programs for students must undergo accreditation. Organizations such as the Commission on Accreditation of Allied Health Higher Education Programs, (**CAAHEP**), the Committee on Allied Health Education and Accreditation (**CAHEA**) and The Commission on Accreditation of Athletic Training Education (**CAATE**) work with allied health/athletic training programs to ensure the level of education meets established standards. Currently the NATA works with CAATE in accreditation of the 350+ entry-level athletic training education programs.

Certification

To become certified as an athletic trainer, the student not only must satisfy the educational and experience requirements but also must pass a national **certification**[1] exam. Applicants first must satisfactorily complete an undergraduate degree at an accredited program; only then can one apply to take the certification exam. The athletic training curriculum subject matter requirements include the following:

- Prevention of athletic injuries/illnesses
- Evaluation of athletic injuries/illnesses
- First aid and emergency care

- Therapeutic modalities
- Therapeutic exercise
- Administration of athletic training programs
- Human anatomy
- Human physiology
- Exercise physiology
- Kinesiology/biomechanics
- Nutrition
- Psychology
- Personal/community health
- Instructional methods

The certification exam includes a written test of didactic information; a practical demonstration of athletic training skills; and a written simulation that tests problem solving, decision making, and critical thinking in the management of selected patient problems. The satisfactory completion of all three exams is required for entering the field of athletic training and earning the designation of ATC (certified athletic trainer). Once certified, athletic trainers must continue their education through any combination of continuing education programs and activities. The certified athletic trainer must verify accumulation of a predetermined number of CEUs during each 3-year term of membership. In addition to CEUs, the athletic trainer must show proof of having a current cardiopulmonary resuscitation (CPR) certificate. Members must adhere to the NATA Board of Certification (NATA BOC) Standards of Professional Practice as well as remain current in the payment of annual professional dues.

Licensure

In addition to becoming certified, practicing athletic trainers often need to become licensed in the state where they work. States with licensure may require an examination, others merely paperwork. Licensure helps to ensure legal practice of athletic training in the state. Techniques of athletic training are often construed as "physical therapy skills."

If a state does not have licensure for athletic trainers, people offering the same techniques as the athletic trainer could claim to be practicing "athletic training." On the other hand, athletic trainers often use the same skills and techniques as other professions; and if they do not have a license to perform those skills, they could be sued by another profession for practicing that profession without a license merely because they offer the same services. Figure I.1 shows the status of the states in gaining licensure for athletic training. Some states have opted for certification similar to the NATA certification. Other states have received an exemption to the practice act of similar professions, usually physical therapy. At the time of publication, only Alaska and California allowed athletic trainers to practice without a license.

Although licensure sounds like a difficult process, often it involves nothing than more than a few forms to complete. Some states do require a licensure examination, which may include, in addition to athletic training questions, questions about state regulations governing athletic trainers.

Code of Ethics

As with other professions, the NATA—the governing body for athletic trainers—has a well-established **code of ethics**. (Visit the NATA website to view its Code of Ethics.) The Code of Ethics was one of the first steps the NATA took as it became organized early in the 1950s. This code was written by athletic trainers and is enforced by fellow members of the organization. A system for evaluating infractions of the code is well established and ready for immediate activation. Infractions of the Code of Ethics may result in loss of certification privileges.

Organization

Although the committee dealing with the Code of Ethics is one of the oldest committees within the NATA, it is far from the only sign of organization. The number of committees, subcommittees, and organizations within the

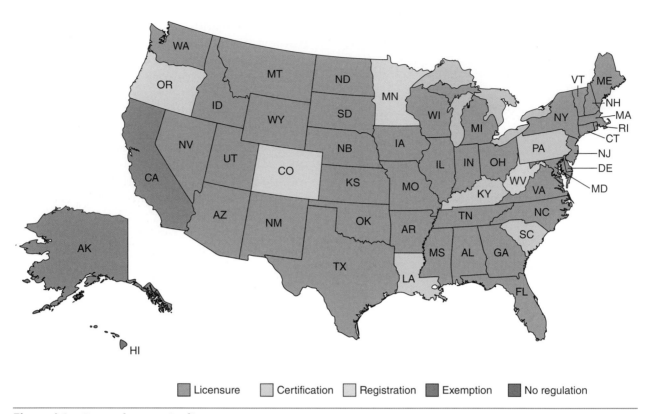

Figure I.1   States that require licensure.

Reprinted, by permission, from NATA. Available: http://cf.nata.org/legislators/map.htm?q=state-government/regulatory-boards

NATA is staggering. No area within athletic training is without representation in the NATA. Each state is represented within one of the 10 NATA districts. Figure I.2 illustrates the division into these 10 districts. A district chair represents each district. The district also has a leadership structure like that of the total organization. Athletic trainers may serve on committees locally in the state organization; they may serve a group of members from neighboring states through the district level; or they may serve a more global group of members through the national organization. A simple reporting structure maintains coordination of the organization from the state to the national level: State organizations report to the district level, and district organizations report to the national level. Research, scholarship programs, educational programs, and a multitude of committees operate throughout the various levels in the NATA. All levels within the NATA are eligible for financial and administrative assistance if

needed. The NATA provides money to state organizations for administrative costs of pursuing **licensure** as well as providing money to the Foundation to aid in the pursuit of its research and education goals (see the sidebar NATA Research and Education Foundation Goals).

History of Athletic Training

Just as familiarity with the early history of the United States helps us understand events that occur today, knowledge of the history of the NATA leads to a better understanding of the profession of athletic training. In the years preceding establishment of the NATA, information regarding the employment and function of the "trainer" was sparse. Not until the early 1950s did athletic trainers develop any organizational structure; then information and communication blossomed. The organization began very small, with only a

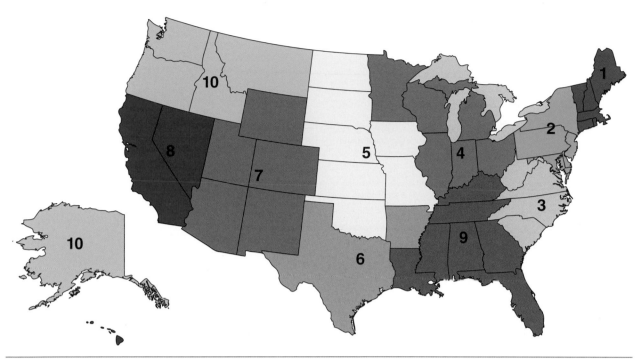

Figure I.2 National Athletic Trainers' Association districts.

Reprinted, by permission from NATA. Available: http://www.nata.org/Districts

NATA RESEARCH AND EDUCATION FOUNDATION GOALS

1. Advance the knowledge base of the athletic training profession.

2. Encourage research among athletic trainers who can contribute to the athletic training knowledge base.

3. Provide forums for the exchange of ideas pertaining to the athletic training knowledge base.

4. Facilitate the presentation of programs and the production of materials pro-

viding learning opportunities about athletic training topics.

5. Provide scholarships for undergraduate and graduate students of athletic training.

6. Plan and implement an ongoing total development program that establishes endowment funds, as well as restricted and unrestricted funds, that will support the research and educational goals of the Foundation.

Courtesy of John Oliver, former NATA Foundation Director

few athletic trainers across the nation—most of whom worked in the college or university setting. Since then the profession has grown to its current size of more than 35,000 people who have earned the ATC credential world-wide, covering a wide range of jobs in clinics, schools, professional sport, industry, health and fitness organizations, and educational institutions, to name just a few. See figure I.3 for a summary of this chronology.

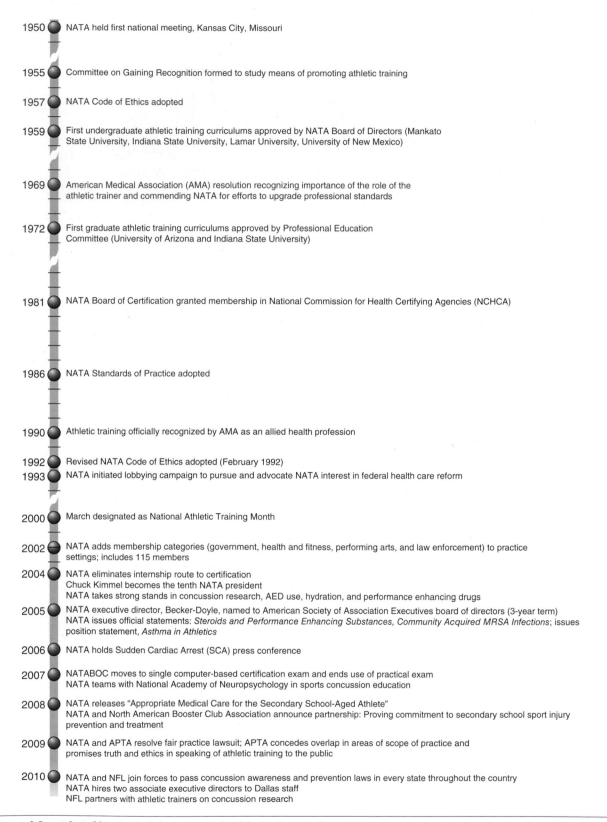

1950 ● NATA held first national meeting, Kansas City, Missouri

1955 ● Committee on Gaining Recognition formed to study means of promoting athletic training

1957 ● NATA Code of Ethics adopted

1959 ● First undergraduate athletic training curriculums approved by NATA Board of Directors (Mankato State University, Indiana State University, Lamar University, University of New Mexico)

1969 ● American Medical Association (AMA) resolution recognizing importance of the role of the athletic trainer and commending NATA for efforts to upgrade professional standards

1972 ● First graduate athletic training curriculums approved by Professional Education Committee (University of Arizona and Indiana State University)

1981 ● NATA Board of Certification granted membership in National Commission for Health Certifying Agencies (NCHCA)

1986 ● NATA Standards of Practice adopted

1990 ● Athletic training officially recognized by AMA as an allied health profession

1992 ● Revised NATA Code of Ethics adopted (February 1992)
1993 ● NATA initiated lobbying campaign to pursue and advocate NATA interest in federal health care reform

2000 ● March designated as National Athletic Training Month

2002 ● NATA adds membership categories (government, health and fitness, performing arts, and law enforcement) to practice settings; includes 115 members

2004 ● NATA eliminates internship route to certification
Chuck Kimmel becomes the tenth NATA president
NATA takes strong stands in concussion research, AED use, hydration, and performance enhancing drugs

2005 ● NATA executive director, Becker-Doyle, named to American Society of Association Executives board of directors (3-year term)
NATA issues official statements: *Steroids and Performance Enhancing Substances, Community Acquired MRSA Infections*; issues position statement, *Asthma in Athletics*

2006 ● NATA holds Sudden Cardiac Arrest (SCA) press conference

2007 ● NATABOC moves to single computer-based certification exam and ends use of practical exam
NATA teams with National Academy of Neuropsychology in sports concussion education

2008 ● NATA releases "Appropriate Medical Care for the Secondary School-Aged Athlete"
NATA and North American Booster Club Association announce partnership: Proving commitment to secondary school sport injury prevention and treatment

2009 ● NATA and APTA resolve fair practice lawsuit; APTA concedes overlap in areas of scope of practice and promises truth and ethics in speaking of athletic training to the public

2010 ● NATA and NFL join forces to pass concussion awareness and prevention laws in every state throughout the country
NATA hires two associate executive directors to Dallas staff
NFL partners with athletic trainers on concussion research

Figure I.3 A brief history of the National Athletic Trainers' Association.

The 1930s and 1940s: Promoting the Exchange of Ideas

The '30s and '40s marked an awakening with regard to the need for an organization for athletic trainers. The original attempt to establish a national association for athletic trainers was undertaken in 1938, at the Drake Relays in Des Moines, Iowa. The athletic trainers working with teams competing at the Drake Relays track meet realized the need for an association of individuals to promote the exchange of ideas and techniques that would be useful in providing athletic training services to participants. Through the originality of thought and the energy of people like Charles Cramer who sought to establish such an organization, the NATA was founded in 1939. This early organization saw the appointment of a president and secretary-treasurer as well as the establishment of a home office for the association in Iowa City, Iowa. Early on, the NATA published a small, mimeographed monthly newsletter called the *NATA Bulletin*. Members received a copy of the bulletin and were encouraged to write articles for inclusion in future issues. The members paid annual dues of $1.00, which allowed them to receive the bulletin and a membership card. The NATA continued until 1944, when World War II caused a great strain on the members of the fledgling association. The difficult years of the association from the late 1930s to the mid-1940s saw several accomplishments. The NATA

- established membership classes (1939);
- published the *Trainers Journal* (1941-1942), written for athletic trainers, and the *Athletic Journal*, written for coaches;
- created an insignia and established a certificate (1941);
- established regional divisions of athletic trainers (1942); and
- held national meetings.

Although the early organization failed, perhaps due in part to financial and communications difficulties, it appears that many lessons were learned and later applied in the creation of what we know as today's NATA.

The 1950s: Establishing the Organization

Beginning in 1947, more and more schools were employing athletic trainers in their athletic departments, giving a renewed focus to the establishment of the NATA. These athletic trainers often had no formal education to qualify them for their positions. Many had learned the skills and techniques from others in the same field and from physicians working with the sport teams.

The new era of the NATA began, and in 1950 the first national meeting was held in Kansas City, Missouri. The various groups of athletic trainers served as regional divisions of the association, providing a strong network throughout the country. In the first 5 years of the decade, the organization achieved success through the financial support of the Cramer Chemical Company, and Charles Cramer was appointed as the first national secretary. The leadership consisted of representatives of each of the 10 "conferences" (now known as districts) who served as members of the board of directors. Members were athletic trainers from universities, colleges, junior colleges, and high schools, as well as coaches. Only athletic trainers from accredited universities could serve as the "national director" for a district. This grassroots approach to the development of the NATA allowed every state and every district to share in the decision-making processes of the association.

The decade of the '50s was one of considerable growth for the NATA. During the decade, schools began offering undergraduate programs in athletic training. Outstanding accomplishments of that era included the following:

- The NATA constitution and bylaws were formed (1951).
- The official logo of the NATA was adopted (1952).
- The first nonathletic trainer was accepted as an "honorary member," signifying cooperation between the athletic trainer and other professionals (1953).
- John Cramer replaced Chuck Cramer as the national secretary (1954-1955).
- W.E. "Pinky" Newell was appointed chair of the Committee on Gaining Recognition (the precursor of the Professional Education Committee and Certification Committee) (1955).
- W.E. "Pinky" Newell was appointed as third national secretary (1955-1968).
- *Journal of the National Athletic Trainers' Association* began publication (1956). The mission of the journal is to enhance communication among professionals interested in the quality of health care for the physically active through education and research in prevention, evaluation, management, and rehabilitation of injuries.
- The NATA Code of Ethics was adopted (1957).
- The first program of undergraduate education of athletic trainers was submitted to and approved by the board of directors (1959).

The 1960s: Continuing the Growth

The 1960s allowed a continuation of the organizational start that had occurred in the previous decade. In 1969, the medical profession fully recognized the significance of the NATA when the American Medical Association (**AMA**) acknowledged the importance of the role of the athletic trainer and commended the NATA for its role in developing professional standards. Gaining this respect was an important development for athletic training programs and the NATA.

During this era the NATA also accomplished the following:

- Establishment of Helms Hall of Fame for Athletic Trainers (1962)
- Appointment of Jack Rockwell (St. Louis Cardinals professional football club) as executive secretary (1969)
- Establishment of Professional Education and Certification Committees (1969)

The 1970s: Developing Standards for Certification

The decade of the 1970s was marked by a spurt in the growth of the NATA. Committees formed in the '60s were developing standards for certification (first NATA certification examination in July 1970) and educational programs. There was a change in the structure of the association when the 1973 NATA Board of Directors changed the title for the leader of the association from executive secretary to president. Bobby Gunn of the Houston Oilers served in this post first, from 1970 to 1974. Educational program development continued through the decade, with a new interest in graduate-level curricula. In 1972, the first graduate athletic training curricula were approved. In 1974, educational interest went beyond curricular issues to continuing education for certified members, and by 1979 the NATA had established continuing education requirements for all certified athletic trainers. In 1975, the 25th annual meeting of the NATA was held in Anaheim, California; here the association adopted official initials for designating the certified athletic trainer (ATC) and, through the generosity of Otho Davis, ATC (head athletic trainer of the Philadelphia Eagles Football Club and then executive director of the NATA), began the first NATA endowment fund.

By the middle of the decade, the attention of certified athletic trainers turned toward state licensure, and in 1978 the NATA and the American Physical Therapy Association held joint meetings to discuss licensure of athletic trainers in an attempt to give athletic trainers legal rights of practice. No nationwide cooperation could be established through these meetings, as each state was asked to remain responsible for its own licensure laws. Most states at that time had an act governing the practice of physical therapy; and in some situations, the athletic trainer was potentially in violation of those regulations. The NATA wanted to assist the state organizations of athletic trainers in establishing licensure of its members. This licensure would serve both to protect athletic trainers and to further define the professional role of the association.

To summarize this very busy decade, the NATA in the '70s stimulated more awareness of and attention to the membership, as well as making a strong statement regarding the proper education of the athletic trainer. Less time was spent on the earlier tasks of bringing recognition to the profession and on other organizational tasks as focus shifted toward the members.

The 1980s: Strengthening the NATA's Role

The 1980s brought heightened interest in the certification of the athletic trainer as well as a continued emphasis on education. During this era, the leaders in the areas of education and certification began to sense a disparity between the information being taught within NATA-approved curricula (see the sidebar Athletic Training Curriculum Model: Suggested Courses) and the information that was tested during the process of certifying the student athletic trainer. In the role delineation study of 1982, members were surveyed to determine the various duties involved in various positions held by athletic trainers. Role delineation studies conducted by the NATA continue to provide information that aids the association in understanding the skills required of athletic trainers.

In 1982, the National Commission for Health Certifying Agencies granted membership to the NATA, evidencing continued respect on the part of other health professions for the athletic trainer.

Throughout the 1980s, the NATA paid respect to educational leaders in the association through the Sayers "Bud" Miller Distinguished Athletic Training Educator Award. This award, named for a respected educator from Penn State University, honors an individual who has made a significant contribution to professional education of the athletic trainer.

The 1990s: Becoming a Recognized Allied Health Profession

The tremendous growth of the association continued in the 1990s, in terms both of membership and of status in the medical community. Among varied accomplishments during this period was the official recognition of athletic training as an allied health profession by the AMA on June 22, 1990. To the leaders of the NATA, this was a monumental achievement for the young profession of athletic trainers.

Mark Smaha of Washington State University started the decade off by serving the second of his two consecutive terms as president of the NATA (1990-1992). In 1990, Otho Davis resigned after 18 years as NATA Executive Director, and the NATA sought the full-time assistance of Allan Smith, whom it named chief executive officer.

In addition to seeking to promote athletic training and its educational programs, the NATA looked to the AMA's Committee on Allied Health Education and Accreditation (**CAHEA**) for curriculum evaluation. A joint CAHEA-NATA committee accomplished this review procedure. One of the developments with the greatest impact was the creation of guidelines for schools to follow to ensure compliance and give them the best opportunity for program accreditation. To further raise the bar, the NATA sought to have all college athletic training programs attain the status of an academic major or its equivalent. The NATA recognized that the conventional role of the athletic trainer had changed; athletic trainers now had positions not only

ATHLETIC TRAINING CURRICULUM MODEL: SUGGESTED COURSES

1959

Anatomy

Physiology

Physiology of exercise

Applied anatomy/Kinesiology

Psychology*

First aid and safety

Nutrition and foods

Remedial exercise

Techniques of athletic training

Advanced techniques of athletic training

Laboratory practices*

Coaching techniques**

Organization and administration of health and physical education

Personal and community hygiene

Laboratory physical science like chemistry or physics*

Additional recommended:

- General physics
- Pharmacology
- Histology
- Pathology

Mid-1970s

Anatomy

Physiology

Physiology of exercise

Applied anatomy/Kinesiology

Psychology*

First aid and safety

Nutrition

Remedial exercise

Basic athletic training

Advanced athletic training

Laboratory or practical experience***

1983-2004

Human anatomy

Human physiology

Exercise physiology

Kinesiology/Biomechanics

Psychology

First aid and emergency care

Nutrition

Prevention of athletic injuries/illnesses

Evaluation of athletic injuries/illnesses

Therapeutic modalities

Therapeutic exercise

Instructional techniques

Administration of athletic training programs

Personal/Community health

2004 to the Present Day

Students interested in becoming an athletic trainer must graduate from an accredited ATEP. The ATEP is charged with providing the courses and the clinical observation and clinical experience required to prepare the candidate for certification.

*Six semester hours (or two courses); **nine semester hours; ***a minimum of 600 clock hours under the direct supervision of a trainer certified by NATA.

in school and team environments but also in clinical and industrial settings. With the change in job opportunities, the educational programs needed to include issues relevant to those nontraditional settings. Today there are schools that offer specialized degrees in athletic training and sport health care.

These programs educate their students in the roles and responsibilities of all aspects of the profession.

During the first 2 years of the decade, the NATA saw several positive developments. On the educational front, the AMA Council on Medical Education accepted the NATA's guidelines for establishing an athletic training curriculum; in another area, the NATA launched its first public relations campaign. Both developments served to further solidify the professional image of the athletic trainer.

Early in the decade, a protégé of the late W.E. "Pinky" Newell was elected the seventh president of the NATA: Denny Miller of Purdue University (1991-1994). As had many other fine leaders, Mr. Miller would go on to serve two consecutive terms at the helm of the association. A landmark study, sponsored in part by the National Collegiate Athletic Association, examined the practice of drug dispensation in college athletics. It was perhaps not a great surprise at the time that the study indicated a need for closer regulation of medicinal drugs dispensed through college athletic training facilities. This study set off an alarm for many athletic trainers when they realized that some of their "accepted" practices—allowed and sometimes even encouraged by team physicians—were illegal and potentially unsafe. Today's strict regulations are an effect of this report by Laster-Bradley and Berger (1991). By the second year of the decade, research and scholarly publication had become an increasingly prominent goal for the profession. The NATA's Research and Education Foundation was established with the aim of promoting both research and the dissemination of information regarding health care of the physically active.

The association became more active politically as it initiated a lobbying campaign relating to the NATA's interest in federal health care reform. On the home front, the NATA governing board voted on revisions to the Code of Ethics, the membership standards, eligibility requirements and membership sanctions and procedures, and the association bylaws. Later in the decade, the NATA was recognized for its excellent code of ethics when it received the Advance America Award of Excellence issued by the American Society of Association Executives. This award served to bring attention and a bit of prestige to the association and began to pave the way toward increased respect for the profession.

Educational issues continued to arise as the AMA dissolved its academic accreditation role and the certifying of athletic training curricula was turned over to the CAAHEP. The NATA Board of Directors, in a proactive step, established the Educational Task Force, charged with studying various perspectives on athletic training education. In an attempt to identify some of the changes in the educational needs of the athletic trainer, the NATA BOC published results of the second role delineation survey as the "Role Delineation Matrix"—thus effectively reflecting suggested changes in educational competencies to meet continued changes in job opportunities for athletic trainers.

As a sign of changes to expect, the AMA issued a recommendation that high schools employ an athletic trainer for coverage of sport activities. The AMA recommendation helped the NATA begin to build a positive awareness regarding athletic trainers and the job they do.

The New Millennium

As the 1990s ended, the NATA moved forward into the 2000s with a progressive stance. In September 1999, the first woman was named president of the NATA. Ms. Julie Max followed the strong leaders preceding her, and the membership voted her into that office for two consecutive terms. In 2004, Mr. Chuck Kimmel took the helm as NATA president, the same year the athletic trainer would no longer be able to become certified through the **internship** route. From 2004 onward, all athletic training educational programs had to be part of at least a bachelor-level sequence with strict guidelines regarding curriculum content.

Throughout the 2000s, the NATA Education Council (now referred to as the NATA Executive Committee for Education) continued to refine and develop the competencies by which all athletic trainers are measured, as well as redefine and structure the clinical education of the athletic trainer. The NATA Foundation entered into a multimillion dollar fund-raising effort to support national and international research and scholarships. Most certainly, the NATA Foundation will continue to work to enhance health care of the physically active through funding and support of research and education. This decade showed a major change in how members participate in the NATA. With "Think Tanks" and short-term service in areas of interest, more members could begin serving their profession. In addition, with the installation of the second female president of the NATA, Marje Albohm, the role of and respect for the services of the athletic trainer continued to grow as third-party reimbursement began to take hold. The next decade will continue to be a time of questioning regarding the proper name for the profession, an ever-present issue in the effort to position the NATA and the athletic trainer for a more prominent role in health care of the physically active.

Employment Opportunities in Athletic Training

Where do athletic trainers work? Probably the first thought of most is that the athletic trainer works with sport teams in a college or other school system. Calling this the conventional setting for athletic training employment may not be entirely correct. The NATA conducts periodic surveys of certified members to establish the practice settings as well as the typical job-related duties of the members. These role delineation studies guide athletic training educators in establishing the special skills and knowledge to which the student athletic trainer should be exposed. Based on the latest NATA BOC data, employment of athletic trainers was highest in the **secondary school** setting (24%), followed by the clinic or hospital setting (19%), with the **university or college** setting coming in a close third with 17% of the total NATA membership (table I.1).

Athletic Training Course Instructors

The instructor of a core content athletic training course should be a certified member of the NATA. In addition to serving as a course instructor, often this individual is an athletic trainer for the athletic department of the school. Obviously, not all athletic trainers teach, and not all teaching athletic trainers work in the athletic training room. But all athletic trainers have had experience on the field and in the athletic training room, doing all the things that every student athletic trainer is asked to do.

Often the athletic training course instructor has served on the athletic training staff for a school before dedicating increasingly more time to teaching and training students. These instructors can be teaching entry-level students or graduate students, depending on their interests and experiences. These educators are frequently on the cutting edge of the research being done in the profession.

As you may know, student athletic trainers range from those in entry-level undergraduate programs all the way to the doctoral candidates who are choosing to specialize in sports medicine education and research. As the profession grows and the educational needs of the members increase, there will be a need for more and more athletic training educators.

University or College Athletic Trainers

College athletics was the setting in which athletic training first gained recognition, and it remains the case that graduating student athletic trainers often seek positions in college athletics. Colleges generally employ a person to take the leadership role in the health care team; this athletic trainer, usually a full-time employee of the school, carries a title such as head athletic trainer or director of athletic training services. Large colleges and universities often employ several certified athletic trainers to assist with the health care of the intercollegiate teams. In addition to performing daily athletic training duties, college athletic trainers may be asked to teach or to perform other athletic department functions such as coordinating the travel or meals for road games, assisting with the laundry and with equipment distribution, or fulfilling other general duties.

Table I.1 Where the ATC Works

	Certified		Requests		Responses	
	N	%	N	%	N	%
Clinic hospital—AT	1244	17.1	862	17.2	144	12.5
Health fitness industry	346	4.8	240	4.8	34	3.0
Industrial, corporate	143	2.0	98	2.0	18	1.6
Military, government, law enforcement	41	0.6	29	0.6	5	0.4
Not currently practicing	233	3.2	146	2.9	26	2.3
Other	945	13	662	13.2	91	7.9
Professional sports & performing arts	212	2.9	151	3	27	2.3
Sales, marketing	80	1.1	56	1.1	8	0.7
Secondary school—AT	2197	30.3	1531	30.6	394	34.2
University, college, junior college—AT	1555	21.4	1042	20.8	353	30.6
Youth sports	37	0.5	27	0.5	7	0.6
Secondary school—Administrative	3	0	3	0.1		
University, college, junior college—Educator	45	0.6	30	0.6	16	1.4
University, college, junior college—Administrative	9	0.1	8	0.2	3	0.3
Clinic, hospital—Administrative	29	0.4	22	0.4	5	0.4
Student	82	1.1	58	1.2	15	1.3
Unknown	37	0.5	29	0.6	2	0.2
Multiple settings	17	0.2	9	0.2	4	0.3
Total	7255	100	5003	100	1152	100

Adapted, by permission, from Board of Certification. 2009, *Role delineation study/practice analysis*, 6th ed. (Omaha, NE: BOC), 21.

High School Athletic Trainers

Colleges are not the only school settings in which the athletic trainer works with a school sport team. Some high schools employ full-time athletic trainers; other high school athletic trainers serve in a dual capacity, as the athletic trainer and also as a teacher. Occasionally a school system contracts with a sports medicine or physical therapy clinic that employs athletic trainers; in this case the clinic provides the schools of the district with athletic training coverage. Regardless of the contract, these athletic trainers play a critical role in the prevention and care of sport injuries: The absence of such a service could hinder an individual's chance of obtaining a college athletic scholarship should an injury occur. The athletic trainer in this setting usually has a team physician who oversees the activities surrounding patients' medical treatment. This relationship allows the athletic trainer to provide immediate care for the injured patient and to manage the situation on behalf of the physician.

Student Athletic Trainer

There are only a few certified athletic trainers who were not formerly student athletic trainers. Most careers begin while the student is in high school or college. The student interested in athletic health care would normally seek out the person or persons providing the athletic training services at her school. Volunteering time as a student athletic trainer is the first step in learning more about and gaining the needed understanding of the profession. High school students fortunate enough to have a full-time athletic trainer at their school can begin observing and learning even before they are able to obtain credit for the experience. But although the high school experience is certainly worthwhile, a student without this early experience is not necessarily disadvantaged. Regardless of previous experience in athletic training, most colleges accept students into the athletic training program if they meet the established grade point requirements.

In the college setting, the student athletic trainer will undoubtedly have a busy course schedule. As students' progress in the ATEP continues, they are often given more and more responsibilities. Ideally, every student athletic trainer will earn the responsibility of working directly with sport teams.

Once the student has fulfilled the NATA requirements for certification, he may apply to take the certification examination. Most often, students take the certification examination at the conclusion of the undergraduate degree, although they may wish to delay the test until a later date. Students who do not satisfactorily complete the certification examination are allowed to repeat the exam at a later date.

Graduate School Opportunities

Students who become certified after completion of their bachelor's degree may elect to pursue a master's degree in athletic training or another related field such as exercise **physiology**, **biomechanics**, or the allied health professions. Many schools contract with an athletic trainer to provide athletic training services for university athletic teams, allowing the student to also pursue an advanced degree. Often, college and universities supplement their full-time staff with these graduate students. But students who wish to pursue an advanced degree in athletic training may do so without serving the school as an athletic trainer. Certified students can often find part-time employment in athletic training in the community.

Athletic Trainers/Coaches

The combination of athletic trainer and coach is not common, mostly because of the somewhat adversarial roles of the two positions. Would an athletic trainer and a coach make the same decision regarding the playing status of a key player injured in the final minutes of a critical game? Who would give the injured patient the needed attention if it were important for the team to have a strategy session?

Clinic Athletic Trainers

Health care clinics also may offer employment opportunities for athletic trainers. These clinics, frequently owned or managed by physical therapists, employ the athletic trainer to assist a licensed health care provider in rendering services to the physically active patient. In some states, the athletic trainer is allowed to provide services and to bill for those services; other states require the athletic trainer's work to be overseen and countersigned by the licensed physical therapist. The same situation applies when the clinic is owned and operated by a licensed physician; that is, the athletic trainer's services must be supervised and countersigned by the physician. Although this may appear to be a somewhat controlling atmosphere, most athletic trainers employed in the clinical setting are quite happy with the work schedule, the job duties, and the learning opportunities the clinic provides. An athletic trainer considering employment in a clinic should examine the athletic training as well as the physical therapy practice legislation of the particular state to achieve a full understanding of the legal limits of employment. As time goes on, third-party reimbursement will continue to be a focus of attention. Third-party reimbursement is a step that gives the ATC additional autonomy, allowing the ATC to bill for athletic training services in the clinic as well as in more traditional settings.

As mentioned previously, a school system, an individual school, or even a sport team may contract with a sport health care clinic for athletic training coverage. This contract is usually made with the athletic trainer's employer, the clinic, or the physician. The employer provides malpractice insurance for the athletic trainer working in an outreach program of health care for the school or team.

Athletic Trainers for Professional Sports

Because of the small size of most professional teams, fewer athletic trainers are employed in this setting than in the others. Some professional teams, however, use students or certified athletic trainers during camps at which the total team size is much larger than during the regular season. Most athletic trainers working for professional teams were once students too! Many of those individuals spent time as volunteers at the professional level during their vacation periods in the summer.

Some professional sports, such as tennis, golf, and even rodeo, hire certified athletic trainers to provide evaluation and treatment at major events. The Professional Golfers' Association has a trailer that travels to the sites of major golf tournaments. The trailer houses exercise equipment and treatment facilities as well as a full-time staff to help the professional golfers with their musculoskeletal health care needs.

Workplace Athletic Trainers

Industry provides a unique opportunity for the athletic trainer interested in working primarily in a health maintenance capacity. Corporate executives have realized the importance of relaxation time during their hectic workdays and have incorporated regularly scheduled periods for exercise into the workday or the workweek. Organizations dedicated to the prevention of cumulative trauma in the workplace have increased corporate attention to the need for frequent scheduled breaks for exercise and stretching activities. Large corporations such as AC Delco, Microsoft, Dial, Motorola, and Intel participate regularly in programs for preventing injury in the workplace. A growing number of companies employ athletic trainers or other health care providers to

care for both work-related and non-work-related injuries, allowing the employee to manage the injury without having to leave the corporate grounds.

The athletic trainer is not often the first health care professional that companies seek to lead corporate injury prevention programs, yet the athletic trainer's background is quite well suited to such a position. Athletic trainers who seek opportunities with corporations are often able to work with a physician in the design of programs—not only programs for the prevention and treatment of acute and cumulative trauma on the assembly line, but also exercise programs and fitness routines for administrative-level employees.

Other Potential Opportunities

The potential opportunities for the athletic trainer are without number. Some athletic trainers have established their own corporations; some have obtained medical degrees and now practice as team physicians; and some have started private sports medicine clinics—the list could go on and on. Job opportunities for the athletic trainer may not appear numerous in certain settings, but few people with initiative are ever without employment.

The Sports Medicine Team

Just as a group of individuals work together to form a sport team, a team of individuals works toward the common goal of health care of the physically active. This sports medicine team includes a variety of individuals from a variety of disciplines.

The Athletic Training Team

Athletic trainers working on a sports medicine team may be categorized according to sport or may be grouped into a total department. For the sake of this discussion we consider the department, rather than the sport team, as the team unit.

Most professional teams and major college programs have more than one athletic trainer on their sports medicine team. Those programs with more than two assistant athletic trainers usually appoint one person to serve as the lead or head athletic trainer. Some programs give this department head another title, most often director. At the college and university level, the head athletic trainer or director of athletic training services has responsibility for a team of trainers. The head trainer reports to the team physician and coaching staff. The team of athletic trainers usually includes any number of certified athletic trainers (full- or part-time people and graduate assistants), as well as a group of student athletic trainers.

Physicians

The typical sports medicine team includes one team physician (either an **allopathic** medical doctor [MD] or doctor of osteopathy [DO]) who is often a family practice specialist or general medicine practitioner. This individual may be employed full-time by the team or school or may be hired jointly by the campus medical service and the athletic department. Occasionally the team physician is a local private physician and is paid a retainer for any and all services needed during a set period of time. These services may include, for instance, the diagnosis and treatment of illness and disease, assistance with the treatment of allergies or asthma and other chronic conditions, and diagnosis and treatment of skeletal and neurological trauma.

Many areas of medicine have some interest in the care of the physically active patient. The medical specialty areas, as outlined next, often establish special committees within their medical organizations to study and discuss sports medicine. The list of specialties and organizations may surprise you, but as you learn more about medical care of the physically active, you will realize that the medical, dental, and psychological needs of the physically active patient are similar to those of other individuals. Those needs are often magnified by the intense physical demands of athletic participation. Specialists who concentrate on the physically active

usually have a good understanding of the physical demands of the sport and also the schedule for the participant's competitive season. Additionally, the highly athletically-trained individual may experience unusual medical problems that must be understood and addressed to allow healthy participation.

Orthopedic Surgeons and Other Specialists

Because of the prevalence of **orthopedic** trauma during sport participation, the orthopedic surgeon is a critical member of the sports medicine team. One or more orthopedic surgeons, like the team physician, may be paid a retainer fee or may receive a fee for services rendered. Sport teams and schools employ few orthopedic specialists full-time.

The orthopedic surgeon, also known as the "orthopod" or the "orthopedist," could be an interested physician from the local medical community or a member of the medical school staff if the school has a medical school. The orthopedic surgeon's job is to care for injuries to bones and joints. If a patient has an injury that requires surgery, the orthopod chooses the hospital where the surgery will take place—often because of regulations that each medical facility places on physicians and also because of the equipment available at a particular hospital. A doctor who is allowed to use a facility is said to have *privileges* at that hospital.

Additional physician specialists, such as the dentist, ophthalmologist, or cardiologist, may be associated with teams or school programs. The number and types of specialists involved often vary with the local interest as well as the philosophy of the sports medicine team and the organization's management. Table I.2 lists the terms commonly used in athletic medicine to identify particular medical specialists.

Rehabilitation Specialists

Often an individual is employed by the busy athletic training department to aid in the care and rehabilitation of patients requiring

Table I.2 Medical Specialists

Profession or specialist	Area of focus	Common reasons for referral
Audiologist	Hearing and balance	Tinnitus, hearing difficulties, vestibular problems
Cardiologist	Heart	Heart murmurs, arrhythmias
Dermatologist	Skin	Acne, skin rashes, contact dermatitis
Ear, nose, throat (ENT)	Ear, nose, and throat	Broken nose or deviated septum, nasal polyps, cauliflower ear, swimmer's ear, tonsillitis
General surgeon	Abdomen and pelvis (or other areas as needed)	Appendicitis, hernia, generally all types of surgery, emergencies
Gynecologist	Female reproductive system	Menstrual disorders, pathology of the reproductive system
Neurologist/Neurosurgeon	Nervous system	Nerve conduction problems, disc rupture, concussions, nervous system disorders
Orthopedic surgeon	Bones and joints	Musculoskeletal trauma
Ophthalmologist	Eye	Diseases of the eye, eye trauma, detached retina
Optometrist	Eye	Visual acuity problems
Podiatrist	Foot	Foot trauma, foot function (biomechanics)
Sport psychologist	Mental training	Problems with confidence or concentration, overcoming fears, goal setting
Vascular surgeon	Circulatory system	Compartment syndromes of the leg or arm, thoracic outlet syndrome, deep vein thrombosis

long periods of absence from team activities. Although certainly within the expertise of the athletic trainer, it may be that this rehabilitation duty can be more consistently carried out by a clinician who does not have daily duties and travel responsibilities with a sport team. Often the logical choice is the physical therapist. This "rehabilitation specialist" would design and implement treatment and rehabilitation programs for the injured patient. Having the rehabilitation specialist available even when the team is at practice or away from campus allows more continuous progress toward returning the injured patient to participation with the team. An additional advantage of the physical therapist in this position is that insurance companies often pay for physical therapy treatments; thus the rehabilitation specialist can generate some income for the athletic department.

Nutritionists

Nutritionists are often employed by the campus medical center or food service but may be called on to supplement the medical staff's attention to the nutritional needs of individual student-athletes or to assist in the management of patients with eating concerns. The nutritionist may give suggestions to the department that provides training-table service to the athletic teams or, if necessary, may help the athletic trainer in designing a pregame meal for a specific team.

Sport Psychologists

In addition to working with Olympic teams, psychologists specializing in athletics are becoming more involved with sport teams at the college and professional levels. The sport psychologist can be an asset to the noninjured student-athlete in the area of enhancing sport performance or even in dealing with emotional pressures of college life and athletic competition. The injured patient may seek out the assistance of the sport psychologist in dealing with the emotional difficulties of losing playing status, coping with the injury itself, or going through the rehabilitation program.

Paramedics and Emergency Medical Technicians

Some athletic trainers are also certified as paramedics (**EMT-P**) or emergency medical technicians (**EMT**). These people may be able to contribute additional emergency care skills to the sports medicine team, but the athletic trainer, though infrequently, may serve in a dual capacity at an athletic event. More likely, the EMT or paramedic is a member of the ambulance squad hired to cover athletic events. These personnel, if assigned to home events, should be familiar with the school's emergency care plan and should discuss any special concerns of their own with the school's athletic training staff.

Other Support Staff

As with any team, other staff members contribute to the smooth operation of the athletic training program. The secretarial and insurance personnel are great assets in the management of the medical program, and it is important to regard these individuals as members of the team. The work of adminis-trative staff and insurance personnel not only keeps the athletic department functioning smoothly but also enables the athletic trainers to concentrate on athletic training concerns.

Coaches and Athletes

Lastly, the coach and the athlete are obviously central to the sports medicine team. The coach can often recognize subtle changes in the athlete's skill performance, academic performance, or general personality that could signal some underlying problem. The coach's critical observation of a decline in performance can save an athlete from exacerbating a small problem. Yet no matter how many individuals there are on the sports medicine team, physically active persons must accept responsibility for their health. Good hygiene, sound nutritional practices, and attention to signs of fatigue or injury are all, ultimately, responsibilities of the individual. Still and all, it is part of the work of the athletic trainer to educate athletes about their bodies and encourage them to take an active role in keeping physically, psychologically, and emotionally healthy.

Learning Aids

SUMMARY

Athletic training is a far-reaching profession serving the physically active population. Prospective athletic trainers should understand the educational and certification requirements before embarking on the profession. The types of workplaces where an ATC can find employment is almost unlimited. Refer to the NATA BOC *Role Delineation Study/ Practice Analysis, Sixth Edition* (RD/PA6) (www.bocatc.org/images/stories/resources/ rdpa6_content_outline.pdf) to discover areas of practice into which other ATCs have ventured.

KEY CONCEPTS AND REVIEW

▸ **Describe the education, training, and licensure and certification of the athletic trainer.**

Athletic training requires at least 4 years of college education plus hands-on practice in evaluation, prevention, and management of athletic injuries. The education must be through a CAAHEP-accredited athletic training program. The student must pass the certification examination through the NATA BOC and may need to satisfy state licensure requirements before working as an ATC.

▸ **Provide a general history of the athletic training profession.**

The NATA began in 1939 as a way to exchange information and ideas. By the 1950s, undergraduate courses and programs were established. Professional education and certification committees were formed in the 1960s. The decade of the 1970s was one of great growth in membership in the NATA, and with that came a focus on certification standards for athletic trainers. In the 1980s, the National Commission for Health Certifying Agencies granted membership to the NATA, giving the association a boost in terms of medical recognition. The 1990s continued the gains in recognition of the NATA as athletic training was recognized as an allied health profession by the AMA. Also, the NATA turned to the AMA's Committee on Allied Health Education and Accreditation (CAHEA) for curriculum evaluation. Through this evaluation, the NATA began revision of the routes toward certification, away from internship and toward having students major in athletic training. The new millennium saw the first female serving as association president. Efforts during the decade centered on the education and certification of members.

▸ **Identify the top three employment settings for athletic trainers in 2009.**

(1) Clinics, (2) secondary schools, and (3) colleges and universities

▸ **Identify various employment opportunities for athletic trainers.**

Clinics, schools, industry, hospitals, professional teams, recreational teams, health clubs, youth sport leagues, military, law enforcement and other emerging work settings—limited only by the ATC's interest and ambition

▸ **Describe five members of the sports medicine team and explain the general duties of each.**

Members include physicians (general and specialists), rehabilitation specialists, nutritionists, sport psychologists, emergency medical providers, support staff, coaches, and athletes.

PRACTICE!

For hands-on practice in this area, go to the web resource and complete the following:

Level 1.1, Module X1: Athletic Training Observation

Level 1.4, Module C7: Medical Services (Health Center, Hospitals, Physicians)

CRITICAL THINKING QUESTIONS

1. You were helping your longtime friend and fellow ATC cover lacrosse practice one afternoon at a local university. You overheard your friend, an assistant ATC at the school, speaking in detail with the soccer coach about the injury status of a lacrosse patient who was sitting out of practice that day. The patient, who was on the sideline at the moment, also overheard the conversation and was very upset with your friend—enough so that he left practice to go find the head ATC at the facility. Look up the NATA Code of Ethics. Which, if any, part of the NATA Code of Ethics did your friend violate? Do you have any professional responsibilities or obligations in this situation to act? Would you be in violation of any NATA policies if you did nothing? If so, which ones, and what should you do?

2. Good sport health care in a time of emergency treatment relies on three basic necessities: proper planning and practice, good communication skills, and good working relationships among all staff and support staff. How would you as the head ATC at any level ensure that things ran smoothly during an athletic emergency with

each of the following support staff groups? Include any preplanning you would do (practice sessions, letters sent out, meetings, and so on).

- Paramedics/EMTs
- Orthopedic doctors (team doctors)
- Student trainers

3. You are in charge of the medical services for your high school. After a year, it is clear to you that you need some help before the start of the next school year. You decide to go to the athletic director and propose two things: (1) You want to begin seeking reimbursement from your patients' insurance companies for the treatment and rehabilitation you are providing, and (2) you want to hire a full-time assistant to help with the day-to-day sport coverage as well as management of the billing for the insurance reimbursements. Prepare a list of five things you want to be sure to express to the athletic director to support each of your proposed points.

Prevention and Health Promotion

Prevention is an area that most medical specialists do not provide the patient. The athletic trainer is in close communication with the patient, often for several successive years, and thus is able to detect aspects of the patient's health that may pose an increased risk to participation.

Prevention is a global term, but the ATC works in many specific ways to prevent athletic injury or communication of illnesses. The NATA Board of Certification (BOC) periodically surveys certified members regarding the skills and knowledge needed to function in their capacity as an athletic trainer. From this information, "domains"—areas or spheres of knowledge—are established that form the blueprint for the ATC examination. NATA BOC (2011) identifies "Prevention and Health Promotion" as a domain.

Chapter 1 addresses the preparticipation exam (PPE) and the ways in which the detection of problems can help correct deficits and prevent injury. In this chapter you will learn about the components of the PPE, administration of the exams, and options there might be for any medical findings that may limit participation.

Chapter 2, which introduces aspects of fitness testing and conditioning, covers testing for strength, endurance, and flexibility, as well as conditioning and reconditioning to bring patients to top levels of fitness. Detecting and rectifying deficiencies in an individual's fitness level helps reduce the chance of injury. Keeping the body in top physical condition helps to prevent injury, and that is the goal of every participant and athletic trainer.

Chapter 3 looks at the nutritional aspects of health and performance. Learning about the nutritional values of foods, monitoring caloric intake, and understanding the MyPlate and USDA Dietary Guidelines will aid you in your job of helping active people stay nutritionally healthy. Good nutrition is essential for good health, and good health essential to good performance. It should be easy to see that nutrition can help prevent injury and illness.

Chapter 4 examines how the environment affects athletic participation. The chapter covers concepts of heat dissipation, which will help you understand factors that inhibit cooling. Severe weather is often region specific, and you should understand the risks of participating in severe conditions. The chapter also discusses the risks associated with various physical hazards found in and around athletic venues, encouraging readers to take a critical look at their local athletic facilities.

Chapter 5 looks at the protective devices used in various sports. Governing bodies for sports impose sport-specific regulations regarding proper and improper equipment that athletic trainers need to understand. Athletic trainers may devise ways to further protect an injured body part to prevent exacerbation of the injury or help prevent an injury. This chapter will look into the legal ramifications of equipment alteration.

Chapter 6 introduces methods of taping and bracing, a skill that is relatively distinc-

tive to the athletic training profession. Taping and bracing can prevent injury, and this is the goal of all applications of tape or braces for use in participation. Some braces and taping techniques can be used for rehabilitation or in treatment of an injury, and the chapter covers these also.

Through study of this part of *Core Concepts in Athletic Training and Therapy*, readers will gain knowledge of preventive measures used in athletic training. Understanding in all these areas—the preparticipation examination, fitness and conditioning, nutrition and good nutritional habits, and the protection of injured or vulnerable areas through use of specialized equipment and techniques—will help prevent injury and illness and keep your patients participating.

COMPETENCIES

Prevention and Health Promotion (PHP): PHP-8-14, PHP-20, PHP-26-38, PHP-40-41

Acute Care of Injuries and Illnesses (AC): AC-36d

Therapeutic Interventions (TI): TI-16

Healthcare Administration (HA): HA-23

The Preparticipation Physical Examination

Susan Kay Hillman, ATC, PT

OBJECTIVES

After reading this chapter, the student should be able to do the following:

- Discuss the importance of a preparticipation physical examination for sport team members or for someone beginning a fitness program.

- Discuss how knowledge of preexisting conditions may help in the medical care of the physically active individual.

- Present the two main ways to conduct a physical examination for athletic sports teams, and list the advantages and disadvantages of each.

- List the types of examinations to be included in the preparticipation physical examination, and identify the members of the medical team needed to conduct these exams in a group physical.

- Compare and contrast aspects of the group physical and the individualized examination.

- Identify problematic areas in conducting a group physical and list ways in which those situations may be managed.

Whenever one works with a group of physically active individuals, it is wise to know the medical conditions existing before the first day of participation. Failure to fully evaluate a patient prior to participation could result in injury or illness if an underlying problem is not known. The goal in establishing a **preparticipation physical examination (PPE)** policy is to control the risk of injury before it occurs. No one wants to learn that a physically active individual has a problem that precludes the person from participation. But working with a known problem is ultimately better than allowing an individual to potentially suffer serious injury or permanent impairment because she has been allowed to play.

Another consideration in evaluating clients for participation is the type of sport in which they intend to participate. Needless to say, some conditions may not pose a problem in particular sports but would be a firm contraindication to participation in others. For example, a patient with spinal steno-sis, a narrowing of the spinal canal, may be fine for participation in swimming but could be restricted from participation in a contact sport such as football. The American Academy of Pediatrics has published recommendations for the classification of sports in terms of contact to help in the evaluation of a patient's relative risk of participation. See the sidebar Classification of Sports by Contact, which shows the American Academy of Pediatrics summary of contact or collision status of various sports.

Essential Elements of the Preparticipation Physical Examination

For athletic patients, the National Collegiate Athletic Association (NCAA) has established guidelines for all member institutions to follow regarding the preparticipation physical examination (PPE). Additionally, many

CLASSIFICATION OF SPORTS BY CONTACT

Contact or Collision

Basketball
Boxing[b]
Cheerleading
Diving
Extreme sports[d]
Field hockey
Football (tackle)
Gymnastics
Ice hockey[e]
Lacrosse
Martial arts[f]
Rodeo
Rugby
Skiing (downhill)
Ski jumping
Snowboarding
Soccer
Team handball
Ultimate Frisbee
Water polo
Wrestling

Limited Contact

Adventure racing[a]
Baseball
Bicycling
Canoeing or kayaking (white-water)
Fencing
Field events (high jump, pole vault)
Floor hockey
Football (flag or touch)
Handball

Horseback riding

Martial arts[f]

Racquetball

Skateboarding

Skating (ice, in-line, roller)

Skateboarding

Skiing (cross country, water)

Softball

Squash

Volleyball

Weightlifting

Windsurfing and surfing

Noncontact

Archery

Badminton

Bodybuilding[c]

Canoeing or kayaking (flat water)

Crew or rowing

Curling

Dance

Field events (discus, javelin, shot put)

Golf

Orienteering[g]

Powerlifting[c]

Race walking

Riflery

Rope jumping

Running

Sailing

Scuba diving

Swimming

Table tennis

Tennis

Track

---

[a]Adventure racing has been added since the previous statement was published and is defined as a combination of two or more disciplines, including orienteering and navigation, cross country running, mountain biking, paddling, and climbing and rope skills.

[b]The American Academy of Pediatrics opposes participation in boxing for children, adolescents, and young adults.

[c]The American Academy of Pediatrics recommends limiting bodybuilding and powerlifting until the adolescent achieves sexual maturity rating 5 (Tanner stage V).

[d]Extreme sports has been added since the previous statement was published.

[e]The American Academy of Pediatrics recommends limiting the amount of body checking allowed for hockey players 15 years and younger in order to reduce injuries.

[f]Martial arts can be subclassified as judo, jujitsu, karate, kung fu, and taekwondo; some forms are contact sports, and others are limited-contact sports.

[g]Orienteering is a race (contest) in which competitors use a map and a compass to find their way through unfamiliar territory.

states have established their own policies for providing the high school PPE for interscholastic patients. These NCAA and state regulations have been written to ensure consistent treatment of patients from the early years of interscholastic sport to the final years of collegiate participation. Many states require a yearly physical examination for all interscholastic patients. This means that each patient must undergo a thorough physical exam each school year of participation in sport. The NCAA, as well as some state high school associations, requires only a "one-time physical examination," meaning that the patient must have a thorough physical examination prior to the first year of participation at a particular school. During subsequent (sequential) years of participation, the patient is required to have an abbreviated physical based on interim medical history as supplied by the patient or the patient's family (or both) and the team's medical staff. (See the sidebar NCAA Guidelines 1B: Medical Evaluations, Immunizations, and Records.)

Preparticipation Medical Evaluation

A preparticipation medical evaluation should be required upon a patient's entrance into the institution's athletics program (See NCAA Bylaw 17.1.5). This initial evaluation should include a comprehensive health history; an immunization history as defined by current Centers for Disease Control and Prevention (CDC) guidelines; and a relevant physical exam with strong emphasis on the cardiovascular, neurologic, and musculoskeletal evaluation. After the initial medical evaluation, an updated history should be performed annually (2010-11 NCAA Sports Medicine Handbook).

The American Heart Association has modified its 1996 recommendation for a cardiovascular screening every 2 years for collegiate patients (American Heart Association 1996). The revision recommends cardiovascular screening as a part of the physical exam required upon an intercollegiate patient's entrance into the intercollegiate athletics program (American Heart Association 1998). In subsequent years, an interim history and blood pressure measurement should be taken. Important changes in medical status or abnormalities may require more formal cardiovascular evaluation.

Medical Records

Patients have a responsibility to report any changes in their health to the team's health care provider. **Medical records** should be maintained during the client's collegiate career and should include the following:

1. A record of injuries, illnesses, new medications or allergies, pregnancies, and operations, whether sustained during the competitive season or the off-season.

2. Referrals for and feedback from consultation, treatment, or rehabilitation.

3. Subsequent care and clearances.

4. A comprehensive entry-year health-status questionnaire and an updated health status questionnaire each year thereafter. Components of the questionnaire should consider recommendations from Maron and Zipes (2005).

5. Immunizations. It is recommended that patients be immunized for the following:

   a. measles, mumps, rubella (MMR);

   b. hepatitis B;

   c. diphtheria and tetanus (and boosters when appropriate); and

   d. meningitis.

6. Written permission, signed by the patient, which authorizes the release of medical information to others. Such permission should specify all persons to whom the patient authorizes the information to be released. The consent also should specify which information may be released and to whom.

Note: Records maintained in the athletic training facility are medical records and therefore subject to state and federal laws with regard to confidentiality and content. Each institution should obtain from appropriate legal counsel an opinion regarding the confidentiality and content of such records in its state. The United States instituted a law to protect the privacy of personal health information. The law is called HIPAA, which stands for Health Insurance Portability and Accountability Act of 1996. This privacy rule regulates who can look at and receive an individual's health information. HIPAA rules apply to all forms of an individual's protected health information, regardless of its format—electronic, written, or oral.

Follow-Up or Exit Examination

Those who have sustained a significant injury or illness during the sport season should be given a follow-up examination to reestablish medical clearance before resuming participation in a particular sport. This policy also should apply to pregnant clients after delivery or pregnancy termination. These examinations are especially relevant if the event occurred before the client left the institution for summer break. Clearance for individuals to return to activity is solely the responsibility of the team physician or that physician's designated representative.

Reprinted, by permission, from National Collegiate Athletic Association, 2010, *NCAA sports medicine handbook*, 21st ed. (Indianapolis, IN: NCAA), 4203.

People wishing to participate on teams or in athletic clubs, or in any strenuous physical activity, should undergo a physical examination prior to the start of participation. Those who participate in school sports may be allowed to provide a copy of the signed school physical examination form as evidence of current health status. For example, the National Youth Sports Program (NYSP) offers structured recreational activities for young people in many metropolitan areas. An individual who plays on the junior high school team and wishes to participate in NYSP may be allowed to bring a copy of the completed junior high sport physical to fulfill the PPE requirement of the youth sport program. What would you suggest if you were in charge of a masters swim team and a 47-year-old swimmer brought a copy of his most recent annual physical provided by his family physician? Would you accept this physical as evidence that there is no reason to restrict this person from strenuous activity? What would you want to be sure was included in this physical examination?

It is important that all individuals participating in organized physical activities undergo an examination to ascertain that they have no additional risks from strenuous exercise. Regardless of the level of participation, nondisabled participants as well as those who are disabled should have their health status checked. This evaluation can vary considerably but should include several essential components (see table 1.1), each of which we will consider later in this chapter.

Before beginning any physical examination, the patient is required to provide certain types of information for administrative purposes as well as for the physician's review.

Health Status Information

Entering the individual's personal information into the medical records is the first step in conducting the PPE. The patient's legal name, date of birth, and some identifying number (social security or other identification number) are essential for the proper recording of medical information and the results from subsequent examinations. Other information collected during this time includes the following:

- Signatures on any legal forms that may be required for participation. If the patient is not of legal age, the parent or guardian's signature must be obtained, usually prior to or at the physical examination.
- Address and telephone information.
- Emergency contact information: name and phone number of the individual to be notified in the event of an emergency, accident, or other medical need.
- Health insurance information.
- Health status information.

Background information regarding the individual's health status can also be termed the medical history. This health status

Table 1.1 Typical Stations Used in Multistation Group Physical Examinations

Station	Examinations used	Purpose of evaluation
Height/Weight	Height, weight, body composition (optional)	Data collection, baseline for future reference.
Cardiovascular	Blood pressure, heart rate, electrocardiogram (ECG), exercise ECG (recommended)	Heart health at rest and with stress, cardiac problems.
Visual screening	Vision test and visual tracking examination	Visual acuity and need for correction.
Blood tests	Complete blood count Hemoglobin/Hematocrit	Acute problems, infections. Look for anemia.
	Lipid profile (patients >40 years of age)	Evaluate cholesterol levels.
	Sickle cell (black patients)	Presence of sickle cell trait or sickle cell anemia.
Urinalysis (UA)	UA using dipstick or laboratory evaluation of urine	Detect protein, sugar, or blood in urine to look for infections, dietary conditions, or other problems. May be used for drug testing.
Ear, nose, and throat (ENT)	Clinical evaluation with specialized equipment (otoscope)	Evaluate inner ear, eardrum; nasal septum position; presence of polyps; general health of tonsils and thyroid.
Cardiopulmonary evaluation	Clinical evaluation using stethoscope	Heart and lung health; detect aortic or cardiac abnormalities, lung conditions such as asthma.
Internal examination	Clinical evaluation	Check males for hernia, evaluation of organ systems.
Orthopedic examination	Clinical evaluation, may use specialized equipment if available	Check bones and joints for laxity or other pathology.
Neurological examination	Clinical evaluation, electroencephalogram, or both	Evaluate nervous system, observe brain waves.
Dental examination	Clinical evaluation, visual inspection	Note dental caries, bridges, other appliances for records.
Flexibility measures	Various clinical tests depending on objective	For research, baseline data, or both.

information is critical to the examining physician's ability to anticipate and understand the need for special examinations and laboratory tests. Medical information can be obtained through simple questionnaires and forms that can be distributed before or at the physical exam and collected at check-in. (For examples of forms, see figures 1.1 and 1.2.)

Medical experts agree that the medical history is the cornerstone of the examination process, potentially capable of identifying a patient's medical problems without further physical examination. As the single most important aspect of the examination, the medical history form should be well thought out and reviewed before it is printed for inclusion in the examination process.

The medical history questionnaire is a document with questions to be answered by the individual being tested, or by a parent or legal guardian if the person is under 18 years of age. The questions should draw out information without putting too many words into the person's mouth. Rather than asking, "Have you ever sprained your ankle badly?" ask, "Have you ever had to miss a practice or game due to an ankle injury?"

HEALTH STATUS QUESTIONNAIRE

This questionnaire identifies adults for whom physical activity might be inappropriate or adults who should seek physician consultation before beginning a regular physical activity program.

Section 1. Personal and Emergency Contact Information

Name: _____ Date of birth: _____

Address: _____ Phone: _____

Physician's name: _____

Height: _____ Weight: _____

Person to contact in emergency: _____

Name: _____ Phone: _____

Section 2. General Medical History

Please check the following conditions you have experienced.

Heart History

☐ Heart attack   ☐ Cardiac rhythm disturbance
☐ Heart surgery   ☐ Heart valve disease
☐ Cardiac catheterization   ☐ Heart failure
☐ Coronary angioplasty (PTCA) ☐ Heart transplantation
☐ Cardiac pacemaker   ☐ Congenital heart disease

Symptoms

☐ You experience chest discomfort with exertion.
☐ You experience unreasonable shortness of breath at any time.
☐ You experience dizziness, fainting, or blackouts.
☐ You take heart medications.

Additional Health Issues

☐ You have diabetes (type 1 or type 2).
☐ You have asthma or other lung disease (e.g., emphysema).
☐ You have burning or cramping sensations in your lower legs with minimal physical activity.
☐ You have joint problems (e.g., arthritis) that limit your physical activity.
☐ You have concerns about the safety of exercise.
☐ You take prescription medications.
☐ You are pregnant.

Section 3. Risk Factor Assessment

Risk Factors for Coronary Heart Disease

☐ You are a man older than 45 yr.
☐ You are a woman older than 55 yr, have had a hysterectomy, or are postmenopausal.
☐ You smoke or you quit smoking within the previous 6 mo.
☐ Your blood pressure is >140/90 mmHg.

Figure 1.1 Health status questionnaire. *(continued)*

☐ Your blood cholesterol is >200 mg/dL.

☐ You have a close male blood relative (father or brother) who had a heart attack or heart surgery before the age of 55 or a close female blood relative (mother or sister) who had a heart attack or heart surgery before the age of 65.

☐ You are physically inactive (you get <30 min of physical activity at least 3 days per wk).

☐ Your waist circumference is >40 in (101.6 cm in men) or >35 in (88.9 cm in women).

Section 4. Medications

Are you currently taking any medications?   Yes   No

If yes, please list all of your prescribed medications and how often you take them, whether daily (D) or as needed (PRN).

_____

_____

List your specific goals for your exercise program. _____

_____

Please inform the fitness professional immediately of any changes that occur in your health status.

Patient Information Release Form

If you have answered yes to questions indicating that you have significant cardiac, pulmonary, metabolic, or orthopedic problems that may be exacerbated with exercise, you agree it is permissible for us to contact your physician regarding your health status.

Signature: _____   Date: _____

Fitness staff signature: _____   Date: _____

To be completed by fitness professional (circle one)

AHA/ACSM risk stratification: Low   Moderate   High

Physician consent: Yes   No

Figure 1.1   *(continued)*   Health status questionnaire.

Reprinted, by permission, from E.T. Howley and B.D. Franks, 2007, *Fitness professional's handbook*, 5th ed. (Champaign, IL: Human Kinetics), 26-27.

The medical history form should include questions such as the following:

- Have you been medically advised not to participate in any sport? If so, what was the reason for such advice?

- Have you been hospitalized or under a physician's care in the past 12 months? At any time in your life? If so, what was the reason for such care?

- Have you undergone any surgery? If so, what was the reason for the surgery and the approximate date of operation?

- Have you had any inoculations or childhood diseases? If so, what and approximately when?

- Have you ever experienced convulsions or seizures? If so, what were understood to be the precipitating factors, if any, and when did they occur?

- Is there a history of heart disease or sudden death in any member of the family? If so, in whom and at what age was the diagnosis or the sudden death?

- Have you had frequent shortness of breath, syncope, or heat intolerance?

PAR-Q & YOU

(A Questionnaire for People Aged 15 to 69)

Regular physical activity is fun and healthy, and increasingly more people are starting to become more active every day. Being more active is very safe for most people. However, some people should check with their doctor before they start becoming much more physically active.

If you are planning to become much more physically active than you are now, start by answering the seven questions in the box below. If you are between the ages of 15 and 69, the PAR-Q will tell you if you should check with your doctor before you start. If you are over 69 years of age, and you are not used to being very active, check with your doctor.

Common sense is your best guide when you answer these questions. Please read the questions carefully and answer each one honestly: check YES or NO.

YES	NO		
☐	☐	1.	**Has your doctor ever said that you have a heart condition <u>and</u> that you should only do physical activity recommended by a doctor?**
☐	☐	2.	**Do you feel pain in your chest when you do physical activity?**
☐	☐	3.	**In the past month, have you had chest pain when you were not doing physical activity?**
☐	☐	4.	**Do you lose your balance because of dizziness or do you ever lose consciousness?**
☐	☐	5.	**Do you have a bone or joint problem (for example, back, knee or hip) that could be made worse by a change in your physical activity?**
☐	☐	6.	**Is your doctor currently prescribing drugs (for example, water pills) for your blood pressure or heart condition?**
☐	☐	7.	**Do you know of <u>any other reason</u> why you should not do physical activity?**

If you answered

YES to one or more questions

Talk with your doctor by phone or in person BEFORE you start becoming much more physically active or BEFORE you have a fitness appraisal. Tell your doctor about the PAR-Q and which questions you answered YES.

- You may be able to do any activity you want — as long as you start slowly and build up gradually. Or, you may need to restrict your activities to those which are safe for you. Talk with your doctor about the kinds of activities you wish to participate in and follow his/her advice.
- Find out which community programs are safe and helpful for you.

NO to all questions

If you answered NO honestly to <u>all</u> PAR-Q questions, you can be reasonably sure that you can:
- start becoming much more physically active – begin slowly and build up gradually. This is the safest and easiest way to go.
- take part in a fitness appraisal – this is an excellent way to determine your basic fitness so that you can plan the best way for you to live actively. It is also highly recommended that you have your blood pressure evaluated. If your reading is over 144/94, talk with your doctor before you start becoming much more physically active.

DELAY BECOMING MUCH MORE ACTIVE:
- if you are not feeling well because of a temporary illness such as a cold or a fever – wait until you feel better; or
- if you are or may be pregnant – talk to your doctor before you start becoming more active.

PLEASE NOTE: If your health changes so that you then answer YES to any of the above questions, tell your fitness or health professional. Ask whether you should change your physical activity plan.

<u>Informed Use of the PAR-Q</u>: The Canadian Society for Exercise Physiology, Health Canada, and their agents assume no liability for persons who undertake physical activity, and if in doubt after completing this questionnaire, consult your doctor prior to physical activity.

No changes permitted. You are encouraged to photocopy the PAR-Q but only if you use the entire form.

NOTE: If the PAR-Q is being given to a person before he or she participates in a physical activity program or a fitness appraisal, this section may be used for legal or administrative purposes.

"I have read, understood and completed this questionnaire. Any questions I had were answered to my full satisfaction."

NAME _____

SIGNATURE _____ DATE _____

SIGNATURE OF PARENT _____ WITNESS _____
or GUARDIAN (for participants under the age of majority)

Note: This physical activity clearance is valid for a maximum of 12 months from the date it is completed and becomes invalid if your condition changes so that you would answer YES to any of the seven questions.

CSEP | SCPE
THE GOLD STANDARD IN EXERCISE
SCIENCE AND PERSONAL TRAINING

© Canadian Society for Exercise Physiology www.csep.ca/forms

Figure 1.2 PAR-Q and You.

Source: *Physical Activity Readiness questionnaire (PAR-Q)* © 2002. Used with permission from the Canadian society for Exercise Physiology. www.csep.ca.

If so, identify symptoms and indicate approximate date of last episode.

- Have you experienced a loss of consciousness? If so, what was the nature of the events preceding the period of unconsciousness and what treatment did you receive, if any?

- Have you had a fracture of any bone or dislocation of any joint? If so, describe the injury.

- Do you take any medication on a regular basis? If so, what is (are) the name(s) of the medication(s) and what are the reasons for use?

- Do you have allergies such as hives, asthma, or reaction to bee stings? If so, what?

- Have you experienced frequent chest pains or palpitations? If so, what was the approximate date of the last episode and what is the frequency of occurrence?

- Have you had a recent history of fatigue and undue tiredness? If so, when did it begin, or how long have you noticed the symptoms?

- Do you have a history of fainting? If so, under what circumstances?

All information obtained during the medical history must be reviewed during the PPE and thereafter if necessary. Subtle information obtained from the individual on the medical history may be as important as the physical examination findings in the remaining portion of the evaluation.

Physical Components of the Preparticipation Physical Examination

As indicated in table 1.1, the physical testing of the patient should include examination of all the major systems of the body—heart and lungs; abdomen; musculoskeletal system; ear, nose, and throat; and eyes and vision—as well as physical measurements and laboratory tests.

Height and Weight

Height and weight measurements are a part of every physical examination, regardless of the athletic involvement of the patient. This information on any patient can signal conditions that may otherwise be overlooked. In addition, height and weight information on patients allows one to notice changes in these statistics that may help in understanding some types of injuries. For example, consider Sara, a junior on the cross country team, who has complaints of pain in her lower back. In looking back at her PPE records, you note that Sara's weight was 23 lb (10.4 kg) less last year. Could this change in physical size play any role in the pain? Without the records, this clue might have been overlooked.

Blood Pressure and Pulse Rate

Elevated blood pressure (hypertension) or increased pulse rate may be a warning of a current medical condition in the patient. Normal pulse rate varies throughout the day; it is usually lowest first thing in the morning and tends to become lower with physical conditioning level. Normal ranges for pulse rates are provided in the sidebar Normal Values for Resting Heart Rate. When blood pressure as recorded in the physical examination is higher than normal (120/80 mmHg for teenagers and young adults), one should consider possible causes of the hypertension. A change in body weight or the use of certain drugs or other medications may contribute to a high reading and should be investigated. For the general population of adults, blood pressure below 140/90 mmHg is considered normal, and a pressure above 160/100 mmHg is considered too high. Elevated blood pressure during the physical examination should be reevaluated to ensure that the initial reading was not merely due to the patient's anxiety about the examination. To ensure that the measurement is valid (that it is correct), a series of repeat readings should be taken over the next several days at various hours during the day. To ensure reliability, it is important that the same clinician perform all of the follow-up pressure measurements. After three to five measurements have been collected, the blood pressure is usually quite consistent, and this should be the reading used for evaluation (see table 1.2).

An unexplained elevated blood pressure could signify the use of anabolic steroids, since one of the side effects of steroid use is hypertension. Should the client's blood pressure be elevated and remain elevated during repeat measures, further investigation into the cause should include evaluation of changes in the client's weight, physical appearance, and performance increases.

NORMAL VALUES FOR RESTING HEART RATE

- Newborn infants: 100 to 160 beats per minute
- Children 1 to 10 years: 70 to 120 beats per minute
- Children over 10 and adults: 60 to 100 beats per minute
- Well-trained clients: 40 to 60 beats per minute

Usually the suspicion of steroid use is heightened as a combination of signs is observed.

Blood Tests

It is not always necessary to do a blood test; such testing may not provide significant information if the patient is in good health. However, if an individual has been ill, the physician may order this test to help explain unusual symptoms or suspicious information contained in the medical history. It is customary to obtain a routine **complete blood count (CBC)** or **hemoglobin/hematocrit (Hb/Hct)**, or both, during the physical examination on individuals new to a program.

Red blood cells (RBCs), called erythrocytes, contain hemoglobin, which is bright red because of the iron it contains. About 60% to 70% of the iron in your body is in the hemoglobin in your blood. The percentage of RBCs in the blood is called the hematocrit. The primary function of the RBCs is to carry oxygen to the cells.

Minimally, each new participant should have an evaluation of Hb/Hct to check for iron-poor blood, or anemia. In addition to evaluating people new to the club or team, it may be desirable to evaluate female and endurance sport participants each year because of the prevalence of iron deficiencies in these groups. For example, consider John, a 31-year-old male who had been participating in a local running club for the past

Table 1.2   Blood Pressure Ranges

Category	Systolic (mmHg)		Diastolic (mmHg)	Follow-up recommended
Optimal*	Less than 120	and	Less than 80	Recheck in 2 years
Normal	Less than 130	and	Less than 85	Recheck in 2 years
High normal	130-139	or	85-89	Recheck in 1 year
Hypertension				
Stage 1 (mild)	140-159	or	90-99	Confirm within 2 months
Stage 2 (moderate)	160-179	or	100-109	Evaluate within 1 month
Stage 3 (severe)	180 or higher	or	110 or higher	Evaluate immediately or within 1 week depending on clinical situation

*Unusually low readings should be evaluated for clinical significance.

several years. In the last 2 years his interests had changed from the shorter-distance 10K race to the longer marathon and the ultra-marathon (100 miles [161 km]). Last year his success at Leadville, an ultramarathon event, had caused John to increase his running in preparation for the upcoming season. During the PPE for the running club, this patient admitted to the physician that he had had several cases of tendon injuries during the last year, as well as a feeling of fatigue with normal workouts. John had convinced himself that the fatigue was a direct result of the tendon problems.

The physician ordered a CBC with Hb/Hct to fully evaluate the oxygen-carrying capacity of John's blood. The Hb/Hct was slightly below the norm for John's age and gender, and the findings indicated a progressive form of iron deficiency anemia. In questioning John about other aspects of his life that could contribute to the blood-work findings, the physician discovered that John had been a vegetarian for the past 2 years and had been on nonsteroidal anti-inflammatory drugs (NSAIDs) off and on for the past year and a half. It was finally found that John lacked iron in his body and that this low iron level was the cause of his blood test results. Both the NSAIDs and the vegetarian diet could have contributed to the problem. The physician made several dietary suggestions for John and asked him to schedule a follow-up visit for another blood test in 4 months (the life span of the RBC is 120 days, so changes would not show up before that time). John left the PPE with mixed emotions; he felt a bit of sadness that he would need to cut back on his ultra-distance training but also relieved to know that something he was doing (and thus something he could change) was what was jeopardizing his health.

Because of the prevalence of sickle cell anemia in the black population, a special test of the blood, the sickle cell test, is important for black individuals. The sickle cell is an unusually shaped RBC (erythrocyte) that, if present, may become trapped and unable to exit the capillary wall because of its shape (figure 1.3). Patients with **sickle cell anemia** or **sickle cell trait** are at risk of complications during exertion. Close monitoring of persons with the sickle cell is necessary during participation, and education and counseling play a critical role in helping the person understand the condition.

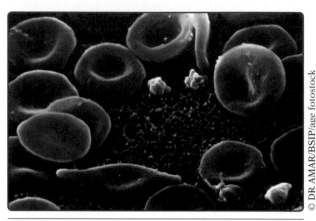

© DR AMAR/BSIP/age fotostock

Figure 1.3   Normal red blood cells and abnormal sickle cells.

Urinalysis

During the physical examination, urine may be collected for use in detecting some medical conditions as well as for random drug testing. Clients must be informed of the reason the **urinalysis** is being done if it is for drug-testing purposes, and in this case legal consent must be obtained; but the routine urinalysis for medical evaluation requires no legal permission. Findings of the urinalysis may indicate urinary tract infection, dehydration, diabetes, or kidney pathology. Urinary tract infection is indicated by an excessive number of white blood cells and the type of white blood cells in the urine. The urine specific gravity is an indication of the level of hydration and could signal impending difficulties with heat tolerance if the patient is not well hydrated. Diabetes is suspected if the level of sugars (glucose) in the urine is elevated to between 80 and 120 mg/100 ml. Red blood cells in the urine may be an indication of kidney disorders and warrant further testing.

Visual Acuity

Changes in the individual's vision could certainly affect performance. A quick and simple visual acuity test using the **Snellen eye chart** (figure 1.4) can provide the sports medicine staff with enough information to determine whether further evaluation might be warranted. In the evaluation of visual acuity using the Snellen eye chart, the patient must read the chart from the chart-specified distance (usually 20 ft [6.1 m]), and the area of the testing should be well lighted.

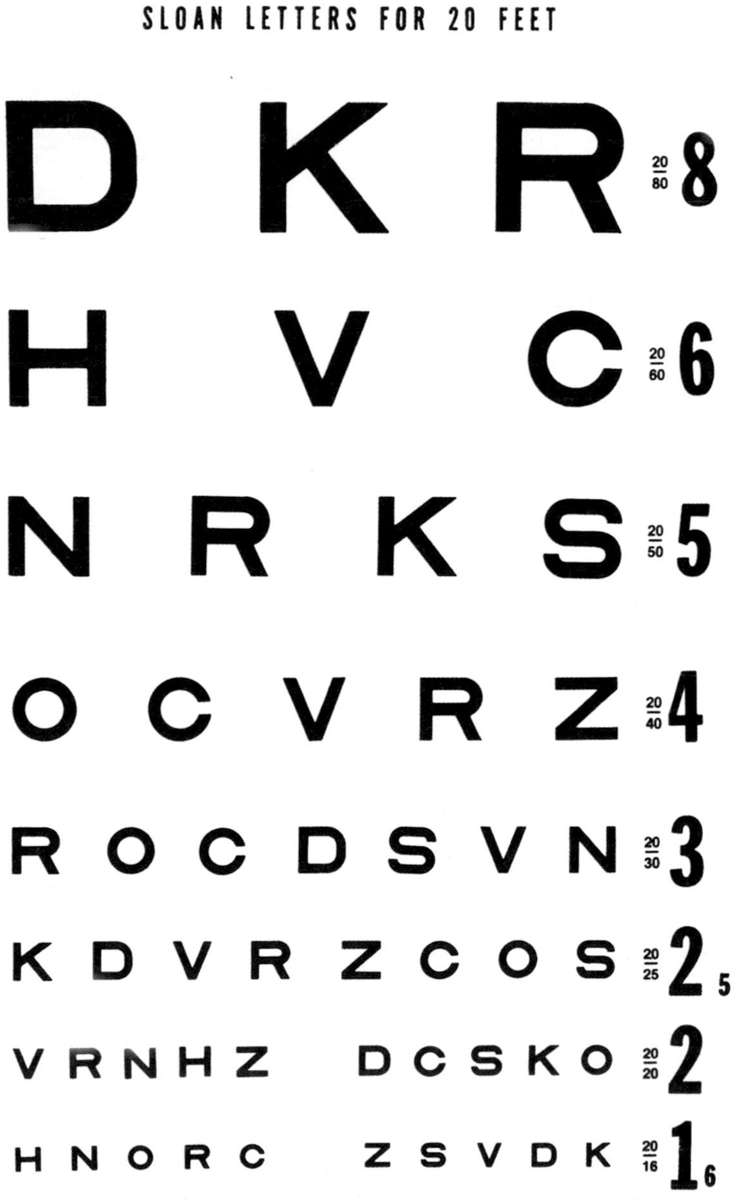

General Medical Examination

The general medical examination includes dental, heart and lung, abdomen and pelvis, **ENT** (ear, nose, and throat), and musculoskeletal examinations. Trained physicians must perform these examinations, and frequently specialists are used in lieu of the general practitioner.

The reasons for evaluation of these areas include detection of pathology as well as the establishment of normative data for the patient. For example, a young individual with an **undescended testicle** may experience no trouble with the condition yet, but if he were struck in the groin during practice or competition, this otherwise undiscovered finding could be a cause for great concern.

Other Testing

The special evaluations to be conducted include, but are not limited to, the items listed in table 1.3. Any physician can perform testing in any of the evaluation areas if a specialist is not available or willing to serve in that capacity.

Specific Tests for Individuals With Disabilities

When providing PPEs for persons with disabilities, it may be necessary to perform additional medical tests to clarify the existing pathologies involved. Depending on the type of disability, more in-depth clinical evaluation may be necessary. Most importantly, laboratory

SLOAN LETTERS FOR 20 FEET

Figure 1.4 Snellen eye chart.

Table 1.3   Special Evaluations

Specialist and area of examination	Specific target of examination
Optometrist or ophthalmologist	
Examination of the eyes	Evaluate visual acuity, use of eyeglasses or contact lenses; examine the sclera for the presence of jaundice.
Examination of the optic disc and retina if examination environment allows	Look for the presence of any abnormal findings.
Ear, nose, and throat specialist	
Examination of the ears	Determine the presence of acute or chronic infection, perforation of the eardrum, and gross hearing loss.
Examination of the nose	Assess the presence of deformity that may affect endurance.
Orthopedic surgeon	
Examination of the skin	Determine the presence of infection; scars of previous surgery or trauma; jaundice; and purpura (to be performed by all examiners).
Assessment of the neck	Determine range of motion and the presence of pain associated with such motion.
Assessment of the back	Determine range of motion and abnormal curvature of the spine.
Examination of the extremities	Determine abnormal mobility or immobility, deformity, instability, muscle weakness or atrophy, surgical scars, and varicosities.
Neurological examination	Assess balance and coordination and presence of abnormal reflexes.
Cardiac specialist or general or family practitioner	
Examination of chest contour	Pay attention to conditions causing constriction of the chest such as scoliosis.
Auscultation and percussion of the lungs	Listen for signs of airway obstruction, wheezing, or abnormal congestion.
Assessment of the heart	Pay attention to the presence of murmurs, noting rhythm and rate before and after exercise.
General surgeon or general or family practitioner	
Assessment of the abdomen	Look for possible presence of hepatomegaly, splenomegaly, or abnormal masses.
Examination of the testes	Determine the presence and descent of both testes, abnormal masses or configurations, or hernia.
Assessment of physiological maturation	Determine normal growth and development.

testing (blood tests and urinalysis) should be delayed until all other aspects of the physical examination have been completed. After the clinical examination is complete, the physician will be more prepared to order the particular special tests that may be needed.

In the PPE of a participant who is physically challenged, it is critical to consider the events or activities that the person will be participating in. There is no reason to withhold a person with a disability from participation if the sport does not create additional risks.

Fitness or Performance Testing

Some teams conduct fitness testing or performance testing as part of the PPE. Other groups use performance testing to serve as a baseline for exercise prescription. It should be an individual organizer's decision what performance tests, if any, to include in the physical exam, yet special attention should be given to older patients. The American College of Sports Medicine (ACSM) recommends that all men over the age of 40 and all women over 50 be evaluated with a graded exercise test (with a physician present) before being allowed to enter into high-intensity exercise. This test is also recommended prior to participation for any patient with a high risk of heart disease. A graded exercise test is used to evaluate cardiorespiratory function and is administered using a bench, cycle ergometer, or treadmill. Complete fitness evaluations are often performed when a new member joins a fitness facility or when someone hires a personal or fitness trainer (figure 1.5).

PHYSICAL FITNESS EVALUATION FORM

Time in: _____   Time out: _____

Student box number: _____   Class of: _____

Department: _____

Name: _____   Date: _____

☐ Male ☐ Female   Resting heart rate: _____   Resting blood pressure: _____

Age (years): _____   Height (inches): _____   Weight (pounds): _____

- -

	Male	**Female**
Skinfolds (mm)	Chest _____	Triceps _____
	Abdomen _____	Suprailiac _____
	Thigh _____	Thigh _____

Hip-to-waist ratio   Waist _____   Hip _____

Sit and reach (in.)   _____   _____   _____

Grip strength (lb)   Right _____   _____   Left _____   _____

Agility run (or jumps/10 s)   _____   _____

Curl-up   _____

Vertical jump (in.)   Reach _____   Jump _____   _____

Bench press reps (male: 80 lb; female: 40 lb)   _____

Bike ride   Workload (kg – m/min) _____   5th min HR _____

                                                              6th min HR _____

Figure 1.5   Fitness evaluation form.

Adapted, by permission, from D. Martin.

Less stressful measurements of physical abilities, such as the sit-and-reach test for hamstring and low back flexibility, can be easily included in the examination, whereas it may be necessary to schedule a cardiovascular fitness evaluation (graded exercise test) for another time, after the other portions of the PPE have been performed. One can establish the number and types of fitness tests on the basis of the time allowed for each individual going through the PPE. Certainly you do not want to include tests that will substantially affect the length of time needed in the physical exam unless you have done prior planning and allotted sufficient time.

Preparticipation Physical Examination Results

Results from the physical examination will assist in the decision-making process through which the physician allows, or more precisely, finds no reason to limit, the patient's participation in the desired activity. One must be careful not to assume that a participant who is cleared for participation in one activity will automatically be suited for a more strenuous event or sport. As an example, consider Jason, who was born with spina bifida, a condition in which the vertebrae fail to fully form around the spinal cord. In Jason's case, the condition caused some muscle weakness in the lower extremities. Jason was able to walk and could even run short distances but fatigued quite quickly, and with the fatigue came a loss of muscle coordination. The family's physician evaluated Jason for the local bowling team and signed the form stating that there was no reason to limit this person's participation on that team. After the season, Jason asked his parents if he could participate in the Athletes with Disabilities Soccer League. Since Jason had done so well on the bowling team, his parents gave their permission. Jason was delighted, but the joy was short-lived; the coach told him that he would not be allowed to play until he had had the proper PPE for youth soccer. Unfortunately, as Jason had

feared, the physician would not clear him to play soccer.

Why wouldn't Jason be allowed to play soccer if he was physically able to participate on the bowling team? The answer relates to the purpose of the PPE, which in turn relates to the most difficult decision—that of approval for participation. The American Academy of Pediatrics' Council on Sports Medicine and Fitness (2008) has identified three categories of clearance: (1) unrestricted clearance, (2) clearance after completion of further evaluation or **rehabilitation**, and (3) not cleared for certain types of sports or, in extreme cases, any sports. Table 1.4 shows examples of clearances for some common conditions.

Each PPE form must clearly state the sport or activity in which the person is to participate. The coach and the patient must realize that the permission applies only to the sport(s) or activities indicated.

In the event that a preexisting condition is found during the PPE, steps should be taken to ensure safe participation of the individual. On occasion, the patient must be held from participation until a condition is corrected and the medical staff determines that participation will not impose an unusual risk. For example, a volleyball player who reports to the PPE with a swollen and ecchymotic (black and blue) ankle may be withheld from running and jumping activities until the swelling is reduced and the stability of the ankle is evaluated as within normal limits (WNL).

Most physicians and organizations attempt to counsel the participant about finding a safe sport and also attempt to provide the rehabilitation or medical assistance needed to allow the patient some level of involvement with the team. Thus, the aforementioned volleyball player may be able to do some volleyball drills of serving or hand skills of setting if jumping is not required.

Medical Referral

In all cases of restricted clearance for activity, the underlying reason for limiting the par-

Table 1.4 Common Medical Conditions Limiting Sport Participation

Condition	Clearance decision	Recommendation
High blood pressure	Pass	Monitor blood pressure (BP) for several days. If BP fails to stabilize, refer for evaluation.
Anterior cruciate insufficiency	Defer for evaluation	Establish baseline strength; fully evaluate joint stability.
Spinal disc pathology	Defer for evaluation	Refer to specialist for magnetic resonance imaging (MRI) and other testing to establish health of disc. Refer to rehab for evaluation and strengthening.
Sickle cell anemia	Fail	Counsel patient regarding high risks of sport participation. Encourage toward alternative involvement (manager position).
Absence of one of a paired organ	Pass with limitations	Patient must be allowed to participate in sport only where there is little to no risk of injury to the healthy organ. If some risk does exist, legal counsel must be involved to establish consent to play.
Diabetes	Pass	Staff and students involved with this patient must be educated on the warning signs of diabetic emergencies. Patient should be closely monitored for blood sugar levels.

ticipation should be fully evaluated, even in cases in which the patient is allowed full participation but only if supervised. One should not only refer the individual to a medical provider but, if possible, should also make the appointment for the participant. Usually the referring party receives notification of the evaluation and treatment rendered by the consultant. This information, an important part of the patient's medical information, should be obtained, discussed, understood, and retained in the individual's medical records. Later follow-up with the same specialist is frequently necessary to allow the practitioner to follow the person's progress.

Activity Clearance With Supervision

Occasionally a participant has a medical condition that is currently under control but warrants supervision. In such instances, the physician may permit the individual to participate in the indicated activity or sport under the stipulation that she have the supervision of a medical or other trained person. Thus the patient is not allowed to participate in sports in which the coach or other supervisors are not present at all times. Conditions such as **asthma**, bronchitis, diabetes, epilepsy, bleeding trait, colitis, and other

treatable ailments may require this type of supervision.

Disqualification of a Participant

The team physician is usually considered the person responsible for determining that a person should not be allowed to participate in a specific sport. As previously indicated, efforts should always be made to find some avenue for participation if a specific sport is not well suited for the client. The responsibility of deciding on total disqualification from a sport sometimes creates a difficulty for the team physician, who does not want to restrict participation unnecessarily but is responsible for protecting the patient's health.

If the person does not receive clearance for the sport, this denial is an indication that participation poses additional risks. In establishing whether a condition warrants restriction from participation, the physician typically addresses the following questions:

- Does the problem place the individual at an increased risk of injury?
- Does the problem place another team member's safety in jeopardy?
- Could the person safely participate with compensations such as medication,

bracing, padding, or specific rehabilitation?

- Could limited participation be permitted during the time in which treatment is being completed?
- If clearance is denied, what activities can the person safely participate in?

Ideally, the decision regarding sport participation should meet with agreement between the team physician and other medical specialists, team officials (athletic trainer, coach, and attorney), and the patient or family or both.

Considerations for Athletes With Impairments

As explained in the *2010-2011 NCAA Sports Medicine Handbook*, collegiate sport participants who are considered impaired include, but are not limited to, the following:

1. Individuals who use a wheelchair
2. Those who are deaf, blind, or missing a limb
3. Those who have only one of a set of paired organs
4. Those who may have behavioral, emotional, and psychological disorders that substantially limit a major life activity

A sport participant who has only one of a set of paired organs and who wishes to participate may do so if the medical specialists agree and, again according to the NCAA, if the following factors are considered and found in favor of the patient:

1. The quality and function of the remaining organ
2. The probability of injury to the remaining organ
3. The availability of current protective equipment and the likely effectiveness of such equipment to prevent injury to the remaining organ

No firm rationale for disqualification can be stated for each sporting activity because each case is individual. It is reasonable to suggest, however, that all individuals should be provided the opportunity to participate if participation will not jeopardize their health or that of teammates.

Administration of the Preparticipation Physical Examination

There are as many different ways of doing the PPE as there are ranks of sport participation and fitness levels. However, all should establish the same thing: that there is no medical reason to prohibit the individual from participation. We consider two main methods of conducting a PPE: individual and group.

Individual Preparticipation Physical Exams

Teams with a limited budget frequently ask the individual to be responsible for his own PPE, but the examination is usually outlined in a form provided to the participant (figure 1.6). This procedure is quite common, especially at the high school and pre-high school levels. An advantage of having participants see their own physicians for the PPE is that the family doctor is usually familiar with the individual and the individual's family. A physician who knows the medical history of the person and the family may question and report medical conditions that might otherwise go undetected. The physician familiar with the individual may be able to discuss sensitive issues and may have a good understanding of the person's motivation for participation. Perhaps the best physical examination would be provided by the family physician who is knowledgeable about the physical demands of the sport and who is skilled in orthopedics as well as general medicine.

Medical costs have skyrocketed in part because of the rising costs of medical malpractice insurance. Although rates vary by state, an orthopedic surgeon might pay anywhere between $30,000 and $200,000 a year for medical malpractice insurance. Some

UNIVERSITY OF ARIZONA INTERCOLLEGIATE ATHLETICS HEALTH HISTORY

Name: _____ Emergency Contact: _____

DOB: ___/___/___ Sport: _____ Emergency Phone: _____ Relationship: _____

This questionnaire is for medical screening only. Your honest and complete answers will help the medical staff better assess your health. The content of this questionnaire is confidential and will be treated as a medical document according to university, state, and federal guidelines. Failure to answer questions fully and honestly may have consequences as noted below. If you do not understand any of these questions please contact medical services or your medical provider.

Please note yes answers in Notes section below	Yes/No		Yes/No
1. Are you taking any prescription or nonprescription medicines, vitamins, or supplements (including inhalers, ointments, birth control, etc.)?	☐ ☐	21. Have you ever had a "ding" (gotten your bell rung), or had an injury that left you with a headache, feeling dizzy, or confused?	☐ ☐
2. Are you allergic to any medicines, foods, pollens, or insect stings?	☐ ☐	22. Do you have a history of head injury or concussions? If yes, how many?	☐ ☐
3. Have you been diagnosed with, or take medication for Attention Deficit Disorder (ADD/ADHD)?	☐ ☐	23. Do you have a history of seizures?	☐ ☐
4. Have you had a medical illness or injury since your last physical?	☐ ☐	24. Do you get frequent or severe headaches?	☐ ☐
5. Do you have any chronic or ongoing medical conditions (diabetes, high blood pressure, sickle cell trait, etc.)?	☐ ☐	25. Do you ever have numbness or tingling in your arms, hands, or feet?	☐ ☐
6. Have you had any surgeries?	☐ ☐	26. Do you have a history of stingers, burners, or pinched nerves?	☐ ☐
7. Has your participation in sports ever been restricted or denied due to heart problems?	☐ ☐	27. Do you have a history of asthma, exercise induced asthma, shortness of breath during exertion, or coughing or wheezing during exertion?	☐ ☐
8. Do you have a history of rheumatic fever?	☐ ☐	28. Do you have a history of heat illness or heat stroke?	☐ ☐
9. Have you ever passed out or been dizzy during or after exercise?	☐ ☐	29. Do you wear any special protective or corrective equipment not usually used in your sport (brace, neck roll, etc.)?	☐ ☐
10. Do you get chest pain during or after exercise?	☐ ☐	30. Do you have any problems with your vision?	☐ ☐
11. Do you get palpitations (skipped or racing heart beats) with exercise?	☐ ☐	31. Do you wear glasses or contacts?	☐ ☐
12. Have you ever been told you have a heart murmur, or had a special test for your heart??	☐ ☐	32. Do you have any current skin problems (itching, blisters, rash, warts, etc.)?	☐ ☐
13. Have you ever been told you have high blood pressure or high cholesterol?	☐ ☐	33. Do you want to weigh less or more than you do right now?	☐ ☐
14. Is there a family history of sudden death or death from heart problems before age 50?	☐ ☐	34. Do you feel pressure to achieve or maintain a particular weight or body composition?	☐ ☐
15. Does anyone in your family have: hypertrophic cardiomyopathy, Marfan syndrome, arrhythmogenic right ventricular cardiomyopathy, long QT syndrome, short QT syndrome, Brugada syndrome, or catecholaminergic polymorphic ventricular tachycardia?	☐ ☐	35. Have you or anyone in your family been treated for a psychological issue (ADHD, anxiety, depression, eating disorder, etc.)?	☐ ☐
16. Have you had a severe viral infection (like Infectious Mono or myocarditis) in the last month?	☐ ☐	36. Do you or anyone in your family have any drug or alcohol problems?	☐ ☐
17. Do you have any missing or broken teeth or do you have braces or a retainer?	☐ ☐	FOR WOMEN ONLY: 37. Have you ever had a menstrual period?	☐ ☐
18. Are you missing any paired organ (eye, kidney, testicle, ovary)?	☐ ☐	38. At what age did you have your first period?	
19. Has your participation in sports ever been restricted due to injuries of the head, bones, or joints:	☐ ☐	39. How many periods did you have in the last 12 months?	
20. Do you have a history of broken bones, dislocated joints, strains, sprains, or abnormal swelling? Please list below.	☐ ☐	40. Are you currently, or have you recently, been pregnant?	☐ ☐

Notes:_____

_____

_____

I, the undersigned, hereby acknowledge, affirm, and represent that all above statements are true and accurate to the best of my knowledge; and that no answers or information have been withheld. If any information and/or statements are false and/or have been omitted in reference to my past and/or present medical history, I fully understand that the University of Arizona, its agents, servants, trustees, and employees disclaim liability, and will not be held liable for any injuries and/or illnesses not noted. **I also accept the responsibility for reporting my injuries and illnesses to the medical staff during my time as a student-athlete at the University of Arizona, including signs and symptoms of concussion.**

Student-Athlete Signature: _____ Date: _____ Provider: _____ Date: _____

Figure 1.6 Preparticipation physical evaluation form. *(continued)*

Name:
DOB:
Sport:

DO NOT COMPLETE BELOW THIS LINE — FOR OFFICIAL USE ONLY

Height: _____ Weight: _____

BP: _____/_____ Pulse: _____

<u>VISION</u>

R20/_____L20/_____ With/Without correction?

Corrective lenses: YES/NO Pupils: R>=<L

[ ] See electronic medical record

Ears: _____

Nose: _____

Throat: _____

Heart rhythm: _____

Heart murmurs: _____

Femoral pulse: _____

Marfan syndrome: _____

Lungs: _____

Abdomen: _____

Skin: _____

Neuro: _____

Immunizations: _____

Laboratory test ordered: _____

Recommendations: _____

_____

_____

Evaluator: _____

Date: ____/____/____

_____
                    Team physician
_____

_____

_____

_____

Approved _____ Deferred _____ DQ _____

Team physician: _____

Date: ____/____/____

Previous orthopedic surgery?

yes _____ no _____ Date: ____/____/____

Head/neck: _____

Trunk/Spine: _____

Shoulders: _____

Elbows: _____

Wrist/Hand: _____

Hips/Pelvis: _____

Thigh: _____

Knees: _____

Ankles: _____

Foot: _____

Flexibility: _____

Special tests: _____

Comments/Recommendations: _____

_____

_____

_____

_____

Deferred pending ortho physician eval _____

Approved _____ DQ _____

Evaluator: _____

Date: ____/____/____

_____
                        Ortho

Comments/Recommendations: _____

_____

_____

_____

_____

Approved _____ Deferred _____ DQ _____

Ortho physician: _____

Date: ____/____/____

Figure 1.6 *(continued)* Preparticipation physical evaluation form.

Reprinted, by permission, from University of Arizona Athletic Department.

medical specialists pay more and others pay less, yet all medical providers must hold this type of insurance to protect them financially in the event of an error in medical care. The net result is increased costs to the consumer. Medical care has become so expensive, in fact, that many families subscribe to large health maintenance organizations (HMOs) rather than receiving health care from a family physician as in the past. All too commonly, an individual visits the HMO physician only when in need of urgent care, and a different physician handles the visit each time. The family physician who knows the entire family and all associated medical histories may be the exception rather than the rule in today's medical system. This lack of familiarity, and perhaps a lack of frequent wellness exams, makes the PPE even more important.

In addition to lacking personal knowledge of the individual and perhaps of the family's medical history, the HMO physician may not be equipped to handle some aspects of the physical exam such as the eye test, body composition measures, or some of the flexibility exams. The coach or another trained team representative can complete these somewhat nonmedical aspects of the evaluation.

Group Preparticipation Physical Examination

When a large group of people must be screened at the same time, a group examination may be an efficient means of accomplishing the task. The group examination relies on a number of health care professionals who staff stations through which the person must pass to complete the physical examination. In situations in which a team or school uses a number of physicians as consultants, it is logical to use these consultants as physicians for the medical evaluations in the group PPE.

Since the group exam uses a number of physicians and other health care specialists, each has only a small portion of the entire exam to complete. In this situation the physician may be able to be more thorough and also more efficient, thereby reducing the

time needed for the examination. Additionally, having the same physician evaluate each member of a team on a given part of the exam provides great reliability (meaning that the same finding is reported in the same way each time). If the team is fortunate enough to have the same medical professionals from year to year, participants remaining with the team over a period of years have the benefit of continuity of care and excellent consistency of medical practice.

The group PPE gives the team's athletic trainer the added advantage of personally knowing the physician and knowing that each individual on the team has undergone the same thorough PPE. However, although peace of mind comes from having a degree of control of the participants' PPEs, problems often arise in conducting a physical examination with a large group.

Problem areas found in group physicals are variable, but often include participants who become excited to re-unite with teammates after the summer vacation and noise levels (and energy levels) can make it difficult to hear at nearby stations. When using various rooms and locations for the group physical, patients can become confused and not know their next station. Sometimes minor problems or physician comments can be overlooked when overall, all specialists "signed off" on the patient. This might be a comment of "needs to continue quadriceps strengthening," but the weakness is not sufficient to limit the patient's participation. Some physicians take more time with their patients, causing a backup of waiting individuals. This often causes an increase in noise level and sometimes increased pressure on the physician. And, due to the large numbers, individual counseling is limited during the exam and must be programmed into the patient's schedule. With proper advanced planning, one may minimize each problematic issue.

To use a school gymnasium as an example, stations may be set up to allow a smooth transition from one test to another in the group physical examination. Group physicals require preplanning of space, equipment,

GROUP PHYSICAL IN A SCHOOL GYMNASIUM

Station 1: Check-In

Participants obtain appropriate forms and progress to chair area to complete required documents. Computers may be used.

Station 2: Height and Weight

Student workers take measurements and record them on medical forms; worker from the sport information office or department records data for use in media relations.

Station 3: Vision and Eye Screening

A well-lighted area 20 ft (6.1 m) in length is needed for the vision screening. The physician supervises the vision screening and then performs individualized eye exams.

Station 4: Laboratory Testing (Urinalysis and Blood Test) and Immunizations

Participants progress to the rest room area. Nurses perform any needed immunizations. Contracted laboratory phlebotomists do blood draws and obtain urine samples.

Station 5: Ear, Nose, and Throat

Physician perform ear, nose, and throat evaluation with the patient in a seated position. A small table, such as a taping table, is usually satisfactory.

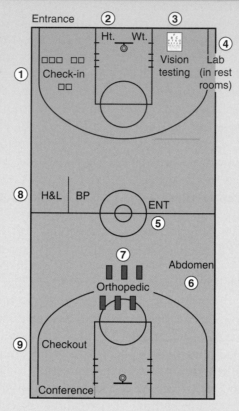

Station 6: Abdominal Area

Physician checks abdomen and pelvis. This location within the examination area must be sectioned off to ensure privacy for the patient.

Station 7: Orthopedic Exam

Because of the length of time required to perform each orthopedic exam, athletic trainers and physical therapists may assist the orthopedic surgeon(s) in the evaluation of bones and joints. This location need not be enclosed, but having some partitions on the periphery of the area is beneficial.

Station 8: Blood Pressure and Heart and Lung Evaluation

These are actually two adjoining stations, both of which require a degree of silence. Several evaluators are needed to obtain blood pressure and pulse, while only one or two physicians are necessary to complete the heart and lung examination.

Station 9: Checkout

Typically the team physician responsible for the medical services performs the checkout duties. The physician must perform a thorough review of all data collected before signing off on the permission to participate.

and personnel needs. Each station may create a unique concern; for example, the station in which blood pressure is measured must remain as quiet as possible in order to allow the examiners to hear. If this station is positioned where patients congregate, noise levels may rise and make the evaluation of blood pressure difficult. See the example of a gymnasium setup in the sidebar Group Physical in a School Gymnasium.

CASE STUDY

Derrick, a transfer student from California, reported to the athletic training staff for the preparticipation physical as directed by his coach. Derrick had been unable to attend the group physical for the football team due to a family medical crisis. Derrick's newborn son had been born with a heart defect, which required emergency surgery. Derrick had spent every day and night at the hospital for the past 4 days. Unfortunately, the baby did not survive the surgery, and the funeral was on the day the team was scheduled for the PPE. Derrick's flight into Phoenix from San Diego arrived at noon the day after the PPE.

Since the rest of the team had already finished the PPE, Derrick was sent to the health center for his physical. He returned from the appointment with the proper forms signed, ready to start practice. He picked up his football gear from the equipment room and went to the team meeting that afternoon. In the meeting he learned that the team would be doing the physical testing in the morning,

starting with the shuttle run, which he was told he had to finish within 120 s.

Derrick was concerned about the run but thought he could make the time. After finishing the run, Derrick collapsed on the side of the field, exhausted and starting to become nauseated. After immediate attention by the medical staff, Derrick was transported to the hospital for treatment of a sickle cell crisis. Derrick carried the sickle cell trait, but not the disease.

Think About It

1. What factors contribute to problems when a participant has the sickle cell trait?

2. What was happening in Derrick's life that could have contributed to dehydration? Would the change in climate have any effect?

3. How could the PPE have prevented this episode? Do you think participation in the group PPE would have been better than the individual exam Derrick received at the local health center?

Learning Aids

SUMMARY

The PPE is an important step in understanding possible limitations to participation for the fitness-conscious individual. Understanding the physical limitations can help to prevent injury or illness that might result from participation. The PPE should be used as a tool to help the patient prevent problems and not as a tool to restrict participation. If individuals can see the positive benefits of a thorough physical examination, they will be much more receptive to it.

KEY CONCEPTS AND REVIEW

▶ **Discuss the importance of a preparticipation physical examination for sport team members or for someone beginning a fitness program.**

The PPE evaluates the medical status of the individual with reference to the requirements of the sport or activity to be undertaken. The PPE differs from an annual physical exam (wellness exam) in that the evaluation focuses on potential areas of increased risk of health hazard during vigorous activity rather on than the health of the sedentary individual.

▸ **Discuss how knowledge of preexisting conditions may help in the medical care of the physically active individual.**

When a preexisting condition is detected before it has caused harm, treatment or adaptations can be instituted to allow safe participation in physical activities. For example, a person who is diagnosed with a small hernia may be cleared to participate in activities but restricted from heavy weight training. Knowledge of the potential for further trouble can help keep the patient and the medical staff alert if symptoms increase.

▸ **Present the two main ways to conduct a physical examination for athletic sports teams, and list the advantages and disadvantages of each.**

Individual examinations cost less for the school or team, and the physician may know the patient or her medical history well. On the other hand, the physician may not know the individual, and the quality of the exam will not be uniform across all patients tested. With a group examination, in which all participants are checked by the same physicians, the exam is concluded during one session (therefore it's fast). The problems associated with group exams are typical of managing a large group: the noise level is high; individuals may become distracted and confused; follow-through on suspicious findings is difficult; and there is less privacy and individual counseling.

▸ **List the types of examinations to be included in the preparticipation physical examination, and identify the members of the medical team needed to conduct these exams in a group physical.**

Administrative forms and history are handled by a department administrative assistant or other staff members. Local emergency

medical technicians, paramedics, nurses or nursing students, and athletic trainers or trained student athletic trainers usually take an individual's blood pressure and pulse. Nurses or phlebotomists (or both) from a laboratory take samples for the blood test and urinalysis. Athletic trainers or trained students measure height, weight, and body composition. Optometrists or trained ancillary staff perform vision screening. Orthopedic surgeons and athletic trainers do an orthopedic evaluation. A general surgeon or other MD, or a doctor of osteopathy (DO), assesses the abdomen and pelvic areas. An ear, nose, and throat specialist or other MD or DO evaluates the individual's ears, nose, and throat. A cardiologist or other MD or DO performs the evaluation of the heart and lungs. Optional tests include dental check by a dentist and an electrocardiogram by an exercise physiologist or other trained ancillary staff.

▸ **Compare and contrast aspects of the group physical and the individualized examination.**

Both methods of PPE evaluate the participant to ascertain that there is no known risk to participation in the desired sport. The group physical uses the same examiner for each participant and thus provides a degree of reliability, whereas a group of individual examinations yields data from a variety of examiners. The individual exam can provide more time for discussion and counseling for the individual participant, while the group exam may become backlogged if one individual needs additional time. The individual examination is as quiet as the examining physician needs it to be, while the group physical can become noisy. The team, at no cost to the individual participant, typically conducts the group physical whereas the individual exam is at the patient's expense.

▸ **Identify problematic areas in conducting a group physical and list ways in which those situations may be managed.**

Problematic areas include the following:

- Noise levels may make it difficult to hear: Arrange stations to limit congregation outside critical areas.

- Participants may become confused regarding where to go next: Provide "ushers" to direct traffic flow and assist people in finding the next station.

- Minor findings may become lost in the numbers: Generate a list of any remarks made on the participant's physical exam form. Assign an ATC for a sport team to ensure proper follow-through and follow-ups.

- Physical arrangement of stations may allow a waiting patient to pressure the examiner: Arrange stations to provide as much privacy as possible, and have a staff member serve as monitor to control situations.

- The large number of patients waiting for evaluation may reduce individual counseling: Have physicians schedule postexam time to speak with patients.

PRACTICE!

For hands-on practice in this area, go to the web resource and complete the following:

Level 3.4, Module 06: Pre-Participation Medical and Physical Examination

CRITICAL THINKING QUESTIONS

1. You recently accepted the position of Director of Sports Medicine at a local community college, and your first challenge is to develop the PPE plan for the fall sports of cross country, soccer, volleyball, and swimming. Discuss your proposal. Include the type of exam you will suggest; and from a local directory, identify the individual(s) you would use to conduct the exams.

2. You are assisting with the group PPE for your college, and the medical director comes to you saying that your station is doing fine with the number of helpers you have, so he wants you to go help elsewhere to keep the flow going. What exam area(s) would you feel prepared to help in? What other thoughts would you have about attempting to improve the traffic flow?

3. You have planned for a group physical for several fall sports. Unfortunately, recent changes were made to one of the team's plans, and the participants will not be reporting to campus until 2 days after the scheduled PPE. The next scheduled group PPE is 2 weeks after the day that team plans to begin practice. Explain what you would do to ensure that all participants in this sport will obtain their physical in time for the scheduled first practice.

Fitness Testing and Conditioning

Susan Kay Hillman, ATC, PT

OBJECTIVES

After reading this chapter, the student should be able to do the following:

- Identify ways in which information from fitness testing can help the athletic trainer.

- Discuss the rationale for conducting fitness testing at various times before, during, or after the sport or training season.

- Explain the method of establishing the 1-repetition maximum in weightlifting.

- Define *aerobic* and *anaerobic* with reference to energy systems and relate each to various activities.

- Define isotonic, isometric, and isokinetic exercise and give an example of each.

- Compare and contrast the two types of muscle contraction: concentric and eccentric.

- Discuss factors to consider in designing an exercise prescription.

- Define the overload principle and explain how it applies to conditioning and strength techniques.

The area of strength and conditioning has grown considerably in recent years: Whereas in the past it was just one of a coach's responsibilities, today we have full-time strength and conditioning coaches. Strength and conditioning coaches have helped to reduce the sport coaches' responsibilities, giving increased attention to off-season conditioning as well as to strength and conditioning during the sport season.

Unfortunately, some schools and teams still rely on the sport coach to provide proper conditioning and strengthening programs for the participants. Regardless of the job description, all individuals working with the team should be familiar with the various aspects of strengthening so that they can advise individuals in this area if necessary.

In addition, there may be times when you work with people who are **deconditioned**. Through inactivity they are not as fit or active as they were at another time in their lives. With attention to proper warm-up, exercise moderation, and a good stretching program, even patients in their eighth decade of life may be challenging one another in physical activities. Because of decreases in **cardiorespiratory** function, these participants may experience "dizziness" and "side stitch." Orthopedic conditions affecting the weight-bearing joints may be related to a loss of bone density or to various stages of **osteoarthritis** in the older patient. Careful planning and exercise selection can help minimize these types of conditions.

The first half of this chapter is devoted to fitness testing procedures and fitness testing parameters, including muscle function, cardiorespiratory function, agility and speed, flexibility, and body composition. The second half of the chapter focuses on developing an appropriate strength training program and the different types of strength training that can be used. Integrating cardiorespiratory training and flexibility programs is also discussed.

Fitness Testing Procedures

Starting a conditioning program requires knowledge of the baseline of fitness. If you ever have begun a strength or conditioning program, you may have had no real idea where to start. You may have found yourself looking at a rack of weights and wondering how much you should start with. This sense of uncertainty reflects one of the reasons the fitness test is so important. A fitness test can allow you to identify the muscle groups or the basic energy sources that need to be trained. Fitness testing can take many forms but usually comprises tests of muscular function (strength, endurance, and power), cardiorespiratory function, speed, and agility, as well as body composition (see table 2.1).

You probably remember fitness tests from your early years in physical education classes. The Presidential Physical Fitness Test may have been one of your earliest exposures to fitness testing. The President's Council on Physical Fitness and Sports works toward promoting physical activity, fitness, and sports that enhance and improve health. In an attempt to promote participation in sport and physical activities for people of all ages and abilities, the council coordinates several programs, including the President's Challenge, the Presidential Sports Awards, and National Physical Fitness and Sports Month (each May). In addition to the national focus on fitness and fitness testing, almost every fitness center, club, and school conducts fitness evaluations either for the participant's information or for preparticipation purposes. Additionally, coaches, to determine the level of conditioning of patients, have almost always used fitness tests. Fitness tests may be done before an individual is accepted for a sport team, during the season, or at the end of the sport season to allow the setting of goals for the next season. Whenever the testing is performed, the goal is to measure the individual's level of fitness. Before we discuss fitness testing, let's consider when the tests should be done.

Table 2.1 **Various Methods to Test Fitness**

Fitness test	Test purpose	Description	Pros and cons	Comments
Run tests for set time or distance	Cardiorespiratory endurance	Various tests use time (9, 10, 12 min) or distance (1 mile, 1.5 miles).	Pros: Easy, inexpensive to conduct; can test large groups. Cons: Affected by motivation.	Well suited to all age groups and fitness levels. Use longer time (10 min) for adults, shorter time or distance for children.
Harvard Step Test	Cardiorespiratory endurance	Subject steps up and down 20-in. height at 30 steps/min for 5 min or until exhaustion. Exhaustion = inability to keep pace for 15 s. Stop, sit, and count heart rate (for 30 s) at 1, 2, and 3 min postexercise.	Pros: Simple test, easy to administer. Cons: Metronome or cadence tape required.	Scoring: (100 × test duration in seconds) divided by 2 × total number of heartbeats in recovery period. Excellent: >90 Good: 80-89 High average: 65-79 Low average: 55-64 Poor: <55
1-repetition maximum tests	Isotonic strength	Subject lifts one repetition of a selected weight. If weight can be lifted properly, heavier weight is selected. Repeat until maximum is identified.	Pros: Equipment is usually available. Cons: Applies only to that particular lift.	Excellent method of determining pre- and postmeasurements of strength.
Vertical jump test	Muscle power	Subject stands next to wall and reaches up with the hand closest to the wall to highest point. That point is recorded. Subject then takes one step into jump to touch as high on the wall as possible. Three jumps are completed. Record the difference between highest jump and reach.	Pros: Simple and easy to administer. Cons: Subjects with low coordination may score poorly.	Raw score is only a distance measure. Calculations can be used to convert to power.
Standing long jump	Muscle power	Subject stands with both feet comfortably placed behind marked line. Using arm swing and leg propulsion, subject launches forward as far as possible, landing on both feet.	Pros: Simple and quick to administer. Cons: May be somewhat traumatic for elderly or previously injured subjects.	Distance jumped is recorded.
Push-up test	Muscle endurance	Subject performs (using tester-defined protocol) push-ups during specified time period (60 s, 2 min).	Pros: No equipment is required. Cons: Subjects with low upper body strength may be unable to perform test.	Number of correctly performed push-ups is recorded.
Abdominal endurance test	Muscle endurance	Subject performs sit-ups (using tester-defined protocol) during set time period (20-60 s, 2 min).	Pros: No equipment is required. Cons: Subjects with low back pain may be unable to perform.	Tester must standardize sit-up test with the methods used to establish norms. Record total sit-ups performed.
Sprint test	Speed	Subject runs (sprints) designated distance for time, typically 10, 20, 30 m.	Pros: Quick and simple. Cons: Requires subjects to warm up. Performance may be influenced by motivation.	Use sprint distance that applies directly to sport or activities in which subject is involved. Norms can be established for individual groups.

Preseason Participation Evaluation

Preseason participation evaluations are often used to assess the individual's level of conditioning to determine areas of weakness and to establish an in-season conditioning or training program. Discovering that an individual's endurance level is less than that of other members on the team may allow special attention to endurance training to help the patient develop better stamina in long bouts of activity or in long competitions. A recreational patient, or anyone entering a fitness program, should consider participating in a fitness testing program prior to the start of the activities. Just like the client on a sport team, the participant will benefit from knowing her level of fitness before beginning the exercise endeavor. In addition to showing the fitness baseline, performance in a fitness test can indicate the person's potential for success or difficulty in the upcoming activities. Knowledge gained from the fitness tests can be used to design the activity level of the participant to allow safe and beneficial participation.

Ongoing Evaluations

Evaluations during a sport season or during training are probably less common than pre- or postseason evaluations. An evaluation may be employed during the middle of the off-season strength and conditioning program to allow the coach to judge the effectiveness of that program. Testing in the middle of the competitive season can be used to demonstrate a particular weakness that has developed during the season because of misuse or disuse. This decrease in strength is often seen during a competitive season, especially in lifts that are not specific to the skills the client uses in the sport. It might be logical to think that an in-season weightlifting program would alleviate this problem, yet increases in conditioning during a long competitive season may place too much physical demand on the individual and prove counterproductive. Many coaches require the participant to continue to lift during the competitive season but limit the exercises to those most applicable to the sport. Evaluation of these in-season programs could allow the coach to better individualize the lifting program of each participant. People participating in less organized teams or groups, as well as those entering an exercise program on their own, benefit from repeating the preparticipation fitness evaluation during the course of the program. This periodic evaluation indicates the individual's progress toward the fitness goals and also when it would be advisable to consider changes in the current program.

Postseason Fitness Evaluations

Postseason evaluations of fitness levels give the coach or participant a baseline for measuring changes that occur during the off-season. These data are also used to better establish the specific areas to address during the off-season training program. Individuals participating in more than one sport in a school year may not be able to participate in a sport-specific off-season training program; in this case the postseason evaluation is very important. Individuals who have undergone an end-of-season evaluation of fitness have a better understanding of the goals they are to reach during the off-season conditioning program.

Fitness Testing Parameters

Sport performance obviously requires unique physical abilities. Different sports necessitate different levels of physical performance; yet in general, fitness testing for any sport includes evaluation of muscular function (strength, endurance, and power) as well as cardiorespiratory function, agility, and speed. If we stop for a moment to examine these parameters, we may conclude that they are the same factors that contribute to injury prevention. Looking at fitness test results to determine areas of weakness could help the athletic trainer and strength and conditioning specialist work together to prepare the participant—and thus take a step closer to preventing an injury. In addition to these strength and conditioning parameters, measures such as flexibility, body composition, and height/weight can be included either in the preparticipation physical examination or in fitness tests. Let's look at why these parameters may be important to measure.

Muscle Function

Muscle strength refers to the maximum force that a muscle or muscle group can generate in a specific movement pattern at a specified velocity of movement. Few would debate the need for muscle strength in sports like wrestling, American football, or gymnastics, yet people often regard sports like swimming and track as speed events that involve little need for muscle strength. Coaches have become more aware of the need for strength in all events and sports and have found that muscle strength evaluation data are very useful.

Muscle endurance refers to the ability of a muscle or a group of muscles to perform a repetitive action. Sports like cross country, some events in track, and most swimming events require a great amount of endurance, both muscular and cardiorespiratory. In tennis, as another example, muscle endurance allows the participant to perform repetitive actions like the backhand swing and overhead serve. Individuals in activities such as cycling or rowing continually repeat the same movement patterns. Repeated movement can cause trauma in weak or unconditioned muscles.

Muscle power is the rate of performing work. You might think of this as how fast you can perform a particular lift, yet the concept is not that simple. Power is a term from physics, where it is defined as work during a unit of time. Physicists further define work as force times distance. Thus, muscle power equals a weight lifted (force) through a range of movement (usually a vertical distance) divided by the unit of time required to perform the lift. One can develop power by lifting the same weight the same distance in a shorter period of time, or by

lifting a greater amount of weight the same distance in the same period of time. Activities that strength and conditioning specialists evaluate to determine muscle power include exercises like the clean and jerk. In the clean, the weight is lifted from the floor to chest level in one smooth motion. This exercise involves carrying a weight bar (force) over a large range of movement (vertical distance from the floor to the chest) in a short period of time—thus power. If someone is lifting 100 lb, if the distance from the floor to the chest is 4 ft, and if it takes 1 s to perform the lift, the power is 100 lb × 4 ft, which equals 400 ft-lb/s.

Evaluating Muscle Strength

To evaluate muscular strength, a baseline measure is first taken. This measurement is typically performed using a technique called 1-repetition maximum (1RM). If a sport requires particular muscle activity, the fitness evaluation may include a 1RM test of a lift that uses those muscles or muscle groups. Traditionally the bench press is used to evaluate upper body strength, and the leg press or squat is used for lower body strength.

A repetition maximum is the maximum number of repetitions per set that a person can perform at a particular weight. Thus a 1RM is the heaviest weight that a person can lift for one complete repetition of an exercise. To determine the 1RM weight, the participant must use more than one lift. The first lift should be at 50% of the anticipated 1RM, and subsequent lifts should be at 75%, 90%, and 100% of the predicted weight. If the individual can lift the full weight, additional weight should be added until he is unable to perform the lift. The final completed lift is the weight to be recorded as the 1RM. Unfortunately, the more trials one must complete prior to establishing the proper weight of 1RM, the more the possible muscle fatigue. This simply means that the 1RM is, at minimum, the maximum weight the individual can lift one time. The individual may be wise to attempt to lift the weight after a sufficient rest and make further adjustments at that time.

A number of other tests of muscle strength may combine various aspects of muscle fitness—for example, a test of how many times you could bench press 100 lb (45 kg). A test such as this, which evaluates fatigue of the muscle, is considered a test of muscle endurance. If we change the test a little to show how much weight you can bench press 12 times, it becomes more a measure of strength; but it may become a test of endurance if you started with too heavy or too light a weight and had to lift many more than 10 repetitions. How much weight can be lifted is a measure of strength; how many times it can be lifted is a measure of endurance.

Testing Muscle Endurance and Evaluating Muscle Power

Muscle endurance uses an energy source different from that needed for muscle strength and must be evaluated independently. One can measure endurance of a muscle group to allow sport-specific evaluation of that muscle group; or one can use a general test such as sit-ups or timed push-ups as a test of muscle endurance generally. As an example, if you wanted to evaluate the muscle endurance of a cross country runner's legs, you might use the squat because its combination of joint movements resembles to some extent the use of the legs in running. The participant would do as many repetitions as possible of the squat exercise at a given weight (a relatively light weight, such as 25 to 45 lb [11.3-20.4 kg]). This test compares performance between participants and also provides a baseline for further individual evaluation as the season or weight program progresses.

A more general test of muscle endurance is the sit-up test. The individual does as many bent-knee sit-ups as possible in a set period of time (usually 60 s). Exact performance issues, such as feet secured or free, are factors to be determined in relation to the abilities of the individual being tested; test-to-test consistency is, of course, essential.

In terms of exercise, power is the ability to exert a maximal force in as short a period of time as possible, as in the vertical jump.

Cardiorespiratory Function

Cardiorespiratory means heart and lungs and, in conditioning, typically pertains to activities that would challenge those systems. The differences in the length of time of the activity tax different metabolic systems. **Anaerobic**—"without oxygen"—power comes into play in activities of very short duration. Activities such as sprints that occur very quickly are often anaerobic; they use a source of energy that does not require as much oxygen. Many sports that entail short spurts of activity involve both the anaerobic and the aerobic systems. The fast break in basketball is typically an anaerobic event, whereas the period of offense or defense in which the ball is moving around the half-court is an aerobic phase. Aerobic power involves the ability to utilize oxygen in performing work. Aerobic power relates to most athletic events that require oxygen consumption during performance. **Aerobic**—"with oxygen"—simply refers to the individual's use of an energy source that is dependent on oxygen.

Measuring Anaerobic Power

A way to measure the anaerobic (without oxygen) system is to have an individual perform an explosive movement such as a vertical jump or a shuttle run. Both of these tests are very short in duration and are usually performed anaerobically. The shuttle run can be designed to replicate some of the anaerobic demands of the sport. The subject is asked to run back and forth between two lines (about 20 yd [18.3 m] apart) in the least amount of time possible. The number of touches of the line can be chosen according to the demands of the sport. Because the performance frequently improves after the first repetition, the testing protocol often allows the participant to perform the run three times, and the best of the three times is recorded.

Evaluating Aerobic Power

We can measure aerobic power without using sophisticated equipment by timing the participant during a run. One common test, the 1.5-mile (2.4 km) timed run, is an accepted standard for measuring aerobic power (table 2.2). Other tests that can measure aerobic power include the step test and the 2-mile (3.2 km) timed run test. The sidebar Aerobic Tests outlines how to administer running tests and step tests.

Agility and Speed

Agility is the ability to start, stop, and change direction; and evaluating agility is very useful in most sports. Sudden changes in direction of movement involve an element of agility. The shuttle run can be used as a test of agility because of the rapid change in direction inherent in the activity. Speed, on the other hand, does not depend on the subject's ability to change direction but reflects only the length of time required to travel a set distance.

Testing Agility

Important factors that permit the performance of agility tests include the absence of injury and the use of proper footwear. Agility tests require rapid acceleration, deceleration, change of direction, and acceleration to the next line or object with deceleration to

Table 2.2 Standards for Maximal Oxygen Uptake and Endurance Runs

Age[a]	$\dot{V}O_2$max (ml · kg^{-1} · min^{-1})		1.5-mile (2.4 km) run (min:s)		12-min run in miles (km)	
	Female[b]	Male	Female	Male	Female	Male
Good						
15-30	>40	>45	<12	<10	>1.5 (2.4)	>1.7 (2.7)
35-50	>35	>40	<13:30	<11:30	>1.4 (2.3)	>1.5 (2.4)
55-70	>30	>35	<16	<14	>1.2 (1.9)	>1.3 (2.1)
Adequate for most activities						
15-30	35	40	13:30	11:50	1.4 (2.3)	1.5 (2.4)
35-50	30	35	15	13	1.3 (2.1)	1.4 (2.3)
55-70	25	30	17:30	15:30	1.1 (1.8)	1.3 (2.1)
Borderline						
15-30	30	35	15	13	1.3 (2.1)	1.4 (2.3)
35-50	25	30	16:30	14:30	1.2 (1.9)	1.3 (2.1)
55-70	20	25	19	17	1.0 (1.6)	1.2 (1.9)
Needs extra work on CRF						
15-30	<25	<30	>17	>15	<1.2 (1.9)	<1.3 (2.1)
35-50	<20	<25	>18:30	>16:30	<1.1 (1.8)	<1.2 (1.9)
55-70	<15	<20	>21	>19	<0.9 (1.4)	<1.0 (1.6)

These standards are for fitness programs. People wanting to do well in endurance performance need higher levels than those listed. People at the *good* level should emphasize maintaining this level the rest of their lives. Those in the lower levels should emphasize setting and reaching realistic goals for cardiorespiratory fitness (CRF).

[a]CRF declines with age.

[b]Women have lower standards because they have a larger amount of essential fat.

Reprinted, by permission, from E.T. Howley and B.D. Franks, 2007, *Fitness professional's handbook*, 5th ed. (Champaign, IL: Human Kinetics), 69.

AEROBIC TESTS

Running Tests

Follow these steps to administer a 1-mile run.

Before Test Day

1. Arrange to have the following elements at the test site:
   - A person to start and read the time from a stopwatch
   - A partner for each runner (perhaps with a sheet to mark off laps)
   - A stopwatch for the tester (with a spare ready)
   - A score sheet or scorecard

2. Explain the purpose of the test (i.e., to determine how fast participants can run 1 mile, or 1.6 km, which reflects the endurance of their cardiorespiratory system).

3. Do not administer the test until participants have had several fitness sessions, including some with running.

4. Have participants practice running at a set submaximal pace for one lap, then two, and so on, several times before the test day.

5. Select and mark off (if needed) a level area for the run.

6. Explain to people being tested that they are to run the mile in the fastest time possible. Walking is allowed, but the goal is to cover the distance as quickly as possible.

Test Day

1. Participants warm up with stretching, walking, and slow jogging.

2. Several people run at the same time.

3. The procedure is explained again.

4. The timer says, "Ready, go," and starts the stopwatch.

5. Each individual has a partner with a watch that has a second hand.

6. The partner counts the laps and tells the individual at the end of each lap how many more laps to run.

7. The timer calls out the minutes and seconds as the runner finishes the mile run.

8. The partner listens for the time when the runner finishes the mile and records it (to the nearest second) immediately on a scorecard.

9. The runner continues to walk one lap after finishing the run.

Harvard Step Test

Description and procedure: The subject steps up and down on a 20-in. (50.8 cm) platform at a rate of 30 steps per minute for 5 min or until she cannot maintain the stepping rate for 15 s. At completion of the test, the subject immediately sits down and records the heart rate either with a heart rate monitor (at 1.5, 2.5, and 3.5 min) or by counting heartbeats for 30-s periods from 1 to 1.5, from 2 to 2.5, and from 3 to 3.5 min.

Scoring: The score is determined as follows: score = (100 × test duration in seconds) divided by 2 × (total heartbeats in the recovery periods). Excellent: 90 or above; good: 80-89; high average: 65-79; low average: 55-64; poor: less than 55.

Equipment required: Step or platform 20 in. (50.8 cm) high, stopwatch, metronome, or cadence recording.

change direction again; thus individuals with ankle or knee injuries will not perform as well as those who are free of injury. Because these tests are unique, the participant often needs to learn the pattern to be timed before actually performing the test. Even though the agility test seems to require excellent coordination and speed, a participant at any level could complete it if given sufficient time. The most critical factor in administering an agility test is that you compare the individual's performance to the performance of others who are on a similar level. Just as it would be foolish to compare the test results for a tennis team with those for a group of same-age football linemen, it would be unwise to compare test data for participants without disabilities with data for persons who have disabilities.

Many other agility tests have been devised for sport-specific purposes. Many variations are possible, depending on the demands of the sport or the skill of the participant. Two quite different tests are the T-test and the Edgren Side Step test. In the T-test, four cones are set up in a "T" (see figure 2.1). The participant, starting at the bottom of the "T" (cone 1), runs 10 yd (9 m) straight ahead to cone 2, touches its base with the right hand, and then sidesteps to the left (5 yd [4.6 m]) to touch cone 3. He then immediately sidesteps toward the right (past cone 2) 10 yd (9 m) to cone 4, touches it with the right hand, sidesteps back to the center to cone 2, touches it with the left hand, and backpedals to the starting point. The timer starts the watch as the subject leaves the starting point and stops the watch as soon as the subject reaches cone 1 on the return.

The Edgren Side Step test uses an area 12 ft (about 3.7 m) wide, marked off in 3-ft (.9 m) sections (figure 2.2). The subject sidesteps from the center line outward to the leftmost line (6 ft [1.8 m] away), immediately changes direction, and sidesteps back past the center line and all the way to the right boundary (12 ft [about 3.7 m] away). This side-to-side movement is continued for as many touches as possible during a 10-s period. Each touch of the boundary line is recorded as a point, and any partial distance is recorded as 1/4 point per 3-ft (.9 m) section completed.

There is a good case for the learning effect in some agility tests, as you may even notice when you are the fifth or sixth

person to go through a drill and have been able to watch the participants ahead of you. The test of agility allows for the learning effect, usually measuring the time for completion three or more times and then using the best of the scores. The examiner can vary these tests by asking the subject to perform a crossover step rather than the side step or by making other footwork changes relevant to the sport.

Measuring Speed

Speed tests involve running, and it is best for participants to perform them in distances similar to those that occur in the sport. Often sports include short bursts of activity with the participant sprinting to a position or location. For these sports, one may use a timed dash such as the 40-yd (36.6 m) or 100-yd (91 m) run. In shorter sprint tests, an area for deceleration should be provided so that the participant is not required to stop suddenly.

Flexibility

Imagine a gymnast bending backward as if there were no limits to the motion, or a football player doing a hamstring stretch that

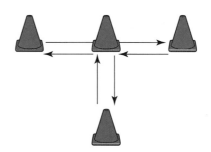

Figure 2.1 The T-test evaluates agility and is good for basketball, volleyball, and other sports that require quick shuffling moves.

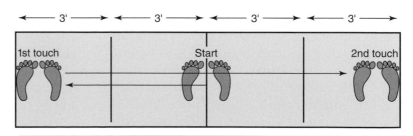

Figure 2.2 The Edgren Side Step test.

enables her to place her head on her knees. We would consider these individuals flexible. **Flexibility** is the result of several anatomical factors: muscle size, ligament and tendon composition, age, and sex. It is also a result of training. Let's look at each of these factors.

Effect of Muscle Size on Flexibility

You have undoubtedly seen people with great muscle mass, so much that it may even appear they can't put their arms next to their sides (adduction of the shoulder joint). Muscle bulk can limit movement. For example, flex your elbow and notice how the bulk of the biceps comes into contact with the forearm. If the biceps is very hypertrophied it could limit the range of elbow flexion. Compare the range of motion in your dominant arm to that of your other arm. Is there any difference? Could that be due to a larger (hypertrophied) biceps on your dominant arm? Compare the angle of flexion in your elbow against that of someone different in size, strength, or gender. Are there differences?

There are two ways in which a loss of flexibility can be limited or avoided: by stretching the muscle (the **agonist**[1]) that is being strengthened and by strengthening the opposite muscles (the **antagonists**[1]). Thus, it is important to (1) always include a stretching program for all muscles exercised and (2) always exercise both the agonistic muscle group and the antagonistic muscle group in any exercise program.

Effect of Ligament and Tendon Composition on Flexibility

Although all connective tissues are made up of a combination of collagen and elastin, some people seem to have more elasticity in their ligaments and tendons than others. A quick and easy test for the elasticity of ligaments is to bend your wrist forward and try to passively pull your thumb down to your wrist. (Careful! Don't do this with much force. Just pull gently.) People who can easily put the entire thumb against the surface of the wrist have greater elasticity in their connective tissues (ligaments and tendons).

Effects of Age and Sex on Flexibility

It is generally thought that females tend to be more flexible than males of the same age and body size, yet these differences are certainly not absolute. People who participate in the kinds of activities that encourage flexibility increase in their ability to stretch regardless of their sex. Likewise, as people age they tend to decrease in flexibility; yet with continued stretching, these individuals can delay or actually reverse these effects of aging. Overall, active people have higher levels of flexibility than sedentary individuals.

Testing Flexibility

Evaluation of the individual's flexibility is an important part of the fitness testing program. A decreased range of motion at a joint may play a role in causing an injury. Take, for instance, an inflexible hamstring muscle. As you run, the hamstring muscle must elongate or stretch to allow the foot to progress to take the next step. If the hamstring is too short or otherwise unable to elongate, it may incur injury during strenuous running. Hamstring flexibility is the most standard flexibility element included in fitness evaluations.

One test of hamstring flexibility, the sit-and-reach test, involves sitting on the floor with legs out straight ahead (figure 2.3). The participant's shoeless feet are placed flat against the back of a sit-and-reach box. If no sit-and-reach box is available you can use a ruler taped to a box. The ruler should be positioned so that you can measure the distance to the right or the left of the edge of the box. The individual slowly leans forward toward the box as far as possible and holds the greatest stretch for 2 s. The fingertips will reach a point on the ruler area either in front of, even with, or behind the front side of the box. The ruled guide helps to quantify the distance. The score is recorded as the distance in front of (positive) or behind (negative) the side of the box (see table 2.3). This test is repeated twice, and the best score of the three trials is recorded.

One can devise similar tests to evaluate flexibility at a particular joint. The key to

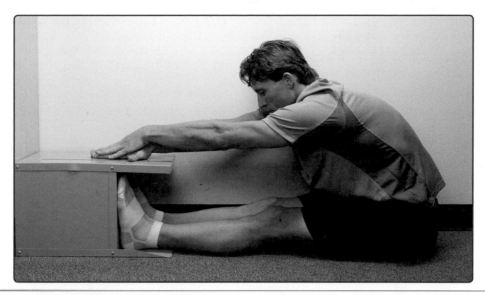

Figure 2.3 The sit-and-reach test for flexibility.

Table 2.3 Sit-and-Reach Measurements for Adults		
Category	Men	Women
Excellent	+17 to +27 cm	+21 to +30 cm
Good	+6 to +16 cm	+11 to +20 cm
Average	0 to +5 cm	+1 to +10 cm
Fair	−8 to −1 cm	−7 to 0 cm
Poor	−19 to −9 cm	−14 to −8 cm
Very poor	<−20 cm	<−15 cm

designing such a test is to position the subject so that other joints are stabilized and there is a way to measure the relative flexibility. For example, for evaluation of the flexibility of the **pectoralis major** muscles, subjects take a supine position (i.e., lie on their back) on a table (figure 2.4). They are asked to clasp their hands behind their head and then relax their shoulders to allow the elbows to move toward the table. The test is considered normal if the subject's elbows can touch the table. If the elbows fail to reach the table, the test is positive for pectoralis major tightness. Measurement of the distance between the elbow and the table would further quantify the evaluation. For other tests of range of motion, see Shultz, Houglum, and Perrin (2010).

Height, Weight, and Body Composition

Measurement of an individual's height or weight is sometimes referred to as **anthropometry**, which means measurement of body size. Body composition has to do with the amount of fat in relation to lean tissue in the body. Levels of fat that are too high affect the ability to move the body optimally. Additionally, obesity has been found to be associated with heart disease, high blood pressure, diabetes, arthritis, and some forms of cancer.

Methods of measuring body composition include the use of skin calipers, body mass index, underwater (hydrostatic) weighing, and electric impedance. The most common method is the skinfold method. With use of this method, one person trained in taking these measurements should be responsible for all individuals being tested in order to maximize reliability. Specially designed skinfold calipers measure the thickness of folds of tissue. Formulas for analyzing skinfold measures provide an accurate means of calculating the percentage of fat using the data from specific body locations. Depending on the measurement device used, body composition can be an accurate way to determine

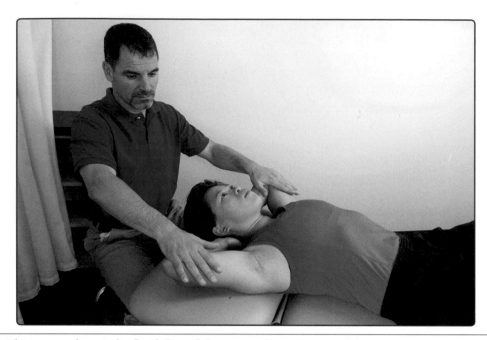

Figure 2.4   This test evaluates the flexibility of the pectoralis major muscles.

the amount of lean body tissue in an individual. The average healthy male should have approximately 12% to 18% fat, and the average healthy female approximately 14% to 20% fat. Table 2.4 shows optimal body fat percentages on the basis of age and gender. These values are generally accepted in sport physiology and reflect the averages used by various medical agencies and research groups.

Hydrostatic weighing is a well-established method of estimating an individual's total body fat, but it may not be totally reliable for all ages, sexes, and ethnic backgrounds. In hydrostatic weighing the individual's lung volume is measured, and the person is then submerged in water and weighed. Lung volume and underwater weight are computed using a special equation that yields the body fat percentage.

Bioelectrical impedance uses **electrodes** attached to the wrists, ankles, or feet. Based on the fact that fat resists electricity, the test measures resistance to the current transmitted by the electrodes. This method of calculating the individual's total body fat can be quite reliable (yielding reproducible data), but it is less likely than other techniques to be the method of choice because it has less

Table 2.4	Optimal Body Composition	
Subject's age	Optimal % fat for male	Optimal % fat for female
<20	15	19
20-29	16	20
30-39	17	21
40-49	19	23
50-59	19	23
60+	20	24

validity (accuracy) and the equipment is less available. Bioelectrical impedance may soon become the preferred method of evaluating an individual's body composition, however, because of the speed with which the data can be collected and because of the test's reproducibility.

Exercise Prescription

You would probably not be surprised to hear that there is some debate about the best exercises to use to develop overall strength, aerobic function, and flexibility. Exercises can be highly specific, taxing only one joint in one motion pattern, or can involve several joints, maximizing use of the large muscle groups. One must consider several factors when establishing an exercise prescription: the results of needs analysis, the setting of goals (including short-term goals, long-term goals, and limitations to the plan), and the exercise plan itself.

Needs Analysis

Before venturing into the development of an exercise or conditioning program, one should complete a needs analysis (see figure

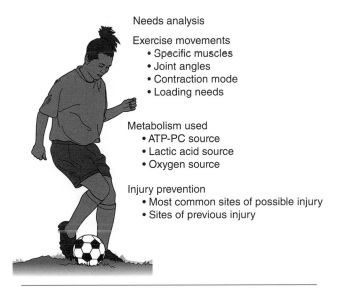

Needs analysis

Exercise movements
• Specific muscles
• Joint angles
• Contraction mode
• Loading needs

Metabolism used
• ATP-PC source
• Lactic acid source
• Oxygen source

Injury prevention
• Most common sites of possible injury
• Sites of previous injury

Figure 2.5 A careful look at what needs to be trained during a conditioning program is called needs analysis.

Reprinted, by permission, from S.J. Fleck and W.J. Kraemer, 2004, *Designing resistance training programs*, 3rd ed. (Champaign, IL: Human Kinetics), 154.

2.5). Whether the individual is young or older, a beginner or a seasoned performer, it is advisable to consider the objectives of the program. In forming the objectives, you should take into consideration the fitness demands of the activity as well as the current fitness level of the individual. In establishing the program objectives, it may be helpful to answer the following questions as suggested by Fleck and Kraemer (2004):

• What muscle groups should be conditioned?

• What energy system (aerobic vs. anaerobic) should be trained?

• What type of muscle activity (concentric, eccentric, or isometric; see figure 2.6) should be used?

• What are the typical sites of injury for the sport? What are the individual's previous injuries?

Muscle Groups

Two factors come into play when one determines which muscle groups should be exercised: the demands of the sport and the abilities of the individual. An understanding of the physiology and mechanics of the sport and the sport skills is essential for designing the exercise program. If you are very familiar with the sport and the skills it requires, this analysis may be relatively easy; but if not, there is always help. The sport coach

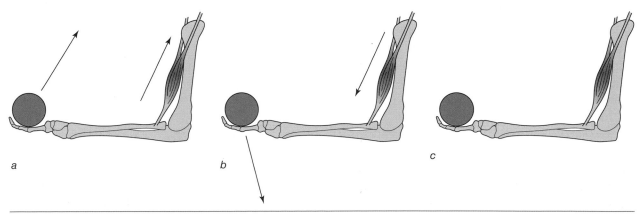

a   b   c

Figure 2.6 *(a)* During a concentric action, a muscle shortens; *(b)* during an eccentric action, the muscle lengthens in a controlled manner; and *(c)* during an isometric action, no movement of the joint occurs and no shortening or lengthening of the muscle takes place.

is generally the most knowledgeable person regarding what is needed in the sport. Videotapes of practices can be helpful for an understanding of the muscle groups used in particular skills, as can textbooks on sport techniques. This **biomechanical** evaluation of the skills of the sport will direct you toward the muscles used in the sport. Often, in investigating the muscle groups needed, you will begin to answer your fourth question for the needs analysis. You will also begin to understand how the muscles work.

Energy Systems

The analysis of the energy systems used in the sport may not be as clear as you would like. Many sports use short bursts of activity during long periods of participation: For example, basketball players often have a burst of speed as they steal the ball and drive to the basket but then immediately afterward have to run (or jog) back to the other end of the court to play defense. This back-and-forth activity is clearly aerobic overall, yet the bursts of activity at various times during the play may actually be anaerobic. When you find such a combination of energy systems in a sport, you will be wise to include exercises to address both energy systems in the conditioning program.

Muscle Activity

What types of muscle activity should be trained? As already mentioned, you will understand the way the muscle works on the basis of the same information you used to select the muscle groups. The analysis of the skills of the sport allows you to understand the way the muscles are expected to work. A skill that demands a "ready" position uses the quadriceps muscles in an eccentric capacity. The quadriceps may also be used in a concentric capacity if the individual is required to jump, for instance. The exclusion of either eccentric or concentric muscle activity would be detrimental to most sport skill development.

Understanding isometric muscle activity is another aspect of understanding how the muscle needs to work—one that is easy to observe. Isometric muscle contraction is used in activities that require a position to be held motionless. For example, gymnasts may be awarded additional points if they are able to hold a position motionless for several seconds. This type of muscle activity—in which there is no joint movement—is isometric activity. Specific training of the muscles involved in an isometric exercise may be needed in a sport skill and should be addressed in the exercise prescription.

Injury Patterns

Understanding the team's injury history may indicate a weakness in the conditioning program. Check with the coach and the team's medical staff to learn the injury trends over past seasons. In addition to the general injury trends for the team, you should understand the injury history of the individual. If a participant in your conditioning program has a preexisting condition, it is necessary to obtain clearance from the person's physician before beginning the exercise program.

Goal Setting

Goal setting plays a critical role within the exercise prescription. A program without objectives and goals will usually not last very long. It is easier for people to develop dedication and motivation to continue in an exercise program if they can achieve success during the process. Since success comes from achieving goals, setting the goals is critical. You should make sure that all program participants have formed a set of long-term goals for their participation. Knowledge of these long-term goals will help you more clearly identify ways of progressing toward the goals, and in doing this you will establish the short-term goals.

Short-Term Goals

After performing the needs analysis for each individual, you can establish the short-term goals of the program. These goals should be the immediate (individual day) and short-range (month) goals of participation in the program. These short-term goals should contribute to the long-term goal of the program. As an analogy, if your long-range goal is to get a college degree, your daily goals (attending classes, completing assignments) and short-term goals (getting an A on each test and project, earning an A in each course this term) will contribute to your long-term goal of achieving your degree. Achieving the long-term goals will be more difficult without achievement of the short-term goals along the way.

Long-Term Goals

Each individual must establish her own goals for the exercise program. It would be unfair to ask you to dedicate yourself to someone else's goals if you had no interest in the outcome that person wanted. If you don't want your college degree but are trying to get it to satisfy your parents, it will be a long, hard struggle. When people take responsibility for establishing their own personal goals, motivation is more likely to remain high.

Most people would desire "success" as a long-term goal, but success must be more clearly defined to serve its purpose as a goal. Encourage all participants to identify specific long-term goals for their participation in the exercise program. Help participants identify exact outcomes they desire through participation. When team members set goals pertaining to their position on the team, you must remind them that the purpose of the exercise program is to prepare the body and that the execution of the skills of the sport has to come from the individual. A solid conditioning program should provide the participant with the muscle strength and endurance to complete sport skill tasks, and it should build the cardiorespiratory system to allow stamina throughout practice sessions; but the conditioning program cannot be responsible for execution of the right play or for hitting the ball at the correct moment. Guide the participant in establishing performance goals that are measurable and that can be attributed to the conditioning program. Improving performance on a specific fitness test at the end of the season, being able to run 100 yd (91 m) in under x seconds

after every practice session, and being able to increase the vertical jump by the end of the conditioning program are measurable long-range goals. Depending on the time of the sport season, various exercise plans may be used to aid progress toward the long-term goals.

Limitations to the Plan

There will always be obstacles to a conditioning program: time constraints, availability of facilities or equipment, travel difficulties, and any number of others. Unfortunately, we cannot always avoid the difficulties associated with dedication to an exercise program. Insofar as possible, alternative plans should be in place that will allow the participant to achieve the daily, weekly, and monthly goals even if difficulties arise.

A key to one common difficulty, "remote participation," is communication and encouragement. With the Internet, daily progress notes can be exchanged, programs modified, and motivation provided typically without additional cost to the participant. If an individual does not have access to the Internet, it is important to achieve daily or at least weekly communication by some other method. Another potential barrier to dedication is boredom. Unless you provide a stimulating and rewarding program, you will hear more excuses about why someone had to miss a workout than you could have imagined. Just put yourself in the position of the other person, and you should soon see ways to make the program more appealing.

Finally, there is a saying used in management: "People support what they help create." Individuals should be involved throughout the development of the goals and the exercise prescription so that they are able to take ownership in the program's success. "Where there's a will there's a way" is often the motivated participant's motto. Your job is to help develop that "will."

Exercise Plans

There are a number of strengthening methods, each having unique benefits. After establishing the needs of the individual, the demands of the activity or sport, the goals of the program, and of course the availability and type of weightlifting equipment, one can develop the exercise plan or prescription. Next we take a look at two concepts associated with various techniques—namely, training volume and exercise order—and at two different types of designs for programs.

- *Training volume.* Training volume is simply the amount of work performed during a workout, during a week, or during a season. To estimate training volume, calculate the total number of repetitions performed or the total weight lifted. If the individual is seeking to increase muscle mass, frequently the training volume is increased as the program progresses.

- *Exercise order.* Two of the standard designs for strengthening programs focus on the order in which exercises are performed: the station approach and the circuit training approach. In the station approach, the participant accomplishes all the sets for a given exercise before moving to the next exercise. This method of ordering exercise is sometimes called horizontal training, while circuit training is sometimes called the vertical training method.

- *The station approach.* The concept behind the station approach is to maximize the overload on one muscle group before moving on to another exercise. This approach appears to impose a more intense load on the given muscle group, yet the length of rest time between sets may offset the benefits of stacking the repetitions.

- *Circuit training.* The order of exercise performance in circuit training differs from that of the station approach in that the participant performs only one set of a particular exercise before moving on to the next exercise. This means, for example, that after the first set on the bench press you would move (quickly) to doing biceps curls for one set, then on to triceps extensions, and so on until you have completed one set of all the prescribed exercises. After the first time through the exercises, you begin the circuit

again by returning to the first exercise and performing the second set. Participants usually follow the circuit—performing one set of each exercise prior to moving to the next exercise—until they have completed three sets of each exercise.

An aim of sport scientists who popularized the circuit training approach was to maximize the body's ability to ward off fatigue. The concept behind circuit training is to work a muscle group to near fatigue and then hurry to the next exercise (maintaining the elevated heart rate from the exercise) to work another muscle group. The muscles in the first group are rested somewhat during the subsequent exercise, but the taxing of the cardiorespiratory system continues.

Developing the Strength Training Program

When developing the exercise prescription it is necessary to incorporate two essentials into every program: resistance and overload. Even minimal exercise equipment can provide resistance to muscle actions. Handheld weights, machine weights, or elastic bands can offer adequate resistance. Thus resistance may take many forms. On the other hand, overload means only one thing: that the stress or load on the muscle is greater than what the muscle is accustomed to moving.

Now program design can begin. The principal factors to consider are exercise intensity, periodization, progressive overload, and rest periods and training frequency. These are the components that are manipulated during a training program and as the individual adapts to the training.

Exercise Intensity

The intensity of the exercise being performed is measured using the 1RM performance of the technique. As described earlier in this chapter, the 1RM can be calculated quite easily. This 1RM is then used to determine the amount of weight prescribed in the training program.

Intensity refers to the percentage of the 1RM. Generally the minimal intensity used in a set is 60% to 65% of the 1RM; so if an individual's 1RM for a leg press is 55 lb (25 kg), the minimum intensity used in training will be 30 lb (13.6 kg). If this person were to perform an average number of repetitions of the leg press (10-15) with a low-intensity weight (say 25 lb [11.3 kg]), he would undoubtedly show no strength gains. There must be an overload. One must keep intensity of a set in mind when designing progressive overloads.

Two general categories of methods of assigning exercise intensity are the hypertrophy method (bodybuilding method) and the high-intensity training (HIT) or neurological method. Each has its specific physiological benefits, and selection of one or the other depends on the activity or sport skill as well as the individual's body structure.

• *Hypertrophy method.* The objective of hypertrophic training is to increase a muscle's mass (achieve hypertrophy). Muscular **hypertrophy** is a general increase in bulk of the muscle through increase in the size of individual muscle fibers (but not the number of cells). The program uses between 5 and 12 repetitions, and the amount of weight is 70% to 85% of the 1RM.

• *High-intensity training method.* In HIT, the intensity reaches up to 100% of the 1RM. The purpose of the HIT method is to improve the recruitment of existing muscle fibers rather than to increase the size of the fibers. Every muscle is made up of muscle fibers. These fibers contribute to the performance of an action depending on the size of the load. The greater the load, the more fibers are used

to perform the task. In HIT, the weight used is from 85% to 100% of the 1RM, and the number of repetitions is between one and four.

In both methods, the intensity or load may be adjusted as the individual improves. Generally, when the individual is able to perform the maximum number of repetitions, the weight should be increased. With use of the HIT method, the amount of weight being lifted should be increased if the individual is able to lift the prescribed weight more than four times. The same concept applies to use of the hypertrophy method; if the individual can perform more than 12 repetitions, the load must be increased.

Periodization

Just as you would use a different strengthening program in the off-season than during the season, you might find it beneficial to use a different training volume or intensity during one part of the week or month than another. This cycling is known as **periodization**. Periodization is a gradual change in the type, intensity, and amount of training to allow the individual to achieve optimal gains in strength and power. Slight but safe variations in the position of the hand or foot can produce strength gains, as can the use of several different exercises that work the same muscle group. Periodization incorporates various types of exercises in a logical progression from general to specific throughout the cycles of the competitive season.

There are many varieties of periodization programs, but all types have the components of hypertrophy training, strength training, development of power, muscle endurance, and muscle recovery built in (table 2.5).

Table 2.5 Differences Between Strengthening Methods

Component	Sets	Repetitions	Weight (% max)
Hypertrophy	3-6	8-20	65-80
Strength	3-6	1-6	85-120
Endurance	1-3	10-30+	15-60
Recovery	3-6	8-20	15-60

Generally the hypertrophy component is trained using three to six sets of 8 to 20 repetitions at about 65% to 80% of the individual's maximum. Strength training in periodization techniques uses three to six sets of one to six repetitions at the 85% to 120% level. Endurance training uses from one to three sets of a higher number of repetitions and somewhere from 10 to upward of 30 reps done at the 15% to 60% level. The recovery component of periodization training techniques incorporates three to six sets of 8 to 20 repetitions at a load of about 15% to 60% of the individual's maximum.

Although varied, all periodization programs also incorporate the timing of implementation of different components in the competitive season and off-season programs. For example, periodization programs use the off-season periods for hypertrophy and heavy strength training and avoid heavy loading during the competitive season.

Progressive Overload

Progressive overload refers to a gradual increase in the stress placed on a muscle as it gains strength or endurance. For instance, once you can easily lift 25 lb (11.3 kg) for 10 repetitions on the biceps curl machine, you should add more resistance so that further changes may occur. Therefore your overload would consist of more repetitions or more resistance. This means you would lift 30 lb (13.6 kg) for the same number of repetitions or lift the 25 lb (11.3 kg) 10 more times.

Rest Periods and Training Frequency

Resting between training sessions as well as between exercises or sets is an important component of training. In this discussion the rest period refers to the amount of time between consecutive sets, while the term training frequency refers to the length of time between exercise sessions.

Rest Periods

The rest period between sets depends on the training volume and exercise order and

should also reflect the needs and goals of the participant. Individuals training with a high volume (1RM loads) for strength require a longer rest period between sets than if they were training for muscle hypertrophy. Rest periods of 3 to 5 min are not uncommon for the individual working on absolute strength by lifting the 1RM weight, while a 30- to 60-s rest is more typical for the individual working on muscle hypertrophy and doing 8 to 12 repetitions of the exercise with a submaximal weight.

When the exercise order uses a longitudinal design as in circuit training, the rest periods should be approximately as long as the period of time spent on the exercise. This 1:1 ratio can help to produce gains in both strength and aerobic endurance but can create a feeling of nausea in some participants. If you are working with someone who is elderly or is deconditioned as a result of illness or other difficulty, it might be wise to begin the circuit training program using a rest period that is longer than the time required to complete the set. As the individual's fitness level increases, the recovery rate will improve, and you may begin to gradually decrease the length of rest time until the ratio gets down to 1:1. The better the individual's condition, the less time the person will require between consecutive sets.

Training Frequency

Training frequency, a highly individualized aspect of the total strengthening prescription, should be planned according to several principles.

- Traditionally, participants have done weight training on alternating days (1 day of rest between exercise sessions). The intent is to allow sufficient recovery from the exercise session prior to the next session.
- Early in the exercise program, people often experience increased muscle soreness, perhaps because of eccentric contraction (negative phase) of the muscles used. This soreness usually abates after

about the second week of the program; but until that time, less frequent lifting sessions may be necessary. If the exercise consists of only concentric muscle activity (isokinetic machines), postexercise soreness is usually not a factor, and the exercise frequency can be increased.

- Sessions of multiple-joint exercises require longer recovery periods than sessions using only single-joint exercises.

- With use of maximum (1RM) or near-maximum loads in multiple-joint exercises, the individual requires more recovery time prior to the next heavy lifting day.

- More frequent lifting sessions can be performed with use of a lower training volume on the days between high-volume exercise sessions.

- Persons who have been weightlifting on a regular basis for a long time (years) may benefit from more frequent exercise sessions than those who do not have a long history of strength training.

Taking the individual's strength training background and short-term goals into consideration, you should be able to devise a suitable training frequency with adequate rest periods in each session.

Types of Strength Training

Various types of strength training are used for conditioning as well as in the rehabilitation of an injured patient. Strength training is only a portion of an individual's overall conditioning program. As one considers the needs of the person and the demands of the sport or activity, specific strength training types become apparent. Some high-level participants have suggested that they have attained their level of performance without formal strength training. This is certainly possible for some gifted performers, but it is not the rule for most people. Some individuals with specialized skills also suggest that

they cannot strength train without adverse effects on their skill performance. This may be partially true, especially if the individual makes gains in strength without simultaneous development of skill patterns; but with attention to skill development, this adverse effect can be controlled. Overall, strength training is an integral part of every participant's training regimen. Discussed in this section are the common strength training methods: isometrics, isotonic training, variable resistance, isokinetics, concentric and eccentric training, and plyometrics.

Isometrics

Isometric contraction occurs when the muscle generates a force but there is no joint movement. This means that the resistance is far greater than the participant is able to move, and thus no movement occurs. There are stories of prisoners who have been able to maintain high levels of strength by performing isometric muscle contractions. Hettinger (1961) published one of the earliest reports of the positive effects of isometric muscle activity, saying that for the best results one should perform multiple sets of maximal or near-maximal muscle contraction held for 3 to 10 s each. One limitation with isometric training is that the strength gains are greatest at the precise joint position at which the contraction was performed; there is only slight overflow of strengthening to the adjacent joint positions.

Isometric muscle activity is not often applicable to sport performance, yet when you analyze the performance of wrestlers and gymnasts, you may see application of isometric muscle strengthening. In addition to the holding of a position as in wrestling and gymnastics, in other sports some muscles act in a very limited range that appears nearly isometric. For example, in swimming, the abdominal muscles are exercised very strongly, yet there may not be large movements of the trunk. Running also taxes the abdominal and back muscles without significant excursions in the range of motion of the trunk.

Although isometric muscle activity can be done in virtually any setting and with virtually no equipment, it may not be a wise choice for a strengthening program, mainly because of the difficulty in measuring the overload. Without some feedback on muscle performance, the participant's motivation may decline and thus directly affect the overload applied. If the participant fails to produce a maximal contraction, an increase in the time the contraction is held may still not sufficiently overload the muscle; thus there will be little or no change in muscle performance.

Isotonic Training

Isotonic muscle activity involves moving the joint through a range of motion with a set amount of resistance applied. Isotonic muscle activity occurs in lifting free weights, as well as in the performance of most activities of daily living. For example, as you stand up from your chair, you may need to reach down and pick up your backpack. As you reach for the pack, you will extend your elbow to its maximum position. As you raise the pack toward your shoulder, your elbow will begin to bend. This activity is an isotonic exercise because the weight does not change while your limb moves through a range of motion.

If you have ever had to move heavy objects from one place to another, you may have found that the loads you can carry are much heavier than the loads you can pick up. You may be able to take a 100-lb (45 kg) box off a waist-high counter and carry it to another counter, but if that 100-lb box is in the trunk of your car, you may not be able to lift it up. This illustrates one of the primary difficulties in isotonic strengthening.

There are points in the range of every joint where the muscle is at its weakest. At other points (usually in the middle of the joint action), the muscle is at its strongest position. These points make up what is called a strength curve, which illustrates why you can carry the box from counter to counter but cannot lift it out of the trunk of the car.

Variable Resistance

Variable resistance was introduced in the 1970s by the Nautilus Corporation. Nautilus used an offset cam to deliver a variation in the resistance to the movement. The cam was designed to maximize strength at various points in the range of motion as suggested in the strength curve. The variable-resistance machines using the cam system tended to be quite expensive, so some manufacturers developed the sliding lever bar systems, and others brought out various forms of elastics or large rubber bands.

The rubber band or elastic tubing provides increased resistance as the band is elongated. These very portable and inexpensive devices gained favor for patients in rehabilitation as well as for persons with a limited budget or limited space.

Isokinetics

Isokinetics refers to a muscular action performed at a constant velocity. In other words, an isokinetics (or accommodating resistance) machine uses shock absorbers, hydraulics, or a braking system to provide a maximum resistance through the entire range of joint movement. Isokinetic (*iso* means "same"; *kinetic* means "movement") machines are typically very expensive and are used most often in rehabilitation. Some isokinetic machines are capable of extremely high angular velocity (up to 1,000°/s). The theory behind isokinetics is that the muscle has a varied capacity (strength curve) as well as being capable of very high speeds of joint movement (see figure 2.7). Some models of

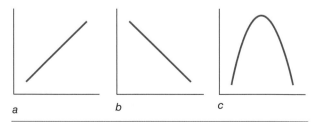

Figure 2.7 The three major strength curves are *(a)* ascending, *(b)* descending, and *(c)* bell shaped. The resistance varies throughout the exercise.

isokinetics even provide ways to adjust the type of muscle contraction being produced.

Concentric and Eccentric Training

If you were to analyze a sport activity, you would probably find that it involves both a concentric phase and an eccentric phase. Are there any sports or sport skills you can name that involve only concentric muscle activity? Consider wrestling, swimming, gymnastics, and golf. Does each involve eccentric muscle activity? If so, what specific motor pattern or what part of the motor pattern produces the eccentric contraction?

Concentric Muscle Activity

Concentric muscle activity occurs when the limb moves through a range of motion with a resistance applied. This concentric phase of the lifting movement involves a shortening of the muscle during the movement. This muscle action is the force-production part of almost every human movement. The only exercises that do not include concentric muscle activity are those exercises designed specifically to tax the muscle in an exclusively eccentric manner—and in those cases the "positive" or concentric movement is accomplished by an external force (another person or, in rehabilitation cases, the uninvolved extremity).

Eccentric Muscle Activity

The lowering of the weight produces a lengthening of the muscle while it is contracting. This lengthening contraction is called an eccentric muscle contraction. Some people describe eccentrics in terms of gravity, suggesting that most weights that are lifted are lifted away from the pull of gravity. This lifting away from the gravitational pull is the concentric phase, while the lowering back to the starting position involves contraction by the same muscle as it elongates. The muscle must generate force, even though it is working with the gravitational pull, to achieve a slow and controlled descent.

Eccentric muscle contraction does not occur in all forms of isokinetic exercise (some isokinetic machines do allow eccentric contractions), nor will proprioceptive neuromuscular facilitation exercises and manual resistance exercises provide eccentric contraction without some specific adaptations. Most other weightlifting machines use an eccentric phase, as do all forms of body weight conditioning (push-ups, pull-ups, sit-ups, etc.).

Plyometrics

Plyometrics, a stretch–shortening cycle exercise, replicates many aspects of physical activity. The stretch phase is an eccentric loading phase of the exercise, while the shortening phase is the force-producing or concentric phase. Most physical activity relies heavily on this type of muscle activity. Imagine for a moment a very slow-motion film of a tennis player hitting a backhand shot. As the ball contacts the racket, the player absorbs the force of the ball (eccentric phase). Then for a split second, the movement stops (isometric); this is followed immediately by a production of force imparted to the ball (concentric), sending it on its way toward the opponent. Every physical activity incorporates the stretch–shortening cycle, making a strong case for the use of plyometrics in the training program.

Stretch–shortening cycle exercise can take many forms. It can be used as part of a rehabilitation program or can be part of an exercise program to prepare for specialized skill performance. The critical feature of this type of exercise is that a concentric force production follows every eccentric load absorption. For example, in-depth jump training is a form of plyometrics that has been used to increase leg power. The technique uses two boxes; the individual stands on one box and steps off it, lands on the ground between the two boxes, and springs back upward to land on the top of the other box. This early form of plyometric training continues to be a cornerstone in many training programs but is not suitable for individuals weighing over 220 lb (100 kg).

The principles underlying the stretch–shortening concept were introduced by two physical therapists named Knott and Voss. They found that when a muscle was stretched prior to the onset of a contraction, the contraction was greater than it would have been otherwise. They used this technique to help weakened patients perform motor activity. The preliminary stretch of a contractile unit (muscle and tendon) stimulates a muscle contraction greater than would be produced by a contractile unit at the normal resting length.

There are many variations of stretch–shortening cycle exercise, making success possible for participants of every fitness level. Low-load plyometrics can be used with individuals who are disabled, allowing them increased power and in some cases increased dynamic stability. A simple exercise on a slide board can be used as a low-load plyometric. If the individual can manage to slide to one end of the board and then slide back, the momentum of the slide will serve as the stretch phase as the exerciser makes contact with the end of the board. After the shock absorption, the kinetic energy is released as the shortening phase produces movement in the opposite direction. Progressively advanced exercises can be found in many texts on plyometrics.

Integrating Cardiorespiratory and Flexibility Parameters

Suppose that you are lifting in the weight room and that friends come by to coax you into playing some basketball. You can probably imagine how your regular jump shot would feel if you had just finished three intense sets on the bench press. The basketball would feel light as a feather, and you would have a tendency to overshoot the basket. This same concept applies to weight training during the season and illustrates the importance of a good balance between lifting and skill performance.

Aerobic Endurance Training

The cardiorespiratory system is a cornerstone of physical activity. Nearly every recreational or sport activity requires some degree of cardiorespiratory, or aerobic, endurance. For decades the positive benefits of exercise have been well understood and accepted by those in the fitness and exercise physiology fields. Efforts to employ those concepts and promote physical activity in the American public have been a challenge undertaken nationally by the Surgeon General as well as the President's Council on Physical Fitness and Sports. As a health care provider, you should make it your goal to help promote physical fitness. The challenge then is to develop a rational program that must start with an understanding of the participant's current fitness level.

When the individual's fitness status is in any way questionable, or, at the other end of the spectrum, when the individual is in top physical condition, the best method for establishing fitness level is to use a cardiorespiratory stress test. One can design an aerobic conditioning program for young, healthy individuals by using data from fitness tests such as the 1.5-mile (2.4 km) or 2-mile (3.2 km) run test referred to earlier. Whichever method you use, you can determine the subject's maximal heart rate and general level of fitness. If the heart rate data are not available, you can estimate maximal heart rate by subtracting the individual's age from 220.

The recommendation in the American College of Sports Medicine (ACSM) position statement is that exercise intensity for aerobic conditioning fall between 60% and 90% of the maximal heart rate (or 50-80% of the $\dot{V}O_2$max obtained in a stress test). The training should be performed at a minimum frequency of 3 days per week and should last for 20 to 60 min each session.

Common sense dictates that if you are working with people who have a very low level of fitness and who are beginning an aerobic conditioning program, you should start them with an activity that allows them to reach and maintain at least 60% of their maximal heart rate and to sustain that pace (and heart rate) for at least 20 min. People who start the program with a higher level of fitness need more intense exercise to reach the desired heart rate; for these individuals, you may want to set a training heart rate goal of 70% of the maximal, or have them sustain this rate for longer than 20 min, or both.

Design of an aerobic conditioning program follows the same principles as for a program for muscle training: An overload is required. Your cardiorespiratory endurance program should encompass a short-term goal (the goal for the day, the week, or the month), as well as a long-term goal (goal of the program), and should move from one goal to the next in a logical and steady progression (see figure 2.8). A key to helping new exercisers stay with a program is to have them start at a low enough level to be training the aerobic system without overexertion; this will help keep them from giving up. Another good way to keep people motivated for cardiorespiratory exercise is to vary the program. Varying the use of the treadmill, stepper machine, elliptical apparatus, pool, or bike in achieving and maintaining the heart rate to gain cardiorespiratory conditioning can do this. Some people can work at a seemingly high effort level for long periods of time and never reach the target heart rate while doing particular exercises. But it is essential to pay attention

to the heart rate responses to exercise, no matter what activity is chosen.

Anaerobic Training

Anaerobic training is not as universally required as aerobic training, yet it plays a critical role in most activities and especially in sport participation. Sport skills often involve both anaerobic muscle activity and anaerobic cardiorespiratory work. Here we consider anaerobic cardiorespiratory training only.

Events that take between 1 and 5 min to complete require use of a combination of the aerobic and anaerobic systems. On the 1-min side of the spectrum, energy is produced by both systems in a 50-50 aerobic-anaerobic mix; as you move closer to the 5-min duration for the event, the aerobic system plays a greater role and the anaerobic system a lesser role in energy production. This means that most physical activity requires some amount of anaerobic metabolism (energy production) as well as some aerobic metabolism. Thus it is important to train both metabolic systems.

Anaerobic cardiorespiratory work means energy production by the body in the absence of oxygen. Training to improve the anaerobic system requires short, intense bursts of activity, and that activity should be sport specific. For example, if you are a water polo player,

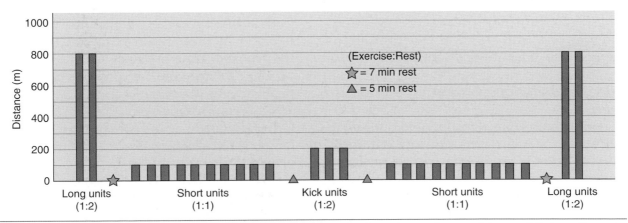

Figure 2.8 A sample power-unit workout for the development of aerobic and anaerobic capabilities. The units are performed on a grass field, four times a week, with a ratio of work time to rest time of 1:2 (i.e., if it takes the individual 20 s to sprint the distance, the rest period would be 40 s).

Adapted, by permission, from S.J. Fleck and W.J. Kraemer, 2004, *Designing resistance training programs*, 3rd ed. (Champaign, IL: Human Kinetics), 140.

you will want to do sprint training to increase your anaerobic endurance. But running sprints will not be as beneficial to your sport performance as swimming sprints.

Anaerobic training can be accomplished by running short, intense sprints or by performing short, intense bouts on the slide board, bicycle, step-up equipment, and so on. High-intensity, near-maximal exercise is impossible to sustain for long periods of time because it leads to exhaustion; therefore some period of rest is needed to allow the body to recover. Interval training does just that. Rather than using total rest between sets, participants can combine aerobic and anaerobic conditioning by alternating easy, submaximal exertion with hard, near-maximal output. Whichever way one chooses to use to train the anaerobic system, a key principle is that high-intensity, short-duration activity builds the anaerobic system but leads to exhaustion and cannot be sustained for long periods of time.

While everyone needs regular, moderately vigorous exercise, high-intensity exercise is primarily for people with a moderate level of fitness who want to improve this aspect of their conditioning. It is not appropriate for older individuals or others who have low fitness levels, or for anyone who might risk injury doing exercise at high intensity. Since high-intensity exercise means very high heart rates, persons at risk for cardiorespiratory disease should be carefully screened by their health care provider before entering into an interval or sprint training program. Many people who have their physician's endorsement for low- to moderate-intensity exercise may not be approved for high-intensity exercise.

People who are well prepared for an interval program must start out at a safe level and then progress, just as with every other part of the fitness program. At the beginning of an anaerobic or interval training program, the participant might run a set distance at maximum capacity (speed) and then jog back to the start. This sprint/jog cycle would then be repeated, say 10 times, before fatigue causes the person to stop. To make the program progressive, you change one of two variables: You can increase the distance sprinted or decrease the rest (jog) time. Interval programs are much easier to do on a track or other continuous path so that as the rest interval decreases, the next sprint can begin regardless of the distance to the starting line. A cross country runner who does intervals could use a trail. Obviously the trail will not have distances marked off, so the work bout would be a length of time rather than a distance.

Often it is advantageous to vary the distance of the sprint during the workout. For example, assume that your physical fitness is fairly good and you have decided to start an interval program. The first day you might run a total of 2,500 m (2,734 yd; half of your average daily run) because you realize that if you are adding interval training to your exercise program, you will be exercising for shorter durations. After warming up and stretching, you may decide to start with 200 m (219-yd) runs at about 80% of your top speed. You run the 200 (30 s) and then jog for about 30 s; you then repeat this pattern seven times (total run is now 1,600 m [1,750 yd]). Next you do 10 intervals of 100 m (109 yd) with a 10-s jog between repeats. That adds another 1,000 m (1,093 yd) to the total—and that is about what your workout was supposed to be. As your conditioning improves, you will increase your speed in the sprints (if possible) or decrease the jog cycle. You can accomplish both in that the faster you run, the less time it takes to achieve the distance and therefore the recovery time does not have to be quite as long. Keeping an accurate record of the number and distance (or time) of the reps will aid you in developing your progression.

In designing a progression in interval training, always increase the training volume gradually in order to avoid injury. A rule of thumb is to increase your training volume (mileage or time spent) by no more than 10% per week. Do not increase at all if injury or signs of overtraining are present. Signs of overtraining include fatigue, depression, irritability, insomnia, increase in resting heart rate, muscle pain, joint pain, overuse injuries, decline in athletic performance, and unexplained weight loss.

Because HIT is physically and psychologically demanding, many participants alternate interval training days with days of rest or with days of more moderately paced exercise.

Flexibility and Stretching Programs

You may have heard a coach or a friend say that good muscle flexibility will decrease the chance of an injury. This concept is not strongly supported by research, yet many people insist that the only reason they have avoided serious injury is that they have an appropriate level of flexibility. When you consider that many injuries occur because a joint is forced beyond the range of motion it is capable of, you might suspect that flexibility could have a role in injury prevention.

In rehabilitation, stretching techniques are often used in achieving objectives of treatment. In addition to the use of stretching for injury management, there are a variety of techniques that coaches and participants employ to increase flexibility to enhance sport performance and prevent injury. Some of the most commonly used stretching methods are passive stretching, active stretching, and contract–relax stretching. Specific stretches should be done for the muscles used in the activity. Suggested muscle groups to stretch and suggested stretching exercises designed for a runner are listed in table 2.6.

Passive Stretching

As the name implies, **passive stretching** entails no work on the part of the individual. The individual relaxes while someone else carries the limb through a particular range of motion. Athletic trainers and physical therapists often use passive stretching to assist in the individual's recovery after injury. The passive stretching technique requires that the assistant understand the meaning of muscle tension. An unskilled person may think that the stretch should be taken farther into the range of motion than is safe, and this can actually damage muscle tissue. Passive stretching requires training and experience in placing the participant in a stretching position.

Active Stretching

In **active stretching**, the individual uses her own body to produce the stretch of the particular area. For example, calf stretching can be done standing up, and the individual's body weight and strength produce the range of motion. This muscle group is stretched more easily with the active technique than with the passive method. All forms of stretching have a place in the total development of the individual.

Contract–Relax Stretching

In contract–relax stretching, the individual works with a partner or therapist who both provides the resistance to the contraction and stretches the muscle group. Contract–relax stretching can be done in any movement plane. For example, contract–relax stretching of the hamstrings is much like the passive stretching except that during the contract phase, the individual activates the hamstrings and gluteals, trying to extend (push down) at the hip joint. People who use contract–relax stretching feel that the contraction of the muscle prior to stretching

Table 2.6 Suggested Flexibility Exercises for Runners

Abdomen and back muscles	Press-up (abdominal muscles)	Back stretch (spine)
Hamstrings	Seated hamstring stretch	Standing hamstring stretch
Quadriceps and hip flexors	Hurdler stretch	Standing quad stretch
Groin muscles (adductors)	V-stretch	Butterfly stretch
Back of leg (gastrocnemius/soleus)	Calf stretch, standing	Bent-knee calf stretch

allows the muscle to more fully relax during the stretching cycle.

Contract–relax stretching is very useful for individuals who have a difficult time relaxing during a passive stretch. The preliminary contraction helps to decrease anxiety and the discomfort of the stretch.

Proprioceptive Neuromuscular Facilitation

Proprioceptive neuromuscular facilitation (PNF) is a specialized technique of therapy that incorporates muscle spindle stretch, resistance to stimulate strength, and specific movement patterns. In the strict sense, PNF requires that three movements occur in the extremity: flexion-extension, abduction-adduction, and rotation. The PNF contract–relax stretching is performed in a diagonal pattern so that all three components of the motion can be performed. This technique requires a good understanding of the diagonal patterns, the points of resistance, and the manual contacts during the stretching. It's important to realize that contract–relax stretching uses a single, straight plane of motion while PNF employs diagonal patterns of movement traversing three planes of movement.

Stretching Methods

In addition to active, passive, and contract–relax stretching, the ways in which a muscle or other connective tissue is stretched are classified into static, dynamic, and ballistic. Static stretching is a technique whereby the joint is moved to the point at which tightness is felt and that position is held. This static position of stretch is beneficial if the stretch can be held for up to about 30 s. If it is possible to hold the stretch for a longer period of time, the deformation of the tissue is greater and the tissue is less apt to return to the previous shortened state. This low-load, prolonged stretch is a mild stretch that is held for a period of minutes or hours (if possible); it is often used in physical therapy to reduce muscle **contractures**. The shorter time period of the hold phase in static stretching increases the elongation of the muscles and

CASE STUDY

Raul was entering junior high and hoping to follow in the footsteps of his older brother and play on the school's soccer team. Raul's brother, Javier, was much taller and weighed almost 35 lb more than Raul. On the first day of tryouts, Raul was asked if he was related to Javier, and when it was discovered he was Javier's brother, the pressure was on. The coaches asked Raul to demonstrate how to dribble through a set of cones and later to perform a free kick. The players all did some footwork drills, a series of runs, and passing drills. Then it was time for Raul to demonstrate the dribble drill. The pressure was on, and Raul could feel his legs getting heavy. Halfway through the dribble drill, he tripped and almost fell flat on his face. When the time came for the free kick drill, Raul was exhausted. He hadn't played all summer and really didn't do much other than ride his bike a couple of times a week.

Think About It

1. Was there anything Raul could have done to better prepare for the tryout day?

2. What are the components of a conditioning program you would suggest to Raul?

3. What would you suggest he do to better prepare his legs? Strength? Endurance?

4. Design an 8-week preseason program for this soccer participant.

provides a feeling of increased "looseness." Static stretching is used extensively by coaches, participants, and athletic therapists to decrease muscle tension.

Ballistic stretching involves a bouncing movement. This stretch is much more difficult to perform safely because the bouncing movement fires the **Golgi tendon organs (GTO)** and causes the muscle to reflexively contract. Stretching a contracting muscle can cause muscle damage and should be avoided. Ballistic stretching is not entirely safe, so when individuals bounce during stretching, the athletic trainer or coach should advise them to stop bouncing and to hold the stretch position.

Dynamic stretching involves movements that are sport specific and can be thought of as part of the sport warm-up. The best example of the dynamic stretch might be the technique of "high knees" that sprinters use. The participant raises the knees above waist level while running (or jogging) 5 to 10 yd (4.6 to 9 m). The objective of the "high knees" is vertical rather than horizontal movement. This technique provides a dynamic stretch to the hamstrings and hip extensors in a sportlike drill.

Learning Aids

SUMMARY

This chapter presents several concepts of strength and conditioning training. Although many colleges and universities employ a full-time strength and conditioning coordinator, the ATC should have a firm understanding of exercise physiology and exercise selection. Reconditioning following an injury is usually the role of the ATC, and understanding the concepts of conditioning and strength training is essential. Take a moment to review the chapter objectives and compare your thinking with the information provided here.

KEY CONCEPTS AND REVIEW

▸ **Identify ways in which information from fitness testing can help the athletic trainer.**

An individual's fitness level can be a strong indication of her performance abilities in exercise sessions. Knowledge of a low level of fitness can help prevent an injury during an exercise session. Additionally, information about an aspect of a person's fitness level assists the athletic trainer in designing an exercise prescription to help get the individual into better shape.

▸ **Discuss the rationale for conducting fitness testing at various times before, during, or after the sport or training season.**

Preparticipation fitness testing should be a standard part of every exercise program. The information helps in establishing the baseline of fitness prior to an exercise program and in determining specific needs of the individual to allow safe participation. Evaluation after the training season aids in the establishment of off-season objectives and gives the individual a better understanding of the progress made as a result of the training program.

▸ **Explain the method of establishing the 1-repetition maximum in weightlifting.**

To establish a 1RM in a particular weightlifting exercise, you would select a weight that is your best guess at the appropriate weight for the individual. If the person cannot lift that weight, the weight is reduced until the individual can accomplish one full lift. If the original weight is lifted easily, additional weight is added until the person cannot perform a full lift, and the recorded weight is the last successful lift or weight.

▸ **Define aerobic and anaerobic with reference to energy systems and relate each to various activities.**

The aerobic energy system depends on the availability of oxygen, whereas the anaerobic energy system can function without oxygen. All activities have some combination of anaerobic and aerobic function. Activities shorter than 1 min are as close to anaerobic as possible; the event lasting 1 min uses energy from both sources equally, and that ratio gradually changes toward aerobic energy supply as the event duration increases. Most sprints use the anaerobic system, while sustained activities can use energy from the aerobic system. Sports often involve a combination of the two—sprints or spurts of high-intensity work followed by periods of lower-intensity work. High-intensity, short-duration exercise uses the anaerobic system and cannot be sustained for long periods of time.

▸ **Define isotonic, isometric, and isokinetic exercise and give an example of each.**

Isotonic exercises are those in which a muscle contraction causes movement of a joint in response to a nonchanging load or weight. This type of exercise is like picking up a bowling ball or any other object. Isotonic exercises involve a joint action, muscle contraction, and accommodating resistance (weight); this type of action is like stretching a very heavy rubber band—the farther you stretch it, the harder it becomes to stretch. Isometric exercises are those in which the muscle force is generated but no movement occurs. This type of exercise is similar to what a football lineman does when he holds his opponent away and to the execution of a hold by a wrestler. Special machines are needed to supply the accommodating resistance in isokinetic exercises.

▸ **Compare and contrast the two types of muscle contraction: concentric and eccentric.**

Concentric muscle contraction involves a shortening of the muscle whereas eccentric contraction involves a lengthening of the muscle during the contraction. Most activities involve both types of contraction, generally with the eccentric activity acting to slow down or decelerate a movement or to act against the pull of gravity.

▸ **Discuss factors to consider in designing an exercise prescription.**

Several factors are essential for establishing an exercise prescription: the results of needs analysis, the setting of goals (including short-term goals, long-term goals, and limitations to the plan), and the exercise plan itself. The requirements of the activity or sport and the abilities and needs of the participant help in designing the objectives for the prescription. The participant and athletic trainer should work together in establishing the goals for the day, the week, and even the month. Based on the objectives and on input from the participant, the long-range goals can be developed. Limitations to the plan can be numerous or few. Each individual must play an active part in developing the exercise prescription to keep small obstacles from becoming large roadblocks.

▸ **Define the overload principle and explain how it applies to conditioning and strength techniques.**

Strength and endurance gains occur only when the system is challenged. Overload, or asking more of a muscle or system than it is used to performing, stimulates growth and development. Overload in strength training can come from an increase in the amount of weight being lifted, the number of times the weight is lifted, or the number of exercises used. Adaptations will always occur; and with adaptation, growth may be hampered. Progressions in the weight program are essential to improvement. In cardiorespiratory training, the same principles apply: The system must be overloaded. The sprint must be accomplished in less time or with less rest between repeats; the distance needs to be increased, or the pace increased on the same distance. Any additional challenge will provide an overload. A key to providing the overload is to do it in a measurable fashion. Subjective changes in performance are not only difficult to quantify; they are difficult to reproduce and thus difficult to use as a basis for overload.

PRACTICE!

For hands-on practice in this area, go to the web resource and complete the following:

Level 2.6, Module G5: Flexibility Training

Level 2.12, Module M7: Muscular Endurance

CRITICAL THINKING QUESTIONS

1. Muscle function is divided into three subcategories: muscle strength, endurance, and power. What are the advantages of testing individuals for each? Develop and describe a testing procedure for each subcategory that you might perform in an athletic preseason, during the season, and postseason.

2. Flexibility involves a combination of several anatomical structures (joint structure, muscle size, ligament and tendon composition). Describe how each of these would play a role in the flexibility differences between a 300-lb (136 kg) freshman lineman on a college football team and a 110-lb (50 kg) gymnast who has been performing since she was 5 years old. In your answer, include any significance their sport histories may have.

3. As you tour the facilities of a prospective new employment opportunity, you notice that the weight room includes only the following equipment:

   - Free weights ranging from 25 lb to 200 lb (11-91 kg)
   - A relatively new treadmill
   - A lower extremity multijoint machine (leg extension, hamstring curls, leg press)
   - A large (10 ft × 12 ft) interlocking rubber mat area that is currently empty

The athletic director asks you, as part of your interview, to suggest changes to the current weight room given the opportunity to buy five new pieces. Discuss the current equipment, including machines you might give away, as well as those you would add. Consider all areas of a workout regimen in your answer, including types of strength training and plyometrics, aerobic conditioning, and flexibility training. Provide rationale for your equipment decisions. Remember that all sports, male and female teams, will be using this weight room.

Nutritional Aspects of Health and Performance

Susan Kay Hillman, ATC, PT

OBJECTIVES

After reading this chapter, the student should be able to do the following:

- Discuss the recommended dietary intake of carbohydrate, fat, and protein and explain how one would calculate the caloric content of a meal or diet.

- Explain the role of carbohydrate as an energy source and list the types of carbohydrate found in foods.

- Discuss the recommended daily intake of water and explain suitable alternatives to plain drinking water for replenishing body fluids.

- Explain the difference between "good" and "bad" cholesterol and suggest the method one might use to minimize the negative effects of cholesterol.

- Discuss the concepts of a preevent meal versus preevent nutrition and explain why some people may feel they are able to eat anything they want prior to competition.

Nutrition has become a concern of almost every physically active individual. The concept that a diet is a program for losing weight is as far from fact as the generalization that individuals should not have to think about the foods that they eat. Good nutrition should be viewed as a method to provide the body with the best tools for growth and development as well as an aid to recovery when injury or illness strikes. When the physically active individual fails to consider the nutritional demands of increased activity levels, both performance and health suffer. Understanding the role that nutrition plays in keeping the body healthy is as important as understanding the need for a regular workout schedule. Nutrition should be viewed as an asset to performance. Every physically active person must attempt to understand the effect of nutrition on performance and health. Good nutrition can help the physically active person prevent injury and illness as well as help improve performance.

Why Study Nutrition?

It seems reasonable that a competitive participant would want to employ as many techniques as possible in the quest for excellence. In this age of athletic competition, the skill levels of the participants are so closely matched that the participant's nutritional practices can make the difference between winning and losing. Not only does nutrition help the individual with performance issues; it is imperative that the physically active indi-

vidual understand the demands that athletic participation places on the body's fluid and fuel supplies. A poorly nourished individual trying to win at sport is similar to a race car driver trying to win races using low-grade or limited fuel sources.

Basic Nutritional Needs of Active Individuals

The basic nutritional needs of the physically active person are quite similar to those of any other individual. A well-balanced diet with protein, fat, and **carbohydrate** at every meal is the key to both optimal performance and health (see table 3.1).

To determine if you are meeting the criteria of a well-balanced diet, first you must understand how to calculate the total calories (energy) consumed and determine the percentages of energy sources provided. Both carbohydrate and protein provide about 4 calories (energy) per gram, while fat contribute 9 calories per gram. To calculate the total calories in a meal, you need to know how many grams of protein, fat, and carbohydrate are in each item. Multiply the number of grams of each energy source by its specific factor (4 or 9) and add the values of the three energy sources together. This total is the total caloric (Kcal) content of the item. Add all the items consumed in a meal, and you can calculate the calories consumed in that meal. (See the sidebar An Example of Calorie Calculations for a Meal for an example.) Adding all foods consumed during a full day can provide the daily intake. If you average

Table 3.1   **Typical Sources of Carbohydrate, Protein, and Fat**

High-carbohydrate foods	Protein-rich foods	High-fat foods
Breads	Meat, fish, poultry, eggs	Fats and oils (used in cooking)
Fruit juices	Dairy products	Meat, fish, poultry
Dried fruits	Cereals	Dairy products
Fresh (or canned) fruits	Fruits, vegetables	Eggs
Grains, pastas, starches	Beans, peas, nuts	Beans

AN EXAMPLE OF CALORIE CALCULATIONS FOR A MEAL

Here are the calculations for a meal of one plain bagel with cream cheese and an 8-oz glass of 2% milk.

Food	Fat (g)	Carbohydrate (g)	Protein (g)
1 plain bagel	2	38	7
1 oz cream cheese	10	1	2
1 cup 2% milk	5	12	8
Total grams	17	51	17

To calculate the calories for this meal, multiply the number of grams of fat by 9, the number of grams of carbohydrate by 4, and the number of grams of protein by 4:

17 g fat × 9 Kcal/g = 153 Kcal

51 g carbohydrate × 4 Kcal/g = 204 Kcal

17 g protein × 4 Kcal/g = 68 Kcal

This calculation gives you 425 Kcal total.

several days' intake, you should come close to your average daily caloric consumption.

Generally, for physically active individuals, 60% of total calories should be derived from carbohydrate foods, 30% or less from fat, and 10% to 15% from protein (see table 3.2). Participants benefit from a fairly high consumption of carbohydrate because the storage form of carbohydrate is glycogen, and glycogen is the source the muscle depends on for energy. Physically active and competing individuals need higher levels of carbohydrate to provide the fuel (glycogen) for workouts and competition. Additionally, physically active people need slightly more protein (about 0.9 to 1.34 g of protein per pound of body weight per day) than the non-athletic individual (0.8 g of protein per pound of body weight per day). When the physically active person follows a well-balanced diet and consumes adequate calories to meet the energy demands of the sport, she can usually obtain the additional protein needed. Many of the foods that contain high amounts of necessary carbohydrate (e.g., breads, pasta, and cereals) also contribute to the protein goals.

Fluid Needs for Active Individuals

In addition to a well-balanced food intake, physically active people must pay close attention to their fluid intake. Some people have the misconception that soft drinks contribute to the goal of providing the body with fluid. Actually, some soft drinks can contribute to fluid loss. The caffeine in many soft drinks acts as a diuretic and depletes your body of fluids. Drinking these beverages increases the need for water. The body's need for fluid is best satisfied by water unless specific electrolytes or carbohydrates are also needed. As a general rule, the average person should consume eight 8-oz glasses of water each day (64 oz). Active people require even more water to make up for the water lost in perspiration. Unfortunately, thirst cannot be used to indicate your need for water. By the time you feel thirsty, you are already slightly dehydrated.

Most people tend to drink more of a particular fluid if it tastes good. If the water from a drinking fountain has a bad odor or taste, you'll tend not to drink it. This comes into play in efforts to get physically active people to drink more fluids. Because of the taste factor, sport drinks are often preferred even if there is little or no need for the extra carbohydrates or electrolytes. The concentration of carbohydrate should be low enough (less than 7%) to allow rapid intestinal absorption if people are using sport drinks for hydration during physical activity. A flavored sport drink with 6% carbohydrate

Table 3.2 Examples of Approximately 60/25/15 Meals (60% Carbohydrate, 25% Fat, 15% Protein)

Food item (size)	Calories	Protein	Fat	Carbohydrate
Breakfast				
English muffin with margarine (1 tsp)	190	6	5	30
Banana (1)	105	1	1	27
Yoplait yogurt, fruit flavored (1 serving)	190	8	3	32
Orange juice, frozen-reconstituted (1 cup)	112	2	0	27
Lunch				
Turkey breast (2 slices)	47	10	1	0
Butterhead lettuce (2 leaves)	2	0	0	0
Whole wheat bread (2 slices)	135	3	1	28
Mustard (1 tsp)	4	0	0	0
Romaine lettuce (1 cup)	10	<1	<1	1
Raw broccoli flowers (1/2 cup)	12	1	0	2
Raw cauliflower (1/2 cup)	12	1	0	2
French dressing (5 tbsp)	290	0	22	23
Peach (1)	37	1	0	10
Snack				
Grapes (1 cup)	116	1	1	31
Dinner				
Baked potato (1) with margarine (1 tbsp)	364	6	11	61
Beef round, broiled (3 oz)	162	25	6	0
Steamed broccoli (1 cup)	44	5	1	8
Snack				
Popcorn, popped plain with margarine (1 tsp)	103	2	5	14
Totals				
Grams		73 g	58 g	296 g
Calories	1,935	292	522	1,184
Percent of total calories		15%	25%	60%

(60 g carbohydrate per liter of drink) is well tolerated and aids in replenishing body fluids as well as providing an additional energy source.

Every physically active person should establish his own fluid replacement schedule based on his individual sweat rate (see the sidebar Sweat Rate Calculation), exercise parameters (availability of rest breaks and fluid, duration of exercise, and exercise intensity), environmental factors, and degree of acclimatization. People unaccustomed to exercise in certain environmental conditions usually require more frequent rest breaks and

SWEAT RATE CALCULATION

To calculate sweat rate, you'll need a few measurements. First subtract body weight (in grams) after exercise from the body weight before exercise. This gives you the difference in body weight (DBW). Next, measure total drink volume in milliliters (DV) consumed during exercise. Then measure the urine volume (UV) in milliliters.

Sweat loss (SL) = DBW + DV − UV.

Sweat rate (ml/h) = SL ÷ duration of exercise (in hours).

For example, Retesha weighed in before practice at 120 lb; following practice she weighed again and found that she weighed only 118 lb. During practice she consumed the entire contents of two sport bottles, each containing 1 L water (total of 2 L or 2,000 ml). The practice lasted 2 h, and after practice Retesha emptied her bladder into a special cup for measuring urine and found that she had eliminated 300 ml. The calculations would be as follows:

Prepractice weight = 54,545 g (120 lb)

Postpractice weight = 53,636 g (118 lb)

DBW = 909 g

DV = 2,000 ml

UV = 300 ml

(Note that 1 ml of water is approximately 1 g.)

Thus sweat loss = 909 g + 2,000 ml − 300 ml = 2,609 ml/practice session or

Sweat rate = 2,609 ml/2 h = 1,3074.5 ml/h or 1.3 L/h.

a greater intake of fluid than indicated by the sweat rate alone. Those who are acclimatized may be able to consume fluids at a rate equal to or slightly higher than the sweat rate without compromising performance. A general rule is that fluids should be consumed prior to the event as well as during the event, and also until about an hour or more following the event.

Caloric Demands of Active Individuals

The major nutritional need of the active individual is increased calories. The obvious reason for the increased need for calories is the increased use of calories as energy to perform. When the number of calories consumed in the diet is lower than the number of calories burned throughout the day, weight loss results. On the other hand, if the number of calories consumed is greater than the number of calories burned, weight gain results. Depending on the sport and the participant's role on the team or in the sport, body weight may be important. A lineman on the football team may be able to gain weight and still perform very well in his position; the distance runner carrying extra pounds may suffer greatly from the added weight.

MyPlate

MyPlate is a system designed by the United States Department of Agriculture (USDA) to teach people to eat a balanced diet from a variety of food groups without counting calories or other nutrients. MyPlate is divided into five food groups: grains, vegetables, fruits, protein, and dairy (see figure 3.1). The recommendation for daily intake of each food group depends on your age, gender, and level of physical activity.

MyPlate is part of a USDA communication initiative based on the 2010 Dietary Guidelines for Americans intended to help people make wise food choices. MyPlate emphasizes three main topics to remind the consumer to make wise choices:

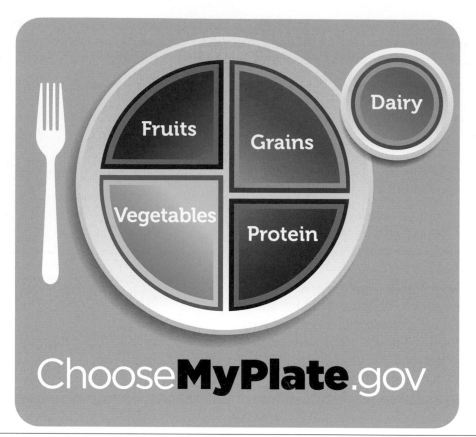

Figure 3.1   MyPlate.

Reprinted from USDA and DHHS.

Balance Calories

- Enjoy your food, but eat less.
- Avoid oversized portions.

Foods to Increase

- Make half your plate fruits and vegetables.
- Make at least half your grains whole grains.
- Switch to fat-free or low-fat (1%) milk.

Foods to Reduce

- Compare sodium in foods like soup, bread, and frozen meals and choose the foods with lower numbers.
- Drink water instead of sugary drinks.

The 2010 Dietary Guidelines for Americans is a downloadable book (see www.cnpp.usda.gov/DietaryGuidelines.htm) consisting of six easy-to-read chapters. The book is the USDA's attempt to educate the population on topics such as the following:

- Balancing calories to manage weight
- Identifying foods and food components to reduce or increase in the diet
- Building healthy eating patterns
- Making healthy choices of food and exercise

Carbohydrates in the Diet

Since carbohydrates are such an important source of energy for working muscles, it should be easy to understand why at least 60% of the calories in an active individual's diet should come from carbohydrates. Some foods may be high in carbohydrate but also high in dietary fat. It is important for people to distinguish carbohydrate calories from fat calories when consuming a combined food. Menu items high in carbohydrate and low in fat include breads, grains (brown rice, oats, barley, and so on), pastas, vegetables, fruits, fruit juices, and juice drinks. Muscles replenish stored carbohydrate most efficiently within the first 2 h following exercise. Therefore, the active person should begin to replenish her carbohydrate stores as soon as possible after exercise and then again a few hours later.

Because carbohydrates are such an important source of energy for short-duration or intense exercise, it is wise to understand the foods that supply the needed nutrients. Carbohydrates can be classified as monosaccharides (fructose, galactose, or glucose), disaccharides (in which two or more of the monosaccharides are chemically linked), or polysaccharides (hundreds or thousands of linked monosaccharides). Simple (monosaccharides and disaccharides) and complex carbohydrates (polysaccharides) are also terms used to describe the types of carbohydrates. Both are outlined in table 3.3.

Different types of carbohydrates are composed of different combinations of monosaccharides. During digestion, carbohydrates are broken down into their component monosaccharides. This process occurs to a limited degree in the mouth and stomach, but most of the digestion happens in the small intestine. In the small intestine, enzymes

from the pancreas (insulin) break the large carbohydrates into fructose, galactose, and, mainly, glucose. After the breakdown, galactose and glucose leave the mucosa of the intestine by a process called active transport, which requires energy. Fructose can pass through the mucosal membrane by diffusion (no energy required) as long as the concentration gradient is low on the opposite side of the membrane.

Once in the blood, the monosaccharides enter the bloodstream and progress to the liver. The liver converts the fructose and galactose to glucose or another product of glucose metabolism. Glucose is stored in the liver in the form of glycogen. Glycogen can also be transported and stored in the muscle, with the kidneys and intestines adding yet other minor storage sites. With up to 10% of its weight as glycogen, the liver has the highest glycogen content of any body tissue. These stores of glycogen can be quickly converted to glucose for use in working muscles.

According to nutritional researchers, although one might assume that simple carbohydrates are absorbed most quickly, digestion and absorption do not happen at the same rate for all carbohydrates in a particular grouping. Nutritionists working with persons who have **diabetes** have used the **glycemic index** to evaluate the rise in blood glucose following ingestion of food. This same concept of the glycemic index has been

Table 3.3 **Types of Carbohydrates**

Carbohydrate class	Type	Source
Monosaccharides (simple carbohydrates)	Fructose	Fruit sugar
	Galactose	
	Glucose	Blood sugar
Disaccharides (simple carbohydrates)	Sucrose (glucose + fructose)	Table sugar
	Lactose (glucose + galactose)	Milk sugar
	Maltose (glucose + glucose)	
Polysaccharides (complex carbohydrates)	Amylose (straight chain of glucose)	Starchy foods like bread, potatoes, corn
	Amylopectins (branched chain of glucose)	

applied to people who do not have diabetes in an effort to understand the types of carbohydrates that are more readily usable during exercise. Current concepts relating to the use of the glycemic index in exercise suggest that carbohydrates that empty quickly into the bloodstream (high glycemic index) should be consumed immediately after training to help replace the glycogen stores in the body. The remaining meals of the day should be derived from other natural complex sources of carbohydrates such as beans, vegetables, grains, and fruits. These yield a slower, steadier flow of glucose into the bloodstream (low glycemic index), promoting glycogen replacement hours after exercise.

Fats in the Diet

The average American's diet may be surprisingly high in fat even with the number of "light," "low-fat," and "fat-free" products available. It would not be unusual to find 40% to 45% of the daily caloric intake represented by dietary fat. Most nutritionists agree that 30% or less of the daily caloric intake should be from fat. Nevertheless, it is very important that we realize how essential fats are in providing energy for exercise. Light to moderate exercise and exercise of longer duration depend on energy from fat stores. Remember, carbohydrates are the main source of energy for short bursts or intense bouts of exercise; less intense or longer-lasting exercise uses fatty acid fuels. In addition to the overall percentage of calories, it is important to understand the types of fats available. As with carbohydrates, fats are grouped into three different categories: saturated, monounsaturated, and polyunsaturated. It is well known that the type of fat is just as important as the total amount of fat you eat.

Dietary fats, or **lipids** (see table 3.4), are found in our bodies predominantly in the form of **triglycerides**. Each triglyceride is a molecule of glycerol bonded to three molecules of fatty acid. The breakdown of the triglyceride occurs mainly in the small intestine. The stomach and pancreatic enzymes

Table 3.4	**Lipid Content of Some Common Foods**
Food	**Percent fat**
Meats	
Veal	10
Chicken	10-17
Beef	16-42 (depends on cut)
Lamb	19-29
Ham, sliced	23
Pork	81
Plant sources of fat	
Potato chips	35
Cashew nuts	48
Peanut butter	50
Margarine	81
Oils	100
Other fats	
Baked beans	31
2% milk	35
Cream cheese	89.5
Hard-boiled egg	61
Cheesecake	63

(working in the small intestine) remove two of the three fatty acids from the glycerol molecule, thus forming a monoglyceride. Some short-chain fatty acids (those with fewer than 12 carbon atoms) are absorbed by the process of diffusion into the bloodstream. However, most of the fatty acids are long-chain fatty acids, which, along with the monoglyceride, require bile for their absorption. These dietary triglycerides reach the bloodstream by dissolving into a tiny sphere called a micelle, which is a carrier of bile salts. The micelles provide a transport service for the fatty acids and monoglycerides, transporting them through the intestine without any change to the micelle. Further along in the process, the monoglycerides (glycerol) and the fatty acids recombine as triglycerides. These triglycerides are transported in the bloodstream as one of three lipoprotein particles: very low-density lipoproteins (VLDLs),

CHOLESTEROL

Almost every adult has heard something about **cholesterol** levels. Blood cholesterol has been studied to attempt to understand its relationship to heart disease and **atherosclerosis**. Blood cholesterol tests often evaluate total cholesterol, **low-density lipoprotein (LDL) cholesterol**, **high-density lipoprotein (HDL) cholesterol**, and triglycerides. Low-density lipoprotein is called the "bad cholesterol" because it deposits fats and cholesterol on the lining of arteries. High-density lipoprotein is called the "good cholesterol" because it carries the fat and cholesterol away.

Knowing this, most of us would want to decrease our LDL and increase our HDL, but how can that be done? The answer is diet and exercise. So, what foods contain this bad cholesterol? Saturated fats contribute to LDL levels and should be reduced in our diets. Generally, meats and dairy products contain mostly saturated fats. Foods that are less apt to increase LDL levels and may in fact lower the blood cholesterol include unsaturated fats: either monounsaturated (canola, olive, and peanut oils) or polyunsaturated (corn, soybean, and sunflower oils). Additionally, whole foods that contain unsaturated fats include avocados, olives, and peanuts. Reducing total fat and replacing some saturated fat with unsaturated fat should be a goal of every healthy person. In fact, nutritionists are finding that if we replace some saturated fat with monounsaturated fat, LDL cholesterol and total cholesterol are lowered without decreasing HDL cholesterol levels or raising triglyceride levels.

low-density lipoproteins (LDLs), and high-density lipoproteins (HDLs). (The sidebar Cholesterol provides more information.) When the individual lacks bile salts because of an obstruction or the loss of the gallbladder, lipid absorption is diminished and the lipids are lost into the feces. If the lipids fail to be absorbed, the excellent source of energy from fats is diminished, as is the absorption of fat-soluble vitamins A, D, E, and K.

This energy from lipids, like the energy from carbohydrates, is in the form of adenosine triphosphate or ATP (ATP is the "energy currency" of the cell). Each gram of triglyceride produces about 9 **kilocalories** of energy. If the body doesn't need the energy immediately, the lipids are stored in **adipose tissue** (fat deposits) throughout the body and in the liver. Adipose tissue (the body's fat layers) stores triglycerides until the individual requires the ATP for work, but adipose tissue also provides insulation and protection in the areas where it is present. The major sites for storage of the unneeded triglycerides are the **subcutaneous** tissue (about 50% of that being stored), the kidneys (12%), the abdominal viscera (10-15%), the genital areas (20%), and the spaces between muscles (5-8%). The triglycerides stored in adipose tissue are exchanged very rapidly, and thus there is a new storage of triglycerides in our adipose tissue every 2 or 3 weeks. At any given time, the triglycerides stored in the tissues the previous month have been used or moved out and replaced by other triglyceride molecules. All triglycerides are continually released from storage, transported in the bloodstream, and redeposited in another storage site.

Remember that triglycerides are an excellent energy value and that about 98% of all energy reserves are from the triglycerides stored in adipose tissue. Glucose is not stored as easily as triglycerides, which makes fats an excellent resource for energy stores. Although many of the body's cells prefer to use glucose, the heart muscle is one of the organs that use fatty acids as its energy source.

Dietary Protein

As mentioned previously, the physically active individual needs only slightly more protein than the average person. Proteins provide our bodies with **essential amino acids** (see table 3.5). "Essential" actually means that the amino acid cannot be manufactured in the body but must be ingested from foods. There are 22 different amino acids in proteins, and various foods supply those amino acids in various amounts. One of the best sources of dietary protein is dairy products such as milk. Meat is a good source of protein, and vegetables such as legumes and grains offer a partially complete protein in that they lack one or more essential amino acids or contain less than the required amount of the amino acid.

Physically active people who choose not to consume animal products should understand the essential amino acids that are lacking in their diets and attempt to find sources of those missing components. A vegetarian often experiences more difficulty in consuming the appropriate number of calories in the diet than in finding the proper nutrients partly because animal proteins usually have a higher caloric value than nonmeats. This may be more obvious to you if you consider the amount of fat contained in most meat products. The total caloric value of the meat is obtained from the number of protein calories as well as the number of fat calories.

Proteins ingested from the diet are broken down into amino acids, which are absorbed into the bloodstream and transported to the liver. Unlike fats and carbohydrates, proteins are not stored to be used later. Amino acids are used by the body to produce ATP or as the building blocks of new proteins used for growth and repair processes. Excess amounts of dietary amino acids are converted into glucose or triglycerides and stored in the adipose tissues of the body.

Excess Dietary Protein

Some dietary fads encourage high protein intake with very low carbohydrate consumption. This type of diet can cause a condition called **ketoacidosis** or ketosis, which is a by-product of metabolism when ketones are excreted from the burning of fats in an attempt to maintain the body's acid–base balance. Actually ketosis designates a pathological condition that is potentially dangerous to one's health. The advocates of the high-protein diets insist that the burning of ketones is a good thing in that the process of breaking down the fat into ketones requires energy, which translates into calories burned. Most dietary specialists agree that short-term ketosis is usually not a problem; long-term ketosis (several weeks) can create an accumulation of uric acid, which can cause **gout** or kidney stones in people predisposed to those conditions. Severely restricting carbohydrate consumption is apt to lead the patient into danger much more quickly than diets allowing greater consumption of carbohydrates.

Planning the Participant's Diet

The nutrition needed for optimal performance does not depend on the meal preceding the event but on the nutritional habits of the individual in the days and weeks prior to

Table 3.5 **Recommended Dietary Allowances (RDAs) of Dietary Protein**

Recommended amount	Adolescent males	Adult males	Adolescent females	Adult females
Grams of protein per kilogram body weight	0.9	0.8	0.9	0.8
Grams per day based on average weight	59 g (145 lb = average weight)	56 g (154 lb = average weight)	50 g (123 lb = average weight)	44 g (125 lb = average weight)

the competition. In choosing food products to be consumed to maximize the energy for training and competition, it is important to understand the energy requirements of the activity. The role of carbohydrates and fats as fuel sources during exercise depends mostly on the intensity and duration of the activity. Generally, carbohydrates are used more as the intensity of the exercise increases and less as the duration increases. Long-duration, low-intensity exercise would be expected to rely on fat as the energy source, but actually there is interplay between fat and carbohydrate use during all exercise. Good daily nutritional habits in the weeks preceding the competition provide the best opportunity to build carbohydrate stores to the maximum while also supplying fatty acids that act to increase the use of fat as an energy source.

Preevent Meals

As just mentioned, when the physically active individual prepares for a competitive event, the nutritional habits of the days prior to the event are more important than the meal consumed immediately before the contest. Endurance participants often begin changing their dietary habits several days before an event. In the common practice of carbohydrate loading, the individual increases the carbohydrate intake from the usual 60% to 70% to 80% of the total caloric intake. The individual usually begins this practice 3 days prior to the event and continues the training schedule as customary. This practice is designed to maximize the carbohydrate stores to allow the participant a greater reserve of energy.

The last meal before the contest cannot significantly alter the energy stores built up in the preceding days, although it should serve two purposes: (1) The foods should be easily digested to allow gastric emptying prior to the start of participation, and (2) the food should satisfy the individual's feelings of hunger. Thus, the high-carbohydrate pre-event meal is beneficial for two reasons: Carbohydrates are easily and quickly digested

and may provide a source of energy for the upcoming physical performance. Proteins and fats, on the other hand, are more difficult to digest and often require a longer period of time to convert to usable energy. Generally, if fats and proteins are included in the preevent meal, 3 to 4 h must be allowed between the time of the meal and the start of the event to ensure sufficient digestive time. Most people become focused, or even anxious, as the start time nears, making it even more important to plan the meal to allow sufficient time for the digestive processes. Individuals who experience gastric upset after ingesting a meal before exercise or competition may find it beneficial to use a liquid carbohydrate drink to build the energy stores with less need for digestive activity. In any case, the preevent meal should be supplemented with fluids to aid the individual in the attempt to maximize physical performance.

When a back-to-back competition schedule limits the amount of recovery time between exercise bouts, it is more imperative for the individual to replenish body fluids than to build energy stores. If the ingested fluids contain carbohydrates as well as water, however, both functions are served. The amount of fluid consumed should exceed the amount of body weight that has been lost during the exercise period preceding the rest break.

The psychological issues surrounding performance come into play with regard to menu selection for the pre-event meal. Some individuals disobey all rules concerning when and what to eat before the contest yet insist that their performance is best when they consume the unconventional diet. This points to the fact that the preevent meal is not as important as the meals on the days preceding the contest. In the preevent meal, it is important to avoid foods that irritate the bowel, pull fluids from the intestine, or cause bloating or other signs of indigestion. You can usually count on individuals to avoid foods that cause distress, because they do not enjoy the consequences of bowel distress. The foods that cause distress are not the same for all people.

Managing Weight: Gaining and Losing

Individuals place considerable pressures on themselves to perform well. These pressures don't end when the individual leaves the playing area but continue in everyday life. One such nonsport pressure comes from body weight. It would not be surprising to you if you overheard a female gymnast talking about needing to lose weight. Equally common might be the football interior lineman who is challenged with ways to keep his weight on during the intense practice sessions.

Changes in body weight can be very difficult for individuals to accomplish during a competitive season; such changes may occur very slowly. It is important for participants to establish and maintain good nutritional habits throughout the season. The diet should remain low in fat and high in carbohydrate, with adjustments in total calories to loose (fewer calories) or gain (more calories) body weight.

Weight Loss and Fluid Levels

Sports that set limits on the participant's weight through the weigh-in process certainly encourage fasting and other undesirable dietary practices. Rapid weight losses are usually the result of fluid loss in the body. This fluid loss can lead very quickly to dehydration and very serious outcomes. Wrestling, for example, sets weight limits for competitors of various weight classes. Intentional rapid weight loss in wrestlers became so unsafe that the Centers for Disease Control and Prevention (CDC) in 1998 issued a report on three collegiate wrestlers whose deaths were related to hyperthermia and dehydration. Unfortunately, it took several deaths to bring about modifications in wrestling weight loss practices.

Participants who are attempting to lose weight during the competitive season should anticipate no more than a 2 lb (0.9 kg) per week loss. The diet should be high in carbohydrates, and plenty of fluids must be consumed. Rapid weight loss is a sure sign of a loss of body fluids and could spell disaster if the fluids are not replenished before exercise begins.

Weight gain is sometimes a difficult issue for the individual because of the lack of access to food at various times throughout the day. The key factor in gaining weight while burning a significant amount of energy is to consume more calories than one is using. The individual who is able to supplement the normal meals should do so with high-carbohydrate food choices to provide a source of energy for the workout. Snacking throughout the day allows participants to consume more calories than if they attempt to increase calories only at mealtimes.

Special Diets, Fads, and Supplements

A fast fix is seldom a good fix. Food fads and supplements that offer an easy way to lose weight, gain weight, or gain performance advantages are seldom able to hold up to their promises in the absence of significant dedication to a workout regimen. People who dedicate themselves to an exercise program for improved performance, weight control, or even bodybuilding can rest assured that the changes brought about by hard work and dedication are much healthier than those brought about through chemical means. Nothing will replace the effect of hard work and good nutrition.

As an example, we might look at the product **ephedrine**. Ephedrine is used in many dietary aids as well as in supplements intended to give you more energy. Ephedrine (ephedra) has been linked to death in otherwise healthy professional athletes. One of the many difficulties in studying the effects of ephedrine-containing products is the fact that batches and lots of these products often have inconsistent levels of ephedrine. Inconsistencies in content not only make product evaluation difficult but also put the consumer at greater risk.

Vitamins, Minerals, and Other Dietary Supplements

Anyone who lacks specific items in the diet can potentially develop a deficiency of a vitamin or mineral. For example, some individuals are lactose intolerant, meaning that they have difficulty digesting dairy products. As you realize, dairy products are an excellent source of calcium; and unless a person who avoids them makes an effort to consume other sources of calcium, he could run the risk of a calcium deficiency. In this situation, supplementing the normal well-rounded diet may be indicated. On the other hand, if the individual is consuming a well-rounded diet with adequate calories, there should be no real need to supplement the diet.

Most vitamin and mineral supplements are actually quite harmless even if there is no physiological need for the added nutrients. When a water-soluble vitamin is consumed in quantities greater than the body needs, the excess is excreted into the urine. On the other hand, if the vitamin is fat soluble, the extra vitamin consumed is stored in the body's fat layers, where it can build up to a point of being harmful to the person's health. The fat-soluble vitamins are A, D, E, and K. These vitamins are stored rather than excreted, so people must take caution in using supplements with these vitamins unless they have a known deficiency or have determined that excess amounts will not be harmful to their general health.

When an individual is diagnosed with a nutritional or **metabolic disorder**, a health care provider may prescribe nutritional supplements. These prescribed supplements should always be taken under the supervision of the physician or other knowledgeable nutritional or health care professional. Unfortunately, supplements may appear to be safe and according to advertisements are not banned substances but in actuality have been outlawed by the individual's athletic conference or league. In addition to the possibility that a particular substance is banned, some chemicals interact with others to produce a

banned substance. Extreme care must always be taken to understand any and all chemicals to be ingested. The best method to ensure a drug-free body is to stay away from fast fixes and instead depend on hard work and good nutritional habits.

Nutritional Concerns in Injury or Illness

Nutrition is often used to help people recover from injury or illness, as rightfully it should be. You probably recall hearing that milk builds strong bones. This is certainly true in that calcium is essential for healthy bones. Milk, an excellent source of calcium, is generally advocated when people experience a fracture. Drinking milk and consuming other products high in calcium help to increase the level of calcium in your body, but drinking milk only after the fracture is not a sound dietary practice. Good nutrition, just like proper calcium intake, should be for every day and not only for after an injury or illness.

Nutritional Aspects of Fractures

Stress fractures are one type of fracture that may be due in part to low calcium levels. Low calcium levels are associated with low bone density (osteoporosis) and thus a higher potential for fracture. Estrogen suppresses osteoclasts, the cells that break down bone. Low levels of estrogen cause a loss of bone mineral density in women. Additionally, Boden and colleagues (2001) correlated low hormone levels in stress fractures in both males and females. Calcium is available in the foods we eat; some common foods contain estrogen-like compounds that may supplement low levels of circulating estrogens. These estrogen-like foods include carrots, yams, cheese, milk, yogurt, cottage cheese, and eggs.

Deficiency Diseases

Specific vitamin, mineral, or amino acid deficiencies are well established and often show a direct relationship to nutrition. Some of the well-known deficiencies are anemia (iron deficiency), **scurvy** (vitamin C deficiency), and **rickets** (vitamin D deficiency). A person may develop a deficiency disease due to diet or because of an inability to absorb the nutrient during digestion, yet recovery is usually very quick once the deficiency is understood and the diet is supplemented. The key to avoiding problems associated with these deficiencies is prevention through good nutrition and early medical evaluation once symptoms are observed.

Nutrition and the Diabetic Participant

When we think of a physically active individual who must observe nutrition closely due to an illness or injury, we naturally think of the patient with diabetes. Although it may be true that participants with diabetes need not alter their diet from what is customary for other competitors, people who have diabetes must pay much closer attention to their nutritional habits. People with some types of diabetes use insulin along with their dietary habits to control blood glucose levels. These individuals require very consistent mealtimes, as they must monitor their blood glucose level throughout the day to ensure that it remains normal. An insulin dose that is not followed by food intake could cause a serious hypoglycemic reaction. People with diabetes must ensure that their insulin dose matches their food intake to prevent extreme highs or lows in the blood glucose level. Keeping the blood glucose levels from dropping too low during exercise often requires considerable planning and discipline on the part of the individual. Anyone working with a diabetic patient must be aware of the possible dangers associated with changes in blood glucose levels. It could be quite dangerous for a diabetic patient to go home after a workout and take an insulin dose but then fall asleep before consuming a meal. The high insulin level pushes the glucose to a dangerously low level. Recognizing the potential problems and being prepared

to prevent them is the best method of care possible.

Nutritional Aspects of Growth and Repair Processes

A well-balanced diet is essential for normal growth and following injury when tissue repair is required. Individuals who experience frequent injuries or who seem to heal slowly should seek nutritional evaluation. Only after evaluation and detection of areas of deficiency can the proper diet and supplements be selected. With the physician's knowledge of the healing difficulties, referral to a nutritionist is often recommended when other medical issues are ruled out. Nutritional evaluation and consultation, however, can be very helpful regardless of any relation to an injury.

Fracture Healing

As discussed earlier, calcium plays a large part in the growth and repair of bones. Additionally, calcium can assist in blood-clotting mechanisms following injury and is also a potential factor in the regulation of blood pressure. Calcium is obtained from most dairy products (including cheeses and yogurt), calcium-enriched tofu, tortillas made from lime-processed corn, dark green leafy vegetables (spinach, broccoli, turnip greens, and kale), and canned fish containing soft bones that are normally eaten. A number of other dietary sources of calcium are certainly important for some individuals. One thing we must realize, however, is that some foods act to reduce the absorption of calcium while other minerals and nutrients can affect how well the body is able to absorb and use the calcium consumed. Adequate vitamin D enhances calcium absorption, while excessive meat, salt, caffeine, or alcohol consumption reduces the absorption of calcium from foods. Anyone who incurs frequent or unusual fractures would be wise to consult a nutritionist to evaluate their diet thoroughly.

Learning Aids

SUMMARY

Nutrition is an important topic for the participant and nonparticipant alike. Understanding the nutritional benefits of various foods helps all of us become better consumers and, hopefully, healthier people. MyPlate is a national effort to instill good nutritional practices in the entire population, making lifelong learning possible. It is certainly good practice to advise friends, family, and clients on proper nutrition rather than allow them to jump from one fad diet to another; and through an understanding of MyPlate and the USDA's Dietary Guidelines, that advice can be provided.

KEY CONCEPTS AND REVIEW

▶ **Discuss the recommended dietary intake of carbohydrate, fat, and protein and explain how one would calculate the caloric content of a meal or diet.**

We can calculate calories from food if we know how many grams of each energy source are in a food serving. Each gram of fat is equal to 9 calories, while carbohydrates and proteins have 4 calories per gram. Of the total number of calories consumed in 1 day, no more than 30% should be from fats, 10% to 15% from protein, and about 60% from carbohydrates.

▶ **Explain the role of carbohydrate as an energy source and list the types of carbohydrate found in foods.**

Carbohydrates are the energy source used during short-duration exercise as well as for intense exercise. Because carbohydrates play a critical role in providing fuel for exercise, it is important that individuals consume adequate amounts of carbohydrates for their exercise program. Carbohydrates exist as monosaccharides (fructose, galactose, or glucose), disaccharides (in which two or more of the monosaccharides are chemically linked), or polysaccharides (hundreds or thousands of linked monosaccharides). All carbohydrates are broken down into monosaccharides during digestion, a process that typically requires energy. The monosaccharides are converted to glucose in the liver. The rate of carbohydrate digestion and absorption varies for different foods and is the subject of continued research.

▶ **Discuss the recommended daily intake of water and explain suitable alternatives to plain drinking water for replenishing body fluids.**

As a general rule, the average person should consume eight 8-oz glasses (64 oz total) of water each day. Active individuals require even more water to make up for the water lost in perspiration. Some drinks, such as caffeine products, can increase a person's need for water because the caffeine acts as a diuretic and depletes the body of fluids. Since people tend to drink more of a beverage that tastes good, sport drinks can serve as a viable alternative to water. A flavored sport drink with 6% carbohydrate (60 g of carbohydrate per liter of drink) is well tolerated and aids in replenishing body fluids, as well as providing an additional source of energy from the carbohydrates.

▶ **Explain the difference between "good" and "bad" cholesterol and suggest the method one might use to minimize the negative effects of cholesterol.**

Cholesterol includes low-density lipoprotein (LDL) cholesterol, high-density lipoprotein (HDL) cholesterol, and triglycerides. The LDL is called the bad cholesterol because it deposits fats and cholesterol on the lining of arteries; HDL is called the good cholesterol because it carries the fat and cholesterol away. Reducing total fat and replacing some saturated fats with unsaturated fats should be a goal of every healthy individual.

▸ **Discuss the concepts of a preevent meal versus preevent nutrition and explain why some people may feel they are able to eat anything they want prior to competition.**

Nutrition in the days preceding the event is more critical to athletic performance than the last meal before the contest. Adhering to a well-balanced meal plan will always prove to be the best option. Preevent meals should be high in carbohydrates due to the body's need for that type of fuel and ease of digestion. This meal should be consumed between 3 and 4 h before the event. Psychology plays a large part of all performance and as such has an influence on the ability to perform regardless of the type of food consumed. As long as the food ingested does not cause gastric distress, some individuals are able to consume very controversial meals without an observable reduction in performance.

PRACTICE!

For hands-on practice in this area, go to the web resource and complete the following:

Level 2.7, Module H4: Basic Performance Nutrition and Supplementation

CRITICAL THINKING QUESTIONS

1. One of your gymnasts is concerned with her body image and feels that she looks terrible in her competition leotard. She wants you to help her in designing a diet to lose weight. She is 19 years old and currently taking in 2,800 calories per day on average; she is 5 ft, 2 in. and weighs 124 lb (56 kg). Make recommendations for the total caloric intake needed during this off-season and design her meals for 1 day.

2. One of your track distance runners returned from summer vacation and confided in you that her mother was on a protein-only diet, and that she herself had followed the same diet program for the past several weeks. Now that the participant is back on campus and responsible for her own meals, she wants to know what you think about the Atkins-type diet in which one tries to eliminate carbohydrate. Explain your view of high-protein, low-carbohydrate diets.

3. The distance runner of question 2 is quite thin, and you suspect that her diet may be partly responsible for the stress fractures in her left foot (last year) and her right foot (this season). Explain the dietary elements you would suggest she include in her diet to help strengthen her bones.

Environmental Conditions

Susan Kay Hillman, ATC, PT

OBJECTIVES

After reading this chapter, the student should be able to do the following:

- List and give examples of the four cooling methods used to rid a body of excess heat.

- List the major symptoms associated with heat exhaustion.

- Explain the concept of windchill and how it may affect the physically active individual exercising in a cold environment.

- List things one should observe when inspecting a playing environment for safety.

You may think that swimming, diving, and water polo are the only sports that involve individuals who train and compete under highly-controlled environmental conditions, especially if the pools are indoors. That may be fairly true, but even an indoor environment could be too hot or too cold. Most sports, indoor and outdoor, add the challenge of coping with the environment to the challenge of participation. Imagine training in an air-conditioned facility but participating in a tournament that is in an open-air arena in a warm, humid climate. The participants will have more difficulty in the tournament if they have not conditioned themselves for the heat and humidity. Conditions of the environment vary dramatically across regions as well as across seasons. When traveling to another region, the environment there should be anticipated and adaptations should be made. Understanding how the body dissipates heat is important in knowing the adaptations that must occur when participating in different environments.

The environment is not limited to heat and humidity; it includes the opposite temperature extreme, as well as a variety of weather conditions that affect participation outdoors. Care must be taken to anticipate and prepare for any weather-related challenge.

Although you may think indoor sports have a better controlled temperature environment, attention also must be paid to the physical environment. Having limitations of space in a gymnasium could produce a very challenging environment for some sports. For example, a wall that is 3 feet from the backboard in basketball poses a problem for layups and baseline play, but that same gymnasium may be quite satisfactory for a volleyball competition. Each and every location must be carefully examined for potential injury-producing obstacles or defects and care must be taken to minimize or eliminate those obstacles. Potholes, curbs, thick grass, and so on are all complications to the outside sport environment. This chapter will address the varied environmental conditions individuals might face.

Temperature Regulation and Heat Exchange

A person's perception of heat may occur internally or externally. The human body has an extremely efficient mechanism for maintaining the internal body temperature, making it difficult for the individual to detect small changes. External perception of heat may occur much more rapidly because of the sensory organs located in the skin.

Although heat is a good thing when the weather is cold and you decide to go for a run or workout, heat in the middle of summer may not be so welcome. Actually, when the temperature of your environment is between 70° and 80° F (neutral environmental temperature) or higher, the heat that your body produces (metabolic heat) can place a huge load on your ability to regulate internal heat. The "normal" body temperature is 98.6°. This may be misleading, however, if an individual's normal body temperature (normal meaning that the person is free of illness) is 99°. Every person has his own "normal" body temperature, and even that temperature fluctuates up and down throughout the day; 98.6° signifies the average normal body temperature for humans, and the normal range is from 97° to 100° F.

Core Temperature and Basal Metabolism

Core temperature, or the temperature of the internal systems, is regulated in the brain via the hypothalamus (see figure 4.1). We can affect core temperature by increasing the heat production (warming the body) or increasing the heat dissipation (cooling the body). Core temperatures are very precise, so that small deviations from the normal core temperature (called the set point) are offset by large adjustments in the body.

There are two major internal sources of heat: basal metabolism and exercise metabolism. Basal metabolism is the caloric expenditure of an individual at rest. Since

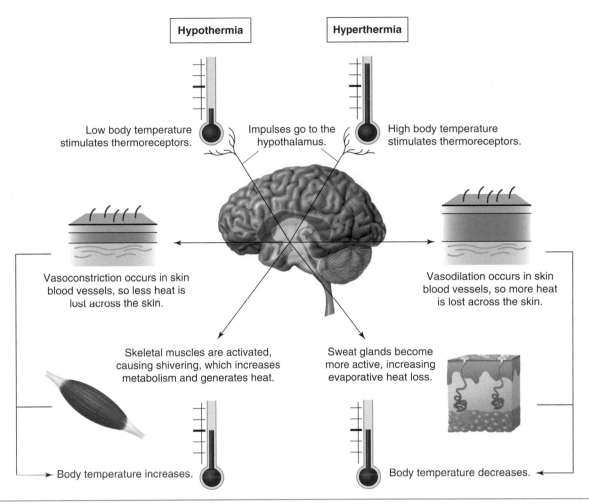

Figure 4.1 Function of the hypothalamus.

Adapted, by permission, from J.H. Wilmore and D.L. Costill, 1994, *Physiology of sport and exercise* (Champaign, IL: Human Kinetics), 246.

caloric expenditure is energy, it represents the minimum amount of energy required to maintain life at normal body temperature. When you start exercising, a second heat source is applied; the heat from exercise (heat is the by-product of metabolism) is exercise metabolism. Strenuous-exercise metabolism may produce 15 to 18 times the amount of heat of basal metabolism, depending on your level of fitness. The human body can also absorb heat from external sources, such as the sun, a fire, and hot drinks. You can end up with far more heat than you need, and in this situation if you were not able to shed the excess, you would experience heat illnesses and even risk death.

Altering Body Temperature

Whether it is hot or cold in your environment, your body attempts to stay at its normal temperature. To do this, it can use four mechanisms: sweat glands (to keep your skin moist and assist with cooling), smooth muscle of the blood vessels (which constrict or dilate the arterioles as needed to control blood flow to the skin), skeletal muscles (which generate heat by working or shivering), and some of the internal organs called endocrine glands (hormones produced by these glands cause cells to increase their metabolic rate). Together, these four systems effectively regulate the internal temperature of your body to keep you in a safe zone.

Physiological Responses to Exercise in the Heat

When we exercise in the heat, our body continually attempts to control its internal temperature. The body burns glycogen for energy, and that process produces heat. As exercise in the warm environment continues, several adaptations occur: The heart rate increases, energy levels decline, and sweating increases.

Increased Heart Rate

The cardiovascular system works to supply muscles with sufficient blood to sustain performance. Unfortunately, when working in a warm or hot environment, the cardiovascular system has an additional, and sometimes competing, function: to pump blood to the skin for cooling. Blood cannot go both places at once, so the cardiovascular system makes an adjustment: It decreases the amount of blood returned to the heart (because so much is shunted to the skin and the muscles). As you might imagine, with less blood available per stroke (called the stroke volume), the heart will have to beat more frequently. This adjustment in the heart rate is usually an obvious consequence of exercise, but the increase in heart rate is even greater during exercise in the heat (see figure 4.2). Unfortunately, there is a limit to the amount of compensation the cardiovascular system can make.

Decreased Energy Levels

As you exercise in the heat, your heart rate increases, as does your need for oxygen. This seems only logical when you realize that the purpose of the blood is to carry oxygen. This increase in the need for oxygen is called oxygen consumption. With the increased oxygen consumption, your muscles use more glycogen and produce more lactate. As glycogen in the muscles is used up and lactic acid builds up, you begin to experience an increased feeling of fatigue. Your energy level is dropping.

Increased Sweating Leading to Decreased Blood Volume

The hypothalamus controls the rate of sweating. As the temperature of the blood rises, the hypothalamus is signaled to start the mechanisms to increase sweating (done through the sympathetic nervous system, see figure 4.3). When working in a hot environment, you can lose more than 1 L of sweat per hour of work per square meter of your body surface. This translates to a loss of 1.5 to 2.5 L of sweat per hour for an average-sized person (110-165 lb [50-75 kg]). At this sweat rate, the person is losing 2% to 4% of her body weight during each hour of work. As fluid (essentially water) is lost from the body, the blood also loses fluid. Since blood is about 80% water, a loss of water in the blood causes a decreased blood volume. Temperature regulation is a critical function for every human being and

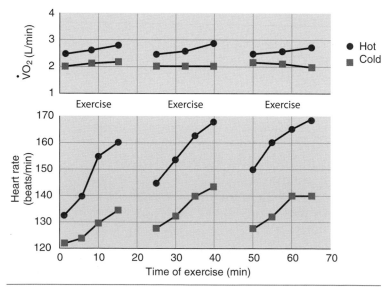

Figure 4.2 Oxygen uptake and heart rate responses during exercise in hot (40° C, 15% humidity) and cold (9° C, 55% humidity) conditions.

With kind permission from Springer Science+Business Media: *European Journal of Applied Physiology*, "Leg muscle metabolism during exercise in the heat and cold," Vol. 34, 1975, pgs. 183-190, W. Fink et al.

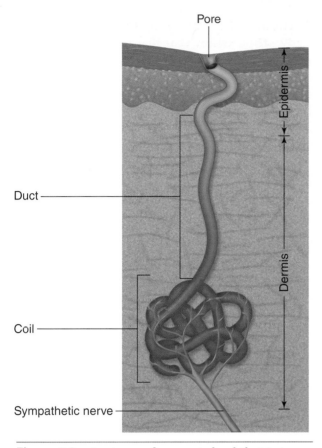

Figure 4.3 Anatomy of a sweat gland that is innervated by a sympathetic nerve.

Adapted, by permission, from L. Kenney, J. Wilmore, and D. Costill, 2011, *Physiology of sport and exercise*, 5th ed. (Champaign, IL: Human Kinetics), 293.

conduction, convection, evaporation, and radiation.

Conduction

Conduction as a method of transfer of heat from the human body to the surrounding environment may take two steps. First there is a transfer of heat from the core of the body to the body surface. We can visualize that mechanism by thinking of blood at normal temperatures. As the blood moves into the muscles, the heat is transferred by conduction from the hot muscle to the blood; thus the temperature of the blood rises. The warmed blood is now taken to the body surface, where the heat is transferred to the skin. Step two in the conduction of heat to the environment is very minimal. As you might surmise, contact between the skin surface and a cooler object must occur in order for heat to be dissipated through conduction. You may observe this scenario readily while watching your dog on a hot summer day. Dogs dig holes in the ground to provide a cooler point of contact; or if in the house, they may lie on a tile floor with all their limbs spread. The animal is attempting to maximize conduction cooling effects. On the other side of the spectrum,

only increases in importance for the physically active individual. Cooling mechanisms, conditioning in the particular environment, and fluid replacement are essential for risk-free physical performance.

Cooling Mechanisms

During exercise, the human body produces heat. This internal heat must be transferred to the environment, or dangerous levels of heat will accumulate inside the body. Under normal conditions, the body is capable of managing this heat, but in extreme conditions, even the best-conditioned participant may be taxed. In the attempt to dissipate heat, the body may utilize one of the four heat transfer methods, shown in figures 4.4:

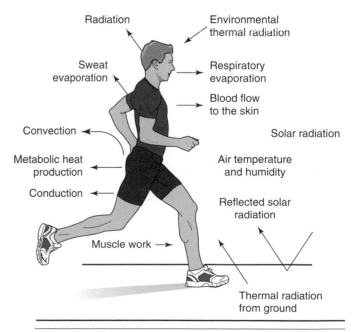

Figure 4.4 Normal methods of heat transfer.

if the air or contact surface is warmer than your skin, the heat will be conducted to your skin, thereby warming it. Heat moves only from the warmer toward the cooler surface or object (second law of thermodynamics).

Convection

Convection is more complex than conduction because it depends on movement of molecules in contact with the body surface. Natural convection occurs when the air that is in direct contact with the body grows warmer (figure 4.5). The warming of the air causes it to expand, and this decreases its density. As the density decreases, the air rises and is replaced by unwarmed, cooler air, and the process starts again. Forced convection occurs not from a difference in temperature but from a difference in external pressure exerted on the air as it flows past the body. If an individual is outside on a hot day with a breeze, the air movement past the body allows forced convection to occur, and the air in the personal air space is warmed and pushed on, replaced by new air to be warmed. On a very windy day, the cooling by convection occurs in the same way, but the efficiency of cooling does not increase.

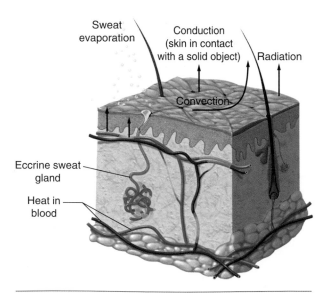

Figure 4.5 Convection.

Reprinted, by permission, from L. Kenney, J. Wilmore, and D. Costill, 2011, *Physiology of sport and exercise*, 5th ed. (Champaign, IL: Human Kinetics), 285.

Without wind, convective heat loss practically stops when you are not moving. It is important to realize that the dissipation of heat by convection is often combined with the effects of evaporation and really cannot be viewed by itself when the person is exercising in a natural environment. In fact, in the exercising person, convection makes an extremely small contribution to the total heat loss.

Evaporation

Evaporation occurs between the skin and the environment as well as between the respiratory tract and the outside environment. The loss of heat from evaporation is our major method of dissipating core temperature to the surrounding environment. We are often quite cognizant of the moisture on our skin after exertion, or even after a shower. How quickly the skin dries is proportional to the rate of evaporation and in turn related to heat being transferred to the environment or the amount of cooling effect. When we are in a very humid climate, we may notice that this dampness on our skin lasts longer. The dampness occurs because the rate of evaporation is low. The vapor pressure (the partial pressure of water vapor in the air) and the air temperature are important factors for understanding how much evaporation is possible. When working with the physically active, one should always consider temperature and humidity and how they relate to the body's heat-response mechanisms. If the air is saturated (high humidity), the body no longer effectively cools by evaporation.

Radiation

Thermal radiation is the exchange of heat energy by electromagnetic waves, a process that occurs at the speed of light. The proportion of the total body heat loss by radiation depends on the temperature difference between the body surface and the environment, but also on the effective radiating area. Some areas of the body, the underarms and the digital web spaces, radiate to other body surfaces and do not contribute to overall heat loss. In a fully extended position, only about 75% of the total body surface is available for radiation. Radiation, in the true sense of the term, requires a very wide difference between the temperature of the object (individual) and that of the environment. Radiation can actually cause absorption of heat from the environment rather than dissipating body heat to the environment. For example, if someone exercises in direct sunlight, significant heat may be transferred to the body.

Adapting to Environmental Heat

In addition to a person's cooling mechanisms, other factors contribute to the body's ability to adjust to exercise in the hot environment: **acclimatization** and hydration. When people pay close attention to preventive measures, prevention of heat illness seems simple (see the sidebar Steps to Remember When Adjusting to a Hot Environment).

Acclimatization

People can gradually adapt to a temperature difference by planning the training program so that their body has the opportunity to adapt to the heat and humidity that are present as the training intensity increases; this is called acclimatization. Without time to acclimatize, a sudden increase in exercise intensity at the same time as a sudden change in environmental conditions could prove too much for the body to handle, resulting in some form of heat illness.

As one might guess, when the air temperature is near or above the body's temperature, cooling is required or performance will deteriorate. Cooling of the exercising body is achieved by various means, depending on the level of activity and the environmental humidity. If the air temperature is above body temperature, cooling through conduction or convection is not possible; the body must depend solely on evaporative cooling. Environmental humidity reduces the ability of the body to cool by the evaporative

STEPS TO REMEMBER WHEN ADJUSTING TO A HOT ENVIRONMENT

- If the temperature is 80° to 90° F and the humidity is less than 70%, just monitor individuals prone to heat illness.
- If the temperature is 80° to 90° F and the humidity is greater than 70%, include a 10-min rest every hour. Have participants change wet clothes frequently.
- If the temperature is 90° to 100° F and the humidity is less than 70%, have a 10-min rest every hour. Have participants change wet clothes frequently.
- If the temperature is 90° to 100° F and the humidity is greater than 70%, schedule short practices in the evenings or early morning. Require only T-shirts and shorts.

Time Considerations

- Acclimatization usually takes 2 to 3 weeks.
- Exercise in the early morning and late evening for the first week.
- Work your way gradually toward midday exercise.
- On very hot or on hot and humid days, exercise early and late in the day only.

Fluid Intake

- Drink at least 3 L of water every day.
- Drink .25 L of cold water every 15 min during intense exercise.

mechanism, and core temperature may reach dangerous levels. Fortunately, adaptation of the human body can occur when the individual is given sufficient time to adjust to exercise in a hot or humid climate or in one that is both hot and humid.

High school and college athletic conferences impose regulations on football teams to allow the participants to adjust to exercise in the particular climate before participating in full football attire. The addition of the heavy pads required in football and other contact sports further reduces the body's ability to dissipate heat.

Different geographic locations throughout the world present specific challenges. Unless you train in the same environmental conditions as those you expect to perform in, serious thermoregulatory difficulties could be associated with strenuous exercise. A college-bound student who lives in a cool climate will find football practice much more difficult if he moves to a hot climate and begins working out in 100° temperatures. This difference in climates will be even greater should the player move to campus during a very humid period of the summer.

Hydration

One method of decreasing the risk of problems from the heat is to keep the participants well hydrated. Exercise accelerates the body's loss of water, making rehydration essential. Coaches must be cooperative in allowing participants to take frequent drinks of water during activity. Participants should be educated regarding the need for water and should be encouraged to drink often during practices and games. People can avoid the feeling of being waterlogged by taking more frequent, small drinks of water rather than less frequent breaks during which they gulp down large quantities. We must remember that the feeling of thirst is not a good indication of the body's need for fluid. Usually, thirst is perceived long after the need for water occurs. Generally, a person does not rehydrate to the full extent needed by the body; thus it is necessary to make a con-

scious effort to hydrate even when thirst is not perceived.

Maintaining Body Fluids

An ideal plan for fluid replacement would allow water (or electrolyte drink) consumption at convenient stopping points during drills and scrimmage. A plan for a basketball practice, as seen in figure 4.6, would position fluid-replacement stations at center court on each side of the gymnasium floor, as well as one station located under one of the basketball goals at a sufficient distance to ensure safety for any participating team members. This plan allows players who are waiting their turn in drills (at the end line) to consume additional fluids; it also provides central locations for fluid replacement for players during periodic breaks, as well as for substitutes during scrimmage sessions.

Team policies should be established regarding the frequency and length of rest breaks during practices in high heat and

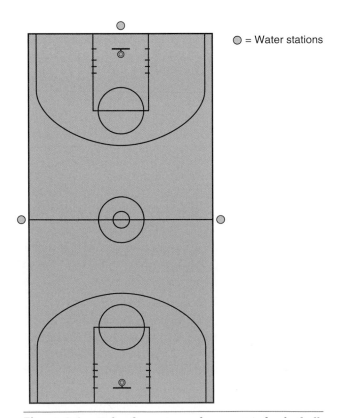

= Water stations

Figure 4.6 A plan for water replacement in basketball.

humidity. Rest breaks should allow time for the individuals to sit down, preferably in a cool location (or if outdoors, in a shaded area), and to consume several cups of water or electrolyte drink or both. Some teams use other methods of cooling the participants, including water misters for increased cooling via evaporation and cooling vests that the individuals may don to help with conductive cooling.

Monitoring Hydration by Weight

Hydration status can be monitored, although roughly, by doing something as simple as recording the individual's body weight. Weight should be taken and recorded before exercise and then after exercise, with the participant wearing the same clothes both times. The process is easier if participants weigh in street clothes before changing into the exercise gear. After they have showered and put on their street clothes, they weigh again. When practice occurs twice in a day, the weight lost during the first practice should be replaced before the second workout begins. The rapid loss of body weight is almost exclusively water loss, which can have a serious effect on the individual's ability to adapt to the heat during exercise. A very small amount (1-2%) of dehydration can compromise performance, and weight loss of more than 3% puts the exercising individual at a much greater risk of heat illness.

An athletic trainer is usually able to observe many participants during practices and workouts. Athletic trainers may spot various warning signs that heat illness is imminent. Individuals who carry extra weight are more prone to heat-related problems than are thinner individuals; extremely hardworking individuals who hustle on every play may experience heat problems more quickly than others; and people who just don't like to drink water during a workout are often the first to experience the initial signs of heat illness—heat cramps. (Realize, however, that an exercising individual will not always have heat cramps first; he may progress directly to more serious forms of heat illness.) Watching each of these types of participants, monitor-

ing their fluid replacement by checking their body weight each practice, and urging them to drink cool sips of water on a frequent basis will aid in the prevention of heat problems. The National Athletic Trainers' Association (NATA) has published a position statement on the prevention of dehydration in the active individual, and your plan should be established on the basis of this information.

Monitoring Hydration Status by Urine Color

The National Research Council's fluid recommendations are individualized based on how many calories are burned each day. Adult women, who may expend 1,600 to 2,200 calories each day, need 6 1/2 to 9 cups of fluid; men, who often need 2,200 to 2,800 calories each day, are advised to drink 9 to 12 cups. To make things a little simpler, studies show that adequate fluid consumption is indicated by pale yellow or straw-colored urine whereas dark urine suggests dehydration.

Heat Illness

As already outlined, human heat is lost in four ways: conduction, radiation, convection, and evaporation. Conduction, or heat loss through direct contact with something cooler than you, does not help much on a hot day. On a very hot afternoon, you may actually take in heat from a hot environment through radiation. Convection is heat loss through the movement of air around your body. Without wind, convective heat loss practically stops when you are not moving. That leaves evaporation, the vaporization of sweat from the skin, as the primary source of heat loss. As your skin heats up, pores dilate and sweat floods out. Evaporation of the sweat cools your skin; heat is drawn from your blood near the surface of your body; and the cooler blood circulates to keep the body's core maintained at an acceptable temperature. Sweat comes from your circulatory system, and it is not uncommon to sweat out a liter of water in an hour during periods of exercise in a hot environment. This water loss may reach 2.5 L/h with prolonged exercise. Sweat contains salt, a critical component of normal body function. It is this—the combined water and electrolyte depletion—that forms the basis of a spectrum of problems with one general name: heat illness.

Heat Syncope and Exertional Hypotension

A decrease in blood pressure can cause fainting. Two main situations in which an individual may faint due to exercise or heat are heat syncope and exertional hypotension. Heat **syncope** occurs when the blood volume decreases and the body is unable to pump sufficient blood to the brain. The brain wants oxygen, and without blood flow it cannot get what is needed and the individual will collapse or faint. The collapse allows the brain to receive more blood since the heart is now at the same level as the brain. Blood volume must be restored as soon as possible.

The second cause of fainting is exertional **hypotension**. This most often occurs when the individual is exercising the large muscle groups in the legs and suddenly stops. The exercising muscles are engorged with blood, and without the pumping action of the leg muscles, the blood pools in the extremities. This in turn causes a decreased blood flow to the brain; and, again, the body collapses to bring the brain to the same level as the heart. This scenario is often seen at the finish line of a long race. The individual finishes the race, comes to a stop in the finish area, and shortly thereafter collapses. Frequently this collapse is thought to be due to heat illness whereas in fact the victim's body fluid levels and core temperature are within safe limits.

Heat Cramps

When we exercise, if the body heat production becomes greater than body heat loss, we are heading toward heat illness. One of the harmful effects of exercise and heat is painful spasm of major muscles that are being exercised, called heat cramps. Those who experience cramps are most often people unaccli-

matized to heat who are sweating profusely. Heat cramps are poorly understood; but they probably result not only from the water lost in sweat, but also from the imbalance between sodium (salt) and potassium once the level of body fluids decreases. That is, as the body's internal water level decreases, the concentrations of sodium and potassium increase, and small imbalances create much bigger problems. Gentle massage of the cramping muscles may provide some relief from the pain associated with the spasm and may even be enough to induce muscle relaxation, especially when combined with gentle stretching of the involved muscle. Drinking water is critical during this time of heat cramps. Heat cramps do not often occur in someone who is adequately hydrated. Once the pain and spasm are gone, exercise may be continued if necessary, but rest is better. Often people experiencing heat cramps rest just long enough to allow the symptoms to abate; as soon as they return to play, the heat cramps also return.

Heat Exhaustion

Prolonged sweating, without proper rehydration, can decrease the body's ability to dissipate heat. A buildup of body heat can lead to **heat exhaustion**, a condition characterized by headache, dizziness, nausea, rapid breathing, and, of course, exhaustion (see figure 4.7). People experiencing heat exhaustion are so sweaty that often they feel cool; they

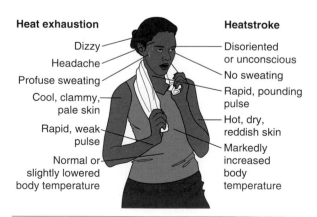

Figure 4.7 Heatstroke versus heat exhaustion.

may have goose bumps and often complain of chills. Treatment should include moving the exhausted person to a shady spot if outdoors, or to a cooler location indoors, and giving the individual fluids. Some experts prefer using an electrolyte-balanced drink, but the drink should be watered down three or four times for more rapid absorption in an exercising person. Maximum absorption ranges from 150 to 250 ml/15 min, so it takes about an hour to get a liter of fluid back into circulation. Heat exhaustion is not physiologically damaging, but it should be treated aggressively and signs and symptoms monitored to protect the individual from core temperature rise.

Heatstroke

The most serious of heat-related illnesses is **heatstroke**, a problem that kills approximately 4,000 people in the United States every year. Heatstroke occurs when the body's thermoregulatory system stops working. Many of the symptoms of heatstroke are the same as for heat exhaustion. However, other indications of heatstroke are cessation of sweating, disorientation, and fainting or unconsciousness. Individuals experiencing heatstroke may be too disoriented to help themselves (see figure 4.7). There are two varieties of heatstroke: typical heatstroke and exertional heatstroke.

Typical Heatstroke

In typical heatstroke, the patient is usually elderly or sick, or both. Usually, environmental temperature and humidity have been high for several days, and people become dehydrated to the point where their heat-loss mechanisms are overwhelmed. It is as if they have run out of sweat; the skin gets hot, red, and dry. They lapse into a coma and, if untreated, usually die.

Exertional Heatstroke

More and more people are succumbing to the second variety of heatstroke, exertional heatstroke. The person is usually young, fit, and unaccustomed to the heat. This patient is actively sweating but is producing heat faster than it can be dissipated. Signs include, primarily, a sudden and very noticeable alteration in normal mental function: disorientation, irritability, combativeness, bizarre delusions, and incoherent speech. The skin is hot and red but may be quite wet with sweat. Rapid breathing and rapid heart rates are often observed. Collapse is imminent. Quick cooling may be required to save this person's life; the best method includes submerging the individual in an ice bath. If total body submersion is not possible, removal of heavy clothing and covering the person with wet cloths, placing ice packs near major arteries (such as those in the neck, groin, and axilla), and vigorous fanning will help to increase evaporative heat loss. A physician should see anyone who has experienced heatstroke as soon as possible, even if the person seems to have recovered. Too much internal heat can cause breakdowns in some body systems that show up later.

It is important to thoroughly evaluate the individual suspected to have a heat illness. Core temperature is the only true measure of the extent of internal body heat and should be used as an emergency evaluation measure. This core temperature is best taken using a rectal thermometer, since other measurements of body temperature fail to adequately reflect the temperature of the body's core (Binkley et al. 2002, p. 334). Frequent questioning of the individual to assess the level of consciousness and mental status is very important.

Factors Contributing to Heat Illness

It is always important to be familiar with factors that could predispose the physically active person to heat illness. When any one of these factors is combined with another, the risk of heat injury increases dramatically. Care must be taken to avoid heat stress when someone with a risk factor is exercising in a hot environment (see the sidebar Factors Contributing to the Risk of Heat Illness). It is important to recognize and understand any

FACTORS CONTRIBUTING TO THE RISK OF HEAT ILLNESS

Avoidable
- Dehydration
- Lack of acclimatization
- Alcohol use
- Inappropriate clothing

Possibly Avoidable
- Drug use such as amphetamines, phenothiazines, and anticholinergics
- Prolonged or excessive exercise (increased exercise demands)

Unavoidable
- Cardiovascular disease
- Sweat gland dysfunction

STEPS TO TAKE WHEN EXERCISING IN A HOT ENVIRONMENT

- Wear loose-fitting, lightweight clothing.
- Avoid headwear or remove it frequently for cooling.
- Take frequent rest breaks to drink fluids.
- Drink abundant fluids prior to, during, and after the workout.
- Avoid overheating if you are taking drugs that impair heat regulation or if you have a fever.

limitations so that one can make appropriate adjustments in the exercise routine.

Prevention of Heat-Related Illness

Heat illnesses can be preventable, but we must take the necessary steps. Children, the elderly, and those who are obese are particularly at risk of developing heat illness. However, even individuals in superb physical condition can succumb to heat illness if they ignore the warning signs.

Several preventive measures can be taken to avoid problems due to heat illness: monitoring environmental conditions and adjusting practice sessions; monitoring individuals' weight loss and replacement between practices; and promoting good hydration habits in participants. In addition, acclimatization must take place before the start of competitive drills and practices. If an individual fails to acclimatize prior to the season, risks of heat illness can be much greater. Educating

people regarding simple steps for exercising in the heat can help prevent heat problems (see the sidebar Steps to Take When Exercising in a Hot Environment). The athletic trainer and coach must pay close attention to individuals who have moved from another climate, those who tend to sweat excessively, and those who have been ill or for any reason are not eating well. Understanding the individual's limitations is more important than the practice, test, or drill on any given day. Although you may understand this concept, it is equally important for you to help the participant understand and agree with it.

Monitoring Environmental Conditions

Taking temperature and humidity readings using a **sling psychrometer** or other heat and humidity device is an important procedure that should be conducted prior to every practice and contest for which there is the potential of temperature or humidity extremes. Taking the readings at the location of the contest is better than assuming that conditions there are the same as at the local weather station, airport, or other weather-forecasting facility. Use web sources of heat and humidity readings only after you establish the validity and reliability of those data in comparison to the data collected on the field. Only after determining the validity of web data should you assume that this is a good source for field conditions. Always be aware of special circumstances affecting the field, such as irrigation of the field itself or surrounding areas and local weather patterns. It is wise to fully understand the environmental conditions under which you are participating.

Heat Index

Physically active people sometimes wish to exercise in an area of the country they are visiting. Since they probably do not have access to a sling psychrometer, they can use local weather data to find out about the local heat and humidity. The **heat index** table (table 4.1) shows how the temperature and dew point combine to produce the heat index value. Exercisers can use the heat index to determine adjustments for workout plans. When heat index reports are 95° to 105°, people fatigue more quickly while exercising and are more susceptible to heat cramps and

heat exhaustion. Above 105°, there is a risk of heatstroke with prolonged activity, warranting appropriate modification of activity. In general, the higher the heat index, the less efficient evaporative cooling is. Whenever possible, practices should be scheduled during cooler times of the day. If a scheduled practice must occur in high heat or humidity, it is wise to provide frequent fluid breaks during which individuals can take several (5-10) minutes' rest in a shaded area.

Local Relative Humidity Readings

Although not recommended if more accurate measurements are available, another method of determining the effect of the hot environment on exercise is to use local relative humidity readings (figure 4.8). Exercise should be modified when the apparent temperature becomes higher, especially if the person is unconditioned or unacclimatized (see table 4.2). Table 4.3 gives apparent temperature (another form of the heat index chart) based on a combination of heat and humidity measures.

Table 4.1 Heat Index Table

Temperature (°F)	Dew point (°F)							
	50	55	60	65	70	75	80	85
65	60.8	62.0	63.3	64.8				
70	70.5	71.4	72.5	73.8	75.3			
75	75.7	76.3	76.8	77.2	77.8	79.3		
80	78.3	79.2	80.2	81.4	83.0	85.5	89.5	
85	82.0	83.2	84.7	86.6	89.1	92.5	97.6	105.2
90	86.5	87.9	89.8	92.2	95.4	99.8	105.8	114.2
95	91.4	93.1	95.3	98.1	101.9	107.0	113.7	112.9
100	96.6	98.5	101.0	104.2	108.4	113.9	121.2	130.9
105	101.9	104.0	106.7	110.2	114.7	120.6	128.3	138.0
110	107.2	109.5	112.4	116.1	120.9	127.0	134.9	145.1
115	112.4	114.8	117.9	121.8	126.8	133.1	141.2	151.4
120	117.4	120.0	123.2	127.3	132.4	138.9	147.0	157.3

Air Temperature and Dew Point = Heat Index

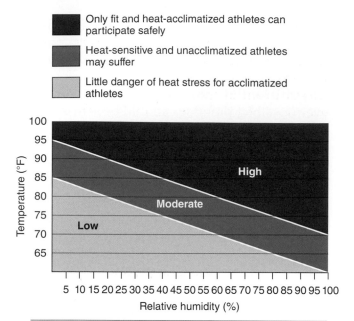

- ■ Only fit and heat-acclimatized athletes can participate safely
- ■ Heat-sensitive and unacclimatized athletes may suffer
- □ Little danger of heat stress for acclimatized athletes

Figure 4.8 Temperature–humidity activity index.

Reprinted from NCAA, 1999, *NCAA guideline 2C: Prevention of heat illnesses* (Indianapolis, IN: NCAA), 30.

Monitoring Participant's Weight Loss

Weight is a commonly used measure of an individual's hydration. It is easy to monitor a participant's weight by weighing her prior to and following each practice. Obviously, the weight should be taken with the individual in the same type of clothing at both weighing sessions. Weight lost during a practice should be replaced prior to the next participation session. If an individual fails to replace the weight lost by the time of weigh-in before the next session, caution is necessary. This ranges from merely providing additional fluids during the practice session to reducing the length of the practice session should the individual show any signs of heat difficulties (cramps, confusion, and so on).

Table 4.2 Suggested Exercise Adjustments Relative to Apparent Temperature Levels

Apparent temperature	Exercise plan
Below 90° F	No need to modify activity plan.
91-104° F	Increase fluid and rest breaks. Monitor participants for heat cramps and signs of heat exhaustion.
105-129° F	Decrease exercise intensity unless participants are well acclimatized. Be aware of danger signs.
130° F and up	Change time of practice or intensity of workout. Have people exercise with caution. High risk of heat illness exists.

Table 4.3 Apparent Temperature Calculations

Relative humidity (percent)	Air temperature (°F)							
	75	80	85	90	95	100	105	110
0	69	73	78	83	87	91	95	99
10	70	75	80	85	90	95	100	105
20	72	77	82	87	93	99	105	112
30	73	78	84	90	96	104	113	123
40	74	79	86	93	101	110	123	137
50	75	81	88	96	107	120	135	150
60	76	82	90	100	114	132	149	
70	77	85	93	106	124	144		
80	78	86	97	113	136			
90	79	88	102	122				
100	80	91	108					

Find the air temperature (°F) across the top of the chart; then read down the column until you find the row of the relative humidity reading (to the nearest 10%). That number is the apparent temperature.

Promoting Good Hydration Habits

Hydration is an extremely important aspect of preventing heat illness but also of general good nutrition. Many options exist regarding the "best" fluid: water or sport drink. The question then is, if a sport drink, which one? Water is an excellent source of fluid replacement, yet when the body is depleted of sodium and potassium (electrolytes), those too must be replenished. A condition called *hyponatremia* occurs when the level of sodium in the body falls too low. This can actually be a result of replenishing fluids with water only, especially if the individual is on a low-sodium diet.

Sport drinks are the common choice of active individuals concerned with fluids and electrolyte replacement. Choosing between the various sport drinks is quite difficult. Two important factors to consider are carbohydrate (CHO) and sodium concentrations of the beverage. According to the NATA position statement on fluid replacement in athletics, "Consuming CHOs during the pre-exercise hydration session (2 to 3 hours pre-exercise), along with a normal daily diet, increases glycogen stores. If exercise is intense, then consuming CHOs about 30 minutes pre-exercise may also be beneficial. Include CHOs in the rehydration beverage during exercise if the session lasts longer than 45 to 50 minutes or is intense. An ingestion rate of about 1 g/min (0.04 oz/min) maintains optimal carbohydrate metabolism: for example, 1 L of a 6% CHO drink per hour of exercise. CHO concentrations greater than 8% increase the rate of CHO delivery to the body but compromise the rate of fluid emptying from the stomach and absorbed from the intestine" (Casa et al. 2000, p. 213).

Although the sodium in the sport drink is not required in most sporting events, the addition of the sodium makes the drink taste much better. Individuals often admit that they would drink more if the fluid tasted good. Part of the battle of hydration is finding a fluid that the participant likes and thus will drink enough of.

To further understand the differences among sport drinks, one would merely need to calculate the content of CHO by dividing the total CHO by the volume of fluid (converted to milliliters, which is equivalent to grams). The following are three of the more popular sport drinks, listed with their CHO content:

Allsport	8% CHO (20 g CHO in 240 ml)
Gatorade	6% CHO (14 g CHO in 240 ml)
Powerade	8% CHO (19 g CHO in 240 ml)

Caring for Heat Illness

Most people think that it is normal to experience some level of discomfort as exercise intensity increases. People may not recognize the degree of this discomfort until they can push no more and some form of heat illness compromises the body. It is essential that everyone working with physically active individuals understand the symptoms associated with heat illness so that proper measures may be taken (see the sidebar Dos and Don'ts of Caring for Heat Illness). Always remember that heat continues to build up and that in the absence of the proper measures, conditions can quickly move from minor to more and more severe.

Heat Cramps

The initial sign of heat illness is often heat cramps. These cramps are difficult to ignore. Often the person experiences such severe cramping that any muscle activity causes another muscle group to go into spasm. A severe cramp in a muscle may actually damage some of the muscle fibers, producing soreness in the muscle(s) that may last for days. Heat cramps are often a sign of excessive exposure to a hot environment and may signal that other more serious problems are to follow if proper care is not forthcoming. The cramps typically related to heat exposure involve the legs and the abdomen. Sometimes people continue to practice despite feeling tightness and cramping in the legs. They

DOS AND DON'TS OF CARING FOR HEAT ILLNESS

What to Do

- Get the victim out of the heat and have him lie down in a cool place with feet elevated about 12 in. (30 cm).
- Apply cool, wet cloths (or cool water directly) to the skin; use a fan to lower temperature. Place cold compresses on the victim's neck, groin, and armpits. Submerge victim in a cool pool of water if available.
- Give the victim sport beverages or cool to cold water to sip. Give a half cup every 15 min.
- For muscle cramps, massage affected muscles gently but firmly until they relax. But do not withhold rehydration to provide massage.
- If the victim shows signs of shock (bluish lips and fingernails and decreased alertness), administer first aid for shock. If the victim starts having seizures, protect him from injury and give convulsion first aid.
- If the person loses consciousness, apply first aid for unconsciousness.
- For serious heat illness, keep the person cool until you get medical help.

What Not to Do

- Do not underestimate the seriousness of heat illness, especially if the person is a child, is elderly, or is injured.
- Do not give the person medications that are used to treat fever (such as aspirin). They will not help, and they may be harmful.
- Do not give salt tablets.
- Do not overlook possible complications resulting from the person's other medical problems (such as high blood pressure).
- Do not give liquids that contain alcohol or caffeine. They will interfere with the body's ability to control its internal temperature.
- Do not hesitate to get medical assistance.

may not think that the feeling is anything serious and may dismiss it as just fatigue. The cramps may intensify by the time the individual returns to the locker room, or even as the person sits in an air-conditioned room or automobile.

It is important to render care as soon as muscle cramps are detected. Since people who are cramping are usually suffering from a low fluid level in the body, they need to ingest water and electrolyte replacements, if available.

Mild stretching of the cramping muscles may help relieve the spasm and associated pain. In some cases the cramping is so severe that most of the major muscles become involved. In this situation people may be so dehydrated that it is not possible to provide the fluids quickly enough through the gastrointestinal tract (oral consumption). Sometimes a trained medical professional decides to provide intravenous fluids to help rehydrate the person's body more quickly. Usually, given appropriate care, the cramping muscles relax; but with a severe case of heat cramps, the likelihood of soreness the next day is very high.

Heat Exhaustion

The individual may enter into more serious stages of heat illness with few outward signs of trouble. Heat exhaustion can occur in anyone working or exercising in a hot, humid environment. Warning signs of heat exhaustion include heavy sweating, paleness, muscle cramps, tiredness, weakness, dizziness, headache, nausea or vomiting, and

SYMPTOMS OF HEAT EXHAUSTION

Late Symptoms

Cool, moist skin

Dilated pupils

Headache

Irrational behavior

Pale skin

Nausea and vomiting

Unconsciousness

Early Symptoms

Dizziness

Fatigue

Muscle cramps

Nausea

Profuse sweating

Thirst

Weakness and light-headedness

If a person faints or becomes unconscious, you will not be able to get him to drink and must get medical help. To get more oxygen to the brain, you'll want to increase the blood available to the head. Elevation of the feet will help to get the blood from the extremities back to the heart for pumping up to the head. Remember: This problem may become worse in the absence of proper care.

Heatstroke

Heatstroke occurs when the signs of heat exhaustion are ignored. Heat overwhelms the body, and the internal systems stop functioning. Heatstroke is life threatening, and one can usually recognize it by the presence of significant symptoms such as those listed here. The extreme confusion and hot skin call attention to the presence of heatstroke. Skin moisture (sweating) is the significant difference between typical and exertional heatstroke: Typical heatstroke means that the person ran out of water and can't cool herself, whereas people experiencing exertional heatstroke have enough water to allow them to sweat but not enough to keep up with the amount of heat they are producing. Don't be confused if you find all the signs of heatstroke in a healthy individual but see that the skin is wet with perspiration. That just may be exertional heatstroke. If you feel you may be prone to errors in judgment in cases of heat illness, it is best to err on the side of caution.

Although heatstroke is less common than other heat illnesses, it is a medical emergency. Proper care of an affected patient involves immediate cooling and transport to a hospital or other emergency care facility. Send someone for help while you get the person into a cold pool or at least a shady area and provide external cooling. Fan the person with cool air; use wet, cool sponges to keep the skin moist; apply cool, wet towels to the major arteries (groin, armpits, neck). Do whatever you can to provide cool airflow over the damp skin to help the person dissipate heat. Because of the decreasing level of consciousness, making the person drink

fainting (see the sidebar Symptoms of Heat Exhaustion). The skin may be cool and moist. The person's pulse rate is fast and weak, and breathing is fast and shallow. If heat exhaustion is untreated, it may progress to heatstroke. You should get the person medical attention immediately if symptoms are severe or if she has heart problems or high blood pressure.

Immediately, the individual needs cooling since the body is not doing a good enough job. The most immediate way to obtain massive body cooling is to submerge the individual in a cold pool of water. If that is not available, get the patient into a cool area, loosen clothing, and allow the skin to be exposed to the cool air. Packing ice in the groin area and axilla can help in the cooling effort. You may help cool the body by fanning, or you may want to wipe the person's body with a cool cloth. Just as with the person who is having heat cramps, anyone experiencing heat exhaustion needs fluid replacement.

is usually not possible. Monitoring the vital signs is important to provide assurance that the airway remains open and the heart continues pumping. This information, as well as knowing the oral temperature, can be a great help to the medical specialists who will assist with the care of the patient in the ambulance and at the hospital or clinic. Additionally, blood pressure should be monitored, and if possible a comparison of blood pressure in supine versus pressure taken immediately upon standing should be recorded. This comparison of blood pressures allows one to see if the pressure is lower in standing than in supine. This drop in pressure is termed *orthostatic hypotension* and may indicate dehydration.

Ultimately all physically active individuals must take responsibility for their own health and safety, because someone else may not always be around during workouts. The individual, the coach, and parents should be educated about the warning signs of heat stress and taught to take prudent and wise steps

to avoid serious problems. Adapting to new or changed environmental temperatures, adjusting the length or intensity of workouts, taking a cooler of water to the workout site, and drinking frequently are all essential practices. For monitoring hydration status, it is important to encourage participants to weigh before and after every workout as well as to be observant of the color of the urine. Physically active individuals must develop a healthy habit of hydrating before, during, and after every workout.

Cold Environments

Although exercise in the cold is not as detrimental to the physiology of the human body as extreme heat can be, cold environments do create performance issues. Exercise in air temperatures below 60° F may lengthen reaction time and reduce manual dexterity and tactile sensitivity. Usually, people who participate in activities in a cold environment

DRESSING FOR COLD ENVIRONMENTS

Selecting clothing and dressing for activity in cold environments should conform to the following guidelines:

- Layer clothing; use several thin layers rather than a single heavy garment. As body heat is generated, layers can be shed.
- Cover the head when outside in cold, damp weather. Use a headband over the ears or a stocking cap if possible. If in a damp environment, the headwear should be water repellant.
- Protect the hands. Use specially designed gloves for the activity. Use insulated gloves if they do not interfere with dexterity.
- Prepare for the rain. Rain capes should be available for participants.

- Stay dry, as water increases body heat loss. Use a vapor barrier next to the skin or a material that will wick moisture away from the skin surface. Cotton does not wick.
- Stay hydrated. Dehydration alters the body's ability to regulate heat.
- Warm up thoroughly. Generate body heat through muscle activity before and throughout the activity period. Stay warm even after the activity, and cool down gradually once finished with the activity.
- Warm incoming air. Use a scarf over the nose and mouth to help prevent bronchospasm from exposure of the airways to severe cold.

dress to retain body heat production and thus reduce the ill effects of low temperatures. (See the sidebar Dressing for Cold Environments for more information on this topic.) The body's natural heat production through muscle activity, as well as sympathetic nervous system activation, is supplemented by the added insulation of clothing (see figure 4.9).

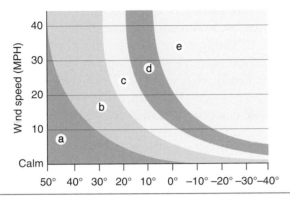

Figure 4.9 Ambient temperatures: *(a)* comfortable—requires normal precautions; *(b)* very cold—travel becomes uncomfortable; *(c)* bitterly cold—travel becomes uncomfortable even on clear, sunny days; *(d)* freezing of human flesh begins, depending upon degree of activity, amount of solar radiation, and character of skin and circulation; *(e)* survival efforts are required. Exposed flesh will freeze in less than 1 min.

Reprinted, by permission, from NCAA, 1999, *NCAA guideline 2C: Cold stress* (Indianapolis, IN: NCAA), 27.

Hypothermia

Hypothermia occurs when the core temperature gets too low. Factors that increase the ill effects of cold include the patient's age, the patient's medical condition, and the ingestion of drugs or poisons. Wet conditions intensify the effects of cold. This is not the dampness from normal sweating during exercise, but a situation in which the participant's shoes are soaked from the moisture on the ground and from water spilled when taking drinks. The wet shoes and cold exposure can increase the likelihood of a local cold injury.

Hypothermia can be local or general, mild or severe. The patient's core temperature drops to between 90° and 95° (normal core temperature is 98.6°). This patient is alert, is shivering, and is maybe moving around in an attempt to produce heat. The key to knowing that the individual is experiencing mild hypothermia and not just feeling cold is increased heart rate and respiration.

The skin is typically red but progresses to cyanotic (showing blueness of the lips and under the nails). As the core temperature drops lower than 90°, the shivering stops and muscle activity decreases. Small muscles of the fingers stop first, and as the core temperature falls more, all muscle activity stops. As the core temperature reaches 85°, the patient becomes lethargic and uncoordinated, and mental functions become disturbed.

Other Cold-Related Injuries

Cold-related injuries usually affect the extremities, especially the nose and ears, the hands, and the feet and toes. The factors that influence the severity of cold injury include length of exposure time, the combination of temperature and wind effects, previous cold injury, impaired circulation, and wet garments.

In most sporting events, participants have sufficient time to cover exposed fingers between plays or series. Rewarming the hands in gloves or with the use of commercial hand warmers is usually sufficient to prevent frostbite; however, recognition of the condition is important for times when prevention has been inadequate. The signs of frostbite are hard, pale, and cold skin and a reduction in tactile sensation. People with atherosclerosis or those taking beta-blocker drugs are particularly susceptible to frostbite because of the decrease in the flow of blood to the skin.

In superficial cold injuries, the affected skin becomes pale (blanches), and normal color fails to return when the skin is palpated. The patient may experience a loss of feeling and sensation, and during rewarming may feel tingling of the affected part.

Deep cold injury, which is much more serious, occurs when tissues are actually frozen. Less severe deep cold injury is called frostbite. In frostbite, the exposed part is damaged but not as severely. Following frostbite, the skin may remain red, tender, and very sensitive to the cold. Deep cold injuries are rare in athletics and should be easy to prevent. Remember, human tissue damages very easily when cold, so take extreme care when touching cold or frostbitten areas of the body.

Windchill

It is necessary to monitor all exposure to cold and to take precautions to avoid cold injury. With good common sense and wise selection of athletic apparel, cold injury should be preventable.

When people engage in sport in very cold environments, the wind may present an even greater risk for hypothermia. Figure 4.10 depicts the **windchill** equivalent tempera-

ture, a relative temperature associated with wind in cold environments. To read the chart, you need to know the wind speed (obtained from the local radio station, weather bureau, or airport) and the air temperature. Read down the left margin for the wind speed and then across the top for the air temperature. Notice that the chart uses the metric scales, so if you know only the Fahrenheit temperature, subtract 32 from the degrees F and then divide that answer by 9. Next, multiply that answer by 5. A temperature of 4° F is about –15° C; thus, according to the chart, if the air temperature is –15° C and the wind speed is 30 km/h, the windchill equivalent temperature is –26° F and freezing is likely when exposure exceeds 30 min. Wind increases the cooling effect of the temperature and can make a cool day feel quite cold.

Wind speed (km/h)	Air temperature (°C)								
	−10	−15	−20	−25	−30	−35	−40	−45	−50
5	−13	−19	−24	−30	−36	−41	−47	−53	−58
10	−15	−21	−27	−33	−39	−45	−51	−57	−63
15	−17	−23	−29	−35	−41	−48	−54	−60	−66
20	−18	−24	−30	−37	−43	−49	−56	−62	−68
25	−19	−25	−32	−38	−44	−51	−57	−64	−70
30	−20	−26	−33	−39	−46	−52	−59	−65	−72
35	−20	−27	−33	−40	−47	−53	−60	−66	−73
40	−21	−27	−34	−41	−48	−54	−61	−68	−74
45	−21	−28	−35	−42	−48	−55	−62	−69	−75
50	−22	−29	−35	−42	−49	−56	−63	−69	−76
55	−22	−29	−36	−43	−50	−57	−63	−70	−77
60	−23	−30	−36	−43	−50	−57	−64	−71	−78
65	−23	−30	−37	−44	−51	−58	−65	−72	−79
70	−23	−30	−37	−44	−51	−58	−65	−72	−80
75	−24	−31	−38	−45	−52	−59	−66	−73	−80
80	−24	−31	−38	−45	−52	−60	−67	−74	−81

Very low	Freezing is possible, but unlikely		**High**	Freezing risk < 30 min		
Likely	Freezing is likely > 30 min		**Severe**	Freezing risk < 10 min		
			Extreme	Freezing risk < 3 min		

Figure 4.10   Windchill equivalent temperature chart showing various combinations of temperature and wind speed that result in the same cooling power as that seen with no wind. For example, a wind speed of 20 km/h at –10 °C would result in the same heat loss as –30 °C with no wind. Also shown in the figure is the risk of tissues freezing as windchill—the cooling power of the movement—increases.

Other Weather Conditions

Other weather conditions that pose a threat to the health and safety of physically active people include thunderstorms and lightning storms. The blowing, gusting winds of a thunderstorm may injure the eyes if dust or dirt is blown about. Lightning storms are nature's deadliest force and are potentially very dangerous. A summer storm may travel very quickly, placing the entire team at risk of injury in the event of a lightning strike. Tornados are usually born out of severe thunderstorms.

Lightning Strikes

Athletic fields are often very large, open areas where the nearest structures are the light poles or, on an athletic club field, the raised stand for the filming of practice. These tall, typically metal structures are more likely targets for lightning than are many other types of structures; and if a bolt of lightning hits such a structure, the arc of the electricity has the potential to injure anyone nearby. If a thunderstorm is occurring in the area, team camera crew members should be advised to stay off any metal towers. A clap of thunder usually follows the appearance of a lightning bolt. The delay between sight and sound occurs as a result of the speed of light versus the speed of sound. An easy and very practical way to figure out your distance from a lightning bolt is to count the number of seconds (one one thousand, two one thousand . . .) between when you see the lightning bolt and when you hear the clap of thunder. Divide this number by five, and that should tell you approximately how many miles away the storm is.

Depending on the speed with which the storm is traveling and the direction of its movement, the team may need to clear the field. The team should remain under cover until about 30 min have passed without lightning. Teams should develop a policy for postponing practice or games in the event of a lightning storm. The National Lightning Safety Institute has published guidelines regarding safety during a lightning storm (see the sidebar Decision Tree for Personal Lightning Safety). All teams should have a person on the staff responsible for watching any approaching storms and for notifying team members when it is time to take cover. Remember: Electricity can be conducted through metal (think of all the things around the field that are metal, including the pipes for the water!), and the electricity from a bolt of lightning that strikes the ground may travel along those pathways. Also, don't assume that lightning doesn't strike twice in the same place; it does.

Tornados

Other types of foul weather are characteristic of specific areas of the country and particular months of the year. People living in the south-central area of the United States often know the devastation that such violent storms can produce. **Tornados** can be stationary or can travel at speeds of up to 70 mph (113 km/h). Although most tornado damage is caused by the violent winds, most tornado injuries and deaths result from flying debris. Clues that a tornado could develop are a dark, often greenish-looking sky; large hail; and a loud roar similar to the sound of a freight train. No matter what area of the country you live in, there is the potential for severe weather. Know the types of weather that are approaching your area, and pay attention to weather reports and to what you see outside. Be wise when subjecting an entire team to bad weather; it's not just you who will be affected.

Other Environmental Factors Influencing Sport Participation

The word "environment" may create in your mind an image of weather conditions—and that's what we have focused on up to now. True, weather is a component of our environment, and weather conditions have been the cause of athletic-related deaths in the

DECISION TREE FOR PERSONAL LIGHTNING SAFETY

The National Lightning Safety Institute (NLSI) recommends that all organizations prepare a Lightning Safety Plan and inform all personnel of its contents. Briefly, lightning safety involves "anticipating a high-risk situation and moving to a low-risk location." Lightning Safety Plans should be site specific, but they all share a common outline:

1. Advanced warning of the hazard. Some options:

   - "If you can see it, flee it. If you can hear it, clear it."
   - TV Weather Channel; NOAA Weather Radio.
   - Fancy lightning detectors; off-site meteorological services.

2. Make decision to suspend activities and notify people.

   - The 30/30 rule says to shut down when lightning is 6 miles away.
   - Use a "flash to bang" (lightning to thunder) count: Five seconds equals 1 mile (10 = 2 miles; 20 = 4 miles; 30 = 6 miles).
   - Notify people via radio, siren, or other means.

3. Move to safe location.

   - A large permanent building or metal vehicle is best.
   - Unsafe places are near metal or water; under trees; on hills; near electrical and electronics equipment.

4. Reassess the hazard.

   - It's usually safe after no thunder and no lightning have been observed for 30 min.
   - Be conservative here.

5. Inform people to resume activities.

Reprinted, by permission, from R. Kithil, 2004, *Decision tree for personal lightning safety* (Louisville, CO: National Lighting Safety Institute). Available: www.lightningsafety.com/nlsi_pls/decision_tree_people.html

---

United States. But weather is not the only factor within the environment that can pose a threat to safe athletic performance. Other important types of environmental risk factors include altitude, the physical characteristics of the facilities and equipment, and potential disease-transmitting organisms in the athletic environment.

Altitude

Just as important as acclimatizing to heat and humidity is the acclimatization to altitude. When an individual changes training or competition venues and begins working out at high altitude (>2,000 m or 6,550 ft), the body must adapt to the thinner air and less partial pressure of oxygen. The immediate change observed is an increase in heart rate and respiration. This occurs both at rest and during submaximal exercise in an effort to overcome the lower levels of oxygen. Due to this lower oxygen level, top performances are impossible until acclimation occurs.

Acclimatization to the new altitude requires sufficient time for the red blood cells to accommodate to the low partial pressures of oxygen, as they both increase in number and acquire the ability to absorb and release oxygen more efficiently. The length of time needed for this and other adaptations varies depending on the level of fitness of the individual.

When faced with a change in altitude, the individual must recognize that the physiological requirements of working at the higher altitude will take a toll on the level of performance. Time for acclimatization is necessary to allow high-level performance.

Facilities and Equipment

Any sport activity may take place in a physical environment that has unsafe or unhealthful characteristics. For each sport with which you are involved, it is wise to spend time analyzing the potential risks in this regard.

Inspecting the Area

Although it may be true that most schools and universities have an office responsible for managing the risks on campus, it is still essential that everyone associated with the institution be alert and observant. Reporting playing field hazards to the risk management department or the facilities manager in the athletic department (or both) usually ensures that the hazard will be corrected.

A careful survey of the playing court or field should be conducted prior to any practice or game. Anticipation of obstructions to safe play such as unpadded supports or walls, fences, and bleachers too close to the area of play helps to avoid problems. Goal supports should be padded before the first practice if the posts are in a position that may cause a collision. Observe the field for potholes, sprinkler heads, or other obstacles. Make sure the court is free of wet spots or other surface hazards. Be very observant and use a critical eye when walking over your practice area.

Physical Obstructions on the Field

It is always crucial to take care to provide as risk free a playing area as possible. Walking over the field or court before a practice or competition gives the coach or athletic trainer the opportunity to recognize any potentially hazardous conditions. Objects to check include posts and standards, building walls, and field-surface obstructions.

Goalposts, standards, and all immovable objects located within the area of play must have sufficient padding to ensure that players will not incur serious injury upon contact

with them. Building walls are another type of structure that may present risk. Occasionally sport activity takes place on a court or field that was constructed without proper attention to the distance required for an individual to stop running before contacting a wall. Obviously the wall cannot be moved, but the court lines may be adjusted to allow a safe stopping distance. Regardless of the potential to adjust the distance from the end line to the wall, walls that may limit the safe deceleration of an individual at full speed must have padding to help absorb the force of the contact.

There also may be obstructions on the field surface itself. Potholes and sprinkler heads in the field of play are common. A careful inspection of the entire field and the 10 ft (3 m) surrounding the field boundary should be undertaken at frequent intervals during the sport season. Sprinkler heads should be flush with or slightly below the level of the playing surface. If at all possible, the athletic field should be designed with watering needs taken into account so that it is possible to provide adequate water coverage with a minimum number of sprinklers within the area of play.

Other Obstructions

Just as a wall that is too close to a sideline or end line may increase the risk of injury, bleachers, benches, and other seating structures may be placed too close to the area of play. The placement of any permanent structure should be considered and thoroughly evaluated before a final location is selected. Movable benches, tables, and seats should be evaluated and repositioned if necessary before the start of every sport session and every practice.

Disease-Transmitting Organisms in Facilities and on Equipment

As a final type of environmental hazard we consider disease-transmitting organisms in facilities and on equipment. The element of the facility most commonly associated with the risk of disease transmission is the wrestling mat. Because of the physical contact between a participant and the mat, bacteria and fungi may be transferred to the mat surface. With the high temperatures typically maintained in most wrestling rooms, the environment becomes conducive to bacterial growth. Disinfecting the mat after every practice should be a priority for every wrestling program. With proper care of the facility, bacterial and fungal growth can be controlled and the risk of transmission of bacteria and viruses between participants is greatly reduced.

In addition to appearing on "community" items such as the wrestling mat, contact dermatoses may occur on one individual but not spread to other members of the team. Rashes, boils, or other skin conditions may erupt as a result of contact between an individual's skin and some part of the protective equipment. When this is the case, the first step to the "cure" is finding the cause and making the appropriate changes. Treatment of the skin condition without changing the offending equipment will only prolong the course of the ailment.

It is important for those responsible to understand how to reduce the likelihood of spreading bacteria via equipment. If skin irritation occurs on a body part that comes into contact with sport equipment, that equipment should be treated to reduce its potential to harbor bacteria. Sometimes it is more effective to dispose of equipment than to attempt disinfection. Items that may harbor bacteria and that should be disposed of if a skin irritation erupts include knee pads used in basketball and volleyball, shin pads used in soccer, and plastic pads used inside the helmet in football. Items that should be cleaned include the larger, more costly items: shoulder pads such as those used in football, the shoes used in any sport. These items should be thoroughly cleaned, and participants should not wear them next to the skin; instead, for skin protection, they should wear T-shirts under the pads and should wear clean, white socks with the shoes.

Finally, and above all else, coaches and athletic trainers must remember that following Universal Precautions is the best means of reducing the risk of transmission of bloodborne pathogens in athletics. The extra time it takes people to perform Universal Precautions and use proper procedures, such as pulling on a pair of gloves, is quite small compared to the time they would lose as a result of contracting a virus.

Learning Aids

SUMMARY

This chapter reviews some of the more common environmental situations individuals may encounter. A safe playing environment requires attention to the playing surface and facility, as well as an understanding of the physiological effects of exercise in temperature extremes. Hazardous weather is always a concern for outdoor sports, and an understanding of weather patterns can help the coach and athletic trainer to maximize practice time while minimizing the risks.

This chapter provides the background for understanding the environmental conditions that can affect athletic participation.

KEY CONCEPTS AND REVIEW

▸ **List and give examples of the four cooling methods used to rid a body of excess heat.**

(1) Evaporation occurs when water is heated and vaporizes into the atmosphere. This takes place when a person sweats. The mois-

ture evaporates, allowing heat to escape and cooling to occur. (2) Conduction takes place when a hot surface is in contact with a cooler surface. Heat moves from the warmer to the cooler area, as when your dog lies on the kitchen floor with all four limbs spread. The contact area of the hotter object (the dog) allows heat to transfer to the cooler area (the floor). (3) Convection occurs when the air surrounding the individual is warmed. The warm air expands and its density decreases, making it lighter, and it then rises. When that warm air moves upward, it is replaced by cooler air. This is what is happening to the football player who is playing on a very cold day. If he removes his helmet, you can see the convection currents as the warm air rises off his head. (4) Radiation comes from a heat source that is not in direct contact with the body; it warms the air by virtue of its temperature. This happens constantly when the sun is shining. The radiant energy of the sun warms us and everything around us.

▶ **List the major symptoms associated with heat exhaustion.**

People experiencing heat exhaustion are usually becoming dehydrated. They often have headache, dizziness, nausea, rapid breathing, and fatigue. They are usually actively sweating, and their skin is cool and pale.

▶ **Explain the concept of windchill and how it may affect the physically active individual exercising in a cold environment.**

Windchill refers to the effects of wind as it combines with cold temperatures. A cold wind is much colder than cold temperature alone. If people consider only the temperature of the air when deciding how to dress or how long to exercise, they may be prone to cold injury if it is also windy.

▶ **List things one should observe when inspecting a playing environment for safety.**

The playing area should be inspected on a routine basis. The inspection should include all areas where potential for injury exists. Observe the condition of the playing sur-

face to ensure that there are no dangerous holes, projecting sprinkler heads, or problems with the floor and that all goalposts or other standards are well padded. Observe the boundaries of the playing area to make sure that all benches and other equipment are well removed from the sideline. If any equipment or parts of the facility appear to be within the path of an errant participant, pad that obstacle to ensure that any contact with the object will be cushioned.

PRACTICE!

For hands-on practice in this area, go to the web resource and complete the following:

Level 1.4, Module C11: Environmental Injury and Illness

CRITICAL THINKING QUESTIONS

1. You were recently hired to coordinate the sports medicine for all middle schools in a school district. The district has five schools, and each school has boys' and girls' soccer, basketball, tennis, and track, as well as girls' volleyball and boys' football. One of your job responsibilities is to review the playing areas and make recommendations for safety measures that may be needed. Visit a school in your neighborhood and evaluate its fields and courts. Write up a summary of each area with recommendations for increased safety. Use drawings or photographs if possible.

2. You are working for a college football team during preseason camp. The participants are practicing twice a day. You are asked to organize a system for monitoring the hydration status for all participants. Explain how you might accomplish this. Discuss the personnel you would need to institute this plan.

3. After a tough soccer practice in the heat, one of your strikers lies down, exhausted, on the field. When you arrive to help him, you fear his body temperature may be a problem because you notice that his shirt is soaking wet but his skin is dry and warm to the touch. Since he is a black individual, you are unable to detect a skin color change, but you think he seems hot. Explain what you can do to help him. Be thorough in your explanation (i.e., tell who will help him and how it will be done).

Protective Devices, Regulations, and the Law

Susan Kay Hillman, ATC, PT

OBJECTIVES

After reading this chapter, the student should be able to do the following:

- Explain the function of a voluntary standards organization and describe how such an organization might affect sport equipment.

- Explain the significance of the National Operating Committee on Standards for Athletic Equipment seal on protective headgear and discuss ways in which that seal would serve to protect the wearer.

- Identify the factors considered in determining legal liability for an injury that occurred after alteration of protective equipment.

- Discuss areas in which product liability might play a role in athletics.

rotective equipment is designed to limit injury due to common occurrences in sport. When a piece of equipment is not sufficient to protect a specific injury, the athletic trainer may use tape and pads (see chapter 6). Although this skill is quite beneficial, a fabricator can be held liable for injuries that are deemed the result of alterations made to manufactured equipment, or may be at fault when an individual is disqualified from competition due to wearing of a brace or splint. Care must be taken to understand the rules and regulations, not to modify existing equipment, and always to keep protective equipment functioning the way it was designed.

Standards for Equipment Design and Reconditioning

Some sports, such as collision sports (American football, ice hockey) and select contact sports (rugby, soccer, lacrosse), use specialized equipment that is considered part of the player's uniform. In many cases, if participants are not wearing the equipment, they are sent from the field to put it on. With the large number of individuals needing protective equipment, many manufacturers produce similar items. Fortunately, the materials used to manufacture protective equipment for sports are governed by various standards, as you will learn in the following sections.

Occasionally individuals find equipment that is optional in another sport quite useful in protecting against injury or reinjury in their own sport. For example, you may see a basketball player wearing volleyball knee pads to protect a bruised knee. A critical evaluation of equipment that has been purchased for all sport teams may allow management of some injuries without special fabrication of protective devices. Not only is manufactured protective equipment easy from a fabrication or modification standpoint; it is often more durable than something you would fabricate in the athletic training room.

Regulating Agencies

Regulation of sport equipment manufacturers is necessary to prevent companies from producing inexpensive equipment that will not stand up to the stress of athletic competition. To ensure that equipment is of the requisite quality, governing bodies have been established to set the necessary standards. Additionally, every piece of athletic equipment must be reconditioned if it is to be used for more than one season of competitive play. Both the manufacturer and the reconditioner must comply with a set of standards.

Protective equipment has long been a concern of both the athletic community and the population in general. Agencies exist to standardize the protective qualities of athletic equipment, as well as of the protective devices used by other active members of the community. For instance, the motorcycle helmet is a piece of safety equipment, as is the bicycle helmet. Both helmets, just like sport helmets, are quality controlled by specific governing agencies. Familiarity with the governing agencies and some of the standards they are empowered with developing is helpful for understanding the criteria and conditions that protective sport equipment must meet.

Several organizations have specific roles in the issuance of standards. These include the International Organization for Standardization, the American National Standards Institute, the Consumer Products Safety Commission, the American Society for Testing and Materials, and the National Operating Committee on Standards for Athletic Equipment (**NOCSAE**). Many of these organizations are voluntary standards development organizations, which means that manufacturers meet the established standards voluntarily. From time to time, a governing body for a particular sport mandates that a piece of equipment must be "NOCSAE approved." This is a rule or mandate imposed by the sport organization rather than by the organization that established the standards.

International Organization for Standardization

On the global scale, there is the International Organization for Standardization (**ISO**: "ISO" is not an acronym, but means "equal"). This is a worldwide voluntary standards committee made up of representatives from most countries. The organization as a whole develops international standards for specific products ranging from microprocessors to swing sets. For example, the format of credit cards, phone cards, and "smart" cards used all over the world is derived from an ISO standard. By adhering to the standard, which defines such features as an optimal thickness (0.76 mm), the manufacturer of the card assures the consumer that the card can be used worldwide. In the area of sport, consider a world without standards; a helmet may be protective if purchased from manufacturer A, but not if a less expensive helmet is purchased from manufacturer B. The ISO ensures that the plastic meets the ISO standard.

American National Standards Institute

Within the United States, the governing agency for standards is the American National Standards Institute (ANSI). This is another voluntary standards development organization, serving as the international connection to the ISO standards network. Organizations wishing to submit a product design, system, or service in order to develop an international standard may do so. The ANSI screens the product design, evaluates it, and eventually presents (if deemed acceptable) the developed standard to the ISO. The ANSI is the American representative to the ISO and also America's liaison from the ISO. Additionally, ANSI works on a more local basis in giving recommendations to many groups, including the Occupational Safety and Health Administration and the American Society for Testing and Materials.

Consumer Products Safety Commission

The Consumer Products Safety Commission (CPSC) is a governmental regulatory agency that deals with the safety of all products (not just athletic goods). Its mission is to protect the public from unreasonable risks of injury and death associated with consumer products. The CPSC's work to ensure the safety of consumer products—such as toys, cribs, power tools, cigarette lighters, and household chemicals—contributed significantly to the 30% decline in the rate of deaths and injuries associated with consumer products over the past 30 years (www.cpsc.gov/about/about.html). Since 1973, the epidemiological research group at the CPSC has operated the National Electronic Injury Surveillance System. CPSC's National Electronic Injury Surveillance System (NEISS) is a national probability sample of hospitals in the United States and its territories. Patient information is collected from each NEISS hospital for every emergency visit involving an injury associated with consumer products. From this sample, the total number of product-related injuries treated in hospital emergency rooms nationwide can be estimated (www.cpsc.gov/LIBRARY/neiss.html).

American Society for Testing and Materials

The American Society for Testing and Materials (**ASTM**), now known as ASTM International, has a number of subcommittees that focus on testing materials and products used throughout industry, recreation, and leisure, among other areas. ASTM International is one of the largest voluntary standards development systems in the world. A not-for-profit organization, ASTM International provides a forum in which producers, users, ultimate consumers, and those having a general interest (representatives of government and academia) can meet to write standards for materials, products, systems, and services. ASTM

International is composed of more than 30,000 of the world's top technical experts and business professionals, representing 135 countries, who publish standard test methods, specifications, practices, guides, classifications, and terminology. The organization deals with all aspects of materials, products, and procedures. Many ASTM International committees focus on the highway and construction industries, but some are concerned with sport products; the most prominent of these is the F08 committee.

ASTM International F08 committee, Sports Equipment and Facilities, is the ASTM committee most involved with sport equipment. Organized in 1969, it includes more than 30 subcommittees. All subcommittees have an interest in some aspect of the materials used in sport. Among the subcommittees are those listed in table 5.1.

National Operating Committee on Standards for Athletic Equipment

In the United States, athletic equipment standards are issued by the NOCSAE. After it was organized in 1969 at Wayne State University, NOCSAE began testing football helmets. Using a replica of a human skull, committee members tested various helmet designs to determine the safety of the model relative to concussion criteria in a severe football impact simulation. They established testing standards, and subsequently their test criteria were accepted as the gold standard for most sport helmets. Each sport has its own set of NOCSAE standards, which include standards for batting helmets for baseball and softball, lacrosse helmets and face masks, and football helmets and face masks. Those interested may obtain copies of all NOCSAE standards free of charge by visiting the NOCSAE website (www.nocsae.org/standards/documents.html).

Manufacturers, medical groups, school organizations, and equipment manager groups are invited to take part in NOCSAE developments. These individuals work to evaluate the standards and make any changes to any sport equipment that they deem necessary. Decisions to change the standards for the manufacture of a type of helmet, for example, would be based on evidence either that the current design is flawed or that some

Table 5.1   American Society for Testing and Materials F08 Subcommittees Involved With Sporting Equipment

Subcommittee no.	Subcommittee title	Sport equipment
12	Gymnastics and Wrestling Equipment	Mats and equipment
26	Baseball and Softball Equipment and Facilities	Protective gear, bats
30	Fitness Products	Exercise bicycles, treadmills, strength equipment evaluation and design
52	Miscellaneous Playing Surfaces	Indoor and outdoor playing surfaces and other facility structures
53	Headgear and Helmets	Helmets worn in football, baseball, equestrian sports, and so on
54	Athletic Footwear	Terminology of footwear and biomechanics, shock-attenuating properties of footwear materials
55	Padding (Body)	Protective padding for all sports
57	Eye Safety for Sports	Protective eyewear
64	Natural Playing Surfaces	Testing of organic matter content, impact-attenuation characteristics; guide for constructing and maintaining turfgrass on fields
65	Artificial Turf Surfaces and Systems	Testing relative abrasiveness, specification for impact attenuation
67	Pole Vault	Landing system construction

additional step could be taken to make the product safer. Each organization is offered two seats on the NOCSAE board. Some of the organizations represented on the board are the following:

- American College Health Association
- American College of Sports Medicine (ACSM)
- American Orthopaedic Society for Sports Medicine (AOSSM)
- American Medical Society for Sports Medicine
- Athletic Equipment Managers Association
- National Athletic Trainers' Association (NATA)
- National Athletic Equipment Reconditioners Association (NAERA)
- Sporting Goods Manufacturers Association International

The NOCSAE symbol indicates that a product design meets NOCSAE standards. The committee also sets the standards for equipment reconditioners to use in evaluating and reevaluating helmets. The NOCSAE itself does not evaluate helmets after they have been manufactured; it only affirms that the design of a helmet meets NOCSAE standards and that the reconditioner's tests meet NOCSAE standards for testing. The organization also does not enforce the standard—it merely approves the use of the NOCSAE seal to be embossed on the helmet. If a helmet later fails to pass NOCSAE testing standards, the evaluating agency has the authority to revoke NOCSAE approval. The NOCSAE is just one of the many voluntary standards organizations for sporting equipment, and its standard in athletic **helmetry** is the one most widely accepted.

Other Regulatory Agencies

There are other agencies that govern the manufacturing of sport equipment. Among these are regional associations such as the European Standards Association, the Canadian Standards Association, and the Swedish Standards Institute, just to name a few. Another agency crosses country borders and governs the testing and certification of equipment used in all forms of the sport of hockey—the Hockey Equipment Certification Council. Realize that these agencies all have one goal: to make equipment safer. If the agency is voluntary, this means that the manufacturer is not required to follow the standards the agency sets. But it is certainly positive for a company to advertise that its product meets standards of several of the pertinent agencies rather than only one or perhaps none.

Reconditioning and Maintenance of Athletic Headgear

Several different standards exist for athletic headgear. The NOCSAE standard is the most widely recognized certification standard, although ANSI and ASTM still control some of the certification procedures.

A yearly inspection of all equipment should be performed by all groups distributing protective gear to participants. Some school equipment supervisors elect to inspect their helmets themselves and to send only certain identified helmets to the reconditioner. Other schools or teams may find it necessary to send all helmets used during the season to the reconditioner.

The National Athletic Equipment Reconditioners Association (NAERA) suggests guidelines for reconditioning helmets as well as other sport equipment. Each area of the country typically has at least one equipment reconditioner. Some companies solicit business nationwide. These companies compete with the local company for the school's helmet-reconditioning business. The reconditioner, usually a member of NAERA, inspects each helmet for defects and deficiencies. Loss of integrity of the helmet shell means an automatic rejection; other problems can be rectified to meet the helmet manufacturer's standards. Upon completion of the reconditioning, the reconditioner places a sticker on the helmet signifying that the reconditioning process has been completed and specifying the date it was completed.

Any helmet worn during practices or games should be evaluated periodically. Naturally, the higher the level of competition, the more abuse the helmet is likely to take. The athletic trainer or equipment manager, or both, should inspect each helmet for structural safety on a weekly basis at minimum. Fit should be inspected daily. Generally, the fit of the football helmet should be snug so that it will not rotate if the face mask is manually moved, and the upper edge of the shell should be approximately two finger widths above the individual's eyebrows. Usually the equipment manager inspects the helmet for fit, but all staff working with football should be knowledgeable in this area.

The NOCSAE helmet test involves mounting the football helmet on an instrumented head model and testing the helmet before and after reconditioning. The testing includes a variety of impact situations at both standard and randomized points on the helmet. Shock measurements are recorded and compared to an established severity index (SI) to determine acceptance or rejection of the helmet. The SI is a scientifically accepted measurement of human injury tolerance (www.naera.net/what_tested.html). Some of the required tests replicate running faster than 12 mph into a flat surface such that the head stops suddenly. Helmets that pass the test get a NOCSAE recertification sticker; those failing are clearly marked "unfit for use" or "reject."

Agencies for Development of Sport Safety Rules

The American Medical Association's Committee on the Medical Aspects of Sports and the NCAA Committee on Competitive Safeguards of Sports have both worked diligently in establishing policies and recommendations on safe sport participation. Among the many issues these guidelines cover are prohibition of athletic participation for an individual with only one of a set of paired organs,

weight loss due to hypohydration, and the procedure for medically disqualifying a participant during an NCAA championship. These policies and recommendations are followed by the majority of schools and athletic clubs, yet individual allowances can be made by teams after careful consideration of the medical problem and the risks of athletic participation.

Many organizations play a leadership role in establishing rules for youth, high school, college, and professional sports. These organizations often include a committee to establish and evaluate rules of the sport with the aim of minimizing the potential hazards of participation. Many organizations, such as the National Federation of State High School Associations and the NCAA, establish guidelines for member institutions yet allow individual states or conferences to amend or add to the recommendations. Generally, all such organizations solicit the recommendations of medical and coaching personnel in changing the rules of games in order to reduce injuries. Careful evaluation of injury statistics is essential in establishing a relationship between a performance technique, a rule of play, or a piece of equipment and the occurrence of injury.

Rules and Regulations for the Use of Protective Equipment

To even begin to understand the rules and regulations concerning the use of protective equipment, we must first be consistent in differentiating between equipment that is required or recommended and equipment that is forbidden for use in a particular sport, which we will term illegal equipment. It is essential for people to be familiar with both the required equipment and the illegal equipment for any sport with which they might be associated.

Certainly there are similarities in the rules for equipment use in a particular sport across the various levels of competition, yet differences also exist. In general, the regulations governing younger players are more strict than those governing the professional athlete.

The intent of the rule difference is to further protect the young, skeletally immature individual.

To understand some of the many equipment rules in athletics, it is wise to concentrate on one level of competition. Here we consider the regulations applicable to intercollegiate athletes. Guidelines for equipment use and regulations are published each year by the NCAA in the *NCAA Sports Medicine Handbook*. This handbook is distributed free of charge to all NCAA member institutions, and any nonmember institution may purchase a copy through the NCAA. Each NCAA-governed sport has a committee designated to review the sport rules on a yearly basis. This means that any sport classified as an NCAA sport, regardless of the division of play, undergoes rule review and potential revision each year. When working with an athletic team, to obtain the latest and most accurate information one would first review the published rule book for the sport; second, review the most current issue of the *Sports Medicine Handbook;* and lastly, contact the NCAA liaison for that sport (obtain the person's name and number from the NCAA).

In the following discussion of the rules regarding equipment use, we consider equipment according to the various classes (headgear, face protection, and so on), as well as the rules that pertain to each sport using that class of equipment.

NCAA-Required and -Recommended Protective Equipment

For participation in athletics, some equipment is required prior to the start of the competition (is mandatory). In addition, some equipment, thought to provide some level of protection from injury, is referred to as recommended. When a player is seen without some part of the mandatory equipment, the referee stops play and requires the participant to leave the playing area to obtain the appropriate protective equipment.

Headgear

Equipment considered headgear includes anything that is worn to protect the cranium or the scalp (see figure 5.1). Most often such an item is called a helmet, and it may be of the hard-shell variety or may be a soft covering of the scalp, ears, or both. Baseball, football, ice hockey, lacrosse, and softball require that all participants wear hard-shell helmets, while wrestling and water polo require protection over the ears by a soft padded material (table 5.2).

Face, Throat, and Mouth Protection

Sports with a risk of laceration of the face often involve use of a face mask to prevent fingers or other objects from coming too

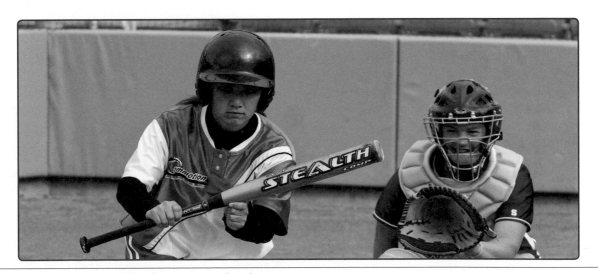

Figure 5.1 Cranium and scalp protective headgear.

Table 5.2	Sports Specifying the Use of Helmets for Participants		
Sport	**Position(s)**	**Type of helmet**	**Comments**
Baseball	Batting and base running	Hard-shell helmet with double ear flaps	Helmets must carry the National Operating Committee on Standards for Athletic Equipment (NOCSAE) mark.
	Catchers	Helmet required to have built-in or attachable throat guard on the mask; hard-shell helmet for fielding the position	Helmets must carry NOCSAE mark.
Football	All players	Hard-shell helmet secured with a four-point chin strap	All players must wear helmets that carry a warning label regarding the risk of injury and a manufacturer's or reconditioner's certification indicating satisfaction of NOCSAE test standards.
Ice hockey	All players	Hard-shell helmet with chin straps securely fastened	It is recommended, but not required, that the helmet meet Hockey Equipment Certification Committee standards.
Lacrosse	Female goalkeepers	Hard-shell helmet with face mask	No standards exist.
	All male players	Hard-shell helmet with face mask and chin pad, secured with a cupped four-point chin strap (high-point hookup)	Helmets must carry the NOCSAE mark.
Softball	Catchers	Protective helmet with face mask and built-in or attachable throat guard	Helmets must carry the NOCSAE mark.
	Batting and base running	Hard-shell helmet with double ear flap	Helmets must carry the NOCSAE mark.
Water polo	All players	Cap with protective ear guards	Cap also differentiates between teams. No standards exist.
Wrestling	All wrestlers	Protective ear guard	Any guard to prevent abrasion of ear on mat (cause of "cauliflower ear").

close to the participant's face. Many collision sports with a potential for concussion and oral trauma use an intraoral mouthpiece. Physically active persons who wear orthodontic devices may also use these mouthpieces to protect both the inside of the mouth and the somewhat fragile wires used in orthodontic bracing. Individuals who incur a risk of contusion to the throat area, such as baseball catchers, may be required to wear protection of this area (table 5.3). These players are usually required to wear a face mask to which an extension for covering the throat can be attached (see figure 5.2).

Protection of the Chest and Shoulders

Thick, open-cell padding material is used often in combination with a hard, plastic outer shell to distribute a local-impact shock

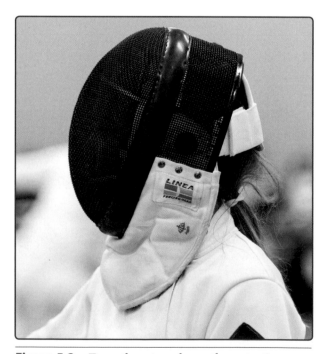

Figure 5.2 Face, throat, and mouth protection.

Table 5.3   **Face, Neck, and Mouth Protection Used in Sports**

Sport	Position	Protection	Comment
Baseball	Catchers	Built-in or attachable throat guard on mask	No standard exists for the design.
Fencing	All participants	Mask with mesh face covering	Usually fits over the sides and front of the face but is open in the back.
Field hockey	All players	Intraoral mouthpiece	Can be colored or clear but must fit over upper teeth.
	Goalkeepers	Throat protector, headgear, and face mask	Permitted, but not required.
Football	All players	Intraoral mouthpiece	Can be yellow or other color (not clear or white) and must cover all upper teeth.
	All players	Face mask	Must be attached to helmet.
Ice hockey	All players	Intraoral mouthpiece	Can be colored or clear but must fit over upper teeth.
	All players	Face mask	Must meet HECC-ASTM F 513-98 Eye and Face Protective Equipment for Hockey Players Standard.
Lacrosse	All players	Intraoral mouthpiece	Must cover upper teeth (women: any color or clear; men: yellow or other highly visible color).
	Goalies	Throat protector	Goalkeeper has the option of using face mask.
Softball	Catchers	Face mask with attached throat protector	Can be detachable but must be worn.
Wrestling	All participants	Protective mouth guard	Recommended.

onto the large surface area of the chest and shoulders (see figure 5.3). Various sports use shoulder pads, and other sports require simple chest protection of only some of the position players. Although both ice hockey players and football players must wear shoulder pads, the difference between the pads used for the two sports is quite dramatic. Since hockey players are seldom "fixed" but instead slide on the ice upon contact with another player, the need for heavy padding is reduced or eliminated in comparison to the situation in football. See table 5.4 for details on the chest protection needed for various sports.

Protection of the Lower Extremities

The joints of the lower extremity are often in contact with the ground or with other players. The superficial location of bony prominences makes protective padding valuable. Baseball catchers, hockey goalkeepers, and football and soccer players incur the risk of contact and are provided special protection

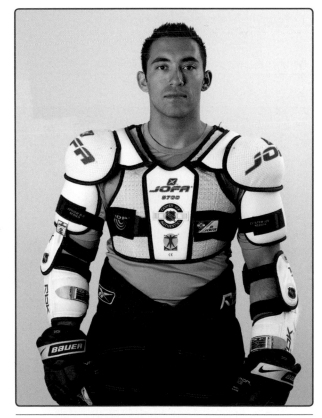

Figure 5.3   Shoulder and chest protection.

(figure 5.4). See table 5.5 for the details of sports requiring lower extremity padding.

Illegal or Restricted Equipment

In an effort to limit unintentional injury to other players, use of some equipment has been made illegal. In general, contact sports attempt to eliminate the potential for contusions or abrasions from casts or braces. Table 5.6 identifies illegal equipment by NCAA sport. In all cases, if a referee or other judge of the sport feels that a piece of equipment or another item (e.g., jewelry) worn by a participant may be dangerous to another player,

the player may be required to remove it or be disqualified from participation.

Fabricating Custom Protective Equipment

Training personnel certainly fabricate custom protective equipment (see chapter 6) in a typical athletic training room, yet the clinician must first evaluate several important variables. First and foremost it is critical to carefully evaluate legal liability issues. If the equipment could cause an injury or worsen an existing condition, it should not be fabricated. If there is no potential of

Table 5.4 **Protection of the Chest and Thorax in Sport Teams**

Sport	Position	Protection	Comments
Baseball	Catchers	Chest protector	Shock-absorbing foam with plastic reinforcement in sternum area
Fencing	All participants	Vest of jacket and metallic lames and underarm protectors	Full coverage of chest with additional protection of vital points
Football	All players	Shoulder pads	Hard outer shell and open-cell foam padding inside
Ice hockey	All players	Shoulder pads	Lighter and thinner pads than for football
Lacrosse	Goalkeepers	Chest protector	Combination of hard and soft outer shell
Softball	Catchers	Chest protector	Similar to protection for baseball

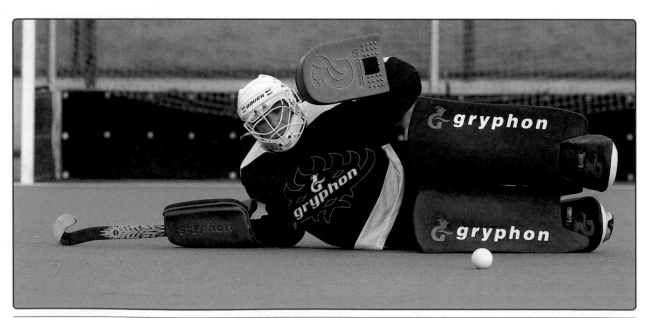

Figure 5.4   Lower extremity protection.

Table 5.5 Lower Extremity Protective Equipment by Sport

Sport	Position	Protection	Comments
Baseball	Catchers	Leg guards covering knees, shins, and top of feet	Should be easily removable for batting and base running
Field hockey	Goalkeepers	Kickers (pads from top of feet to groin area)	Optional equipment
Football	All players	Soft knee pads 1/2 in. thick	Must be covered by pants
	All players	Hip pads, tailbone protector, and thigh pads	Pad must fit into uniform, covered by pants
Soccer	All players	Shin guards	Must meet NOCSAE standards
Softball	Catchers	Protective leg coverings	Similar to baseball gear

Table 5.6 Illegal or Restricted Equipment and Materials

Sport	Equipment	Specifications
Basketball	Braces or casts below the elbow	Must be pliable (no plaster, metal).
	Casts or braces of other body parts	May be used but must be padded.
Football	Protective braces between elbows and hands (to be used only to protect recent fracture or dislocation)	Must be covered on all sides with closed-cell, slow-recovery foam padding at least 1/2 in. thick.
	Hard thigh pads	Must be covered front and back with soft padding material.
	Knee braces unless entirely covered	No additional padding is necessary.
	Projection of metal or other hard substance	Any functional braces used for protection must be covered if made of hard material.
Ice hockey	No equipment that could endanger other players	"Noninjurious" protective equipment must be used.
Women's lacrosse	Any special equipment	Must be approved by umpires.
Men's lacrosse	Any "dangerous" equipment	As evaluated by official.
Soccer	Hard or dangerous equipment on the head, face, or body (braces, casts, and so on)	No hard materials can be used for protection if they may be harmful to an opponent.
	Knee braces	Must be covered, no metal exposed.
	Casts	Permitted if covered and not considered dangerous.
Softball	Plaster or other hard substances	Any hard material that could cause harm to another player.
	Exposed metal	Must be covered by soft material and taped.
Track	Taping of any part of the hands or fingers for hammer, discus, javelin, and shot put	Not permitted unless an injury, cut, or wound requires protection by tape.
Wrestling	Anything that prohibits normal movement of the joints	Equipment cannot prevent the opponent from applying normal holds.
	Hard and abrasive materials	Must be padded and covered.
	Loose pads	May allow an opponent an unfair hold.
Volleyball	Any object that may cause an injury or give an artificial advantage to the player	Hard splints worn on the arms or hands must be padded on all sides with at least 1/2-in.-thick slow-rebounding foam.
		Earrings must be removed.
		Religious medallions or medical identifications must taped or sewn under the uniform.

increased harm, the design of the equipment must adhere to the rules and guidelines for the sport. Fabric selection should take into account the factors mentioned in chapter 6, and those factors should be considered in relation to the sport and playing style of the individual. When fabricating protective devices, always consider all factors before spending time, money, and energy on a misguided effort.

Legal Concerns About Equipment Use in Sport

Since the purpose of protective equipment is to safeguard the player from harm, it should be easy to understand why the consumer (or the family of the consumer in some cases) might think there has been a legal wrong when an individual suffers an injury due to failure of the protective equipment. Carry this thought just a bit further and realize that spectators or workers in the athletic facility also expect proper protection from injury. Spectators attending a practice or game certainly do not attend with the thought that a flying bat, ball, stick, puck, or any other piece of equipment may injure them.

The majority of legal cases brought against an athletic department or its staff entail tort. **Tort** cases usually involve an individual's seeking to blame someone other than herself for an injury or resulting condition. A tort must be classified into one of seven areas, meaning that the person filing the suit (the **plaintiff**) must show one of the following seven reasons for issuing the legal action:

1. Intentional harm to the person
2. Intentional harm to tangible property
3. Negligence
4. Strict liability
5. Nuisance
6. Harm to tangible personal interests
7. Harm to tangible property interests

In a tort case in sport, the injured person would probably attempt to show **negligence**.

This means that the plaintiff attempts to show that the responsible person (the **defendant**) failed to take the action that another person of equal abilities and training would have taken in the same circumstances. For example, if an athletic trainer stops to help the victim of an accident, the care the athletic trainer provides should be the same as what any person of the same level of knowledge would provide. If the care failed to meet that standard of care, the athletic trainer could be held negligent. Each case involving an attempt to show negligence is considered by the court on the basis of its particular set of circumstances; if the circumstances indicate some negligence, a liability issue will result. Specifically, **liability** results from five factors:

1. Ignorance of the law
2. Ignoring the law
3. Failure to act
4. Failure to warn
5. Expense

These five factors are all considered when an injured person tries to establish a tort liability case with a charge of negligence. First, let's define the factors. Later in the chapter we'll look at liability, or *who* is responsible.

Ignorance of the Law

You may have heard your parents say something like "Ignorance is no excuse," and this is never more true than in cases of sport liability. Consider, for example, a situation in which a diving coach decides to have the divers work on the trampoline to perfect some of their diving skills. Let's suppose that the coach fails to supervise the divers on the trampoline, that two of the divers get on the apparatus at the same time, and that during their trials at doing simultaneous flips they collide. Assume also that the collision results in some permanent disability of one of the divers.

Now, realize that in 1977 the American Academy of Pediatrics issued a statement opposing the use of the trampoline in physical education, recreation, and sport programs. This statement was issued not because the number of injuries resulting from trampoline use was great, but rather because of the number of injuries that were serious and debilitating. Safety guidelines have since been established through the combined effort of several organizations; and all supervisors, as well as all participants using the trampoline, must follow these guidelines. Now, this is not to say that the statement of opposition to the use of the trampoline is a law; but the court would expect the coach to be aware of this decision by the national association. The fact that neither the coach nor the divers were aware of the recommendations against the use of the trampoline does not make those individuals less responsible or less liable.

It is certainly expected that coaches know the regulations and laws that pertain to their sport and to the equipment used in training for their sport. When you look at a piece of equipment, do so with a very critical eye regarding the potential for injury. If you are unaware of rules and regulations associated with equipment, check with the manufacturer, attorneys, or other coaches or administrators to gain knowledge of any and all potential ramifications associated with the use of that equipment.

Ignoring the Law

Since everyone is expected to know the law, the next step is to obey the law. Unfortunately, some people still believe that "rules are made to be broken" and consequently ignore rules, regulations, and laws until they are forced to pay attention. Some people may suggest that a school or coach will continue to get away with disobeying a rule or regulation until something serious happens. Examples of ignoring the law or ignoring the rules can be found in every sport and probably in every school or team. It is not difficult to think of injuries that could have been avoided if an individual had been wearing the proper protective equipment. People who decide to ride a bike without a helmet can hardly complain

of the concussion that occurs when their tire catches a pothole and they are thrown to the ground. The same concept applies in a high-contact sport like football when players fail to wear protective thigh pads that are provided and required. A contusion to the quadriceps muscle can incapacitate the individual for several days or even weeks. Although quite minor compared to a life-threatening injury, a quadriceps contusion resulting from inappropriate athletic equipment could be the start of a negligence case citing "ignorance of the law" as the grounds.

Failure to Act

A person who is aware of a rule or regulation and consciously elects to ignore it is guilty of "failure to act." This typically applies when adherence to a rule or regulation is intended (stated in writing or in some other manner) but for some reason the intention has not been carried out. It is expected that regulations will be followed regardless of financial concerns or other issues that may delay the intended action. You may have heard stories about players or spectators who were injured when a flying object hit them in the head. If the incident occurred because the injured person was permitted to come too close to the practice or competition area, there may be negligence on the part of the athletic department.

As an example, if regulations specify that protective barriers must be placed between the hockey rink and the spectator area but the athletic department—failing to act on the regulations—allows visitors to watch practices and attend games in that facility, liability is assumed by the athletic department. A flying puck that strikes an inattentive fan in the head, causing a fractured skull, would become a much different case if it became known that the request for funds to erect a protective barrier in front of the spectator area had been denied. Failure to act can take many forms, but the bottom line is that the proper procedures were not carried out. In contrast to the issue of ignoring the law, this failure to act is a failure to provide or prevent rather than a failure to comply (as when a rule or law is ignored).

Failure to Warn

Some sports have unique associated dangers, regardless of how safe the participants might attempt to stay. The actor Christopher Reeve was an accomplished horseman, yet all his training and skill could not prevent the spinal cord injury that rendered him quadriplegic when he was thrown from his horse. Accidents can and do happen; and the coach, trainer, or other person responsible must fully warn the individual of the potential dangers. It is not only important to provide printed information regarding the risks of participation; in addition, those risks must be conveyed verbally and must be well understood by all participants.

A widely publicized case involving the failure to warn occurred in Seattle in 1982—*Thompson v. Seattle Public School District* (Appenzeller 1985). The plaintiff, Thompson, was awarded $6.3 million when the court found the coach and the school district liable for failure to warn of the dangers inherent in football. Thompson had been injured in 1975 as a sophomore football player. He suffered a fracture of the spine when he lowered his head to ward off a tackle.

Prior to this landmark case in the early 1980s, warning participants of potential dangers was not considered very important. Today, not only must the coach explain the dangers of football participation; the player will see a warning sticker inside his helmet, and he may be asked to sign a statement saying that he has been informed of, and that he understands, the risks of permanent injury associated with football participation.

Expense

Although expense is not as easy as the other issues to immediately relate to liability in sport injury, you might recognize the element of expense in other situations. For example, let's say that you wanted to learn to skydive. You are a starving college student and don't have much money. You save and save and

finally have enough money to take the lessons. You love it. You want to go again and again, but you can't afford the parachute rental. Would you accept a "deal" offered in the classified ads if the parachute was substandard? Budget concerns may cause teams or individuals to use old equipment that they have repaired and refurbished. As discussed earlier, if the equipment must be used over and over again, it is critical that it be reconditioned and its safety recertified. There are agencies that provide the reconditioning service for athletic equipment; and when budgets are limited, the expense of reconditioning must be allowed even when funds are insufficient for new equipment.

Other forms of expense issues could look the same as those discussed in connection with failure to act. When a proposal for providing some protective equipment or improving the safety of a facility is declined for budget reasons, the issue of expense comes into play. One lost life or one serious injury may be far more expensive than the preventive measure would have been.

Liability Negligence

When a healthy, athletic person leaves home to go to school in the morning, the parents naturally expect that their son or daughter will return home that evening healthy and happy. When a catastrophic injury occurs, changing that young person's life forever, it may appear to the community only as a tragic consequence of participation in sport. To the family and the injured individual, it is obviously much more than a consequence of sport; neither the participant nor the parents will want to admit that they did in fact accept the risk of athletic participation. Too often, the injured person and the family are overwhelmed with grief and feel the need to shift blame to some other person in order to explain the tragedy.

In the attempt to shift the focus of responsibility onto someone else's shoulders, the injured party may name any number of athletic department employees as defendants or codefendants: the administrators, athletic trainers, equipment managers, coaches, and even teammates.

Determination of Liability

First and foremost, the courts want to see the degree to which the injured person was responsible (liable) for the actions that resulted in an injury. When an individual chooses to play a sport, the knowledge of potential risk is in most cases clearly understood. This knowledge is termed "assumption of risk" because every person must take responsibility for her own safety. In the unusual case in which the individual is not warned of the dangers of participation, she assumes none of the risk. On the other hand, in the situation in which individuals have no knowledge of the dangers but make no effort to determine the hazards, there may be "contributory negligence."

In a 1979 case *(Brahatcek v. Millard School District)*, the plaintiff (Brahatcek) brought a wrongful death action against the defendant school district after her son David died following an accident in a physical education class. David, a ninth-grade student, was fatally injured when he was struck in the head by a golf club swung by a fellow student. The class was being conducted in the gym because of inclement weather. David's class consisted of 58 students supervised by two teachers. David had missed the first day of indoor instruction but had returned to school the next day and participated without the benefit of the first day's safety instructions. The trial court found the school negligent and therefore ruled in favor of the plaintiff. The school board appealed, asserting that both David and the classmate who struck him were in some way responsible for the mishap. This attempt to diminish the level of negligence of the teacher would shift some of the responsibility for preventing the injury onto the injured person (contributory negligence).

Contributory negligence may prevent the injured person from recovering damages (collecting on a legal liability suit) because it means that the person was in some way responsible for her own injury. It is up to the court to decide the level of responsibility and what action is appropriate. Factors that help the court determine the amount of negligence the injured person is responsible for include the person's age, physical capabilities, level of training, and other factors. In *Brahatcek v. Millard*, the state supreme court upheld the trial court's decision that the 14-year-old was insufficiently prepared to anticipate the dangers of the situation, rejecting the school district's contention that David was guilty of contributory negligence.

In some states, a level of negligence is determined, and that percentage is used to calculate the award. This prorating of damages reflects "comparative" negligence and may mean that both the plaintiff and the defendant are partially responsible. A person who lives in a contributory negligence state would receive nothing if he were found to be partially at fault, while the same circumstances might yield a partial award in a state that observes comparative negligence.

An injured individual may try to point a finger toward the person or persons who issued protective equipment, those who provided medical care, or those who did coaching on particular techniques. Usually, if the equipment person or the coach is named in a lawsuit, the employer is also named. Two reasons for naming two or more persons in a lawsuit are the "deep-pocket" concept and the doctrine of "respondent superior."

The deep-pocket concept seems self-explanatory: When the plaintiff is seeking to recover a large amount of money (damages) for a serious injury, the effort is of little use if the defendant cannot afford to pay the full amount of damages. Thus, more people may be named in the suit, or the school system may be named, to ensure that it will be possible to recover the total damages awarded by the courts.

The respondent superior doctrine allows the plaintiff to name additional defendants due to the established covenant that the employer may be held responsible for actions committed by its employees if they are acting within the scope of their employment. When the employer is named in the lawsuit the employee may, and usually is, still named as a codefendant. An employee named in a lawsuit in which negligence is claimed often suffers a great deal emotionally and perhaps financially. If the employee is considered negligent for her actions, there may be reason to question that employee's abilities. The employer may discontinue the service of the employee, and other potential employers evaluating this person for the same position in which negligence was found may not want to take the risk of employing the person. When the court finds the employee guilty of negligence and damages are awarded, insurance may offset some of the costs of the lawsuit; but if insurance does not fully cover the damages awarded, the employee must come up with the money out of pocket (or out of future wages), and this debt cannot be alleviated by declaring bankruptcy. Overall, negligence and liability are devastating to the individual and, with proper care and attention, should be totally avoidable.

As we realize, the coach, athletic trainer, and equipment person work directly with the participants, and their actions or lack of actions may have a direct relationship to an individual's injury. The person who hires or supervises these employees can be held equally responsible for the employees' actions. The courts expect supervisors to have control of the actions of their staffs; the athletic director is expected to have control of the actions of the coaches, trainers, and equipment people. We see this in an example from New York in which a young man with a heart condition died during participation in the school football program. It was found that the school district had a preparticipation physical examination policy but that the school, and other schools in the district, failed to follow the policy. The administrator responsible for the school district athletic programs was sued and subsequently removed from his position as a supervisor of the athletic programs because he had failed to make sure that his member schools followed the policy (*Monaco v. Raymond*).

Administrators must take an active role in the selection, hiring, and supervision of coaches, volunteers, and all department employees associated with the health and welfare of the participant. If a person is hired and it is found that the individual committed negligence but was insufficiently qualified for the position, the person responsible for the hiring would be guilty of vicarious liability.

Product and Manufacturer Liability

If a product is found to be defective for the purpose for which it was intended, the manufacturer is held liable. The "product" need not be a piece of equipment like a football helmet or shin guards; it could be a diving board, a pool, or even the land upon which an athletic field is constructed. If there is some defect in the product—that is, some reason that the product was not adequate for the purpose intended—the manufacturer (or seller in the case of the land) is liable.

Facility or Playing Surface Problems

Manufacturers, architects, and construction firms can be held responsible for the manufacture, design, construction, and consumer support related to playing surfaces. The manufacturer must ensure that the consumer uses the product in the manner in which it was intended and also must issue warnings to the consumer if the product has any chance of being dangerous. This comes into question as we look at the Centers for Disease Control Health Advisory issued in June, 2008, stating that an unsafe level of lead had been found to be associated with some artificial turf fields. Questions would arise if the manufacturer has a responsibility for the decomposition of the materials used in the manufacture of the original surface. As another example of this area of liability, an architect might have designed a basketball gym with the outer walls of the court too close to the court boundary. This might leave insufficient boundary behind the basket for a player to perform a layup without the risk of collision with the wall. Certainly, there are many people beyond the manufacturer and the architect who would play a role in preventing problems caused by the facility or playing surface, yet if a serious injury occurs, the plaintiff looks for anyone at fault.

Sporting Equipment

As we have noted, products are expected to be safe for the purpose for which they were designed. Litigation has been a great financial burden in American football over the years. Lawsuits between manufacturers and sport participants have attempted to show that equipment was improperly designed or defective in some way. One of many examples of this type of suit is *Austria v. Bike Athletic Co.* Austria, a junior on the high school football team, was hit on the front of the helmet by another player's knee during football practice. The plaintiff was initially dazed but seemed to be fine. Two weeks later, Austria was complaining of severe headaches, and one day at practice he collapsed on the field. He underwent a special radiograph evaluation and subsequent surgery to relieve a subdural hematoma (blood clot on the brain), and although his life was saved he was left with permanent disability.

The court found no reason to think that the blow to the helmet was unusual for the sport and therefore concluded that the injury was due to a defective helmet. The court ruled in favor of the plaintiff. Cases such as this were quite frequent especially in the early 1980s, when suits against helmet manufacturers cost various companies over $20 million. After these cases were settled, usually at great expense to the defendant's insurance company, the cost of premiums to insure the manufacturers of football helmets averaged $2.5 million a year (Appenzeller 1985). The higher cost of insurance had to be offset in the price of the helmet, which jumped from $40 per helmet in the 1980s to between $100 and $200 today. The fact that legal action against a manufacturer ultimately affects the consumer is unfortunate but is a part of athletics that is well recognized and reasonably well accepted.

Improper Care or Modification of Manufactured Products

It is not uncommon for an individual to attempt to alter a piece of protective equipment to make it lighter, less bulky, or generally more comfortable to wear. It is important to realize that any modification of equipment will void any legal liability the manufacturer would have due to failure of the product. In 1985, Marc Buoniconti was rendered paralyzed after a tackle in a Citadel football game. Originally, Buoniconti sued the Citadel (Mitten 2002) because the athletic trainer had modified the player's helmet to prevent him from excessive neck extension. The modification included a strap, attached from the shoulder pads to the face mask of the helmet, that would tighten as the player's neck was forced into extension and hyperextension. The plaintiff held the athletic trainer liable because the strap seemed to actually cause the player's neck to be held in a flexed position—a vulnerable position for the cervical spine that increases the potential for vertebral injury in the event of impact with the top of the helmet. This modification of the helmet negated any responsibility of the helmet manufacturer, shifting the blame to the athletic trainer and the Citadel.

Manufacturer's Liability

Only equipment that is unaltered and regularly inspected and reconditioned can be considered within the scope of the manufacturer's responsibility. In *Rawlings Sporting Goods Co., Inc. v. Daniels,* Rawlings attempted to convince the court that a defect in the helmet worn by the injured plaintiff (Daniels) could be due to the failure of the school to inspect and recondition the football helmets. Unfortunately for the sporting goods company, the helmet did not have warning labels to inform the wearer of the potential for injury while playing football.

The defendants tried to demonstrate that the school was partially negligent for not reconditioning all of the helmets and not keeping proper records on each helmet in its inventory. The court found no fault on the part of the school but found the defendants guilty of gross negligence, influenced in part by the company's attitude toward the matter.

Protecting Oneself From Legal Misfortune

The best protection people have from legal misfortune is prevention, yet it is virtually impossible to avoid injuries in athletics. In an effort to protect themselves from the financial drain of attorney fees and court costs, all professionals should consider liability insurance coverage. In some states, liability insurance is referred to as errors and omissions insurance. Often the employer provides this insurance. In addition to any protection offered by the employer, an athletic trainer may also wish to obtain professional liability insurance from a private insurance company. Just as with your auto or health insurance, the policy will not change things that happen, but it will assist you in paying the various fees that will be incurred.

Learning Aids

SUMMARY

The goal of the athletic trainer and the coach should be to keep the individual participating safely and without injury. Although this is not possible, we hope that the risks of participation can be reduced and the chance of injury controlled by the proper use of protective equipment. Not only knowing what equipment is required, but also understanding the significance of an ISO standard in the manufacturing process or of the NOCSAE symbol on a reconditioned helmet, is essential. When products or people fail and an individual is seriously injured, legal liability may become an issue. Understanding legal terminology is helpful in understanding how you can protect yourself in caring for physically active patients and in equipment selection and maintenance.

KEY CONCEPTS AND REVIEW

▶ Explain the function of a voluntary standards organization and describe how such an organization might affect sport equipment.

Many standards organizations exist, each with the common goal of establishing consistency in the manufacture of specific items. The voluntary nature of these organizations means that manufacturers voluntarily follow the standards; if the product does not follow the standards, the manufacturer cannot display the symbol of that standards organization. Certain standards have been adopted in sport and recreation, and equipment not meeting those standards is not accepted for use. Often a product bears the symbols of various standards organizations, signifying that the product is of specified size, shape, and quality.

▶ Explain the significance of the National Operating Committee on Standards for Athletic Equipment seal on protective headgear and discuss ways in which that seal would serve to protect the wearer.

The NOCSAE sets standards for various pieces of athletic equipment, and the seal indicates that the particular product (headgear) design meets the NOCSAE standards. This organization also sets the standards for equipment reconditioners to follow in evaluating helmets. When a used helmet passes the recertification process, it again meets the

NOCSAE standards—this time the standards for a reconditioned helmet.

▶ **Identify the factors considered in determining legal liability for an injury that occurred after alteration of protective equipment.**

If the alteration of the protective equipment is found to have been a causative factor in the injury, the person who altered the equipment may be found liable. This assignment of responsibility for the injury is moved away from the manufacturer as soon as the product design or structure is altered; the person making the adjustments then becomes responsible. The five factors that help to establish this liability include ignorance of the law, ignoring the law, failure to act, failure to warn, and expense.

▶ **Discuss areas in which product liability might play a role in athletics.**

Liability results from five factors: Ignorance of the law, Ignoring the law, Failure to act, Failure to warn, and Expense. In terms of product liability, we would consider each of the five factors and how those relate to the product. Using the sport helmet for example, if one were to have ignorance of the law he may not realize that a specially designed helmet is required for each sport. Using a hockey helmet for football would be ignorance of the law. If one were to ignore the law he may disregard the helmet rule for the sport and attempt to play without proper head protection. Failure to act in this case would involve the coach, equipment manager, or athletic trainer. It is the responsibility of the athletic staff to enforce the rules of the sport and insure the individuals are wearing proper protective equipment. Failure to warn will again involve the athletic department staff. It is the responsibility of the staff to warn of the risks of participation and certainly of participation without proper protective equipment. Expense in this case may be most easily recognized when thinking of the young participant who is expected to buy his own protective gear. Buying a used helmet may be less expensive, but if the helmet is found faulty and the individual is injured, the expense cannot be used as the reason a proper helmet was not used.

PRACTICE!

For hands-on practice in this area, go to the web resource and complete the following:

Level 2.1, Module X5: Football Team Experience

Level 2.1, Module X10: Women's Individual Sport Experience

CRITICAL THINKING QUESTIONS

1. Your athletic director tells you that the athletic budget has suffered a severe budget cut and that all reconditioning of the football, softball, and baseball helmets will have to be done in-house and not sent out this year. Formulate your response explaining why this is not a wise decision.

2. You have witnessed circumstances that you feel may be putting participants at risk of injury, but they are not within your power to change. You decide to approach the athletic director to discuss the situation and what you think should be done about it. What legal concerns are involved in this discussion? What legal issues are in play if the athletic director suggests that you just "ignore" the situation? Discuss what you would do if you were asked to ignore the problem.

Athletic Taping, Padding, and Bracing

David H. Perrin, PhD, ATC, FNATA
Kirk Brumels, PhD, AT, ATC

OBJECTIVES

After reading this chapter, the student should be able to do the following:

- Identify the types of tape commonly used in athletic taping.

- Explain the "check reign" used in athletic taping and identify different styles or shapes.

- Describe the five different taping techniques (spiral, figure 8, teardrop, herringbone, and horseshoe) and give an application of each.

- Identify the points to consider when developing preventive and protective pads.

- Identify six basic products used in the construction of pads and braces for injury protection or prevention.

- Explain why a fiberglass cast on a football lineman's wrist should be padded for practice and games, regardless of rules.

- Identify the three categories of knee braces and when each might be used.

Athletic taping is one of the many **psychomotor** skills required of the athletic trainer and can serve to prevent injury or facilitate an injured person's return to physical activity. Taping can be applied to support the ligaments and capsule of unstable joints by limiting excessive or abnormal motion and enhancing proprioceptive feedback from the injured limb or joint. Indeed, the sensory cues (proprioception) received from tape or a brace may be more important than the restriction of excessive or abnormal range of motion. As with any psychomotor skill, taping requires a great deal of practice; but proficient application of tape quickly earns the confidence and admiration of the patient.

Anatomy and Injury Mechanism as the Foundation for Taping and Bracing

A sound understanding of human anatomy and mechanisms of injury is necessary for mastering the art and science of taping and bracing. It is essential to be able to visualize the anatomical structures that you are attempting to support with the application of tape or a brace. While anyone can learn the psychomotor skills required to apply tape, understanding the link between the anatomical structure, mechanism of injury, and purpose for which the tape is being applied is a distinguishing characteristic of the accomplished athletic trainer. Human anatomy is the foundation for everything you learn about athletic training and is an important component of your curriculum. Indeed, you will probably take at least one course in human anatomy as part of the athletic training curriculum. Part II of this book, "Clinical Examination and Diagnosis," introduces you to mechanisms of injury.

Materials for Taping and Wrapping

The standard materials used for taping and bracing include elastic and nonelastic athletic tape, elastic wraps, and any number of commercially manufactured braces. Nonelastic tape is used to provide optimal support to joints and to strategically restrict abnormal or excessive joint motion. It is normally **porous** and available in 15-yd (13.7 m) rolls with widths of 1, 1.5, or 2 in. (2.5, 3.8, or 5.1 cm).

Elastic tape or wraps are used to support body parts that require greater ranges of motion than are permitted with nonelastic tape. Elastic wraps can also be used to apply compression to an acutely injured body part to minimize the swelling that accompanies soft tissue injuries. Elastic tape is normally available in widths of 1, 2, 3, or 4 in. (2.5, 5.1, 7.6, or 10.2 cm). Elastic wraps usually have widths of 2, 3, 4, or 6 in. (5.1, 7.6, 10.2, or 15.2 cm).

Braces can be used to prevent injury (or reinjury) and support unstable joints. A wide array of braces are commercially produced, primarily for the ankle, knee, shoulder, elbow, and wrist. Braces can also be used to supplement or replace athletic tape, which can reduce cost since they are reusable. However, some braces are very expensive.

Prerequisites to Taping and Bracing

Use of the injury evaluation techniques explained in parts I and II of this book should always precede the application of tape, padding, or braces. A thorough understanding of the nature and mechanism of injury is essential to the correct application of tape or a pad or brace.

Taping, padding, and bracing should also be applied in conjunction with appropriate stretching and strengthening exercises. Taping, padding, and bracing are not a substitute for a fully rehabilitated body part ready for safe return to physical activity. An understanding of the principles presented in part IV of this book is essential to helping patients maintain optimal strength and flexibility.

The final prerequisite to taping and bracing is to confirm that the criteria for return to physical activity have been met. These criteria include normal strength, flexibility, and range of motion; successful performance of functional tests such as running and cutting without limping (in the case of lower extremity injuries); and psychological readiness to return to physical activity.

Preparing for Taping

The taping area should be **ergonomic** in design, should be kept clean, and should be free of clutter and personal items. Taping tables should be approximately 48 in. long (122 cm) and 35 in. high (89 cm). The area should have optimal **illumination** and ventilation and should be free of excessive heat and humidity. The area should be coeducational, and your patient should be a willing and attentive participant during the application of tape. The area and body part to be taped should be clean and shaven for optimal support, or pretaping underwrap should be used. A tape adherent can be applied, and friction pads should be used when the tape is to be placed over bone prominences or muscle tendons.

Applying Tape

The following sections describe methods of tape, wrap, or bandage application that are foundational for the athletic trainer and can be used in many different situations and on many body parts to achieve the outcomes desired. The various application techniques can be used individually, in combination with each other, or with additional more specific **methodology** depending on the injury, reason for application, and desired effect. Creativity with taping techniques and supplies is a valuable skill for athletic trainers as they encounter various injuries and the need to fulfill various taping objectives.

Spiral

Spiral taping is typically used when the athletic trainer feels that pad application, compression, or general support of joints or soft tissue is the taping objective. Spiral taping or wrapping, also used in bandaging and wound care, consists of overlapping layers of tape or wrapping material. The amount of overlapping is dependent on the taping objectives. Spiral taping for compression and support can be applied either over a joint or over long bones or muscle tissue between joints. In most cases it should be applied in a **distal** to **proximal** fashion to aid in venous return and function. Spiral taping is commonly used for thigh, hamstring, quadriceps, lower leg, and wrist injuries but can be applied to many situations in which the benefits of spiral taping meet the treatment objectives. Figure 6.1 illustrates techniques for spiral taping.

Check Reigns

The **check reign** method of taping uses strips of tape that typically cross over a joint in an effort to limit or modify joint movement and provide protection to soft tissue structures. The use of a check reign typically involves **anchor strips** placed proximal and distal to the involved joint. These anchor strips, which serve as attachment points for the check reign, can take on various shapes or styles, such as stacks, "Y," double "Y," fan, or "X." The main premise behind the use of a check reign is to limit either normal or excessive movement. Length and type of the check reign, application technique, and joint

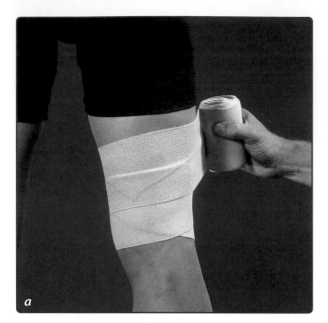
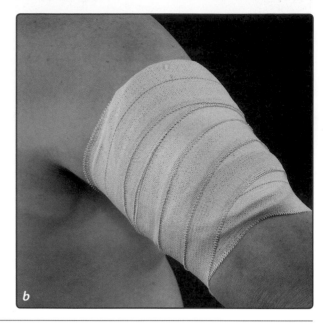

Figure 6.1 Elastic wrap to *(a)* support the hamstring muscle and *(b)* secure a protective pad to the arm.

position can all be chosen by the athletic trainer to produce the desired effect of modifying movement and protecting soft tissue.

Stacks

A stack check reign is made when strips of tape are placed directly on top of each other in an attempt to add strength to the application. The number of strips and thus the strength of the check reign are based on the taping objective. Stack check reigns for use in taping the knee should typically be stronger than those used on the wrist but can be modified to each situation encountered by the athletic trainer. Stacks can be made from various materials, including cloth tape, elastic tape, neoprene rolls, elastic bands, and cotton or nylon strapping. Toes, knees, elbows, ankles, and fingers are common sites for this application. Figure 6.2 depicts the application of stack check reigns using cotton tape and elastic tape for the taping of the Achilles tendon. Complete Achilles tendon taping procedures are described in *Athletic Taping and Bracing, Second Edition* (Perrin 2005).

Fan

The fan check reign is similar to the stack check reign except that one end is wider than the other. Overlapping the tape to form a fan

allows taping over a joint where the proximal aspect is larger than the distal or vice versa. Use of the fan technique allows for greater contact area, thus creating greater control of motion and support.

The "X"

This technique uses a crisscross method for the stack or fan to obtain greater contact and control of the joint and soft tissue. This method is often used on areas such as the wrist where the joint itself is smaller than its distal and proximal aspects. Narrowing the check reign in the middle allows for less bulk over the movement area and increased control as the ends of the tape are able to adhere to and control more tissue. Examples of the use of an "X" check reign for the taping of a knee and an elbow are shown in figure 6.3. Complete taping procedures that incorporate the "X" technique are described in *Athletic Taping and Bracing, Second Edition* (Perrin 2005).

The "Y"

The "Y" style of check reign consists of a stack check reign that is cut or split at one end to facilitate attachment to the anchor strips. The split end of the "Y" check reign can be long enough to be placed in a circular fashion around the anchor strip and body

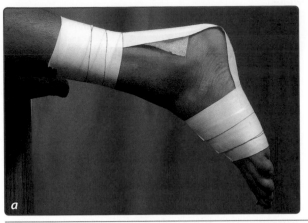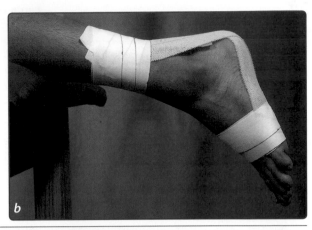

Figure 6.2 Taping procedures *(a)* as proximal and distal anchors and *(b)* to limit dorsiflexion.

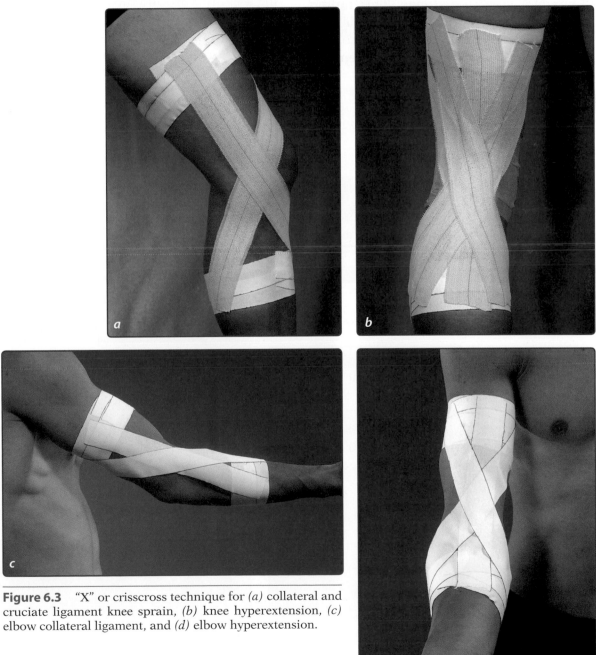

Figure 6.3 "X" or crisscross technique for *(a)* collateral and cruciate ligament knee sprain, *(b)* knee hyperextension, *(c)* elbow collateral ligament, and *(d)* elbow hyperextension.

part and taped in place. This helps to keep the check reign from moving or loosening during activity or participation. The "Y" check reign is often applied during taping procedures with the aim of limiting ankle movement.

The Double "Y"

The double "Y" stack check reign (figure 6.4) is split on each end for the purpose of improving attachment at both anchor sites. It is different from the "X" check reign in that the middle section is more elongated and spans a greater distance. This taping procedure is typically done with elastic tape products for greater comfort and control and is commonly used for elbow **hyperextension**

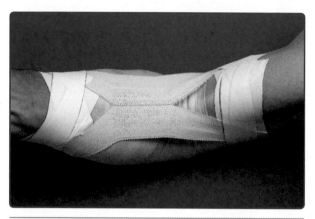

Figure 6.4   The double "Y" taping technique.

taping, as well as taping for Achilles tendon pathology.

Figure 8

The figure 8 taping technique, a foundational technique that can be applied in numerous situations to benefit multiple joints, is used for limiting motion or providing support to a joint. It involves continuous circular and angular placement of the tape so that it crosses over itself and the joint while forming a figure 8 around the proximal and distal aspects of the bones that compose that joint. Tape tension, joint placement during taping, and type of tape are factors that influence the restrictive and supportive characteristics of the application. The technique is used for taping the ankle, wrist, fingers, elbow, shoulder, hip, and knees. Figure 6.5 provides examples of the figure 8 taping procedure on various body parts and joints. Full descriptions of the taping procedures for these body parts are presented in *Athletic Taping and Bracing, Second Edition* (Perrin 2005).

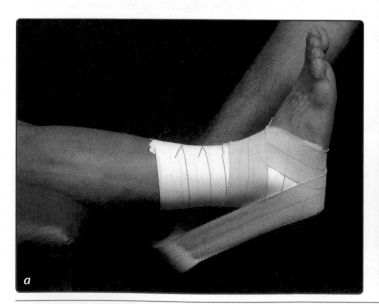

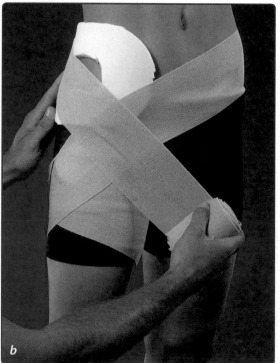

Figure 6.5   Figure 8 taping procedures for the *(a)* heel, *(b)* iliac crest, *(c)* shoulder, *(d)* elbow, *(e)* wrist, and *(f)* thumb.   *(continued)*

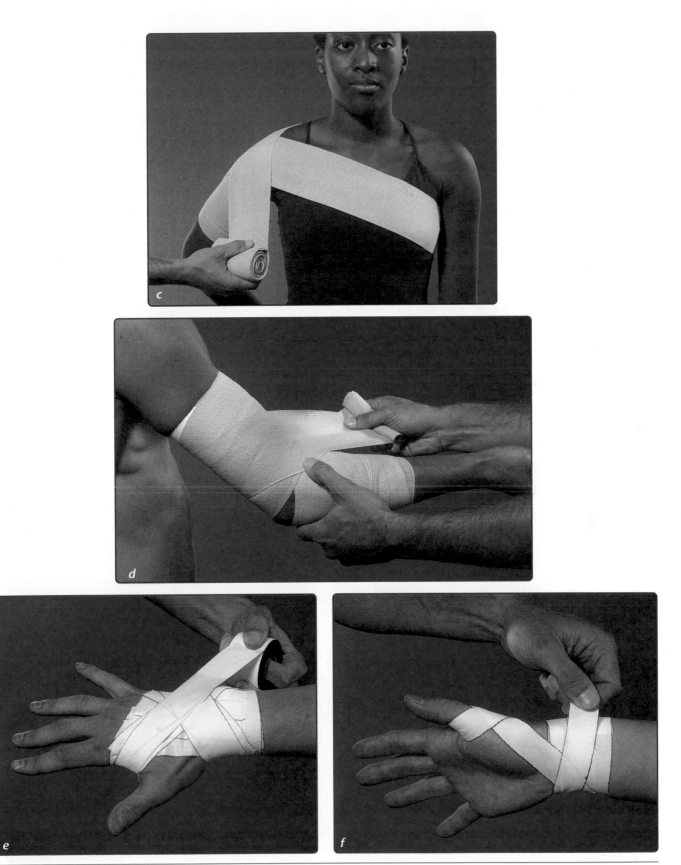

Figure 6.5 Figure 8 taping procedures for the *(a)* heel, *(b)* iliac crest, *(c)* shoulder, *(d)* elbow, *(e)* wrist, and *(f)* thumb. *(continued)*

Teardrop

Another taping technique that is commonly used is the teardrop technique (figure 6.6). A strip of tape originates and ends at or near the same spot to create an oval or teardrop shape. The ends of the strip can cross over each other depending on body part and purpose. A very common location for teardrop taping is on the foot during supportive taping of the longitudinal arch. Complete taping procedures are explained in *Athletic Taping and Bracing, Second Edition* (Perrin 2005).

Herringbone

A classic in the fashion industry, the **herringbone** pattern is also a classic athletic taping technique. The herringbone pattern consists of overlapping strips of tape that are crossed over each other in alternating and opposite directions. The benefit of the herringbone taping technique is sequential support from the overlapping tape strips as well as compression and support due to directional pull applied during the taping process. Common areas for use of the herringbone taping pattern are the lower extremity (lower leg, hamstring, quadriceps), the ribs, and the low back. Figure 6.7 depicts herringbone taping on the lower leg and the quadriceps. Full descriptions of the taping procedures for these body parts are presented in *Athletic Taping and Bracing, Second Edition* (Perrin 2005).

Horseshoe

The horseshoe taping technique is used during taping of the ankle, heel, and shoulder. A strip of tape is placed on a body part where circumferential tape application is not possible. Direction of pull, amount of tension, percentage of overlap, and type of tape all affect the benefits of the technique. The horseshoe technique is used during prophylactic taping of the ankle as a way to limit ankle motion (figure 6.8a). Use of the technique for the heel and shoulder is shown in figure 6.8b and 6.8c, respectively. Other depictions and instructions for use of the horseshoe technique as part of athletic taping

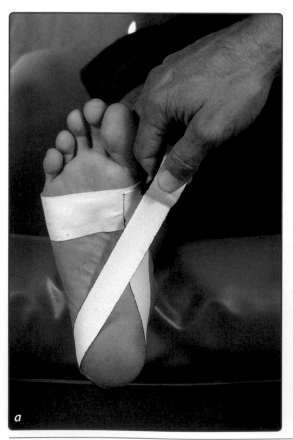

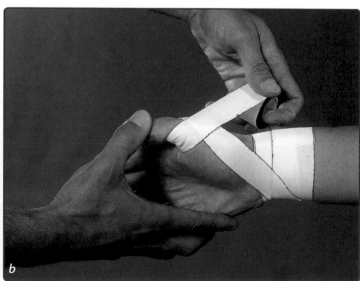

Figure 6.6 Teardrop taping for (a) longitudinal arch and (b) wrist.

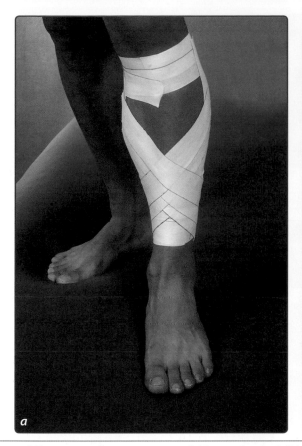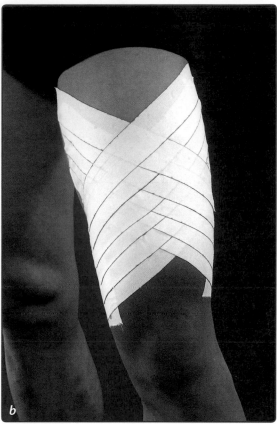

Figure 6.7 Herringbone taping on *(a)* lower leg and *(b)* quadriceps.

procedures for the ankle, heel, and shoulder are presented in *Athletic Taping and Bracing, Second Edition* (Perrin 2005).

Padding

Individuals involved in medieval jousting, American football, bull riding, and other sports have developed an understanding of how valuable padding and protective equipment can be in either preventing or lessening the severity of injuries from sporting competition. From the first chest protector, helmet, or nose guard to the modern equipment used today in football and other sports, the development of various protective products has become a big business. Specialized products manufactured for baseball, football, basketball, softball, soccer, lacrosse, volleyball, extreme sports, outdoor activities, and many

other sports can fill many pages of sports medicine–related product catalogs.

Many different types of pads and protective equipment have been developed by athletic trainers and those interested in protecting individuals from injuries that are an inherent part of many sports. These products have been developed or designed as a response to an observed need for prevention of or protection from athletic injuries. Pads and protective equipment may have been designed or conceptualized on a napkin or on scrap paper before being constructed in a workshop, garage, or athletic training room. We can never be completely sure how some of these items originated, only that they were in response to a need for the prevention of and protection from harm due to competition. **Evolutionary** changes to these items may have occurred slowly over time as materials and circumstances changed. Formal credit

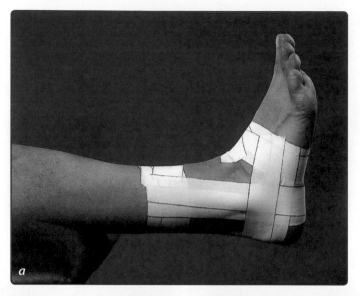

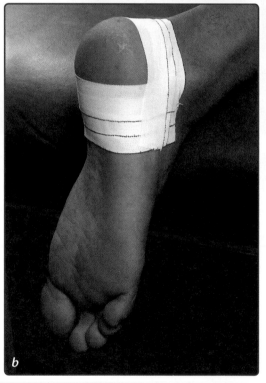

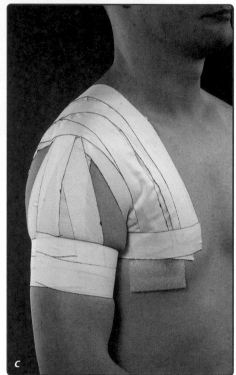

Figure 6.8   Horseshoe technique for the *(a)* ankle, *(b)* heel, and *(c)* shoulder.

may never be given to those involved in the development of the products, though a word of thanks or a look of satisfaction may come from an individual after a successful competition in which a fabricated pad or piece of protective equipment was used. As athletic trainers, those words or glances are all the recognition we need.

Pad Fabrication Considerations

As mentioned previously, numerous commercially developed products meet the many padding and protective equipment needs of sport participants; however, in special and individual situations, athletic trainers might be required to manufacture a pad from materials available commercially or found around the athletic training room, at home, or in a retail store. Not all commercially available pads work for every situation; therefore the athletic trainer must be aware of the different types of materials, shapes, and sizes of pads and of the theories that might apply to their specific situation. In addition, not every employment situation gives athletic trainers the financial wherewithal to purchase commercially manufactured products; in this case they must rely on their own construction of pads. These pads may be used alone or in combination with taping procedures or commercially available products.

The process of developing preventive and protective pads should include consideration of density, strength, rigidity, conformability, self-adherence, durability, ease of fabrication, and cost. The athletic trainer must decide on the desired properties and then choose the specific material or product that best suits those needs.

Density

The main material property that one should consider when making preventive or protective pads is density. Density of a product refers to the weight of the product as compared to its size. In some situations, a dense

pad is needed for its protective qualities and the weight of the product is not a major factor. In other situations, the weight of a dense material may affect performance, so the athletic trainer must consider whether the higher-density pad is the correct choice. In each situation that warrants protection or prevention by means of padding, consideration must be given to the type of material used and its properties relating to protection, weight, and size (see figure 6.9). Table 6.1 provides an overview of materials and properties of products used in the construction and fabrication of various pads. Typically

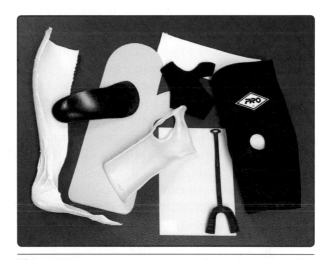

Figure 6.9 In choosing a particular density, consider the type and velocity of contact a participant may experience and match these to the level of protection needed.

Table 6.1	Protective Materials and Their Densities	
Density	**Type of material**	**Examples of products**
High density	Silicone elastomer "casting" material, viscoelastic materials, some foams	• Silicone: various vendors' silicone elastomer liquid • Viscoelastic: Smith & Nephew, Akton, and others • Felts and foams: open-cell foams such as Smith & Nephew Carve-It or Sorbothane, Langer Biomechanics PPT, various orthopedic felts
Medium density	Fiberglass splinting materials, polyethylene and other thermoplastic moldable plastics, most orthopedic felt, some foams	• Fiberglass: 3M Scotchcast, Smith & Nephew Dynacast • Thermoplastics: J & J Orthoplast, Smith & Nephew Polyform, Polyflex II, Air-Thru, Ezeform, Aquaplast, and many others • Felts and foams: Spenco silicone pads, various felts and foams
Low density	Some foams, cotton padding, neoprene rubber	Foams: Smith & Nephew Polycushion or Contour Foam

the products that boast higher density offer greater protection and are more resistant to **deformation** and impact but also have corresponding increases in size and weight. Lower-density foams usually compress more easily under pressure and impact and therefore have less shock-absorbing capability.

Strength

Strength refers to the maximum external stress or load that a material can withstand. The strength of a material is important to ensuring that the splint will function as intended. Some materials are strong enough for normal daily activity but not capable of withstanding the stresses of high-impact athletic participation. If you wanted to provide a splint or support to help prevent inversion ankle sprains, you could select an elastic sleeve, a formed plastic stirrup with air bladder, a lace-up ankle brace, or even a custom-formed hard plastic ankle brace. If the individual had a sedentary job and did not intend to participate in physical activities, the elastic sleeve might provide sufficient support and protection. However, if the person wanted to continue going to basketball practice after work, you might need to consider one of the other devices. The elastic provides compression, but the strength of the material is too low to prevent the ankle from inverting during physical activity.

Rigidity

Rigidity or stiffness refers to the amount of bending or compression that occurs in response to a measured amount of applied stress. Stiffness is measured and evaluated using the concept of *modulus of elasticity*. A product with a high modulus is of a stiffer material, while a product with a low modulus affords greater flexibility (less stiffness) and can absorb shock better (see figure 6.10). A fiberglass splint has a high modulus of elasticity; once "set," the fiberglass is very rigid and nonbending. A splint made of aluminum is an example of a splint with a low modulus.

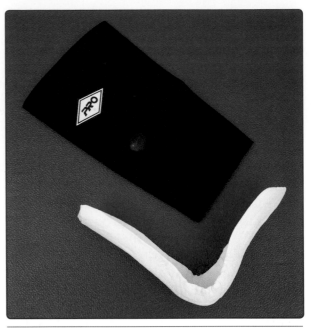

Figure 6.10   A product classified as low modulus (top); material with a high modulus (bottom).

To protect the broken hand of a person who is highly physically active, the fiberglass splint or cast might be the best choice; for someone whose activity level is less apt to lead to contact with the healing hand, an aluminum hand splint may be sufficient. High-modulus fiberglass does not yield and provides rigid immobilization, whereas the aluminum splint can actually be bent if that is desired. Strength becomes an important factor in working with physically active people when one is attempting to limit the movement of a joint or area.

Rigidity depends on the type of material used as well as on the thickness and shape of the material once it is formed into the protective device. Again, the bulk of the finished product may be the limiting factor, requiring use of a stiffer or more rigid material.

Conformability

Conformability is the ease with which material forms to fit the body part. Most participants in most sports want to wear a well-fitting uniform, and they have the same attitude about any protective device they may need to wear. Even if the product is sufficiently strong, dense, and stiff, it may fail to provide the proper protection if it does not bend or conform to the body part to be protected. For example, a dense foam that is 0.5 in. (1.27 cm) thick may be an excellent choice for its ability to disperse the force of contact; yet when you try to adapt that foam to fit snugly around a bruised knee, you find that it is too inflexible to conform. A nylon or Lycra sleeve with a Sorbothane pad may prove to be more conforming and to provide excellent protection.

Self-Adherence

Self-adherence refers to the strength with which the material bonds to itself. This factor determines the integrity and durability of a splint. A splint would be of little value if it uncoupled or separated as the player performed the sport. One product frequently used to ensure self-adherence is Velcro. One surface of this material sticks to almost nothing except its own other surface. This type of material is very useful in binding nonadherent materials together around a limb or joint. A brace or splint with internal padding glued inside is an example of a device that might have poor self-adherence. The glue is often the point of failure for this type of brace. The heat and moisture inside the brace often destroy the bonds of the glue so that the padding pulls away.

Durability

Durability is the material's ability to withstand repeated stress during the sport activity. This simply means that a more durable material will last longer. Although the desirability of this characteristic seems obvious, it becomes even more so when one is working within the limited budget of a club or school team where supplies and equipment are not plentiful. Materials that can be used only once or twice are not cost-effective if the same protection is required at every practice session over a prolonged period of time.

It is common for athletic equipment to wear out or break down; materials eventually stop doing their job if used repetitively. You would want to consider this, for example, if you needed arch support. You might have three main options: tape the arch, use a fabricated orthotic of soft neoprene or felt support with special pads to support the arch, or use a custom-made orthotic device constructed of special materials shaped and reinforced to support the arch (see figure 6.11). The tape is a one-time-use solution. Once wet, it will no longer work. The neoprene or felt can be used over and over again but needs to be replaced from time to time. The most durable of the options is the more expensive custom-made support. This device could serve the purpose well for several years.

Ease of Fabrication

Ease of **fabrication** relates to the time, equipment, and skill needed to shape the material into a form suitable for both protection and comfort. Forming some materials requires heat and thus access to an oven or other heating unit. These materials may be superior for the specific use you intend but are obviously unsatisfactory if you do not have the heating element. In this situation you are left to improvise with other off-the-

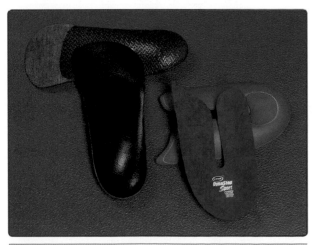

Figure 6.11 Custom-formed orthotic (left) and a prefabricated orthotic (right).

shelf products that may not fit as well. The protective mouthpiece is an example. Many football players wear mouthpieces because of safety requirements. You may have seen or even used a "boil-and-bite" mouthpiece (figure 6.12), a protective device that is designed to be molded by the individual. Molding is quite easy if you have a hot pot, a hydrocollator, or another way to make very hot or boiling water. If you are traveling, you may not have access to water this hot. Unfortunately, individuals have sometimes played while wearing the unformed mouthpiece because of the problem of finding a heat source.

Fabrication of other types of protective devices can be difficult for various reasons; the special soft cast is an example. The equipment and supplies, as well as the special skills needed to fabricate the rubber soft cast, may lessen its attractiveness for daily use. If as an athletic trainer you become interested in such products, it is important to learn the skills needed to fabricate the devices if the supplies are within your budget and you choose to have them on hand. If you don't have the necessary materials or skills, you may need to send patients to another health care provider to obtain a particular device or find an alternative method of protection.

Availability and Cost

Availability and cost are the two factors that pose the greatest obstacles for many athletic programs. Sometimes you know of a material that would work well in a particular situation, but it is not available; in this case you will need to devise an alternate solution using another material. In other cases a material that would be appropriate is expensive, and you would probably not expect to use that material at a school where the budget is limited. Some programs have sufficient capital resources to purchase all the materials one might want to use to fabricate various types of protective devices. It is more realistic, however, to understand the limitations imposed by the particular facility's budget and to plan to work within those limitations. If it is not possible to provide adequate protection of an injured part, the only sound decision may be to withhold the individual from participation until the condition resolves enough to make protection unnecessary.

Pad Construction Materials

Several basic products are used in the development and construction of pads and braces that are designed for injury protection or prevention during athletic activity (Beam 2006; Hillman 2005; Perrin 2005).

Closed Cell Foam

- Has a higher density
- Regains original shape quickly after deformation
- Provides better protection for higher levels of impact
- Is usually stiffer foam, which is less comfortable to wear

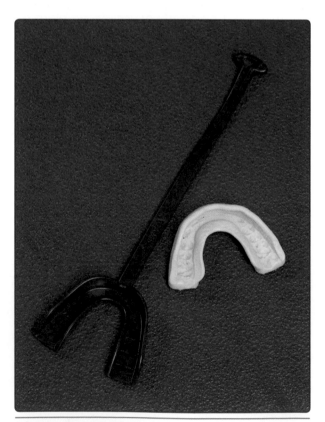

Figure 6.12 Boil-and-bite mouthpieces are designed to give a custom fit.

- Can be purchased with adhesive backing for ease of application

Open Cell Foam

- Has a lower density
- Slowly regains shape after deformation
- Provides better protection for low levels of impact
- Is more comfortable to wear
- Can be purchased with adhesive backing for ease of application

Note: Pads can be and often are manufactured using combinations of both types of foam to achieve a "best of both worlds" scenario.

Thermoldable Foam

- Is closed or open cell foam that can be heated and subsequently molded to the body part
- Improves conformability
- Is great for padding of casts and braces prior to competition

Felt

- Comes in varying thicknesses
- Can be used in conjunction with foams and other bracing and padding materials
- Can be purchased with adhesive backing for ease of application

Gel

- Is typically made entirely or partially of silicone or sorbothane.
- Is effective in dispersing different levels of impact
- Is comfortable to wear due to increased ability to conform to body part
- Can create some adherence problems due to texture

Heat-Moldable Plastics or Fiberglass

- Are activated by heat or water
- Provide hard covering used over foam or felt to increase absorption of high level impact
- Have elevated strength levels
- Can also be used for immobilization or range of motion restriction

In addition to utilizing one of the six product types by itself to provide padding or protection, an athletic trainer may also choose to combine two or more products and create a pad that addresses a specific injury situation. Examples would include using a softer material next to the skin and adding a harder outer layer consisting of plastics or fiberglass. These type of pads would resemble soccer shin guards and many forms of shoulder pads or helmets. Both materials would assist in the dissipation of external forces via their own separate mechanisms thus improving the protection afforded to the patient. Further modification of the materials may consist of making "doughnut" or "bubble" pads where either a hole is cut out or the padding is elevated directly superior to the injured area. The idea is to dissipate forces to tissue adjacent to the injured structures, thus protecting the injured area and allowing for appropriate healing conditions.

Role of Bracing

Braces prevent injury to healthy joints and support unstable joints. A variety of braces are available in the athletic marketplace. In fact, you can find a brace for every joint of the body, although for athletic purposes, you will most commonly need to apply braces for the ankle, knee, shoulder, elbow, and wrist. Braces can supplement or replace athletic tape. Some braces, such as those for the ankle, can save money because unlike athletic tape they are reusable. Braces, however, can be expensive. Some knee braces, for example, cost from $500 to $700.

Ankle Braces

Lace braces have become a popular substitute for ankle tape, especially when a clinician is unavailable (figure 6.13). These commercial supports can also supplement the taping procedure. The brace, normally applied over the sock, often uses **lateral stays** for reinforcement.

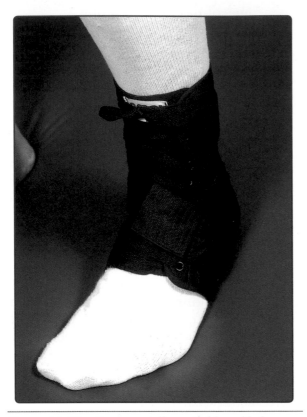

Figure 16.13   Commercially available ankle brace.

Knee Braces

Knee braces fall into three categories: preventive, rehabilitative, and functional. Preventive braces guard the knee from injury during athletic participation by protecting the medial collateral ligament from excessive valgus force. Speculation abounds concerning the potential of these braces to reduce injury to the medial collateral ligament, and they are used far less frequently than they were in the past. Although participants, coaches, and athletic trainers offer **anecdotal** reports that the brace has saved a ligament, scientific research is less conclusive on the value of the preventive knee brace. Many athletic trainers are wary of prescribing a preventive device because of its questionable clinical value and excessive cost.

Rehabilitative braces protect the knee immediately after injury or surgery (figure 6.14). Clinicians can control the range of motion of the knee by adjusting dials on the medial and lateral aspects of the brace.

Functional knee braces may be used on individuals who experience **rotary** instability because of injury to the anterior cruciate ligament (figure 6.15). Some physicians recommend or require a functional brace following surgical reconstruction of a knee with a defi-

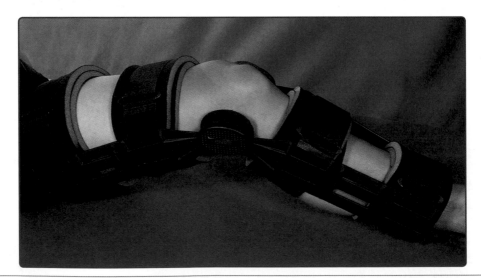

Figure 6.14   A rehabilitative brace with flexion and extension stops that can be used to control the degree of knee motion.

cient anterior cruciate ligament. Individuals have found functional knee braces effective for some anterior cruciate ligament injuries; others require surgical reconstruction before the return to competition. The functional knee brace has the disadvantage of costing at least several hundred dollars.

Shoulder Braces

Commercially produced braces are available to provide support to unstable glenohumeral joints (figure 6.16). These braces limit shoulder abduction and external rotation, which are the common mechanisms of injury for anterior dislocation of the glenohumeral joint.

Elbow Braces

Valgus and varus instabilities of the elbow joint are difficult to support with commercially produced braces. More commonly, a brace can be used to alleviate the pain associated with tennis elbow, known as lateral epicondylitis (figure 6.17).

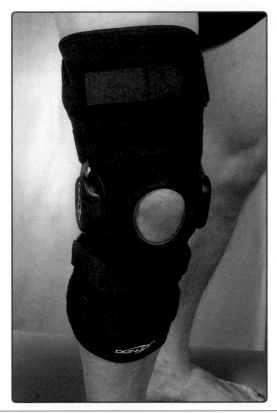

Figure 6.15 A functional knee brace with flexion and extension stops that can also control the amount of knee motion.

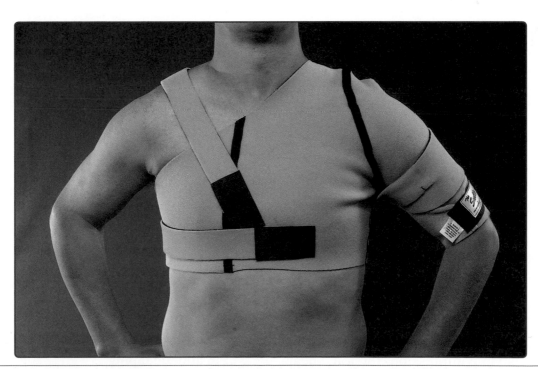

Figure 6.16 Shoulder; a commercially produced brace can limit shoulder abduction and external rotation.

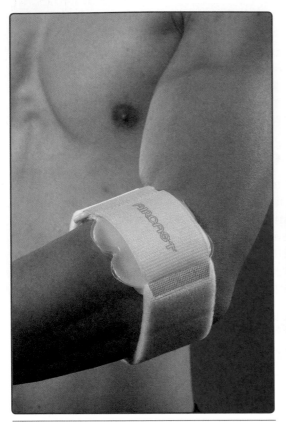

Figure 6.17   Elbow; a commercially produced brace can alleviate pain associated with lateral epicondylitis.

Wrist Braces

Braces can support the wrist and aid in recovery from injuries to the many bones, joints, and muscles essential to normal function of the hand. One common commercially produced brace is designed to protect and rest the wrist from the repetitive stress that produces carpal tunnel syndrome (figure 6.18).

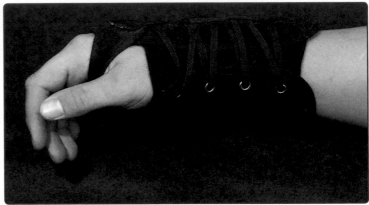

Figure 6.18   Wrist; a commercially produced brace used to relieve the signs and symptoms of carpal tunnel syndrome.

Learning Aids

SUMMARY

Tapping, padding, and bracing are important elements in the prevention of injuries as well as in the protection of injuries. The basic concepts presented in this chapter should serve as foundational knowledge for the athletic trainer to use and apply in the specific cases affecting patients. The basic premise of taping, padding, and bracing is to reduce the amount of excessive force applied to various body parts via compression, torsion, shearing, bending, or distraction. Being aware of the demands of the sport—and how they affect the tissue you are trying to protect—is critical for effective use of taping, padding, and bracing.

KEY CONCEPTS AND REVIEW

▶ **Identify the types of tape commonly used in athletic taping.**

Nonelastic tape is used to provide optimal support to joints and to strategically restrict abnormal or excessive joint motion. Elastic tape or wraps are used to support body parts that require greater ranges of motion than are permitted with nonelastic tape.

▸ **Explain the "check reign" used in athletic taping and indentify different styles or shapes.**

The check reign method of taping uses strips of tape that typically cross over a joint in an effort to limit or modify joint movement and provide protection to soft tissue structures. The use of a check reign typically involves anchor strips placed proximal and distal to the involved joint. These anchor strips, serving as attachment points for the check reign, can take on various shapes or styles, such as stacks, "Y," double "Y," fan, or "X." The main idea behind the use of a check reign is to limit either normal or excessive movement.

▸ **Describe the five different taping techniques (spiral, figure 8, teardrop, herringbone, and horseshoe) and give an application of each.**

- The spiral technique is used for pad application, compression, or general support of joints or soft tissues. Spiral taping consists of overlapping layers of tape or wrapping material, and the amount of overlapping is dependent on the taping objectives. Spiral taping is commonly used for thigh, hamstring, quadriceps, lower leg, and wrist injures.
- The figure 8 technique is used for limiting motion or providing support to a joint. It involves continuous circular and angular placement of the tape so that it crosses over itself and the joint while forming a figure 8 around the proximal and distal aspects of the bones that compose that joint. It is used in taping the ankle, wrist, fingers, elbow, shoulder, hip, and knees.
- With the teardrop technique, a strip of tape originates and ends at or near the same spot, creating an oval or teardrop shape. The ends of the teardrop may cross over each other depending on the body part and purpose. A very common location for the use of the teardrop technique is on the foot during a supportive taping of the longitudinal arch.
- With the herringbone pattern, overlapping strips of tape cross over each other in alternating and opposite directions. The benefit of the herringbone taping technique is sequential support from the overlapping tape strips, as well as compression and support due to directional pull applied during the application process. Common areas for use of the herringbone taping pattern include the lower extremity (lower leg, hamstring, quadriceps) and the ribs and the low back.
- The horseshoe taping technique is used during the taping of the ankle, heel, and shoulder. A strip of tape is placed on a body part where circumferential tape application is not possible. Direction of pull, amount of tension, percentage of overlap, and type of tape all affect the benefits of the horseshoe taping technique.

▸ **Identify the points to consider when developing preventive and protective pads.**

The process of developing preventive and protective pads should include consideration of density, strength, rigidity, conformability, adherence, durability, ease of fabrication, and cost.

▸ **Identify six basic products used in the construction of pads and braces for injury protection or prevention.**

Six basic products include the following: closed cell foam, open cell foam, thermoldable foam, felt, gel, and heat-moldable plastics or fiberglass.

▸ **Explain why a fiberglass cast on a football lineman's wrist should be padded for practice and games, regardless of rules.**

As an athletic trainer, it is your responsibility to protect not only your players, but also those participants with whom your client comes in contact.

▸ **Identify the three categories of knee braces and when each might be used.**

- Preventive braces guard the knee from injury during athletic participation by protecting the medial collateral ligament from excessive valgus force.

- Rehabilitative braces protect the knee immediately after injury or surgery. Clinicians can control the range of motion of the knee by adjusting dials on the medial and lateral aspects of the brace.

- Functional knee braces may be used on individuals who experience rotary instability because of injury to the anterior cruciate ligament. Some physicians recommend or require a functional brace following surgical reconstruction of a knee with a deficient anterior cruciate ligament. Individuals have found functional knee braces effective for some anterior cruciate ligament injuries; others require surgical reconstruction before returning to competition. The functional knee brace has the disadvantage of costing at least several hundred dollars.

PRACTICE!

For hands-on practice in this area, go to the web resource and complete the following:

Level 2.5, Module F1: Ankle Taping, Wrapping, and Bracing

Level 2.5, Module F2: Knee Taping, Wrapping, and Bracing

CRITICAL THINKING QUESTIONS

1. For padding your football lineman's fiberglass cast, discuss the kinds of materials you might use. Explain the pros and cons of each selection.

2. Your women's soccer goalie got her leg tangled in a play at the goal. She came off at halftime and asked you to check out her knee. She has slight tenderness over the MCL (medial collateral ligament) but no instability and no pain with stress testing. She is very functional and there is nobody else on the team who can play this position, so you decide to give her some added protection. Since you are on the road, you have only a knee sleeve, tape (elastic and nonelastic), and a knee immobilizer. What ideas do you have to protect the goalie's knee for the second period?

Clinical Examination and Diagnosis

etermining the nature and extent of an injury is a critical role of the athletic trainer. The NATA BOC (2011) states that, "Athletic trainers must possess strong clinical examination skills in order to accurately diagnosis [sic] and effectively treat their patients." Part II of *Core Concepts in Athletic Training and Therapy* addresses this area.

As you learn the plethora of skills and techniques needed to perform the clinical examination, you will find that organization is important. Some techniques remain the same across areas of the body, such as palpation of a joint, and some techniques are very joint specific. The chapters in this part of the book are organized by body areas to help give you a full understanding of the pathologies and evaluation techniques for each joint.

Chapter 7 introduces injury mechanisms and the ways in which injuries are classified. It includes a discussion of the anatomical reference position and presents terminology that is important in communication between the athletic trainer and others. The chapter also discusses acute and chronic conditions and the classification of injuries to soft tissues, bones and joints, and nerve tissue.

Chapter 8 focuses on the principles of examination. Topics include the primary and secondary surveys and the differences between them; the major steps in performing the on-site examination, the acute injury examination, and the clinical examination; and the differences between the subjective and objective segments of an examination.

Chapter 9, on typical injuries and conditions affecting the upper extremity, discusses how to recognize pathologies of the shoulder, arm, elbow, forearm, wrist, and hand. The chapter differentiates between various conditions and explains predisposing factors and injury mechanisms.

Chapter 10 covers injuries and conditions that affect the lower extremity. Mechanisms, differential diagnosis, and evaluation techniques are presented for the hip, thigh, knee, leg, ankle, and foot.

Chapter 11 focuses on injuries and conditions affecting the spine, head and face, thorax, and abdominal regions.

Chapter 12 discusses general medical conditions of the body. The chapter covers specific conditions of the heart and the respiratory system, as well as systemic conditions such as eating disorders, infections, and sickle cell anemia.

COMPETENCIES

Prevention and Health Promotion (PHP): PHP 21, 22

Clinical Examination and Diagnosis (CE): CE-16, 20a-20e

Acute Care (AC): AC-4, 36a-c, e, f, h, i, k, l, and o

Therapeutic Interventions (TI): TI-16

Injury Mechanisms and Classifications

Sandra J. Shultz, PhD, ATC, CSCS, FNATA
Kirk Brumels, PhD, AT, ATC

OBJECTIVES

After reading this chapter, the student should be able to do the following:

- Describe the anatomical reference position.
- Use appropriate anatomical terminology to describe the location and position of a structure relative to the rest of the body.
- Identify characteristics relating to the various stages of physical maturity.
- Explain the distinctive qualities of the various types of musculoskeletal tissue.
- Differentiate between elastic and plastic tissue properties.
- Classify injuries as either acute or chronic based on the onset and duration of symptoms.
- Define the common chronic inflammatory conditions, including signs and symptoms.
- Define the various classifications of closed soft tissue wounds, including degrees of severity.
- Define and classify closed and open wounds of the bone and joint articulations.
- Classify nerve injuries according to mechanism, severity, and signs and symptoms.
- Identify the classifications of open (exposed) wounds.

lear communication is fundamental to your clinical practice. Proper reference to anatomical positions, as well as knowledge of injury terminology and mechanisms, is essential for communicating effectively with other health care professionals. This knowledge will help you accurately document the findings of your examinations, convey history information during medical referrals, and collaborate with health care professionals regarding continued care of your patients. This chapter discusses anatomical reference terminology, physical maturity classifications, tissue types and properties, injury forces and mechanisms, and injury classifications. Knowledge in these areas will help you understand many concepts in this text and also help you clearly articulate via oral or written communication your findings and observations to other health care professionals. With few exceptions, these terms and concepts apply consistently to the various joints and body regions.

Anatomical Reference Terminology

All anatomical descriptions and references are based on a standardized position of the body called the anatomical position. The anatomical position allows us to reference specific body regions in relation to the body as a whole and also one anatomical landmark to another (Moore, Dalley, and Aqur 2009). Whenever you refer to a body region or anatomical structure, you should describe it relative to an anatomical reference position. Doing so will help avoid confusion and misinterpretation of your findings. The anatomical position can be specified with the body either standing erect or lying supine ("on the spine"); standing is the most common and easiest to visualize.

To place or visualize someone in standing anatomical position, it is important to start with the person's feet together, flat on the ground, and toes facing forward. The legs and knees are straight and in line with the hips, torso, and head, which are also straight and facing in a forward direction. The upper limbs are positioned at the person's side, with elbows straight, and shoulders are rotated so that the palms face forward. Figure 7.1 illustrates the anatomical position.

Once the patient is either physically placed into or visualized in anatomical position, we can begin to refer to specific structures using various anatomical terms. Table 7.1 lists terms that describe the position of body parts with reference to other parts of the body and to the body as a whole in the anatomical reference position. For example, we can clearly describe the location of the tibial tubercle by indicating that it is anterior on the proximal tibia, just inferior to the patella. The table also includes synonyms that are usually reserved for particular body regions. For example, *anterior* describes structures on or near the front of the body, while *posterior* describes structures on or near the back. The anterior surface of the hands is also commonly referred to as the palmar or ventral surface, while the posterior surface is also referred to as the dorsal aspect, or dorsum, of the hand.

From the anatomical reference position, we can also define three anatomical planes of movement useful in describing postural

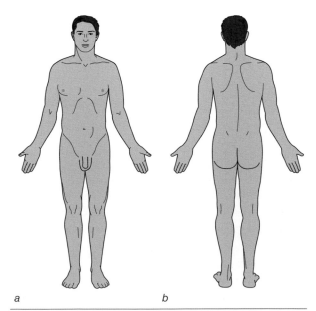

a　　　　　　　　　　b

Figure 7.1　Anatomical position from (a) front and (b) back.

Table 7.1		Anatomical Terms
Term	**Synonyms**	**Term defined**
Anterior	Ventral Palmar	Toward the front of the body
Posterior	Dorsal	Toward the back side of the body
Superior	Cranial Cephalic	Toward the head
Inferior	Caudal	Moving away from the head toward the feet
Medial		Toward the midline of the body
Lateral		Away from the midline of the body
Proximal		Referring to a position or attachment on the body that is closer to the trunk or origin of reference
Distal		Referring to a position or attachment on the body that is farther away from the trunk or origin of reference
Superficial		Nearer to the surface of the skin
Deep		Farther from the surface of the skin
Central		Nearer or closer to the center of a structure or system
Peripheral		Farther away from the center of a structure or system
Visceral		Referring to the covering of an internal organ
Parietal		Referring to the external wall of a body cavity

Adapted from K.L. Moore, 1992, *Clinically oriented anatomy*, 3rd ed. (Baltimore: Williams & Wilkins).

positions, motion, and function of various muscles and joints (figure 7.2). Anatomical planes are imaginary planes that separate the body into left and right (sagittal or median), top and bottom (transverse), and front and back (frontal or coronal). We can describe movement or posture by using the planes that the motion or position occurs in. For example, the motion that occurs when you nod your head "yes," or when you bend (flex) your elbow from the anatomical position, takes place in the sagittal or median plane. Shaking your head "no" or rotating your palm so that it is facing backward from the anatomical position is movement that occurs in the transverse plane, while moving your head so that your ear is closer to your shoulder or lifting your arms out to the side is motion that occurs in the frontal or coronal plane.

Patient positioning terminology is also important and is helpful for understanding starting positions for various medical tests

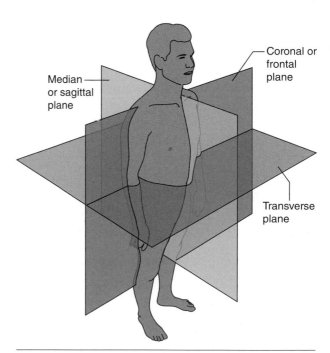

Figure 7.2 Anatomical planes.

Reprinted, by permission, from J. Watkins, 2010, *Structure and function of the musculoskeletal system*, 2nd ed. (Champaign, IL: Human Kinetics), 26.

and procedures. **Supine** and **prone** refer to a patient who is lying down. In prone positioning, the patient lies facedown; in supine positioning, the patient lies face up, or on the spine. The rhyming phrase "supine on the spine" is an easy way to remember these positions. **Short sitting** refers to a sitting position in which the knees and lower legs are hanging off the edge of a table, whereas in **long sitting**, patients have their legs straight out in front of them, as if they were sitting on the floor.

Physical Maturity Classifications

Physical maturity classifications allow us to define stages of physical growth. This standard classification system describes normal anatomic and physiologic development from infancy to older adulthood. These classifications are particularly relevant to this text in that they deal with the maturity and strength of the musculoskeletal system, but they are also used for differentiating physiological findings where appropriate (e.g., normal vital signs for child vs. adult, growth plate vs. bone injury). Physical maturity is defined by the following classifications:

- *Infancy* (0-12 months) is the period when physical changes occur most rapidly. Usually the infant gains three times the birth weight by 12 months and progresses from a totally dependant neonate to a child learning new motor skills such as turning, sitting, crawling, and often walking.
- *Childhood* (1-11 years) spans infancy to the onset of puberty and is characterized by steady growth and development. The skeleton is immature, with the **epiphyseal plates** open to allow bones to elongate. The age range of 1 to 5 years is considered young childhood, and 6 to 11 years is considered middle childhood.
- *Adolescence* (11-13 through 18-20 years) spans the onset of puberty through full skeletal maturity. The onset of puberty is marked by the development of secondary sexual characteristics (pubic hair, **menarche**, and increased breast development in females; pubic hair, deepening voice, and facial and body hair in males) and peak height growth and weight gain (growth spurt). Skeletal maturity is marked by full closure (**ossification**, the formation of bone) of the epiphyseal plates and cessation of further growth in height. The age at which different bones complete ossification differs widely, ranging from the early teens to the early 20s. Because growth and development vary among individuals, it's difficult to give exact age limits. Adolescence begins approximately 2 years earlier in females than in males.

- *Adulthood* (18-40 years) indicates full physical maturity and development. Young adults are those aged 18 to 40 years. In this stage, bone and muscle mass increase through 25 to 30 years of age, after which mass levels off and then slowly declines.
- *Middle adulthood* (40-60 years) is marked by a gradual decline in strength, coordination, and balance.
- *Older adulthood* (greater than 60 years) spans the rest of the human being's life. This stage is marked by accelerating decline in strength, coordination, and balance. However, the degree of decline is highly individual, depending on lifestyle, activity, nutrition, and disease.

Injury Mechanisms

The foundation of body movement is made up of several simple machines that we learned about in middle school. By using levers, pulleys, and wedges among other more complex systems, our bodies are capable of performing very intricate and detailed work along with incredible feats of strength, power, and endurance. However, like other many machines, the "machines" in the body can be influenced by both internal and external mechanical forces that can negatively affect performance. In this section we discuss the different types of tissue in the musculoskeletal system, the physical properties of musculoskeletal tissue, the internal and external mechanical forces that can cause injury to those tissues, and time categories associated with the mechanism of injury to the musculoskeletal system. All of these components are critical to an understanding of injury mechanisms in their entirety.

Musculoskeletal Tissue

The musculoskeletal system consists mainly of five tissue types. They can be classified into soft tissue and skeletal tissue. Soft tissue structures consist of muscles, tendons, ligaments, and cartilage, while skeletal tissue consists of bone. Musculoskeletal injuries can be classified as soft tissue injuries or skeletal injuries and even further classified by exact anatomical structure, location, and extent of injury. Table 7.2 lists descriptions and characteristics of musculoskeletal tissue.

Musculoskeletal Tissue Properties

The degree and location of injury are often determined by tissue strength and the fact that musculoskeletal tissue has elastic and plastic (inelastic) properties that are manifested in response to load or stress. Elastic properties of musculoskeletal tissue are manifested as a response to loading, stress, or mechanical forces that cause stretching or deformation of the tissue; but after the stress is removed, the tissue returns to a relatively normal state. Plastic properties, on the other hand, are manifested at the end range of elastic properties, rendering the tissue unable to return to its normal state. Thus the tissue retains some amount of deformation due to structural injury.

The point at which tissue deformation moves from elastic to plastic is called the yield point and is determined by a specific amount or level of **stress**, called yield stress. Visualize grasping the ends of a small rubber band with your thumbs and index fingers and holding it between your hands. Slowly move your hands apart, stretching the rubber band until you feel resistance, and then return your hands and the rubber band to the starting position. You have just observed the elastic properties of the rubber band. Now move your hands apart much faster and force the rubber band past the resistance point. In doing this you are exploring the upper limits

Table 7.2	Properties of Musculoskeletal Tissue
Tissue type	**Description and characteristics**
Skeletal muscle	Striated contractile tissue composed of multiple individual muscle fibers and myofibrils. Its primary function is to provide stability and mobilize joints through connections to tendons at each end. The proximal portion of the muscle attachment is called the origin, whereas the distal attachment portion is referred to as the insertion.
Tendon	Fibrous tissue connected to bony tissue on one end and to the striated contractile tissue of a muscle on the other. Consists of collagen fibers and fibrocytes. Joined to skeletal muscle at the musculotendinous junction.
Ligament	Fibrous tissue that lends support and stability to joints, muscles, and bones. Ligaments take on various shapes according to their purpose, including, but not limited to, cordlike shapes, bands, fans, or thickened areas of joint capsules.
Cartilage	Firm, essentially nonvascular connective tissue composed of collagen, **chondrocytes**, and ground substance. Three types of cartilage in the musculoskeletal system, **articular cartilage**, **hyaline cartilage**, and **fibrocartilage**, help to increase joint stability, shock absorption, and protection of underlying bone tissue.
Bone	Hard connective tissue that forms the skeletal system. Consists of collagen, ground substance, and minerals in a matrix that provides strength and support. The distal and proximal ends of the bone are covered by articular cartilage, whereas the shafts are covered by the **periosteum**.

Adapted from *Stedman's medical dictionary for the health professions and nursing*, 6th ed. (Philadelphia: Wolters Kluwer/Lippincott, Williams, & Wilkins).

168   Shultz and Brumels

of the elastic properties of your rubber band. If the force or stress is high enough, you may even cause the rubber band to tear or rupture, at which point you have forced it into its plastic property zone. The point at which the rubber band breaks is the yield point, and the yield point is reached if you are able to apply enough **force** (yield stress) to eliminate the possibility of elastic property recovery and cause the rubber band to undergo **plastic deformation**.

Athletic injuries occur much the same way. If the amount of tissue stress, as determined by the amount of mechanical force divided by the total area affected, is low enough that the musculoskeletal tissue remains in the elastic property zone, the patient may incur a relatively minor injury or even none at all. If the stress is high enough to force the tissue into the plastic property zone, the ramifications for injury severity and tissue damage are more significant.

Individuals and individual musculoskeletal tissues have an ability to respond to and resist a certain amount of load or stress before deformation (tissue damage) occurs. This principle is shown in figure 7.3; notice how as the load or stress increases, the potential for tissue deformation also increases. Individual variations in tissue structure play a role in determining where each person's yield point is and where deformation occurs. The type of force applied, along with the surface area acted upon by the force, also affects the injury. Given the same velocity, a localized force can result in substantially greater tissue damage than the same force applied over a broader surface area; but regardless of tissue type and surface area, the chances of deformation increase as stress and load increase.

One of our responsibilities as athletic trainers is to care for, treat, and rehabilitate patients with tissue complaints. Complaints may be the result of a nonpredictable accident or injury, overuse, overload, poor posture, skeletal immaturity, lack of conditioning, improper mechanics, fatigue, inflexibility, muscle imbalance, and genetics. Regardless of the cause, it is important for athletic trainers to understand the physical properties of tissue, the forces that act upon it, and the ways in which it responds to force.

Mechanical Forces

The stress or load applied to the body to cause injury or tissue deformation is a result of one of five types of mechanical force. The mechanical forces of excessive compression, shear, torsion, tension, and bending cause many of the musculoskeletal injuries seen by athletic trainers. The following are definitions of these forces and examples of injuries that they may produce (for illustrations, see figure 7.4).

- *Compression* occurs following a squeezing or condensing of tissue due to external forces that are applied directly opposite each other. These external forces are directed toward each other and cause the tissue in between to compress and thus to increase in density. Examples of compression injuries are bruises (contusions), crushing injuries such as a compression fracture of the cervical spine, pinching, and injuries due to direct impact.

- *Shear* results not from external forces applied directly opposite each other but rather from forces that cause tissue to "slide" over adjoining surfaces or structures in a parallel fashion. Examples of injuries caused by shearing are brain injuries, blisters, lumbar spine injuries such as spondylolisthesis, and tibiofemoral translation injuries such as anterior cruciate ligament (ACL) and posterior cruciate ligament (PCL) sprains.

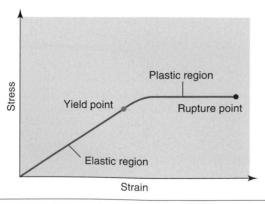

Figure 7.3   Effect of stress and strain on tissue.

- **Torsion** is a twisting mechanism that causes rotation along the long axis or fixed point. Torsion occurs when opposite ends of tissue structures are rotated in opposite directions. Injuries to bones and ligaments that occur following rotation of the body over a fixed foot or lower leg are a result of torsion.

- **Tension** is the stretching or lengthening of musculoskeletal tissue due to stress or strain caused by pulling or drawing apart. Forces involved in tension injuries are pulling in opposite directions, thus causing the tissue in between to stretch. Muscle strains or ruptures are often caused by tension within the **musculotendinous unit**.

- **Bending** is the deformation of tissue into convex and concave shapes due to **axial loading**, forces acting in opposite directions at different ends of tissue, or significant impact to the middle of tissue while the ends

are stable. During the bending mechanism, the convex side of the tissue undergoes tensile forces, while the concave side incurs compressive forces. Fracture of the fibula following a direct blow in sports, as when a player is kicked during a soccer match, is an example of bending force causing injury.

It would be incorrect to think that these mechanical forces act in isolation to cause athletic injuries. In many cases, there are at least two and maybe more forces (combination forces) acting on tissue at one time. For example, let's suppose a football running back is tackled near the lateral side of his knee while his foot is planted. Lateral force moving the knee toward midline in the frontal plane is known as **valgus stress**, whereas **varus stress** moves the knee away from midline in the frontal plane. In the case of the running back, just prior to impact the

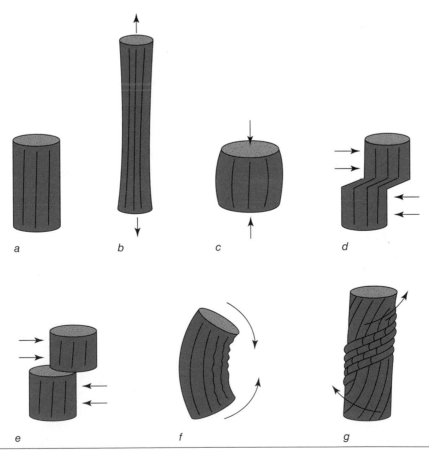

Figure 7.4   Types of load: *(a)* unloaded, *(b)* tension, *(c)* compression, *(d)* shear, *(e)* shear producing friction, *(f)* bending, *(g)* torsion.

Reprinted, by permission, from J. Watkins, 2010, *Structure and function of the musculoskeletal system*, 2nd ed. (Champaign, IL: Human Kinetics), 11.

knee joint undergoes compression due to axial loading of the femur on the tibia. Immediately upon contact from the tackler, tissue compression occurs at the site of impact along the lateral side of the knee; and if the forces from the tackler are great enough, the knee may start to undergo some valgus stress. During the valgus stress, the medial side of the knee takes on a convex shape, placing the medial collateral ligament and joint capsule under tension. The lateral side of the joint becomes concave; and compressive forces are acting between the articulating surfaces of the tibia, femur, and lateral meniscus. If the force generating the valgus stress is great enough to cause the joint capsule and medial collateral ligament to undergo plastic deformation, the knee becomes unstable. Tension and shear forces are transferred to the ACL and other structures due to the momentum of the runner, the external force of the tackler, and ground forces since the runner's foot is planted. The shear and tension forces could potentially cause injury to the ACL; meniscus; articular cartilage; and possibly other musculoskeletal knee tissue, vascular, or nervous tissue structures.

As we can see, there are complex mechanisms and forces that come together to cause musculoskeletal tissue injury. It is important for us as athletic trainers to understand the mechanical forces associated with these injuries and recognize how they may affect the tissue of the musculoskeletal system.

Time Classification Relating to Mechanism of Injury

You should now have a better understanding of musculoskeletal tissue and the mechanical forces that cause injuries to that tissue. The next topic we need to discuss is how and when these forces create tissue injury. The mechanism of injury (injury mechanism) refers to the means by which musculoskeletal tissue is injured. Bonfiglio and colleagues (1998) have described four mechanisms of injury initiation: blunt force trauma, dynamic overload, overuse, and repetitive or cumulative trauma. These mechanisms

have been further categorized into acute and chronic, according to the time needed to produce the associated tissue trauma. The following sections explain these concepts.

• *Acute injuries* are conditions that have a sudden onset, have a shortened duration, and occur via an episode of mechanical force that instantly exceeds the elastic properties of the tissue at a specific time and place and causes tissue deformations. They typically result from a single traumatic event or mechanism such as blunt force trauma or dynamic overload of muscle, tendon, joint capsule, or ligamentous tissue. Usually, the patient knows and clearly recalls the mechanism of injury, as the signs and symptoms associated with the injury typically arise immediately. Examples of acute injuries are dislocating the wrist in a fall, spraining the ankle during a basketball game, and suffering a fracture of the tibia during a tackle in American football.

• *Chronic injuries*, on the other hand, usually have a gradual onset, have a prolonged duration, and occur as a result of an accumulation of minor insults or repetitive stresses that would not be sufficient to cause injury if they occurred in isolation. Often the exact mechanism or time of injury is not known. Overuse, accumulative **microtrauma**, repetitive overloading, or abnormal friction at a rate greater than the body's ability to heal and recover before the application of additional stress causes the tissue to undergo the plastic property deformation associated with injury. These injuries may also be referred to as overuse injuries.

Chronic or overuse injury can also occur following periods of inadequate rest, recovery, or training and may be related to doing "too much, too soon, too often"; in these cases, injury is caused by submaximal stresses and loads that were previously tolerable. Chronic injuries are often more difficult to treat than acute injuries, as the longer the pathologic state continues, the longer it takes for healing to occur and symptoms to subside. Common inflammatory conditions are listed in table 7.3.

Table 7.3	Common Chronic Inflammatory Conditions	
Condition	**Description**	**Signs and symptoms**
Apophysitis	Inflammation of a bony projection or outgrowth that serves as a muscle attachment	Pain, tenderness, swelling, increased bony prominence, pain with muscle tension
Bursitis	Inflammation or swelling of a bursa (synovial-filled membrane that lies between adjacent structures to limit friction and ease movement)	Pain, redness, heat, palpable fluid accumulation, crepitus or fluid thickening or both
Capsulitis	Inflammation of a joint capsule	Pain, localized joint inflammation and swelling, decreased range of motion
Myositis	Inflammatory response in a muscle or its surrounding connective tissue; can lead to ossification	Pain, inflammation, tenderness, decreased range of motion; possible calcium deposit
Neuritis	Inflammation or irritation of a nerve or nerve sheath	Local and referred pain, pain with percussion, tenderness, impaired sensation and motor function
Periostitis	Inflammation of the membranous lining of a bone	Pain, palpable swelling or "bumpiness" and tenderness along the bone; pain with attaching muscle action
Tendinitis	Inflammation of a tendon attaching muscle to bone	Pain, swelling, palpable tenderness and crepitus; pain with active and resistive muscle action
Tendinosis	Microscopic tearing and degeneration of tendinous tissue from repetitive trauma	Chronic pain, palpable tenderness, decreased range of motion, pain with passive stretch, pain and weakness with active and resistive muscle action
Tenosynovitis	Inflammation of the synovial sheath covering a tendon	Pain with palpation and movement of the tendon within the sheath; swelling or thickening, snowball crepitus, and decreased range of motion

Injury Classifications

To this point, we have discussed the importance of proper and appropriate use of medical terminology for record keeping, referral procedures, and continued communication about care among health care professionals. We have considered anatomical reference terminology, tissue types, properties of musculoskeletal tissue, mechanical forces, and injury mechanisms. Athletic trainers also need to understand injury classifications used to describe types of injuries. Athletic trainers classify injuries based on observation and communication as they look for and observe signs and listen to patients' characterization of their symptoms. A **sign** is a finding that is observable or that can be objectively measured, such as swelling, discoloration, deformity, **crepitus**, or redness. A **symptom** is a subjective complaint or an abnormal sensation the patient describes that cannot be directly observed. Complaints or perceptions of pain, nausea, altered sensa-

tion, and fatigue are symptoms that patients commonly report. A later chapter in this book provides more detailed information to help you improve your ability to observe signs and symptoms; but at this point, learning the major injury classifications will enhance your ability to communicate as a health care professional.

Closed (Unexposed) Wounds

Closed wounds include any injury that does not disrupt the surface of the skin. Although closed wounds are not always visually obvious, most result in noticeable signs (e.g., swelling, discoloration, and deformity) that aid in injury examination. Common examples of closed wounds include contusions, ligament sprains, muscle and tendon strains, inflammatory conditions, some bony fractures, joint dislocations, and neurovascular injuries. Closed injuries to soft tissue can occur as contusions, sprains, or strains. These types of soft tissue injuries are further classified according to the degree of severity or the extent of injury. Let's take a closer look at closed injuries to soft tissue.

Contusion

A contusion, or bruise, is characterized by the compression of soft tissue due to a direct blow or impact sufficient to cause disruption or damage to the small capillaries in the tissue. This trauma causes local bleeding or hemorrhage, resulting in ecchymosis, or discoloration of the tissue. There will also be localized pain and tenderness. Ecchymosis and swelling may occur immediately or may be delayed, depending on the severity of injury. The severity of a contusion can be described as first degree, second degree, or third degree, usually according to the extent of tissue damage and functional impairment.

- *First degree.* A first-degree contusion involves only superficial tissue damage, causing minimal swelling and localized tenderness and no limitations in strength or range of motion.

- *Second degree.* A second-degree contusion is characterized by increased pain and hemorrhage caused by increased area and depth of tissue damage, resulting in mild to moderate limitations in range of motion, muscle function, or both.

- *Third degree.* A third-degree contusion is a severe tissue compression, resulting in severe pain, significant hemorrhage, and **hematoma** formation. In addition, these severe injuries may cause significant limitations in range of motion and muscle function. With third-degree contusions, you should strongly suspect that deeper structures (e.g., bone, muscle) may also have been damaged but that such damage may be masked by the signs and symptoms associated with superficial soft tissue damage.

Sprain

A sprain is an injury to a ligament or capsular structure. Because ligaments attach one bone to another, sprains are associated with joint injury. Sprains result from forces that cause two or more connecting bones to separate or go beyond their normal range of motion, subsequently stretching and tearing the attaching ligament(s) or capsule. To describe the severity or extent of injury, a sprain is further classified as first degree, second degree, or third degree.

- *First degree.* A first-degree sprain is characterized by mild overstretching and does not cause any visual disruption in the tissue. Signs and symptoms include mild pain and tenderness over the involved ligament and little or no disability. Active and passive ranges of motion are usually not limited in first-degree sprains, but the patient typically experiences pain at the end of the range as the ligament becomes taut. When the joint is stressed, the patient will complain of pain, but you will notice a firm or definite **end feel**, without any joint laxity. With first-degree sprains, inflammation and discoloration are usually minor and may be delayed until the next day. However, in some body regions, such as the lateral ankle, a relatively minor sprain can cause considerable and rapid swelling if a major capillary running adjacent to the ligament is disrupted. In other words, the degree of swelling and discoloration is not always a good indication of injury severity.

- *Second degree.* With a second-degree injury, further stretching and partial disruption or macrotearing of the ligament occur. Second-degree injuries represent the broadest range of injury; therefore the severity of signs and symptoms and disability vary considerably. Signs and symptoms range from moderate to severe pain, point tenderness, ecchymosis, and swelling. Range of motion and normal function are usually limited secondary to pain and swelling. **Stress testing** will show varying degrees of joint **instability** or **laxity**, but the ligament is still sufficiently intact that you can feel an end point where joint motion ceases.

- *Third degree.* A third-degree sprain is characterized by complete disruption (rupture) or loss of ligament integrity. The patient may have felt or heard a "pop" at the time of injury. Signs and symptoms include immediate pain and disability, rapid swelling, ecchymosis, and loss of function. Stress testing of the ligament will reveal moderate to severe joint instability, and there will be no firm end feel or end point to joint motion. Third-degree injuries can be initially deceiving in that range of motion and stress testing are typically less painful than with second-degree injuries, since no tension is placed on the injured structure if it is completely torn.

Strain

Whereas sprains involve stretching or tearing of a ligament, strains involve stretching or tearing of a muscle or tendon. Muscle and tendon strains occur most often as a result of a violent, forceful contraction or overstretching of the myotendon unit. Fatigue, lack of proper warm-up, **muscle strength imbalance**, and **dyssynchrony** are common predisposing factors. Similar to sprains, strains are classified by severity as first-degree, second-degree, and third-degree injuries.

• *First degree.* A first-degree strain is characterized by overstretching and microtearing of the muscle or tendon, but there is no gross fiber disruption. The patient complains of mild pain and tenderness but typically has full active and passive range of motion and little or no disability. Pain usually accompanies resisted muscle contraction. Following a first-degree strain, it is not uncommon for an individual to continue to practice or compete, as pain and tenderness are often delayed until the next day.

• *Second degree.* Second-degree strains involve further stretching and partial tearing of muscle or tendon fibers. As with sprains, second-degree strains represent the broadest range of injury, and signs and symptoms can vary considerably. These include immediate pain, localized tenderness, and disability. Varying degrees of swelling, ecchymosis, decreased range of motion, and decreased strength are also present. The patient will complain of pain with active muscle contraction and passive muscle stretch. Depending on injury severity, there may or may not be a **palpable** defect.

• *Third degree.* In third-degree strains, a muscle or tendon is completely ruptured. Signs and symptoms include an audible pop, immediate pain, and loss of function of the myotendon unit. Superficial muscles exhibit a palpable defect. Muscle hemorrhage and diffuse swelling are present. Depending on the function or the contribution of the injured muscle or tendon to a given movement, range of motion and strength may or may not be affected and may or may not be painful.

Open (Exposed) Wounds

Open, or exposed, wounds are injuries that involve a disruption in the continuity of the skin, caused by friction or by blunt or sharp trauma. The classifications for open wounds are listed in table 7.4.

There are several types of soft tissue open wounds, and recognition is important in evaluating and caring for them. Open, or exposed, wounds are also susceptible to infection and should be monitored for signs and symptoms of pus, increased pain, redness, swelling, heat, and red streaks running from the wound toward the trunk. If signs or symptoms of infection are present, the patient should be referred for medical treatment and possible antibiotic therapy.

• *Abrasion.* An abrasion, or "strawberry," is particularly painful because of the large surface area that is exposed. Abrasions most commonly occur in soccer, baseball, and softball as a result of sliding. Floor burns are also abrasions, a consequence of sliding or of friction against a wooden floor as commonly occurs in basketball and volleyball. The use of knee pads in such sports is effective in preventing these minor but painful superficial skin wounds. Signs and symptoms include a burning or stinging pain and minimal bleeding. It is important to cleanse these wounds thoroughly, making sure to remove all the dirt and debris to avoid infection.

• *Blister.* A blister—common in people of all levels of activity—is an area of skin that

Table 7.4   Classification of Open (Exposed) Wounds

Classification	Description
Abrasion	Broad scraping or shearing off of the superficial skin layers with sliding of the skin against a rough or high-friction surface.
Blister	Separation and accumulation of fluid or blood between superficial skin layers secondary to repetitive friction or shearing movements.
Incision	A cut through all layers of the skin by a sharp object or instrument (e.g., knife), resulting in smooth, even wound edges.
Laceration	A tearing of the skin by blunt trauma to the skin over a bony prominence, resulting in jagged, uneven wound edges.
Puncture wound	A small disruption in the skin, caused by a sharp, penetrating object. Puncture wounds should be carefully examined for possible injury to underlying structures.
Avulsion	A tearing off or complete disassociation of a portion of skin.
Compound fracture or dislocation	Disruption in the skin surface secondary to penetration by a displaced fracture fragment or joint dislocation.

is exposed to excessive friction or rubbing. Friction from new or ill-fitting shoes in the heel or toe region is a common cause of blisters in physically active people. Gymnasts and baseball and softball players commonly get blisters on the hands as a consequence of repetitive friction and rubbing between the hands and the bar or bat. Signs and symptoms include pain, redness, and accumulation of fluid (may be clear, serous, or blood filled) between the superficial skin layers. Although the injury the blister creates is usually minor, the pain can be extremely limiting. It is important to avoid puncturing or removing the superficial skin layer, as pain and chance of infection are often significantly increased with exposure of the deeper tissue layers. Early examination and recognition of "hot spots" on the skin showing areas of friction, as well as the use of proper padding, can help prevent a blister from forming.

• *Incision.* An incision is usually caused by a knife or sharp object that makes a clean cut through the full thickness of the skin. Signs and symptoms include an observable disruption in the skin, possible separation or gapping of the wound edges if the skin is under tension, immediate bleeding, and minimal pain. Even small incisions in areas that are highly vascularized, such as the face,

can cause considerable bleeding initially, although such bleeding can be quickly controlled with direct pressure.

• *Laceration.* A laceration differs from an incision in that the cause is a blunt, rather than a sharp, trauma. With a laceration, the skin basically ruptures when a blunt force is exerted against a bony prominence. An elbow hitting an opponent's cheek during a rebound, a ball striking the eyebrow region, and a blocker making contact with an opponent's chin are common mechanisms for lacerations. Signs and symptoms are consistent with those of an incision except that because the tissue is torn rather than cut, the wound edges are more jagged, and the blunt force may result in greater pain.

• *Puncture wound.* A puncture wound can result when a pointed, sharp object penetrates the skin. These injuries can be deceiving in that there seems to be little observable tissue damage, and bleeding is often minimal. Evaluating and caring for puncture wounds should involve two primary concerns. If the depth of penetration is beyond the thickness of the skin layers, deeper structures that are not visible may be injured or damaged. In addition, puncture wounds are particularly susceptible to infection because they are difficult to clean given the limited exposure of the involved tissue.

• *Avulsion.* An avulsion is characterized by the complete tearing away of a portion of skin. The range of severity and signs and symptoms can be great, depending on the structures involved and the amount of tissue damage. A simple skin avulsion, the most common type, typically results when the skin is either caught on an unyielding object or pinched between two objects. Depending on the mechanism and the offending trauma, underlying tissues such as muscle, tendon, bone, and even an entire limb (amputation) can be torn away along with the skin, but these severe injuries rarely result from trauma incurred during physical activity.

• *Compound fracture or dislocation.* Compound fractures or dislocations occur when a displaced fracture or joint penetrates the surface of the skin so that the bone or joint is exposed. Compound fractures and dislocations are most common in the fingers but can occur with any joint dislocation or displaced long bone fracture.

Bone and Joint Injuries

The general classifications of closed wounds involving disruptions in a bone, joint surface, or joint **articulation** include fractures, dislocations, and subluxations.

Closed Fractures

Simple, or closed, fractures involve disruption in the continuity of a bone without disruption of the skin surface. Traumatic fractures are caused by direct impact or by an indirect force that exceeds the tensile strength of the bone. The direction of force or impact often dictates the type of fracture that results. Repetitive forces or impact at lower applied loads can also cause chronic weakening or failure of bone tissue, resulting in a stress fracture. Table 7.5 presents the common classifications of closed fractures.

• *Traumatic (acute) fractures.* Signs and symptoms of a traumatic fracture include immediate pain, rapid swelling, bony tenderness, crepitus with movement of the bony fragments, and possible deformity if the fracture is displaced. False joint movement may also occur when the fracture is near a movable joint. With displaced fractures (misalignment of the bony fragments), there is always a danger of secondary injury (compression or tearing) to the surrounding soft tissue and neurovascular structures. Therefore, the examination process should always include determination of neurovascular status distal to the suspected fracture site.

• *Stress fractures.* Signs and symptoms of stress fractures are not usually quite so obvious, and often the patient initially dismisses them. The onset of pain is often gradual, but may appear suddenly once bone failure occurs. Pain or a deep ache may at first be noticeable only during activity and may subside with rest, progressing to more constant pain if the offending activity continues. Swelling is minimal, and localized tenderness is present over the fracture site.

Epiphyseal Injury

Epiphyseal injury or fracture involves the disruption or separation of the epiphysis or epiphyseal plate (growth plate). Epiphyseal injury is a concern in children and in adolescents before the cessation of growth, as disruption can cause premature closing and growth abnormalities in the involved bone. The most widely accepted classification system is the Salter-Harris classification system (Harris 1983) (see table 7.6). Signs and symptoms are consistent with those previously mentioned for closed fractures.

Dislocation

Joint dislocation, or luxation, is a complete disassociation of two joint surfaces. Joint dislocation most commonly results from forces that cause the joint to exceed its normal range of motion, forcing the bony articulation to separate. Consequently, joint dislocation usually involves severe stretching or complete disruption of the capsule and one or more of the supporting ligaments (third-degree sprain). Signs and symptoms include immediate pain, rapid swelling, deformity, and loss of function.

Table 7.5 Classification of Closed Fractures

Classification	Illustration	Description
Comminuted		Fracture resulting in multiple fragments or shattering of the bone at the site of injury.
Compression		Failure of the bone and subsequent compression or impaction of the fracture ends due to axial compression forces.
Greenstick		Incomplete fracture through the bone, most often occurring in young bones. Resembles the breaking of a "green stick."
Oblique		The fracture line extends obliquely or diagonally in relation to the long axis of the bone.
Spiral		An S-shaped fracture line twists around and through the bone due to rotation or torsional forces.
Transverse		The fracture line runs transverse or horizontal to the long axis of the bone. Usually caused by direct lateral impact or stress failure.
Avulsion		The pulling away of a piece of bone secondary to tensioning of an attaching ligament, tendon, or muscle.
Osteochondral		A fracture that extends through the articular cartilage (i.e., joint surface) and into the underlying bone.
Stress or "fatigue"		Complete or incomplete failure of a bone due to repetitive stress or loading. Weakening and failure occur when bone breakdown or absorption exceeds bone production.

Table 7.6 Salter-Harris Classifications of Epiphyseal Fractures

Classification	Illustration	Description
Type I		Complete separation of the epiphyseal plate (epiphysis from the metaphysis). No associated fracture.
Type II		Separation of the epiphysis with associated fracture of the metaphysis.
Type III		Fracture of the epiphysis extending from the epiphyseal plate through the articular surface.
Type IV		Fracture extending through the epiphysis, epiphyseal plate, and metaphysis.
Type V		Crushing or compression of the epiphyseal plate. This injury has a high incidence of premature closure.

Descriptions adapted from R.B. Salter, 1999, *Textbook of disorders and injuries of the musculoskeletal system,* 3rd ed. (Philadelphia, PA: Lippincott, Wilkins & Wilkins).

As with displaced fractures, signs and symptoms associated with neurovascular impairment (impingement or tearing) may also be present and should be monitored. In some instances, dislocation may not be obvious if the joint spontaneously reduces immediately following the injury. In the case of a spontaneous reduction, the patient may complain of a feeling of the joint slipping or "giving out," or a sensation of the joint "going out and coming back in." Chronic joint instability often follows an acute dislocation, precipitating recurrent episodes of dislocation or subluxation (see the next section) at lower forces and applied loads. This is particularly true of the patellofemoral, glenohumeral, and phalangeal joints.

Subluxation

Subluxation of a joint is an incomplete disassociation of two joint surfaces. Depending on the degree of subluxation, these injuries widely vary in signs and symptoms of pain, disability, swelling, and joint instability. Often, subluxations are difficult to identify, as deformity may be minimal and they often spontaneously reduce. History becomes important for identifying these injuries, and the patient may complain of a sensation of the joint's slipping or momentarily giving out at the time of injury.

Nerve Injuries

Nerve injury can result from compression or tensioning of the neural structure. Nervous tissue is very sensitive to compression and **ischemia**, and injury may occur secondary to a direct blow, acute swelling of tissue within an enclosed space, or any pathology that compromises the space through which the nerve courses. Laceration of the nerve can occur secondary to fracture, dislocation, penetrating trauma, or excessive tensioning or stretch. Signs and symptoms of pain, sensation, and motor function can vary considerably depending on the extent of nerve injury. Sensory impairment can range from anesthesia (no sensation) to paresthesia (tingling, burning, or numbness) to hyperes-thesia (hypersensitivity), and motor function can range from no loss in muscle strength or function to weakness to complete loss of muscle function (paralysis).

Classifications for the extent of nerve disruptions include neuropraxia, axonotmesis, and neurotmesis.

- *Neuropraxia.* The least severe nerve disruption is a neuropraxia, a transient and reversible loss in nerve function secondary to trauma or irritation. Neuropraxia entails mechanical deformation of the nerve but no disruption of the nerve fibers. Signs and symptoms of sensory and motor deficits are short-lived, ranging from a few seconds to 2 weeks depending on the extent of nerve trauma. A direct blow over the peroneal nerve at the proximal fibular head or the ulnar nerve at the medial elbow is a common mechanism for a neuropraxia.

- *Axonotmesis.* Axonotmesis denotes a partial disruption in the nerve. With an axonotmesis, sufficient nervous tissue is intact to allow eventual regeneration. However, signs and symptoms of sensory and motor deficits are prolonged, lasting anywhere from 2 weeks to up to 1 year, so that considerable atrophy and weakness may result.

- *Neurotmesis.* Neurotmesis, the most severe nerve injury, is characterized by complete severance of the nerve, resulting in permanent loss of function of the innervated structures distal to the point of injury. With a neurotmesis, no regeneration is evident 1 year after the injury.

Other terms used to refer to nerve pathology are neuralgia and neuroma.

- *Neuralgia.* Neuralgia is an achiness or pain along the distribution of a nerve secondary to chronic irritation or inflammation. Neuralgia is a common symptom in nerve compression syndromes such as tarsal tunnel syndrome, ulnar nerve compression, carpal tunnel syndrome, and disc herniation. These syndromes are discussed later in this text.

- *Neuroma.* A neuroma is a thickening of a nerve, or "nerve tumor," secondary to chronic irritation or inflammation.

Soft Tissue Wounds With Associated Bone or Joint Injury

Open wounds may be associated with an underlying (unexposed) injury. Paying careful attention to the mechanism by which the injury occurred, as well as to signs and symptoms that may be in addition to or out of proportion with what you would expect of the open wound, is important to evaluating these injuries. An obvious example is a compound fracture or compound dislocation. Crushing injuries that compress the soft tissue against the underlying bone and deeper tissue are another example of an open wound with an associated unexposed tissue injury.

Learning Aids

SUMMARY

Understanding anatomical reference terminology is an essential skill for effective communication between health care professionals. Standard medical terminology has been developed to aid communication between health care professionals of varying specialties. Being able to use a "common language" allows for dissemination of knowledge for both academic study and patient care. Understanding anatomical position and the more common anatomical terms goes a long way toward helping athletic trainers learn to describe location of injuries and pathologies. In addition, knowledge about basic injury mechanisms and classifications facilitates the ability to understand and recognize the various injuries and pathologies that are presented for examination. Appreciating the types of injuries that occur due to the various injury mechanisms and then applying that knowledge to the various anatomical nuances and structures within the human body will make your examination, recognition, management, and rehabilitation more effective.

KEY CONCEPTS AND REVIEW

▸ **Describe the anatomical reference position.**

In the anatomical reference position, the body stands erect or lies supine, with the head, eyes, and trunk facing forward; the arms at the sides and palms facing forward; and the legs straight and together with the feet pointing forward.

▸ **Use appropriate anatomical terminology to describe the location and position of a structure relative to the rest of the body.**

A variety of terms describe the position and location of a body part. To define the position of a body part in relation to the body as a whole, positional terms such as anterior, posterior, superior, and inferior are used. To compare the position of one body part to another, terms such as lateral, medial, proximal, and distal are used. The use of these universally acceptable terms will help you communicate the findings of your examination to other health care professionals.

▸ **Identify characteristics relating to the various stages of physical maturity.**

- Infancy (0-12 months) is characterized by rapid physical changes, significant increase in percentage of body weight, the beginning of learning motor skills, and using major muscle groups.
- Childhood (1-11 years) is characterized by steady growth and development. The skeleton system allows for continued growth. Motor skill refinement is observed along with the learning of fine motor skills.
- Adolescence (11-13 through 18-20 years) is characterized by continued skeletal development along with the

development of secondary sexual characteristics and peak height growth and weight gain (growth spurt).

- Adulthood (18-40 years) indicates full physical maturity and development with skeletal maturity occurring during the earlier stages of this age range.
- Middle adulthood (40-60 years) is marked by a gradual decline in strength, coordination, and balance.
- Older adulthood (greater than 60 years) is marked by accelerating decline in strength, coordination, and balance.

▶ **Explain the distinctive qualities of the various types of musculoskeletal tissue.**

- Skeletal muscle is striated and is made up of individual muscle fibers and myofibrils. It provides stability and helps to mobilize joints.
- Tendons are fibrous tissue, which connect bones to muscles.
- Ligaments are fibrous tissue, which connect bones to other bones.
- Cartilage is nonvascular connective tissue that increases joint stability, shock absorption, and protection of underlying bone tissue.
- Bone is hard connective tissue that forms the skeletal system and provides strength and support.

Table 7.2 (p. 167) summarizes this information.

▶ **Differentiate between elastic and plastic tissue properties.**

Elastic properties of musculoskeletal tissue are manifested as a response to loading, stress, or mechanical forces, causing stretch or deformation of the tissue; after the stress is removed, the tissue returns to a relatively normal state. Plastic properties, on the other hand, are manifested at the end range of elastic properties, rendering the tissue unable to return to its normal state. Thus the tissue retains some amount of deformation due to structural injury.

▶ **Classify injuries as either acute or chronic based on the onset and duration of symptoms.**

Injuries are classified as either acute or chronic. Acute injuries have a known mechanism and sudden onset; signs and symptoms usually surface immediately or shortly after the injury. Chronic injuries have a gradual onset and long duration. Often the person does not recall a specific mechanism of injury, and injury results from a repetitive stress over time.

▶ **Define the common chronic inflammatory conditions, including signs and symptoms.**

Chronic inflammatory conditions can result from repetitive overuse, mechanical loading, and friction. A variety of tissues are susceptible to chronic inflammation, including bone, bursa, capsule, muscle, and tendon. Terms used to describe inflammatory conditions of various structures contain the suffix "itis"—for example, bursitis (inflammation of the bursa) and tendinitis (inflammation of the tendon).

▶ **Define the various classifications of closed soft tissue wounds, including degrees of severity.**

Closed soft tissue wounds are generally classified as contusions (soft tissue compression), strains (stretching or tearing of muscle or tendon), and sprains (stretching or tearing of ligament). They are further classified by severity as first, second, or third degree. First-degree injuries, the least severe, are characterized by minimal pain and tissue disruption and no loss of function. Second-degree injuries are injuries with moderate or partial tissue disruption. The signs, symptoms, and functional impairment associated with second-degree injuries can vary considerably, depending on the extent of tissue disruption. Third-degree injuries are the most severe; these are characterized by complete tissue disruption and severe functional impairment.

▶ **Define and classify closed and open wounds of the bone and joint articulations.**

Injuries involving the bone or joint articulation include fractures and dislocations. A fracture occurs when the continuity of a bone is disrupted. Fractures are typically classified by the type, location, and extent of bony disruption, which is often dictated by the impact mechanism. When disassociation of two articular surfaces of a joint occurs, the injury is classified as either a dislocation (complete disassociation) or subluxation (partial disassociation), and is often accompanied by varying degrees of disruption in the supporting ligaments. Fractures or dislocations can be classified as open (compound) or closed wounds, depending on whether the displaced bone or joint segment penetrates the surface of the skin.

▶ **Classify nerve injuries according to mechanism, severity, and signs and symptoms.**

Nerve injury can result from either compressive or tensioning forces imposed on nerve tissues. Classifications for the extent of nerve disruption include neuropraxia, axonotmesis, and neurotmesis. Terms used to refer to more chronic nerve pathologies include neuralgia and neuroma. When an injury involves the nerve, transient or permanent alterations in sensation and motor function are present, with signs and symptoms varying widely depending on the extent of injury.

▶ **Identify the classifications of open (exposed) wounds.**

Open wounds, or injuries that disrupt the continuity of the skin, are classified by the type of tissue disruption. Because the wound is exposed, athletic trainers must use proper precautions when examining and treating these injuries and should always closely monitor the wound for signs of infection.

PRACTICE!

For hands-on practice in this area, go to the web resource and complete the following:

Level 1.3, Module B6: Basic Health Care Nomenclature

CRITICAL THINKING QUESTIONS

1. A friend has come to you asking for your help. He was riding his dirt bike and wrecked on a downhill curve. Explain the types of tissue injury that you suspect he might have.

2. You are working with a new coach of the soccer team in your community. In the past, the team, one of 10 in the conference, has been in second and third place. The coach wants to move the team to first place. Over the initial month and a half of team workouts, five of the 20 players have reported to you with "shin pain" and "knee pain." Both problems seem to have been caused by repetitive drills that the coach uses all the time. Explain how too many repetitions of a drill could cause injury.

Principles of Examination

Sandra J. Shultz, PhD, ATC, CSCS, FNATA
Kirk Brumels, PhD, AT, ATC

OBJECTIVES

After reading this chapter, the student should be able to do the following:

- Explain the difference between the primary survey and the secondary survey in the evaluation of an injured person.
- List the main steps in performing a complete on-site examination.
- List the main steps in performing a complete acute injury examination.
- Explain the term "SINS" as used in acute and clinical examinations.
- Explain the difference between the subjective and the objective segments of the examination.
- List the elements one should include in the objective component of the clinical examination.
- Explain the importance of documenting an examination.

njuries that require medical attention are relatively common among people who are active in their job or who participate in sports. No matter how much attention is given to the prevention of injuries, athletic trainers often need to address injury complaints; it is critical that they understand the nuances of performing a complete and thorough examination. An accurate working diagnosis facilitates appropriate referrals and proper care of injuries. This chapter discusses the components of examinations and the requirements that athletic trainers must fulfill as they examine injuries over the course of their careers as health care professionals.

Examination Components

Before clinicians can make a diagnosis, they must thoroughly examine the injury by sequentially performing tasks involved in specific examination components. The necessity of these components is dictated by the location and timing of the examination. Injury examinations occur in three different environments: on the field (on-site), on the sideline (acute), and in the athletic training facility (clinical). Each environment demands a different examination, but all examinations should begin with an evaluation to eliminate any critical or life-threatening concerns. This process is called the injury survey. The injury survey is divided into two components, the primary and the secondary surveys.

Primary Survey

A primary survey determines the status of life-threatening or limb-threatening conditions using the "ABCs" of emergency medical care: examination of Airway, Breathing, and Circulation. Your first goal is to tend to life-threatening conditions by examining the patient's airway, breathing, and circulation for respirations and pulse. Evaluation of other vital signs and checking for severe bleeding should also occur at this time. Depending on the results of the primary

survey, you will either tend to the emergency conditions or move on to the secondary survey. Chapters 13 and 14 provide information on rendering care in acute and emergency situations.

Secondary Survey

The remainder of this chapter introduces the elements of the injury examination that begins when you have completed and acted in accordance with the findings of your primary injury survey. The secondary injury survey takes place when the injured individual is breathing and you have any bleeding under control. It is at this time that you perform an examination to determine the presence of other injuries. The term *secondary* indicates that the primary survey either has been concluded or been deemed unnecessary. A secondary survey is a rapid examination of the seriousness of the injury, and the conclusions you formulate determine how you should remove the patient from the injury site. A secondary survey and an on-site secondary evaluation are essentially the same, with the primary goal of determining the nature of the injury or illness and identifying positive

WHEN TO REFER FOR FURTHER EVALUATION (EMERGENCY ROOM OR PHYSICIAN)

Refer the patient when any of the following occurs:

- The patient fails to regain consciousness within a few minutes.
- You cannot determine the cause of unconsciousness, even if consciousness is regained.
- You observe any abnormal vital signs.
- You note any signs of serious or limb-threatening or life-threatening injury or illness.

signs that will help you make decisions about referral (see the sidebar When to Refer for Further Evaluation [Emergency Room or Physician]) and emergency care or first aid.

Use figure 8.1 to guide your primary and secondary on-site examinations when you encounter an unconscious patient.

On-Site Examination

On-site examinations are performed when the patient cannot continue full participation during an athletic practice or competition or while performing his job. You may examine the patient on an outdoor field, cross country

---

Primary Survey

As with any emergency situation, you should begin your examination with a primary survey:

- ☐ Attempt to arouse patient; call name
- ☐ Check airway (cervical spine precautions)
- ☐ Check breathing (look, listen, feel)
- ☐ Check circulation

Secondary Survey

If you rule out the need to call emergency medical services, you may proceed to your secondary survey:

History

Try to obtain from bystanders or the surroundings as much information as possible about the following:

- ☐ The cause (trauma or no apparent trauma)
- ☐ Whether loss of consciousness was gradual or rapid in onset
- ☐ Duration of unconsciousness
- ☐ Level of consciousness or behavior prior to loss of consciousness
- ☐ Any complaints made by the patient prior to losing consciousness
- ☐ Any medical history that might have contributed to the loss of consciousness

Observation and Inspection

- ☐ Note position of head, neck, and extremities for deformities
- ☐ Note any unusual body posturing (decerebrate or decorticate rigidity)
- ☐ Note presence of seizure and take appropriate action to protect the patient
- ☐ Determine presence of and note any irregularities in rate, depth, and rhythm of respirations
- ☐ Inspect skin for temperature, color, and moisture
- ☐ Check pupils for size, equality, and reaction to light
- ☐ Check mouth for bleeding (seizures) or unusual odors (diabetes)
- ☐ Inspect for swelling, deformity, or discoloration around the head, neck, or scalp

- ☐ Inspect for otorrhea and rhinorrhea
- ☐ Inspect for swelling, deformity, or discoloration of the chest wall, trunk, and abdomen
- ☐ Inspect for swelling, deformity, or discoloration of the extremities

Palpation

- ☐ Determine presence, rate, and strength of pulse
- ☐ Record blood pressure
- ☐ Palpate head, neck, and scalp for deformity, crepitus, and swelling
- ☐ Palpate chest, trunk, and extremities for deformity, crepitus, and swelling
- ☐ Palpate abdomen for distension and muscle rigidity

Determine Level of Unconsciousness (Glasgow Coma Scale)

Determine whether the patient exhibits any of the following:

- ☐ Drowsiness (individual is aroused by verbal stimuli)
- ☐ Stupor (individual is aroused by painful stimuli such as a pinch to the trapezius or inner arm or thigh)
- ☐ Coma (no response to any stimulus, verbal or painful)

Referral If Necessary

Figure 8.1   Checklist for the examination of an unconscious patient.

course, or indoor floor or in a warehouse, a construction site, or any other work location. Before performing an on-site examination, put in place an emergency plan for managing and transporting the patient based on your findings from the secondary injury survey. Such plans are beyond the scope of this chapter, but whatever the emergency care plan, instruct all participants and coaching staff or coworkers not to move the patient before you have attended to her. Instruct anyone who suffers a significant injury to remain still until adequately examined.

When caring for participants in game situations, you should know the rules regarding on-site examination for each sport for which health care coverage is provided. Many sports have specific rules for injuries. Some sports won't allow you onto the field or court until the official has beckoned you, and other sports have very specific time frames within which a decision for care must be made before the team or patient is penalized (charged with a time-out, removed from play, or disqualified). While such rules should never compromise your care of and attention to the patient, knowing them will help you avoid unnecessary conflicts.

Goals and Purposes

Use on-site examinations to rule out life-threatening and serious injuries, determine the severity of the injury, and ascertain the most appropriate method of transporting the patient or worker from the scene. Your goals are to perform a quick, accurate examination and to treat the injury to minimize its effects. These initial decisions are among the most critical you must make, since an incorrect decision can have dire, even deadly, consequences.

In an on-site examination, the victim is either conscious or unconscious. On-site examination of an unconscious patient is one of the most serious situations you may find yourself in. Unconsciousness is an emergency situation that requires specific steps to ensure an optimal outcome. Although unconsciousness may result from traumatic injury, it may also result from a variety of general medical conditions or drug interactions. Systematically examine patients who are unconscious for no known reason, proceeding from searching for life-threatening conditions to identifying potential signs and symptoms that may reveal the cause for unconsciousness. Most of the techniques you will use in a general examination of the unconscious patient are described in other chapters. If your primary survey shows that the patient is breathing, conscious, and coherent and does not have severe bleeding, use the secondary survey to determine injury severity and the most appropriate method for removing the patient from the area of play or work (see figure 8.2).

Even though an on-site examination often demands rapid decision making, you must stay calm, take your time, and yet be focused and efficient. Good examination skills and judgment along with knowledge and experience are essential. If you are ever unsure of the severity or nature of the patient's condition, it is better to err on the side of caution and refer the patient rather than assume that referral is unnecessary. Always remember to stay within the scope of your practice and training. Hippocrates said that those in medicine should do no harm. Adhere to that advice, and never hesitate to call for assistance if the best course of action is unclear or the demands of the situation exceed your training or knowledge. You must make all decisions with the person's safety in mind. The components involved or the steps that must be taken during an on-site examination include obtaining a history, observing and screening for physical symptoms, monitoring for shock, implementing your emergency action plan, and communicating your findings.

Obtain a History

When taking an on-site history, quickly determine the mechanism, location, and severity of the injury. An on-site history is a focused history in which you investigate only the patient's major complaint and any problems

---

Goals

☐ Rule out emergency conditions
☐ Assess severity of injury
☐ Determine transport method

Primary Survey

Begin every on-site examination with a primary survey. Sometimes it is immediately obvious that there is or is not a problem in one or all of the areas listed here, but whether examination simply involves moving through a checklist in your head or involves a more thorough process, never shortchange assessing

1. consciousness,
2. ABCs (airway, breathing, circulation), and
3. bleeding severity.

Secondary Survey

Once you have examined and cared for any immediate life-threatening problems, you may proceed with a secondary survey.

Essential History

☐ From patient, if he is conscious
☐ From bystanders, if patient is unconscious

Observation

☐ Position or posturing
☐ Respirations (rate, depth, rhythm)
☐ Trauma
    ☐ Observable signs of head injury
    ☐ Gross deformity, swelling, or discoloration of the extremities
    ☐ Signs of shock (wet, white, weak)
☐ Patient's response to injury

General Screening

☐ Sensory and motor testing for suspected spinal or nerve injury
☐ Neurovascular tests for suspected fracture or dislocation
☐ Assessment for head injury if suspected
☐ Orthopedic assessment
    ☐ Palpation
    ☐ Range of motion
    ☐ Strength examination
    ☐ Special tests
☐ Continued monitoring for shock

Figure 8.2 General checklist for on-site examination.

---

that are readily apparent and in need of attention before the individual is transported off the field.

If you were an eyewitness to the event, you may already have vital information regarding the mechanism and the forces involved. Witnessing the patient's initial response to the trauma can provide valuable information as well. If you did not see the injury and the patient is unconscious, ask bystanders what happened and how long the person has been unconscious. In some cases questioning the victim may be a challenge, but it may also calm her and shift her focus off the pain or fear, allowing you to proceed more easily with your examination. To establish the mechanism, ask how the injury occurred and what happened. You may find that the patient has a different perspective from your own or from that of bystanders. For example, although observers on the sideline may not have heard a sound, the patient may have experienced a pop or snap. A patient may also have experienced torque or rotational forces that are not readily observable.

Questions regarding the location and intensity of symptoms help you determine injury severity and decide on the method of transport off the field. Does the patient experience pain? Does she complain of neck or back pain so that you suspect a spinal injury? Is there any complaint of dizziness, light-headedness, or nausea? This type of questioning helps you quickly focus on the area of injury and make appropriate decisions about the direction of your examination. Completing the entire history on-site is unnecessary. Gather the information you need to determine the general nature and extent of the injury and the best course of immediate action, and defer the rest of the history to the acute examination.

Observe and Screen

As you approached the patient on the ground and while you were obtaining the patient's history, you should have been observing the patient's movement ability and patterns. Continue to check for abnormal positioning of the head, neck, or extremities. How is he reacting to the injury? Is he able to move the injured part, is he protecting it, or is he not moving it at all? Do his facial expressions show pain, fear, or panic? Does he show no expression? Is his skin pale, flushed, or normal? Is he bleeding from the head or showing other signs of head trauma? If he suffered a severe blow to the trunk, especially the abdomen and chest, immediately suspect internal injuries and evaluate the patient as indicated. If you suspect a spinal injury, stabilize the patient's head while bilaterally examining peripheral nerves for sensory and motor innervations. For a suspected head injury, proceed with a head injury examination and ask the patient to ascertain his orientation to time, place, and person, which helps you determine the seriousness of the condition. If the injury involves a bony region, palpate for possible fractures or dislocation. With confirmation of either, proceed with proper immobilization and splinting. If the limb exhibits deformity, test for neurovascular compromise. Muscle injuries require a quick **palpation** for muscular defects and a gross examination of range of motion (ROM) and strength. For suspected ligament injury, perform immediate stress tests before transporting the patient, as muscle spasm quickly sets in and precludes accurate stress tests,

especially once you move the patient and pain increases. You may use other special tests to determine the patient's disposition or whether it is safe to move him off the field. These tests depend on the body region and are briefly discussed in chapters 9, 10, and 11; a more thorough discussion is provided in the text *Examination of Musculoskeletal Injuries* (Shultz, Houglum, and Perrin 2010).

Monitor for Shock

Patients with severe injuries, severe pain, first-time injuries of any severity, or poor tolerance for injury are most susceptible to shock. You must understand the signs and symptoms of shock, monitor them throughout the exam, and be prepared to take immediate action if necessary. Look for pale, cool, clammy skin; rapid, shallow breathing; and a weak, rapid pulse. Also look for nausea and falling blood pressure. Treat patients exhibiting any of these signs immediately and have them transported to an emergency medical facility.

Implement Immediate Action Plan

If the previous steps reveal any serious or life-threatening signs or symptoms, refer the patient for further examination and treatment as needed. If you find that her injury does not require immediate medical care, appropriately transport her off the field or out of the work environment and proceed with a more detailed examination in a quieter environment such as the sideline or a treatment facility. Select the method of transporting the patient on the basis of the injury, its severity, and the patient's response. Choose the method that aggravates the injury the least and optimizes the outcome with efficient and safe removal of the patient from the field. The staff responsible for transport must be well rehearsed in the various methods so that transportation proceeds efficiently and effectively. Procedures for immediate treatment to minimize and control the injury, procedures for immediate medical referral when indicated, and appropriate communication systems must be in place in advance so that the patient's care is optimal, efficient, appropriate, and correct. All facilities should have an Emergency Operating Plan (EOP) (Ray and Konin 2011) to ensure clear role delineations and smooth execution when speed is essential.

Communicate On-Site Examination Results

If you suspect that an injured patient requires stretcher transport off the field, it may take several minutes to prepare the equipment and personnel for the transport. Although most officials understand this, occasionally an official may pressure you to move more quickly. You should either address the official or ask someone involved in the examination but not in the transportation to explain to him the importance of careful preparation and transport. The value of ensuring safety before resumption of work or athletic play is often more readily apparent when it is calmly explained.

Acute Examination

The acute examination either follows the on-site examination or is the initial examination of an injured patient who has walked off the field or from the workplace on his own. Both the acute and clinical examinations include a subjective and an objective segment, each of which is divided into other elements. Both segments focus on investigating the SINS—**severity**, **irritability**, **nature**, and stage—of an injury. The SINS of any injury are identified through a thorough and accurate injury examination. You should identify the SINS during both the acute and clinical examinations. Use the subjective examination segment to create a profile of the injury's SINS and the objective segment to confirm or disprove your suspicions.

The purpose of the acute examination is to determine more precisely the nature and severity of the injury so that you can administer appropriate treatment, provide referral, or return the patient to participation (figure 8.3). As with an on-site examination, you may have seen the injury occur and already know what segment was injured and whether the

Goals
- Determine nature of injury
- Determine severity of injury

Subjective Segment
- History
  - Current
  - Past

Objective Segment
- Observation
  - Skin coloration
  - Swelling, deformity, ecchymosis
- Palpation
- Special tests

- ROM
  - Active
  - Passive
- Strength tests
  - General isometric manual muscle tests
  - Specific manual muscle tests
- Neurological tests (as appropriate)
  - Sensory
  - Motor
  - Reflex
- Circulatory tests
  - Pallor
  - Distal pulse
  - Capillary refill
- Functional tests (as appropriate)

Figure 8.3 General checklist for acute examination.

symptoms are referred from the injury site or are localized. For this reason, you usually perform palpation early in the acute examination. Because you already have a good idea of the segment injured, you also use special tests early in the examination to confirm or disconfirm your suspicions and to determine injury severity. Depending on injury severity, special tests can be used before or after ROM tests.

Perform an acute examination in the following order:

1. History
2. Observation
3. Palpation
4. Special tests
5. ROM tests
6. Strength tests
7. Neurological and circulatory tests (if necessary)
8. Functional tests (if necessary)

Subjective Segment

The first step in an injury examination is obtaining a history. It is very important to determine the stage of the injury at this time. Injuries typically fall into one of two major stages or classifications: acute and chronic. An acute injury results from a sudden onset of macrotrauma or a situation in which symptoms develop quickly. Conditions are classified as chronic if they have a more gradual or insidious onset and continue to interfere with activity 6 to 8 weeks after their onset. In some cases, chronic injuries may have been present for some time, but exacerbation during competition or activity will prompt the patient to report his symptoms to you.

You may have already obtained a partial history during the on-site evaluation, but the acute and clinical examinations typically afford you more time to gather additional information from the patient and other observers that will help you in your examination. After the initial primary examination, patients are often less agitated and able to recall information that they could not remember while on the field. Also obtain relevant medical information and previous injury history at this time. Once you have removed a patient from the field, ask again about the chief complaint and injury mechanism. These complaints commonly change within minutes after injury, and you often get a clearer impression of a patient's condition once she has had the opportunity to calm down. Likewise, if you are unaware of an injury until the patient walks into the athletic training room after practice, you will want to get a detailed picture of the chief complaint, mechanism of injury, and current signs and symptoms. Ask questions that will help you develop a good picture of the injury so that you can pay attention to the correct body segment during the objective examination.

Taking a history is the process of learning or knowing through questioning the facts and events associated with an injury or illness. This is an opportunity for patients to describe what happened and what they are feeling or experiencing. Obtaining an accurate record of a patient's injury or illness requires a systematic approach to learning about the events leading to the injury or illness and getting a clear description of the associated signs and symptoms. This history provides an initial impression of the severity, irritability, nature, and stage (SINS) of the condition. You can learn a tremendous amount about a patient's condition simply by listening to the individual describe the injury. When you carefully select your questions, you obtain a useful picture of the patient's complaint and a sense of the direction your objective examination should take. This is the patient's opportunity (or the bystanders' opportunity if the individual is unable to communicate) to describe the injury or illness, the patient's response to the injury or illness, and previous events that may affect the current situation.

Your questioning should be efficient and thorough—pertinent to the moment, but complete enough to allow you to formulate a plan for the remainder of the examination. History questions should not be leading and are used to gain useful information that will guide the rest of your examination. The history helps you focus on specific segments and determine how much force you should use when performing tests. You should ask questions that seek information in the following primary categories: chief complaint, mechanism of injury, nature of illness or injury, signs and symptoms, and previous history or contributing factors. Additional information regarding history taking is presented in *Examination of Musculoskeletal Injuries* (Shultz, Houglum, and Perrin 2010).

Objective Segment

While the patient is reporting his history, use your observation skills to notice how he moves and holds the injured part, and check for any evidence of swelling, deformity, and abnormal skin coloration. During the objective segment, you perform tests to help you establish the severity and nature of the injury. These tests involve palpation, ROM, strength tests, stress tests, special tests, neurological tests, circulatory tests, and functional tests. As the name implies, this part of the examination focuses on impartial evidence provided by the various tests you perform. At this stage of injury management, your objective evaluation is typically more thorough than your on-site examination, but it may not be as complete as your future clinical examination. If the patient is in severe pain, do not perform a complete examination but instead only one or two tests that can establish appropriate immediate treatment or referral. You may defer complete examination until pain has lessened and the injury is less irritable. However, if the patient is able to tolerate a more extensive examination, proceed—as return to participation decisions may need to be made in a timely manner. But continue your examination only as necessity and the level of pain dictate; otherwise you may aggravate the injury and lose the patient's confidence in your ability to help him. The information you gathered in the subjective examination determines which tests you choose to perform. It is crucial that common sense, the subjective report, and your understanding

of the situation dictate how aggressively to perform the objective tests during the acute examination. If previous segments of the examination have shown that the patient will not be able to participate in the sport, defer functional tests until after the injury has been treated. Perform functional tests during acute examination only if there is a possibility that the patient may return to full function.

Clinical Examination

Often, you do not evaluate an injury immediately after it happens. A patient commonly reports to the treatment facility complaining of an injury that occurred within the past few hours or days, or an injury that had no acute onset but has progressively worsened over time. If you did not witness an injury or did not perform an acute examination, your detective work must be broader and yet more detailed, as determining the severity, irritability, nature, and stage can be much more complicated. An injury's profile changes over time, so findings at the onset and upon reexamination may be different, and all findings must be taken into account as you perform your examination.

General Principles of the Clinical Examination

In some cases the clinical examination is a continuation of the on-site or acute injury examinations, and previous observations and findings can be reexamined or tested further. In other cases, the clinical examination may be the first encounter with a particular patient or complaint. In these situations, all components of the examination must be conducted during the visit.

Although the procedures for a clinical examination follow a specific routine and include many of the same components as the acute examination, some components are slightly altered and others are added. Both the acute and clinical examinations include subjective and objective segments, but the on-site and acute examinations are typically not as thorough. The clinical examination does include all the components of the subjective and objective segments.

Subjective Segment

History taking during a clinical examination involves a more in-depth and complete line of questioning. You will ask many of the same questions during the clinical examination that you ask at the sideline regarding the mechanism of the injury and any history of prior injury and treatment. However, allotted time in a clinical examination is usually greater, allowing you to ask additional history questions to obtain the most accurate and detailed injury history possible.

With acute injuries, many of the questions asked during the on-site and acute injury examinations are applicable at this time. Additional questions regarding contributing factors or relevant injury and medical history are helpful. With chronic injuries, inquire also about onset, symptoms, pain profile, and treatments. Use medical questions to rule out general medical problems and internal injuries, some of which could be serious and refer pain to the extremities.

Objective Segment

The objective examination segment of a clinical examination can be quite extensive. It is during this examination that you are attempting to obtain an accurate diagnosis and design a treatment plan and rehabilitation progression, or to determine ability to return to sport or work. You will need to perform a detailed and thorough examination in the areas of palpation, ROM, strength tests, stress tests, special tests, neurological tests, vascular tests, and functional tests to determine extent of injury. The objective segment of an examination is a routine process, requiring specific tests and the identification of responses to confirm your suspicions regarding the patient's diagnosis. Since a goal of the objective examination is

to define the injury, you must know what reproduces the patient's symptoms and what is normal for that patient. You can obtain this information by producing a comparable sign and by comparing the injured segment to the contralateral extremity. The examination process presented here is recommended since it follows a logical sequence. Whether you implement this system or develop your own, you should use a consistent, sequential system each time you perform an examination. Such a system will make you less likely to forget a test and more likely to perform a thorough examination.

- *Comparable sign.* With each test you perform, you are seeking a response. All objective tests should elicit a negative response if the tissue or structure is not injured and a positive response if it is. A positive response results from either a reproduction or an alteration of the patient's symptoms. The reproduction of the patient's complaint of pain through testing is called a comparable sign (Maitland 1991). It is desirable to produce a comparable sign because a test that produces the sign will reveal the problem. A negative response, on the other hand, is seen when the test yields a normal result. One or more of these tests will produce a comparable sign. The information you obtain from these procedures and the procedures of the subjective segment provides a total picture of the injury: a diagnosis or clinical impression.

- *Bilateral comparison.* You should perform all of the objective tests bilaterally (bilateral comparison). To obtain reliable information from the tests, you need to understand the purpose of each test, compare the injured side with the uninjured side, and know the normal response for each test. You must also realize how changes in the patient's position can affect results. For example, the results of strength testing of shoulder flexion may depend on whether the patient is sitting or supine. It is important to examine the patient efficiently. If you do not understand the purpose of each test, you will use more tests than necessary, prolonging the examination and perhaps aggravating the condition.

Tests by themselves do not completely profile the injury. During the examination, every question, observation, and test progressively focuses the picture and narrows the injury possibilities. Be careful not to make unfounded assumptions or rush the investigation by prematurely focusing on one or two tests. Before conducting the objective examination on a postacute or chronic injury, caution the patient that the examination may aggravate the symptoms. The patient may complain of pain and discomfort during the examination, but if she is able to tolerate these effects, proceed, because timely recovery depends on an accurate and complete diagnosis. It is not unusual for symptoms to increase following the examination; assure the patient that these effects should quickly subside. Instruct the patient to inform you at the next visit whether or not symptoms increased.

The objective component of the clinical examination should include the following:

1. Observation
2. Palpation
3. ROM tests
4. Strength tests
5. Stress tests
6. Special tests
7. Neurological tests
8. Vascular tests
9. Functional tests

Observation

Observation is a valuable skill that is used throughout all phases and types of examinations and treatments. Observing how the patient responds provides useful information about the patient's perception of the injury, as well as clues about its nature and severity. Observation begins as soon as you see the patient and continues throughout the subjective and objective segments of an examination. Facial expressions and the eyes are windows into a patient's true response;

thus you should carefully watch them during the objective tests. You also should observe the patient's general posture, the way in which he holds or protects the injured part, and his willingness to move the injured segment. Observe for contour, alignment, and discoloration, and compare the right and left sides—they should be symmetrical.

Palpation

Your sense of touch is critical to the objective portion of the examination. A palpation exam consists of feeling with your hands for changes in tissue size, contour, organization, texture or consistency, tension or tone, and temperature or moisture, as well as checking for pain, swelling, muscle spasm, and tissue thickening. The goal of each palpation is to locate all pertinent structures, determine their characteristic feel, and examine them for the presence of pathology. With concentration and practice, your sense of touch will develop just as your other clinical skills do. In addition to palpating for swelling, pain, and temperature, you will palpate for spasm, deformity, moisture, pulse, and general contour of soft tissue and bony prominences (Shultz, Houglum, and Perrin 2010). As with the acute examination, palpation in the clinic proceeds systematically, moving from superficial to deep structures and traversing the body segment in a specific routine such as from anterior to posterior or superior to inferior. Likewise, palpation of the structures is the same in the acute and clinical examinations. Carefully note differences between the involved and uninvolved sides in soft tissue tension, spasm, restriction, temperature, moisture, swelling, thickness, texture, bony and soft tissue contours, and tenderness.

Range of Motion

Normal ROM is influenced by strength and active and passive tissue integrity. The goal of examining ROM is to objectively quantify the amount of active and passive motion available at and around the injury site. Range of motion examinations assist in confirming or eliminating your suspicions of the structures involved in the injury; help demonstrate the extent of the injury; and determine the integrity of active and passive elements that produce, support, and restrict joint movement. As you test ROM, you should identify the injury's SINS (severity, irritability, nature, and stage) throughout your examination to assist in forming a diagnosis.

Active range of motion (AROM) testing, which is performed first, examines the integrity of the active or contractile tissue of the musculotendinous unit. Active range of motion is produced solely by the patient and is contingent upon adequate strength and structural integrity of the tissue involved. If a patient needs assistance to complete the requested movement, the test changes into an active-assisted range of motion (AAROM) exam.

Passive range of motion (PROM) testing examines inert structures around the joint. It is important to observe how motion is affected by an injury; thus, it is important to perform all the active motion tests first and then follow with all the passive motion tests. Observing the quality of movement is an important purpose of ROM measurement, for it may tell you areas of pain or difficulty. If pain makes the injury very irritable, less active motion is possible. If little active motion but full passive motion is possible, the musculotendinous structure is the likely site of injury. On the other hand, if passive movement is restricted, you will want to evaluate for the possibility of a fracture or some form of internal derangement within the affected joint that is causing a block to movement.

It is recommended that you perform the active and passive motion tests by muscle or muscle group to limit patient movement from one position to another. During ROM testing, you examine both the quality and quantity of physiological and accessory motion and also test for pain. You may also test how the joint feels at the end of the ROM (the joint's end feel). Abnormal end feels are suspicious for the presence of injury. For more information regarding the various elements of ROM testing, see Shultz and colleagues (2010).

Strength

Strength examination follows the active and passive ROM tests that are typically performed in the ROM examination. Some professionals include resistive range of motion (RROM), or strength, in the ROM category; however, in this text we categorize strength separately, since if the patient has significant pain it may not be possible to perform a strength test. If this is the case, you will have to defer strength examination to a later date.

Strength tests examine the musculotendinous resistive ability, the neuromuscular integrity of the contractile tissue, and the pain level of the contractile elements. The method you use to examine strength depends on the type of injury, available equipment, time, and place of examination.

Manual muscle tests are the most convenient method of examining strength as performance requires only your hands and your knowledge. Strength tests typically begin with isometric screening for gross discrepancies in muscle function within the cardinal planes of motion, proceeding to specific muscles or muscle groups if bilateral differences are noted. Isometric tests, or "break tests," are efficient and are usually performed with the joint in a neutral midrange position for multiple-joint muscles and in an end-range position for single-joint muscles. Conduct these tests by asking your patient to maintain a predetermined position while you attempt to move or "break" the given body part away from this position. These static positions and tests limit the amount of stress applied to a joint and ensure that you test for strength without interference from inert joint structures.

If you discover a strength deficit with a break test, you may consider further examination of the muscle's strength throughout its entire ROM using instrumented equipment. Strength testing equipment is extensive and can range from isometric **tensiometers** to free and machine weights (isotonic equipment) to isokinetic equipment. Equipment selection depends on availability, your preference, the muscle or muscle group being tested, and the patient's condition. While manual muscle tests are the most efficient and readily available means of examining muscle strength, instrumented strength testing provides a more objective and reproducible measure.

For an extensive presentation of strength examination, see Shultz and colleagues (2010).

Stress Tests

Stress tests are special tests that specifically examine capsular and ligamentous tissue of injured joints in an attempt to determine whether structural damage has occurred to those structures. These tests are used to evaluate whether a ligament or capsule exhibits laxity and should not be confused with ROM tests, which evaluate for tightness or mobility. Laxity (or looseness) determined by stress testing is an indication that there has been actual structural damage to the structures surrounding a joint, and this is defined as a sprain. Sprains are classified as first, second, or third degree or Grade I, Grade II, or Grade III, respectively. This classification is based on the level of severity. Grade I (first degree) sprains are the least severe and are characterized by pain but no laxity. Grade II (second degree) sprains are partial tears in capsular or ligamentous tissue; pain and laxity are present, but the laxity subsides and becomes firm after the "slack" is taken up. Grade III (third degree) sprains are complete tears of tissue and exhibit severe pain and significant laxity with no firmness at end ranges of stress.

Stress tests should be used in the examination process after the history, observation, palpation, ROM, and sometimes strength tests have been completed. They should be used to eliminate or confirm suspected injuries based on information previously gained during the examination. Techniques for stress tests are specific for each joint; they involve stressing the tissue being examined in such a way that they provide clinical information about the extent and severity of the injury without causing additional irritation. Stress test force is typically applied across the joint and often perpendicular to the ligament or capsule in such a fashion that it stretches the ligament. Presence of pain, increased laxity between involved and uninvolved sides, and increased instability of the joint are all indications of a positive stress test and ligamentous or capsular damage.

Special Tests

Many of the special tests used during the acute examination are also used in the clinic. However, other special tests may be appropriate during the clinical examination depending on the patient's history, your preliminary findings from other objective tests, and the simple fact that you may have more time available. Special tests are unique to specific joints, body segments, or structures. Each body segment requires unique tests for examining the degree of injury to its distinctive soft tissue structures and bones. By the time you are ready to use special tests in your examination, the history, palpation, ROM, and strength tests have narrowed the range of injury possibilities. Use special tests to eliminate or confirm a suspected condition as well as to quantify the integrity of a structure or the extent of an injury. Special tests should stress the structure enough to allow you to either grade an abnormal response or reproduce the patient's symptoms. The stress must be great enough to elicit an accurate response but not so great that it aggravates the injury. In the beginning, finding this balance can be difficult. Special tests do not provide a complete profile of the injury. Throughout the examination process, you progressively focus the picture and narrow the possibilities of what the injury is. You must be careful not to rush the investigative process by making assumptions or focusing too quickly on one or two special tests. Remember to keep an open mind until your understanding of the injury, or the injury presentation, becomes certain. Chapters 9, 10, and 11 of this text present further discussion of special testing, and Shultz and colleagues (2010) provide excellent information for further study.

As noted earlier, deciding on the degree of stress or on which special test to use requires good judgment. It is sometimes neither necessary nor appropriate to use a special test to stress an injury, for example in the case of an elbow dislocation. A patient may simply be in too much pain to undergo a stress test; in this case, it is better to defer the special test. Special tests confirm the severity and nature of the injury. The special tests presented throughout this text are those that clinicians most commonly use because of their accuracy and demonstrated reliability. You must remember, however, that some special tests do not have demonstrated reliability or may not be appropriate for some clinicians because of individual circumstances. You will need to determine the most suitable tests for your examination based on the specific injury situation and your knowledge and skills.

You should perform special tests only after you have explained to the patient what will occur. The special tests are performed on the uninvolved extremity first for two reasons: (1) to familiarize the patient with the procedure so she is less apprehensive, encouraging relaxation that will achieve better test results, and (2) to learn what response to the test is normal for that patient. Since many special tests produce different results from one patient to another, you must establish a baseline for each person to determine whether a test is positive or negative. Depending on the test, the result is considered positive if it produces abnormal results compared to the uninvolved side in terms of laxity or stiffness, stability or instability, presence or absence of sounds, restriction or ease of movement, strength or weakness, normal or abnormal function, and presence or absence of pain.

Always remember that negative or positive results of a single special test do not necessarily indicate the absence or presence of a specific injury. This is why all the factors in your examination are used in combination to provide a full and consistent profile of the injury. Sometimes a result is false positive and complicates your examination results so that other tests are necessary for providing accurate results. Your skills and ability to perform the tests reliably can make a big difference in the test results, and thus experience plays an important role in the accuracy of special tests. Another factor to consider is the accuracy of the specific special tests themselves, as some are more sensitive than others. However, though for some injuries there are several tests, it is not necessary to use all that are available. Remember, a special test is intended to reproduce the patient's symptoms or create a comparable sign; so unless you require additional confirmation, one or two tests per structure are usually adequate and are better tolerated by the patient.

Neurological Tests

Because neurological compromise can have serious and even life-threatening consequences, it is crucial to determine if the nerve structures are intact and functioning normally following an injury. The goal of the neurological examination is to rule out any brain, spinal, or peripheral nerve pathology. Although clinical neural tests are the same as those used during the acute examination, they serve a dual purpose in the clinical examination. Since you may not have been a witness to the injury, it may be difficult to determine if the injury is musculoskeletal or neural in nature. Neurological tests examine the integrity of the central and peripheral nervous systems and should be performed if you suspect a nerve injury or if the patient's symptoms include sensory changes (radiation of numbness, tingling, shooting pain, deep pain, or burning pain), weakness, or paralysis. Radiating, or referred, symptoms can result from pathology in the spinal cord, nerve roots, or peripheral nerves secondary to disc herniations, fractures, or dislocations; impingement or compression syndromes; nerve tensioning or stretch; or other nerve trauma.

Neurological symptoms vary with the level of injury. Because nerve roots from the cervical and lumbar spine send branches to more than one peripheral nerve, the symptom profile is more diffuse with a nerve root lesion than with a peripheral nerve lesion. Unilateral symptoms indicate a nerve root or peripheral nerve lesion (lower motor neuron), whereas bilateral symptoms often result from central cord or brain pathology (upper motor neuron). Although there are specific neurological tests for specific body areas and pathologies, the three primary neurological tests involve examination of sensory, motor, and reflex responses. These tests are designed for spinal cord and nerve root exams, but sensory and motor examination results can also produce peripheral nerve conclusions. Specific neurological tests and their implications are explained in chapters 9, 10, and 11 as well as by Shultz and colleagues (2010).

Vascular Tests

Circulatory tests examine the integrity of the vascular system. You will often palpate pulses to determine the presence of blood flow. If the pulse weakens or disappears following an injury, the situation is a medical emergency, and you must provide for immediate and emergency medical referral to prevent loss of a limb or worse. You will note pallor or lack of capillary refill in areas of decreased blood flow or ischemia. Shock

may also cause some of these pathological signs. Circulatory status along with tests and methods for recognizing vascular conditions are presented in chapters 9, 10, and 11 and also by Shultz and colleagues (2010).

Functional Tests

Functional tests are used only when the patient is ready to return to former participation levels. These final tests determine not so much the nature or severity of an injury but rather the patient's ability to safely and fully resume all activities. Most commonly, you will perform these tests after a course of treatment following an injury rather than at the time of injury. Only in cases of minor injuries—if symptoms have subsided and all previous tests have demonstrated that the patient is able to return to participation—is functional testing a part of the acute examination process. In these cases, you must perform functional tests before permitting the patient to return to full participation. Table 8.1 gives examples of specific functional tests by sport position.

Table 8.1 Examples of Functional Tests for Different Sports and Positions

Sport, position	Examples of functional tests
Football quarterback	Throwing short and long distances; scrambling via sudden cuts, lateral runs, sprints
Football lineman	Thrust from set stance; lateral runs; sprints forward; blocking maneuvers
Football receiver	Sprints forward, laterally, and backward; sudden changes in direction; catching while running; running and jumping
Soccer goalie	Sudden lateral moves; jumping; diving
Soccer forward	Sprints forward, laterally, and backward; dribbling and passing; overhead throws; tackling
Female gymnast	Handstands; jumping; sprinting forward; back and forward walkovers; handsprings; dismounts from bars and beam
Male gymnast	Handstands; jumping; sprinting forward; iron cross on rings; dismounts from bars, rings, and pommel horse
Basketball forward	Sprinting forward; lateral cuts; backward sprints; layups; free throws
Basketball guard	Sprinting forward; lateral cuts; backward sprints; dribbling while running and cutting; 3-point shots
Baseball or softball outfielder	Sprinting 50 to 100 ft; base sliding; running and catching; hitting
Baseball or softball catcher	Squatting; sudden squat to stand; throw to second base; catching; sprinting 20 ft
Volleyball front-line player	Jumping up; jumping laterally; jumping and hitting the ball; approaching the net for a hit or a block and jump
Volleyball setter	Sprinting forward and laterally 15 ft; dive; set and pass

Functional testing helps you determine the patient's confidence and physical readiness to return to participation beyond what you can learn from other aspects of the subjective and objective examination segments. Functional testing requires specific tasks and controlled skill movements that mimic the physical demands and joint stresses inherent to the patient's sport or work activity. By having the patient perform these functional movements, you can also determine the quality of his performance in a more controlled environment and identify any apprehension or compensation with other movements in an effort to protect an area or avoid pain. Specific functional tests are numerous and many are unique to the specific demands of each case or sport. Therefore, you should have a working understanding of the physical demands and stresses that a patient will experience so you can provide an appropriate functional examination. Generic lower and upper extremity functional tests are included in the sidebar Lower and Upper Extremity Functional Tests.

Documenting the Examination

A final ingredient of utmost importance in your examination procedures is accurate and thorough documentation of your findings. Injury documentation is essential for a number of reasons. From a legal standpoint, you may need to reproduce records for a legal dispute or for verifying an insurance claim. From a more practical standpoint, other colleagues may care for your patient when you are not available; and accurate examina-

LOWER AND UPPER EXTREMITY FUNCTIONAL TESTS

Lower Extremity

1. Balance in standing such as the stork stand or tandem stand
2. Walking forward
3. Walking up and down stairs
4. Jogging forward
5. Running forward
6. Sprinting forward
7. Hopping forward
8. Jogging backward
9. Running backward
10. Sprinting backward
11. Jogging side to side
12. Running side to side
13. Sprinting side to side
14. Hopping forward
15. Hopping side to side
16. Hopping alternate feet
17. Hopping involved leg only
18. Skipping forward
19. Skipping backward
20. Skipping side to side
21. Jumping forward
22. Jumping backward
23. Sport-specific activities

Upper Extremity

1. Tossing
2. Throwing
3. Pitching
4. Hitting
5. Batting
6. Catching
7. Receiving
8. Standing on hands
9. Supporting body weight on arms
10. Sport-specific activities

tion, injury, and treatment records ensure continuity of care. Injury documentation also proves useful for reexamining injuries, allowing you to compare your findings from one examination to the next. It is never wise to rely on your memory, as you may forget critical findings.

Your documentation should be thorough but concise. It is likely that you will perform multiple examinations or treatments in a single day, so efficient documentation is essential if you wish to avoid getting bogged down in paperwork. Many computerized systems for tracking injuries are now available. Whether in written or computerized form, the same information is recorded. Excellent information on documentation, record keeping, storage requirements, and **HIPAA** (Health Insurance Portability and Accountability Act) regulations is presented by Shultz and colleagues (2010) and Ray and Konin (2011).

Learning Aids

SUMMARY

This chapter outlines and describes the differences between a primary and secondary survey and provides details on the components of the on-site, acute, and clinical examinations. The principles of examination call for the use of procedures that accurately and thoroughly examine the patient complaints and set the groundwork for further treatment. Developing a routine for injury evaluation and examination is critical for appropriate emergency care and subsequent management of your patient's injuries.

KEY CONCEPTS AND REVIEW

▶ **Explain the difference between the primary survey and the secondary survey in the evaluation of an injured person.**

A primary survey determines the status of life-threatening or limb-threatening conditions using the ABCs of emergency medical care: examination of Airway, Breathing, and Circulation. The secondary injury survey occurs when the injured patient is breathing and any bleeding is under control. It is at this time that the athletic trainer performs an examination to determine the presence of other injuries.

▶ **List the main steps in performing a complete on-site examination.**

The on-site examination includes the primary survey and the secondary survey. The main steps in the primary survey are determination of consciousness, ABCs, and bleeding. The secondary survey comprises history; observation; and general screening, which includes sensory and motor testing for nerve injury, neurovascular testing for suspected fracture or dislocation, assessment of head injury if suspected, orthopedic assessment (palpation, ROM, strength examination, and special tests), and continued monitoring for shock.

▶ **List the main steps in performing a complete acute injury examination.**

The two steps are the subjective segment and the objective segment: subjective segment—history; objective segment—observation, palpation, special tests, ROM, strength tests, neurological tests (as appropriate), circulatory tests, and functional tests (as appropriate).

▶ **Explain the term "SINS" as used in acute and clinical examinations.**

SINS stands for severity, irritability, nature, and stage of the condition.

▶ **Explain the difference between the subjective and the objective segments of the examination.**

In the subjective segment of the examination, the examiner obtains feedback from the patient regarding perception, opinion, feelings, pain level, and so on. It is an opportunity for the patient to explain what happened and what she is feeling or experiencing. In the objective segment, the athletic trainer obtains measurable facts and attempts to decide on an accurate diagnosis, treatment plan, and rehabilitation progression or to determine ability to return to sport or work. The objective segment requires performance of a detailed and thorough examination in the areas of palpation, ROM, strength tests, stress tests, special tests, neurological tests, vascular tests, and functional tests to determine extent of injury.

▶ **List the elements one should include in the objective component of the clinical examination.**

The components include observation, palpation, ROM tests, strength tests, special tests, neurological tests, vascular tests, and functional tests.

▶ **Explain the importance of documenting an examination.**

Injury documentation is essential for a number of reasons. From a legal standpoint, the athletic trainer may need to reproduce records for a legal dispute or for verifying an insurance claim. From a more practical standpoint, other colleagues may care for the patient when the athletic trainer is not available, and accurate examination, injury, and treatment records ensure continuity of care. Injury documentation also proves useful for reexamining injuries, allowing one to compare findings from one examination to the next. It is never wise for athletic trainers to

rely on memory, as they may forget critical findings.

PRACTICE!

For hands-on practice in this area, go to the web resource and complete the following:

Level 1.4, Module C2: Principles of Initial Assessment

Level 2.8, Module I1: Orthopedic Injury Assessment Principles

CRITICAL THINKING QUESTIONS

1. You have been asked to assist with the coverage of soccer practice during preseason training. As you mentally prepare for this activity, what steps of evaluation will you review to prepare for anything that may happen?

2. During the preseason soccer training practice, a patient begins to suffer from a heat illness. You are asked to obtain vital signs on the patient. What vital signs would be extremely concerning to you, and what tests would you perform to ensure that the patient is not going into shock or heart failure?

3. In the initial stages of learning evaluation skills, some tests may be beyond your level of knowledge. Assuming you do not have extensive experience in special tests, list the steps in both the acute and clinical evaluation that you would be able to perform at this point in your education.

Upper Extremity Injury Recognition

Sandra J. Shultz, PhD, ATC, CSCS, FNATA
Kirk Brumels, PhD, AT, ATC

OBJECTIVES

After reading this chapter, the student should be able to do the following:

- Describe the difference between shoulder dislocation, subluxation, and separation.
- Detail the signs and symptoms associated with subacromial impingement syndrome.
- Explain the similarities and differences between golfer's elbow and tennis elbow.
- Give details about structures involved, predisposing factors, and signs and symptoms of little league elbow.
- Identify the mechanism and structures involved in gamekeeper's thumb.
- Detail differences between jersey and mallet finger.
- Identify the location of boxer's fracture.

To accurately examine and subsequently manage injuries, the clinician must be aware of the injuries that can occur to various structures, as well as able to recognize them when they are present. This chapter outlines the more common injuries to the anatomical structures of the upper extremity and the associated pathologies; knowledge in these areas will help you later when you study examination strategies in more detail. The chapter focuses especially on injuries of the shoulder, elbow, wrist, and hand. The information on basic injury mechanisms, classifications, and examination strategies presented in chapters 7 and 8 should be used in examination of shoulder, elbow, wrist, and hand injuries. This chapter does not provide details of tests or specific techniques for examination of the shoulder, elbow, wrist, and hand. Complete examination strategies for these body regions and parts are presented by Shultz, Houglum, and Perrin (2010).

Shoulder and Arm Injury Recognition

The shoulder complex is characterized by a high degree of mobility with limited skeletal stability to allow for the large range of motion (ROM) necessary to perform overhead activities. The shoulder complex as a whole is unique in that it relies very little on bony and ligament structures for stability, with the majority of support coming from the 18 muscles acting on the shoulder complex. The only direct attachment of the upper extremity to the axial skeleton is through the sternoclavicular joint. Statically, the glenohumeral joint is supported by the capsule, capsular ligaments, and glenoid labrum. Knowledge of shoulder anatomy (figures 9.1 and 9.2) is critical to effective injury recognition and examination strategies. Because the shoulder relies so heavily on muscular support for stability, injuries associated

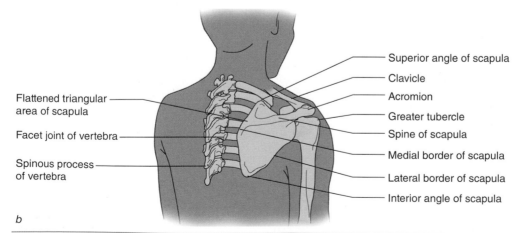

Figure 9.1 Skeletal anatomy of the shoulder complex: *(a)* anterior and *(b)* posterior views.

Reprinted, by permission, from J. Loudon et al., 2008, *The clinical orthopedic assessment guide*, 2nd ed. (Champaign, IL: Human Kinetics): 166.

with muscle weakness, dysfunction, and imbalance are common. In addition, soft tissues of the shoulder complex are chronically exposed to repetitive high-velocity and eccentric forces over a large ROM; therefore the joint is particularly susceptible to chronic instability and repetitive stress injuries.

The shoulder joint is particularly susceptible to injuries because of its great mobility and inherent instability. The heavy reliance on soft tissue structures and balanced muscular control for stabilization during large ROM activities leads to both acute and chronic injuries. Injury recognition is sometimes difficult

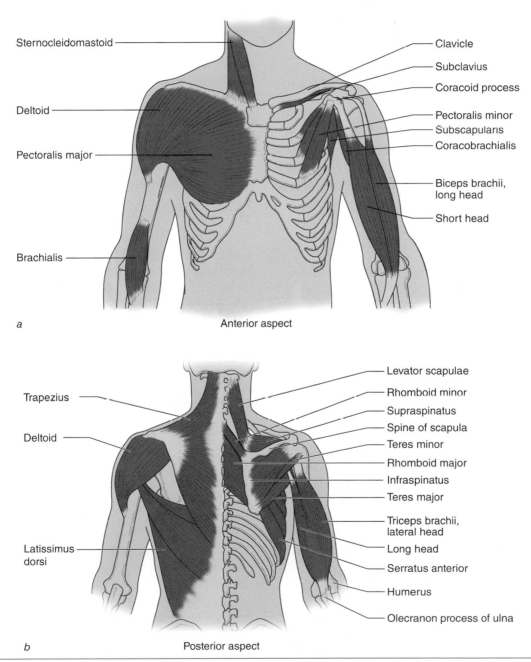

Figure 9.2 *(a)* Anterior and *(b)* posterior aspects of the muscles that act on the shoulder. The rotator cuff includes the subscapularis (anterior aspect), teres major, teres minor, and infraspinatus (posterior aspect) muscles.

Reprinted, by permission, from J. Loudon et al., 2008, *The clinical orthopedic assessment guide,* 2nd ed. (Champaign, IL: Human Kinetics): 87.

because of the interplay of the muscles acting on the shoulder during functional activity. The following sections outline some basic shoulder injury categories.

Acute Soft Tissue Injuries

Acute soft tissue injuries can result from direct trauma, movements forcing the joint beyond its normal range, and forceful muscle contraction during activity. This section describes several of the more common acute soft tissue injuries.

Contusions

During sports such as American football, wrestling, and soccer, direct contact with other players and the ground can result in contusions to superficial bony anatomy and the surrounding musculature. The clavicle, acromion, and lateral arm are bony structures with little soft tissue protection.

Bone Contusions

Contusion of the acromion is often referred to as a "shoulder pointer." **Blocker's exostosis** (also known as tackler's exostosis or blocker's spur), on the other hand, results from repetitive insult to and irritation of the bone, causing excessive bone formation and at times a palpable spur on the anterolateral surface of the humerus. Contusions to these isolated bony structures are rarely disabling, with signs and symptoms typically limited to localized swelling, pain, and point tenderness.

Muscle Contusions

Contusions to the musculature can be more disabling, since hematoma formation and pain can severely limit muscular function. A complication of biceps muscle contusion is **myositis ossificans**, or calcification within and around the biceps. Myositis ossificans can result from an unresolved hematoma in cases with large hematoma formation, repetitive insult, or continued use following the initial contusion.

Sprains and Dislocation

Sprains involving the ligaments and capsule of the shoulder complex vary in frequency and severity depending on the structure involved. Ligamentous and capsular disruption can result from both compressive and tractional forces that force the joint beyond its normal ROM. Sprains of the glenohumeral and acromioclavicular joint occur more frequently than sternoclavicular joint sprains. **Dislocations** and **subluxations** can result from both acute traumatic events and chronic shoulder instability in which the ligamentous tissue is damaged to the extent that it is unable to stabilize the joint.

Glenohumeral Joint Sprains

In order to provide the mobility inherent in the glenohumeral joint, the joint's capsule and ligaments are comparatively lax throughout most of glenohumeral motion. This means that the capsule and ligaments are minimally involved in maintaining joint stability throughout most of the ROM. Forces exerted at the end ranges of motion that are sufficient to tear the glenohumeral ligaments can cause subluxation or dislocation of the humeral head because of its shallow articulation with the glenoid. Signs and symptoms include pain, point tenderness, and limited motion in multiple planes.

Anterior Glenohumeral Dislocation

Anterior glenohumeral dislocations represent the large majority of glenohumeral dislocations. Anterior subluxations and dislocations typically occur with the arm in an abducted and laterally rotated position. Hyperextension of the joint in this position, or a force applied to the posterior or lateral aspect of the humerus, can stress the anterior and inferior glenohumeral ligaments and capsule and cause them to fail. At lower applied forces the capsular ligaments may be partially stretched, and the patient feels a slipping or giving sensation that indicates a subluxation or spontaneous relocation. A patient with an anterior dislocation typically presents with the arm slightly abducted and supporting the injured extremity. Because of its close proximity to the humeral head in the axilla, the axillary nerve may also be injured. In this case, sensation and motor function in the deltoid are impaired. Figure 9.3, *a* and *b*, shows an anterior glenohumeral dislocation.

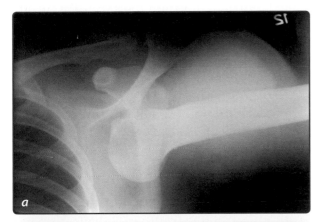

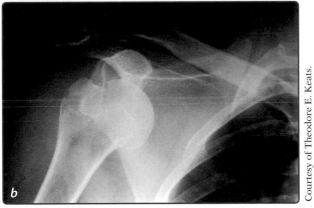

Courtesy of Theodore E. Keats.

Figure 9.3 *(a)* Anterior–inferior and *(b)* anterior glenohumeral dislocation.

Posterior Glenohumeral Dislocation

Posterior dislocations (figure 9.4) are less frequent but can occur if a posteriorly directed force is applied along the length of the humerus while the arm is flexed forward. Straight-arm blocking and falling on the elbow with the shoulder in a forward and flexed position are examples of this type of mechanism. The patient also has signs and symptoms of pain and swelling and an unwillingness to move the extremity.

Acromioclavicular Joint Sprains

Within the shoulder complex, the acromioclavicular (AC) joint is the most commonly sprained or "separated" joint. Ligament injuries to this joint typically result from a fall or from direct contact to the point of the shoulder. Forces transmitted through the arm with a fall on an outstretched hand may also produce an AC sprain. First-degree sprains are characterized by localized pain, point tenderness, and swelling over the joint. The patient may complain of mild to moderate pain during shoulder motion. Second-degree injuries involve partial tearing of the AC or the coracoclavicular ligament or both. The patient has increased complaints of pain, swelling, and disability with arm motion above horizontal. The distal end of the clavicle may or may not be elevated, depending on the extent of disruption of one or both of the associated ligaments (AC and coracoclavicular). Third-degree injuries are characterized by complete disruption of the AC and coracoclavicular ligaments. The patient will complain of severe pain at the time of injury and demonstrate an unwillingness to raise the arm, typically protecting it at her side. Elevation of the distal end of the clavicle is observable and produces a characteristic "bump" at the end of the shoulder.

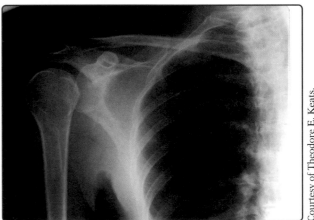

Courtesy of Theodore E. Keats.

Figure 9.4 Posterior glenohumeral dislocation.

Sternoclavicular Joint Sprains

The sternoclavicular (SC) joint is quite stable, and sprains are infrequent. Sternoclavicular joint injury involves disruption of both the SC and costoclavicular ligaments. Injury can result from an anteriorly directed force, or direct blow, but more commonly results from forces transmitted along the long axis of the clavicle. Signs and symptoms of SC sprains include localized pain, swelling, and point tenderness directly over the joint. Pain increases with forward rotation of the shoulders and horizontal adduction, which act to compress the joint.

Strains

The muscles of the shoulder complex provide much of the stability for the shoulder through most of its normal ROM. Consequently, acute muscle and tendon strains frequently occur with overstretch during ballistic arm activities, forceful concentric contractions during limb acceleration, and excessive eccentric loading during limb deceleration. Improper warm-up, poor conditioning, and muscular fatigue can also make the muscles more susceptible to acute strain. Any of the 18 muscles acting within the shoulder complex may be injured; some of those that more commonly sustain injury are discussed here.

Rotator Cuff

The rotator cuff muscles are among the most commonly injured. Acute rotator cuff injuries can result from a fall on the shoulder or an outstretched hand that forces the humeral head into the acromion. These compressive injuries result in contusion and inflammation of the underlying surface of the rotator cuff tendons. Conversely, falling on the top of the shoulder and driving the humeral head downward can traction and tear the supraspinatus muscle. Signs and symptoms of acute rotator cuff injury resulting from these mechanisms include anterolateral shoulder pain, point tenderness, decreased ROM, and loss of strength consistent with the severity of injury. Pain may radiate down the lateral arm but usually stops at midhumerus.

Biceps Tendon Injuries

An acute rupture of the biceps tendon may be caused by a single traumatic event, such as rapid, forceful elbow flexion against heavy resistance, or by repetitive microtrauma over time. Rupture of the proximal biceps tendon is easily observed as a bulging of the muscle in the anterior arm, particularly when contracted. When the proximal biceps tendon is ruptured, the patient complains of experiencing a sudden sharp pain in the anterior shoulder and may experience a "pop" or snapping sensation. You will note palpable tenderness in the anterior shoulder, along with muscular weakness and eventual swelling and discoloration.

Glenoid Labrum Tears

Glenoid labral tears are usually associated with glenohumeral instability and can result from either acute trauma or dislocation or chronic instability. Stresses related to throwing can also disrupt the labrum, particularly near the attachment of the biceps tendon. Patients complaining of pain and a sensation of catching or clicking with overhead motions may have sustained an injury to the glenoid labrum.

Chronic or Overuse Soft Tissue Injuries

Given the repetitive nature of overhead motions that physically active individuals typically perform, the rotator cuff, biceps tendon, and associated bursa are particularly susceptible to chronic inflammatory and degenerative conditions.

Biceps Tendinitis

Tendinitis can result from repetitive overloading and friction as the long head of the biceps passes through the bicipital groove and under the transverse humeral ligament on its way to its proximal attachment on the superior glenoid labrum. Signs and symptoms may include diffuse anterior shoulder pain with point tenderness specifically over the bicipital groove and proximal tendon.

Rotator Cuff

The rotator cuff acts both as a prime mover for shoulder rotation and as a primary stabilizer for normal glenohumeral function, so it is prone to overuse. Signs and symptoms include pain during throwing, tenderness over the supraspinatus or infraspinatus, and mild weakness of the lateral rotators.

Impingement Syndrome

Impingement syndrome is caused by encroachment in the subacromial space that decreases the area through which the supraspinatus and subacromial bursa pass underneath the subacromial arch. Impingement is most commonly seen in occupations and sporting activities involving overhead activities. The patient typically complains of a dull or deep pain underneath or near the acromion. Point tenderness may be noted just anterolateral to the acromion and at the insertion of the supraspinatus tendon. The patient may also complain of pain radiating down the anterior (biceps) and lateral (supraspinatus) aspects of the upper arm.

Chronic Glenohumeral Joint Instability

Chronic glenohumeral instability is commonly seen in physically active persons because of the inherent mobility and weak static stabilizing structures of the shoulder. **Chronic instability** is also classified by the direction of excessive humeral head translation (anterior, inferior, posterior, and multidirectional). Chronic instability can result from an initial traumatic event but also may be unrelated to any previous trauma or dislocation. Signs and symptoms include pain and a sensation of joint slippage while the glenohumeral joint subluxes during overhead activity. The patient may also complain of weakness, numbness, and tingling following the subluxating event.

Traumatic Fractures

Fractures within the shoulder and upper arm are usually caused by traumatic forces; stress fractures are rare. Traumatic fractures can result from both direct contact and indirect forces.

Clavicle Fractures

Within the shoulder complex, the clavicle is the most commonly fractured bone. The clavicle can fracture as a result of a direct anterior blow—or more often as a result of a force transmitted through the shoulder such as those resulting from a fall on an outstretched hand or from landing on the shoulder with the arm adducted. Signs and symptoms include pain, point tenderness, crepitus, and possible deformity.

Humerus Fractures

Fractures of the proximal humerus and humeral shaft are usually caused by a direct blow but may also result from a fall on an outstretched hand. Signs and symptoms include severe pain, swelling, and disability. There may also be deformity and crepitus near the fracture site. In cases of anatomical neck fracture, the deformity may resemble a glenohumeral dislocation.

Epiphyseal Fractures

Epiphyseal fractures of the proximal humeral growth plate, or **little league shoulder**, are usually associated with skeletally immature throwers. These injuries occur most often during the deceleration phase of throwing. The primary sign of impending epiphyseal injury is severe shoulder pain during hard throwing.

Scapular Fractures

The scapula is one of the least commonly fractured bones of the upper extremity, primarily because of the numerous muscles protecting the bony surfaces, as well as the scapula's mobility on the posterior chest wall. Initial signs and symptoms include diffuse aching over the posterior shoulder region and musculature and an unwillingness to move the arm. The pain may become more localized, with tenderness and swelling over the scapula. Patients with this injury typically hold their arm to the side and demonstrate significant weakness when attempting abduction.

Nerve and Vascular Injuries

Because of the close proximity to the shoulder of the brachial plexus and axillary vessels, both nerve and vascular injuries are a concern with significant shoulder trauma (figure 9.5). Most of the nerve injuries in the shoulder are associated with direct blows or traction that affects the nerve's ability to function properly. Associated nerve injuries are more common than vascular injuries at the shoulder. However, any time you observe changes in skin coloration, diminished distal pulses, numbness, tingling, weakness, and loss of motor function, you should suspect neurovascular trauma or compression, which may include the suprascapular, long thoracic, or spinal accessory nerves.

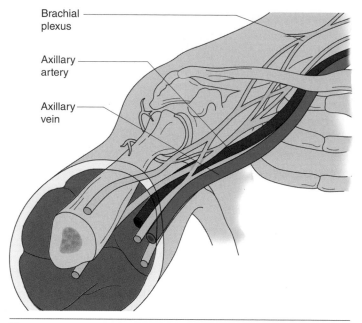

Figure 9.5 Note the close proximity of the brachial plexus (yellow) and axillary vessels (blue) to the shoulder joint.

Summary

Due to the extensive motion and function of the shoulder, recognition of the various injuries that may occur in this area is vital for proper treatment and management. The high level of mobility in the shoulder is offset by its inherent lack of stability, which leads to many of the soft tissue injuries mentioned earlier. With the few exceptions of fractures and acute dislocation types of trauma, an individual with shoulder pain does not seek treatment or examination immediately following injury. Soreness may not set in until hours later or even the next day. Signs and symptoms related to repetitive stress also appear gradually over time. Therefore it is likely that the majority of shoulder examinations will be for postacute and chronic injuries; details of those examinations are presented in chapter 12 of Shultz, Houglum, and Perrin (2010).

Elbow and Forearm Injury Recognition

The elbow plays a critical role in positioning the hand to perform physical and daily living activities. Specifically, the musculature surrounding the elbow (figure 9.6, *a* and *b*) extends and retracts the length of the limb, rotates the forearm, and manipulates the wrist and hand to effectively position the hand and fingers for particular tasks. Consider how difficult it would be to perform simple activities such as combing your hair, brushing your teeth, or opening a door without the elbow. Because of the importance of the elbow, even minor elbow injuries can be disabling. Again, accurate and timely recognition is very important to the recovery process.

The performance of the upper extremities depends on the integrity of the bones, ligaments, and muscles of the elbow and forearm that help position the hand. To allow full mobility at the elbow joint, the elbow and forearm are typically left unprotected during

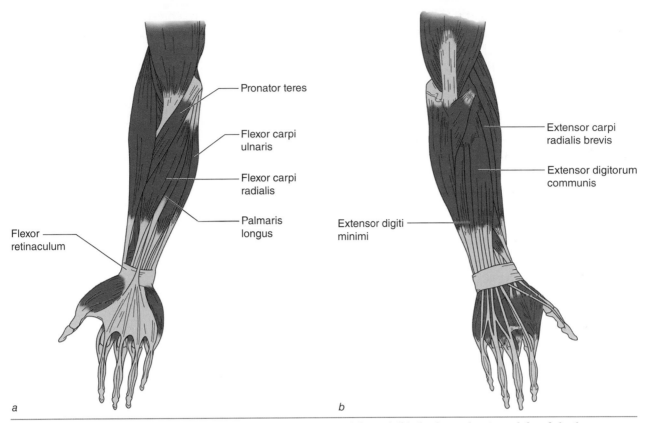

Figure 9.6 Muscles originating from *(a)* the medial epicondyle and *(b)* the lateral epicondyle of the humerus.

athletic activity and thus are exposed to a variety of contact injuries. The follow sections outline some basic injury categories.

Acute Soft Tissue Injuries

Acute soft tissue injuries at the elbow and forearm include contusions, ligament and capsular sprains, and muscle and tendon strains. Signs and symptoms include point tenderness localized over the contact area and ecchymosis. Even though the elbow is a relatively stable joint because of its bony configuration and strong collateral ligaments, acute stretching or tearing of ligament and capsular structures can occur in sport due to excessive joint loading resulting from rotational, hyperextension, and varus and valgus forces imposed on the elbow.

Contusions

During sport activity, contusions frequently occur to the muscles of the forearm and the superficial bony surfaces of the elbow. Signs and symptoms include point tenderness localized over the contact area and ecchymosis. Direct blows to the olecranon process of the ulna frequently cause inflammation or bleeding in the overlying olecranon bursa, resulting in significant bursal swelling, mild to moderate pain, and limited elbow flexion.

Because of the superficial course of the ulnar nerve between the medial epicondyle of the humerus and the olecranon process of the elbow, this nerve is vulnerable to contusions. With a direct blow to the ulnar nerve, the patient will complain of radiating pain down the medial aspect of the forearm, the hand, and into the fourth and fifth fingers. Contusions to the extensor or flexor muscle masses of the forearm may produce symptoms of decreased ROM and pain during muscular stretch or active motion.

Sprain

The elbow is a relatively stable joint because of its bony configuration and strong collateral ligaments. However, acute stretching or tearing of ligament and capsular structures can occur in sport due to excessive joint loading resulting from rotational, hyperextension, and varus and valgus forces imposed on the elbow.

▶ Ulnar (Medial) Collateral Ligament Sprains

Acute stretching or tearing of the ulnar collateral ligament (UCL) most often occurs as a result of a traumatic valgus force. Signs and symptoms of UCL sprains include sudden pain following a valgus force to the elbow. Depending on severity, there may be significant swelling and decreased ROM, with the patient holding the elbow in a flexed position for comfort.

▶ Radial (Lateral) Collateral Ligament Sprains

Lateral collateral ligament injuries occur much less frequently than medial collateral ligament injuries, since direct traction or varus forces to the lateral aspect of the elbow are rare during athletic activity. Signs and symptoms associated with injuries to the lateral collateral ligament include pain, point tenderness, and swelling of the lateral aspect of the elbow.

▶ Anterior Capsular Sprains

Anterior capsular sprains can occur due to a hyperextension mechanism at the elbow, in actions such as using an outstretched arm to stop a ball or an opponent or falling with the arm outstretched and elbow extended. Signs and symptoms include pain and tenderness in the anterior compartment, with the patient often apprehensive of fully extending the joint. The patient may also complain of pain

posteriorly where the olecranon process has been jammed or forced into the olecranon fossa.

Strains

Acute muscle and tendon strains around the elbow joint can result from a one-time episode of excessive overload or stretch. Common areas for strains are the triceps, biceps, and flexor–pronator or extensor–supinator muscles or groups. If the force applied to the elbow musculature is too great, complete ruptures of the muscle or tendons can occur, creating a need for referral and possible surgical intervention.

▶ Flexor–Pronator and Extensor–Supinator Mass Strains

Strains to the wrist flexor–pronator muscle mass can occur with any activity that produces a forceful movement into hyperflexion, extension, pronation, or supination. Excessive eccentric loads that force the wrist into flexion, extension, pronation, and supination can also lead to strains of muscles and tendons that act on the wrist. Signs and symptoms of acute strains in the forearm muscles include acute pain and tenderness over the involved muscle mass, typically near its proximal attachment and the myotendon junction.

▶ Distal Biceps Tendon

Injuries to the distal biceps tendon near or at its insertion at the radial tuberosity are rare in comparison to injuries at its proximal attachment. Signs and symptoms of tendon strain include immediate burning or pain in the anterior cubital area with point tenderness near the insertion on the radial tuberosity.

▶ Distal Triceps Tendon

Strains and rupture of the distal triceps tendon are extremely rare but can occur with forced flexion during active extension. Signs and symptoms include localized pain, palpable defect, swelling, ecchymosis, and a diminished capacity or an inability to extend the elbow against resistance.

Chronic or Overuse Soft Tissue Injuries

Chronic or overuse soft tissue injuries, the most commonly occurring elbow injuries, are typically associated with overhead throwing motions or racket sports. During these activities, the soft tissue structures of the elbow are susceptible to repetitive overuse and microtrauma that can result in chronic inflammatory conditions, fibrotic changes within the tissue, or instabilities due to stretch or weakening of the joint-stabilizing structures.

▶ Bursitis

Olecranon **bursitis** is an inflammatory condition of fluid accumulation in the subcutaneous bursa overlying the olecranon process, often caused by repetitive friction and direct trauma. The patient presents with a large, localized, fluid-filled bursa (figure 9.7); a pressure increase within the bursa during elbow flexion may limit motion.

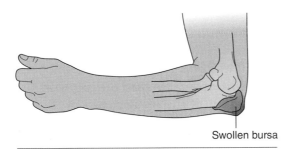

Swollen bursa

Figure 9.7 Olecranon bursitis.

▶ Tendinitis and Epicondylitis

Tendinitis and epicondylitis are overuse injuries to the tendinous attachments of the flexor–pronator group at the medial epicondyle and to the extensor–supinator group at the lateral epicondyle. Whereas tendinitis is a simple inflammatory response, epicondylitis is a degenerative condition.

• *Lateral epicondylitis (tennis elbow).* In most cases, lateral epicondylitis (also referred to as **tennis elbow**) involves primarily the extensor carpi radialis brevis and usually results from activities that tense and stress the wrist extensor and supinator muscles. Signs and symptoms include gradual onset of pain over the anterior aspect of the lateral epicondyle with the majority of tenderness localized to the origin of the extensor carpi radialis brevis tendon. Pain can be reproduced or aggravated with gripping and wrist extensor activities, as well as passive wrist flexion with forearm pronation while the elbow is extended.

• *Medial epicondylitis (golfer's elbow).* Medial epicondylitis occurs much less frequently than the lateral condition. Repetitive wrist flexor and pronator muscle activity, as in baseball pitches, golf swings, overhead tennis serve and forehand racket motions, and pull-through swimming strokes, causes medial epicondylitis (also referred to as **golfer's elbow**) (figure 9.8). Signs and symptoms include pain and mild swelling over the medial epicondyle. Resisted wrist flexion and forearm pronation, along with palpation just distal and lateral to the epicondyle over the flexor–pronator muscle group origin, reproduce pain. Passive wrist extension and forearm supination with the elbow extended may also produce pain.

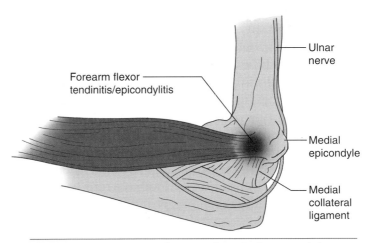

Ulnar nerve

Forearm flexor tendinitis/epicondylitis

Medial epicondyle

Medial collateral ligament

Figure 9.8 Anatomical sites of medial epicondylitis or tendinitis at the common flexor–pronator muscle origin.

Traumatic Fractures

Traumatic fractures at the elbow, relatively uncommon in adults, occur much more frequently in children and skeletally immature adolescents. Traumatic fractures can occur anywhere within the elbow complex from either direct or indirect forces imposed on the bony structures. Signs and symptoms common to all fractures include significant pain, swelling, crepitus, and tenderness over the fracture site. Due to the close proximity of various neurovascular structures in and about the elbow, injury to and compromise of these structures should be a concern with any suspected or confirmed fracture. Suspected injury to these structures is a medical emergency, as serious complications and permanent disability can result if the injury is not recognized and treated immediately.

Distal Humeral Fractures

Condylar fractures can result from a direct blow, a fall on an outstretched hand, or a traumatic valgus or varus force applied to the elbow. Supracondylar fractures (transverse fractures just superior to the condyles), which occur more frequently in children than in others, typically result from a fall on an outstretched hand with the elbow extended.

Radial Fractures
Radial head and neck fractures usually result from a fall on an outstretched arm with the forearm pronated. Signs and symptoms include swelling and pain over the lateral elbow. The patient complains particularly of pain with forearm pronation and supination and when you palpate the radial head.

Olecranon Fractures

A direct blow to the posterior elbow is the primary cause of traumatic olecranon fractures (figure 9.9). Fracture may also occur secondary to a violent triceps pull, although this is rare. Signs and symptoms include pain, point tenderness, and swelling, as well as crepitus and deformity over the posterior elbow.

Forearm Fractures

Fractures of the forearm result from forces transmitted along or across the shaft of the radius or ulna. Axial forces, a consequence of falling on an outstretched hand, may fracture

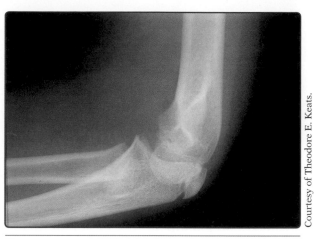

Courtesy of Theodore E. Keats.

Figure 9.9 Traumatic fractures of the olecranon process.

one or both bones. In addition to the typical signs and symptoms of fracture, active wrist motion may cause pain and crepitus.

Bony Lesions Secondary to Repetitive Stress

Chronic, repetitive valgus forces at the elbow joint can result in progressive bony lesions, particularly in skeletally immature youth. As discussed previously, these forces are typically associated with throwing.

Traction Apophyseal and Epiphyseal Injuries (Little League Elbow)

The medial apophysis is a nonarticular growth plate in adolescents that serves as the attachment site for the flexor–pronator muscle group as well as the UCL. In skeletally immature people, valgus traction forces applied during the late cocking or early acceleration phases of throwing stress the apophyseal plate rather than the tendon or ligament. The resulting injury, commonly known as **little league elbow**, may start out as an inflammatory response, or apophysitis, and progress to an avulsion of the apophysis if the repetitive stress continues. Patients with this condition report a prolonged history of pain with throwing. Signs and symptoms include point tenderness and swelling over the medial epicondyle and pain with valgus stress localized directly over the medial apophysis (Andrews and Whiteside 1993).

Dislocation and Subluxation

Elbow joint dislocations are among the more common dislocations seen in sport. Elbow dislocations can range from simple cases involving isolated ligament disruption to more complicated cases involving associated fractures, neurovascular complications, or both. In simple cases, conservative treatment of elbow dislocations produces excellent results, and recurrent dislocation or chronic instability is rarely a concern.

Humeroulnar Joint

In athletics, posterior dislocations of the ulna and radius on the humerus are significantly more common than anterior dislocations. The prevailing mechanism associated with a posterior dislocation of the humeroulnar joint is hyperextension during axial loading, typically resulting from a fall on an outstretched or extended elbow. Signs and symptoms of elbow dislocation include immediate pain, swelling, deformity, and an unwillingness to move the extremity.

Radioulnar Joint

Isolated dislocation of the radioulnar joint is rare in adults, and subluxations are more commonly seen in children. Dislocation is typically preceded by tearing of the annular ligament, distal radioulnar joint capsule, and interosseous membrane. Signs and symptoms include pain, limited ROM, elbow effusion, tenderness over the antecubital region, and inability to supinate the forearm.

Nerve and Vascular Injuries

Always suspect and carefully examine for nerve or vascular injury with factures, dislocations, and other severe trauma to the elbow and forearm. Signs and symptoms of arterial injury and resulting ischemia include pain out of proportion to what is expected for the injury, diminished or absent distal pulses, poor skin coloration, and decreased skin temperature. Signs and symptoms of nerve trauma include loss of sensation and motor function over the involved nerve's distribution.

Arterial injury as well as severe posttraumatic swelling can lead to a compartment syndrome in the forearm. In this condition a muscular compartment, enclosed by its relatively inelastic surrounding fascia, is subject to excessive swelling and increasing pressure. As pressure exceeds that of the vessel walls within the compartment, vascular collapse occurs, compromising circulation to the muscles and nerves. Signs and symptoms of a compartment syndrome include the five Ps (pain, pallor, paresthesia, paralysis, and pulselessness). The earliest and most reliable symptom of a compartment syndrome is unrelenting pain, often out of proportion to the injury.

Nerve Compression Syndromes

Nerve compression syndromes are common around the elbow, frequently resulting from repetitive compression or traction mechanisms seen in sports such as throwing and tennis. This section deals with the more common compression syndromes of the major peripheral nerves of the forearm.

Ulnar Nerve

The ulnar nerve passes the elbow superficially between the medial epicondyle and the medial border of the olecranon. Because of its superficial course and anatomical constraints as it passes the medial elbow, it is prone to contusions, subluxation, traction and frictional forces, compression syndromes, and irritation caused by surrounding chronic or degenerative conditions. Regardless of the underlying cause, ulnar neuropathy typically exhibits pain or aching originating at the medial elbow and radiating down the lateral forearm into the fifth digit and the medial surface of the fourth digit. Radiating pain or paresthesia may be reproduced with light tapping over the inflamed nerve (**Tinel's sign**).

Median Nerve

Compression of the median nerve at the elbow, or **pronator teres syndrome**, can occur between the two heads of the pronator teres secondary to muscle hypertrophy or tight fibrous bands. Pronator teres syndrome is most often seen in sports such as weightlifting, rowing, golf, tennis, and racquetball as a consequence of repetitive pronation and sustained gripping. Achy pain, paresthesia, and motor weakness over the median nerve distribution of the thumb and the second and third digits may indicate median nerve irritation.

Anterior Interosseous Nerve

The anterior interosseous nerve is a motor branch off the median nerve that runs along the interosseous membrane. Occasionally this nerve is compressed by the forearm muscles or overlying fibrous bands secondary to forceful muscle contractions. The prevailing sign is loss of pinch strength between the tips of the thumb and index finger.

Radial Nerve

Radial tunnel syndrome is typically caused by repetitive or vigorous wrist extension and forearm pronation and supination. It is often incorrectly identified as lateral epicondylitis, but careful examination can differentiate the two conditions. Symptoms include pain radiating into the forearm extensors and pain reproduction with resisted supination or extension of the middle finger.

Summary

Injuries to the elbow can be quite debilitating because of its importance in positioning the hand for activities of daily living and sporting activities. Recognition of the various elbow pathologies occurs most often in a clinical examination, but on-site examinations have a heightened urgency due to possible injury to the neurovascular structures that are so important to the hand and wrist. The need for on-site examination of an elbow injury most often arises from direct contact, a fall on an outstretched hand, hyperextension, or a severe valgus or varus mechanism. As always, your goal is to quickly determine the nature and severity of the injury and check for any conditions indicating a medical emergency. As soon as you arrive at the patient's side, conduct a primary survey and observe his response to the injury, his willingness to move the injured limb, the position of the limb, and the neurological and vascular status of the limb. Many elbow assessments are performed in the clinic setting in lieu of an on-site examination, and details of procedures are presented in chapter 13 of Shultz, Houglum, and Perrin (2010).

Wrist and Hand Injury Recognition

Since the purpose of the shoulder and elbow is to position the hand for a variety of tasks, the hand and its functions are the ultimate reason for upper extremity design. The hand is a complex tool used for a large assortment of activities, ranging from fine motor activities such as writing, threading a needle, and picking up small objects to gross motor tasks such as throwing a baseball, gripping a tennis racket, or swinging on the uneven parallel bars. Proper wrist and hand functioning is vital for performing these tasks, and thus even minor injuries can be quite disabling. The structure of the wrist and hand represents a complex network of multiple bones (figure 9.10), joints, ligaments, and intrinsic and extrinsic muscles that function together to provide the precision, coordination, mobility, and strength required to perform various tasks. Because of the anatomical complexity of the wrist and hand, you are encouraged to review the structures and functions of this body region before continuing.

The dexterity and precision that the wrist and hand require for fine motor control often leave them unprotected and vulnerable to injury during sport activity. Contact with the

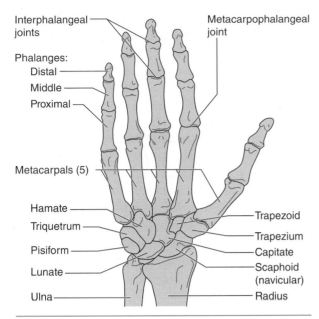

Figure 9.10   Skeletal anatomy of the wrist and hand.

ground (falls), opponents, and balls and other sporting implements is the primary mechanism for acute injury of the wrist and hand. The hand and wrist are also prone to repetitive stress injuries as well as other chronic conditions that may result from ignored or untreated acute injuries.

Acute Soft Tissue Injuries

Physically active people commonly experience contusions, sprains, and strains, primarily as a result of direct contact, falls, and other forces that either compress or place tension on the soft tissue structures of the hand and wrist. Because of the many bony prominences and superficial tendons exposed in the wrist and hand, contusions resulting from direct contact may be bothersome.

Sprains

Because of the multiple bones and joints in the wrist and hand, ligament injuries are quite common. In addition to varus and valgus forces, flexion or extension beyond the normal ROM is often the cause of sprains to the wrist and fingers. Signs and symptoms associated with wrist sprain include pain, swelling, and point tenderness over the injured joint consistent with the degree of injury. The patient often experiences pain with both active and passive ROM.

▶ Collateral Ligament Sprain

Collateral ligament sprains of the fingers are among the most common injuries resulting from physical activity. Collateral ligament injuries (figure 9.11) can occur at either the metacarpophalangeal (MCP) joint, the proximal interphalangeal (PIP) joint, or the distal interphalangeal (DIP) joint. Signs and symptoms associated with collateral ligament sprains include pain, swelling, point tenderness over the injured joint and ligament, and increased pain and possible instability with valgus or varus stress. Pain and swelling commonly persist for a significant amount of time.

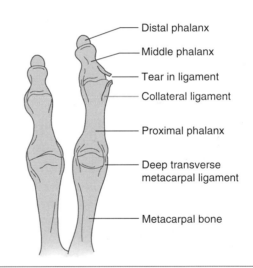

Figure 9.11   Injury to the collateral ligament of the finger.

▶ Gamekeeper's or Skier's Thumb

A collateral ligament injury that can be particularly troublesome, known as **gamekeeper's thumb** or skier's thumb, involves the ulnar (medial) collateral ligament (UCL) of the MCP joint of the thumb (figure 9.12). The injury results from forced abduction and hyperextension of the thumb away from

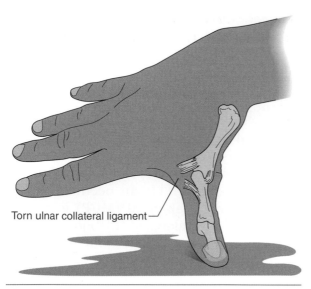

Figure 9.12   Gamekeeper's thumb.

the hand that stretch and tear the UCL. It has been termed skier's thumb because the mechanism often occurs when skiers fall on an outstretched hand while holding on to a ski pole. Signs and symptoms include pain, point tenderness over the medial aspect of the MCP joint of the thumb, swelling, and varying degrees of instability consistent with the degree of ligament injury.

Strains and Tendon Avulsions

Finger tendon injuries are quite common in the physically active. Tendon injuries can result from a direct blow but more often result from abrupt forces applied in the direction opposite to the one in which a joint is contracting. This mechanism can create considerable tensioning of the tendon, causing it to tear away from its distal attachment.

▶ Flexor Tendon Avulsion (Jersey Finger)

Flexor tendon avulsion injuries involve the flexor digitorum profundus tendon; they occur when the distal phalanx is forcefully extended while the finger is flexing. This injury is often called a **jersey finger** because it is frequently seen in patients such as football players who get a finger caught while trying to grab and pull at an opponent's jersey. Signs and symptoms include immedi-

ate pain, swelling, and point tenderness at the attachment of the flexor tendon on the distal phalanx. With complete rupture (figure 9.13), the patient is unable to flex the distal phalanx while the proximal joint is held in extension.

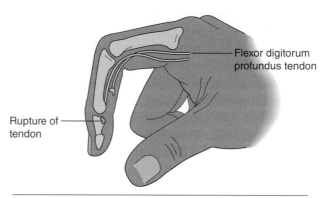

Figure 9.13   Jersey finger.

▶ Extensor Tendon Avulsion (Mallet Finger)

Mallet finger, or baseball finger, occurs when the extended distal phalanx is suddenly and forcefully flexed. A common example is seen when a patient attempts to catch a ball and the ball hits the tip of the extended finger. Rupture of the extensor digitorum longus may or may not include avulsion of a bony fragment (figure 9.14). Signs and symptoms include pain, point tenderness over the distal attachment, flexion deformity of the distal phalanx, and an inability to actively extend the distal phalanx.

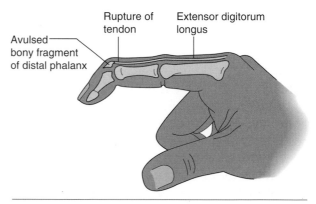

Figure 9.14   Mallet finger.

Chronic or Overuse Soft Tissue Injuries

Because of the repetitive nature of many hand movements, as well as the excessive use of the hands in many sport and occupational activities, chronic inflammatory conditions of the wrist, hand, and fingers are common. These include ganglion cysts, tendinitis, and tenosynovitis. In addition, complications from unrecognized or untreated acute injuries can result in chronic and potentially disfiguring conditions such as contractures.

Wrist Ganglion

A wrist ganglion, or synovial cyst, is characterized by herniation of synovial fluid through the joint capsule or synovial sheath of a tendon. Minor sprains and strains often precipitate a wrist ganglion and are thought to weaken the capsule or synovial sheath, allowing fluid to escape and accumulate. Signs and symptoms include an observable and palpable localized mass over the wrist (figure 9.15). The mass may or may not be painful and may or may not restrict ROM or impede function. Symptoms may be more related to the location of the cyst and the motions it may restrict.

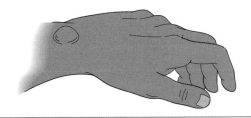

Figure 9.15   Wrist ganglion.

Tendinitis and Tenosynovitis

Inflammation of the tendon or its surrounding synovial sheath is common in physically active people. Overuse or repetitive motion, direct trauma, and continual use following tendon injury are all common mechanisms of tendinitis and tenosynovitis. Signs and symptoms include point tenderness over the involved tendon, swelling, palpable crepitus, pain with active and resistive motion, and pain with passive stretching of the tendon.

Bony Pathology

Fractures and dislocations of the wrist and hand are among the most common injuries in sport. The use of the hands for reaching, blocking, catching, and grabbing increases their vulnerability to injury during sport activities.

Traumatic Fractures

Traumatic fractures of the wrist and hand most often occur due to axial loading forces or falls on an outstretched hand. Other mechanisms include compression, torsion, and repetitive trauma.

Distal Radioulnar Fractures

Fracture of the distal radius and ulna is typically caused by a fall on an outstretched hand with the wrist flexed or extended. Signs and symptoms include immediate wrist pain, rapid swelling, tenderness, and deformity. Loss of wrist and hand function may result both from an unwillingness to move the extremity because of pain and from restrictions caused by the displacement.

Bennett's Fracture

A Bennett's fracture (figure 9.16), involving the base of the first metacarpal bone

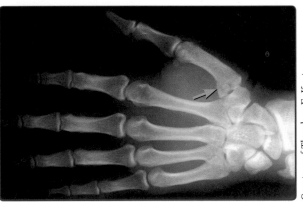

Figure 9.16   Bennett's fracture with metacarpal displacement.

Courtesy of Theodore E. Keats.

(thumb), is most often caused by striking an object with a closed fist, making contact specifically with the thumb. Signs and symptoms include immediate pain, rapid swelling, tenderness, and crepitus at the MCP joint of the thumb, as well as function loss.

Carpal Bones

Among the eight carpal bones, the navicular or scaphoid bone is the one most commonly fractured (figure 9.17). It can also be the most troublesome and slowest to heal. Navicular fractures typically occur when the bone is compressed against the radius during direct contact with the palm of the hand—for example, during blocking with the hands or in a fall in which the thumb and wrist are extended and the wrist is abducted. The patient complains of pain, swelling, and tenderness over the radial side of the wrist. A hallmark of a navicular fracture is point tenderness specifically over the navicular when you palpate in the anatomical snuffbox.

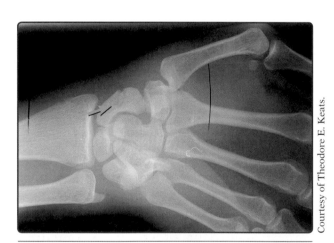

Figure 9.17　Navicular fracture.

Metacarpal Bones

Fractures to the neck, shaft, and base of the metacarpal bones often result from axial loading of the metacarpal bone secondary to an indirect force such as striking an object with a closed fist. Other common causes

are direct trauma or crushing injuries to the hand, as when the hand is stepped on or landed on during sport activity. Signs and symptoms include pain, diffuse swelling over the dorsum of the hand, and tenderness over the metacarpal. You may note bony crepitus and also deformity if the bone is displaced. When the fracture specifically involves the neck of the fifth metacarpal, the injury is commonly referred to as **boxer's fracture** (figure 9.18).

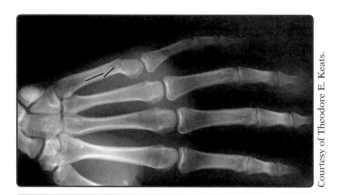

Figure 9.18　Boxer's fracture.

Phalanges

Fractures of the phalanges can be caused by a variety of mechanisms, including direct contact, axial loading to the tip of the finger, torsion, and other indirect trauma. Fractures may also occur with sprains and dislocations. Signs and symptoms include pain, swelling, and point tenderness over the fracture site, as well as loss of function, deformity, and crepitus.

Dislocation or Subluxation

The same forces and mechanisms responsible for wrist and hand fractures may also result in joint dislocation or subluxation. In the wrist, the most commonly dislocated carpal bone is the lunate. Lunate dislocations can be caused by a fall on an outstretched hand or with hyperextension of the wrist. Dislocation of the MCP and interphalangeal (IP) joints (figure 9.19) is consistent with

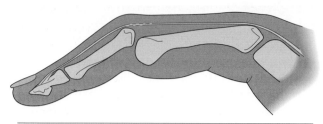

Figure 9.19 Interphalangeal joint dislocation.

third-degree sprains in which the ligaments and joint capsule are stretched or torn sufficiently to allow joint displacement. Unless the joint spontaneously reduces following injury, these injuries are quite obvious. Signs and symptoms of dislocation include obvious deformity, pain, rapid swelling, and loss of function. Often, the patient or coach reduces the dislocation and the patient does not seek medical attention. However, a physician should examine all first-time dislocations to rule out any associated articular fractures or volar plate disruptions.

Nerve and Vascular Injuries

Most cases of nerve or vascular compromise at the wrist and hand are attributable to chronic inflammatory conditions that compress these structures. On occasion, severe fractures or dislocations can also result in secondary injury or compression of the nearby nerve or vascular structure. Signs and symptoms include pain, numbness, tingling, and atrophy of the areas affected by the innervation of the median, ulnar, and radial nerves.

▶ Carpal Tunnel Syndrome (Median Nerve Compression)

Carpal tunnel syndrome is a common wrist and hand condition, although not often seen in athletes. It is characterized by compression of the median nerve as it passes through the carpal tunnel on the palmar aspect of the hand and wrist. The compression can be caused by direct trauma, fluid retention, inflammation, or anatomical abnormalities. Signs and symptoms of carpal tunnel include pain, tenderness, and sensory changes (over palmar aspect of the medial thumb and the first and second fingers). In addition, in severe and prolonged cases, motor weakness of the wrist and finger flexors can be present.

▶ Ulnar Nerve Compression

Prolonged or repetitive pressure, as well as acute trauma such as fractures involving the pisiform and hamate bones in the hypothenar eminence, may produce symptoms related to ulnar nerve compression. Cycling, racket sports, and other implement sports may give rise to irritation of the ulnar nerve as it passes superficially through the tunnel of Guyon, found between the hamate and pisiform. Signs and symptoms associated with ulnar nerve compression include pain, paresthesia, and muscle weakness directly over the area or involving the fourth and fingers.

Summary

Patients commonly delay reporting wrist and hand injuries, so you may not have the opportunity to examine the injury until several days after it has occurred. This often has ramifications for proper treatment and management, as periods of time have passed during which necessary intervention has not occurred. Chronic or overuse injuries are typically not reported until they begin to interfere with work or performance. Therefore the history portion of the examination is critical to an understanding of the injury and in turn to proper examination and management. The recognition and management goals for wrist and hand injuries focus on returning function to as close to preinjury levels as possible. Specific techniques and details of the hand and wrist evaluation are presented in chapter 14 of Shultz, Houglum, and Perrin (2010).

CASE STUDY

Beth is a junior on her college swim team. The team is participating in 2 weeks of very difficult swim practices in preparation for the upcoming season. Many of the swimmers are very tired at the end of these long and intense practices. One day Beth reports to the athletic training room before practice and tells the team's athletic trainer, Kevin, that for the past 6 days she has noticed increasing pain located toward the tip of her shoulder. She does not remember a specific injury episode but tells Kevin that the pain has become increasingly worse over the past couple of days and is most heightened during harder practices and sets that involve overhead strokes. In fact, the symptoms can become so severe that she has to alter her stroke, and she feels that she does not have the power she needs to complete her strokes correctly. The symptoms typically lessen when she is not swimming but are painful whenever she raises her arms over her head. In addition to her pain, Beth complains of some "snapping and popping" and pain radiating down into her biceps and lateral upper arm.

Think About It

1. What pathologies should Kevin consider in evaluating Beth's complaints?

2. What diagnostic tests can he use to help evaluate Beth's upper extremities?

3. What treatment options should he consider to help Beth with these complaints?

4. How should Beth's practice be modified to assist in the resolution of her symptoms?

Learning Aids

SUMMARY

The bones, joints, ligaments, muscles, tendons, nerves, and vascular structures of the upper extremity are common locations of injuries and pathologies. This chapter provides examples of the more frequently seen upper extremity pathologies and also identifies common signs and symptoms to aid in quick recognition. The athletic trainer must be aware of the various pathologies and how to recognize them to facilitate a quick and satisfactory recovery in patients with these injuries and pathologies.

KEY CONCEPTS AND REVIEW

▶ **Describe the difference between shoulder dislocation, subluxation, and separation.**

• Dislocation. Occurs when the bones of the glenohumeral joint (humeral head and glenoid fossa) become dissociated and remain that way until manually reduced and returned to their anatomical position. Dislocation occurs due to force that results in stretching of the glenohumeral joint capsule, thus causing the humeral head to "fall off" the glenoid fossa.

- Subluxation. A temporary and spontaneously reduced partial or complete dislocation. In a subluxation, the humeral head becomes partially or completely disassociated from the glenoid fossa but spontaneously reduces back to the correct (or near correct) anatomical position. Patients often characterize a shoulder subluxation by saying "My shoulder slipped out and went back in." Shoulder subluxations can be either acute episodes caused by a new injury or chronic conditions caused by repeated dislocations or subluxations that cause the joint capsule to become stretched, thus decreasing its ability to restrain the humeral head.

- Separation. In the shoulder, an injury to the AC joint and the associated joint capsule and ligaments. Typically this injury occurs during a fall on the "tip" or "point" of the shoulder and results in localized pain and occasional deformity, depending on how much the joint stability is affected.

▶ **Detail the signs and symptoms associated with subacromial impingement syndrome.**

Subacromial impingement leads to dull or deep pain underneath or near the acromion and to difficulty producing arm movement above the head. Point tenderness may be noted just anterolateral to the acromion and at the insertion of the supraspinatus tendon. The patient may also complain of pain radiating down the anterior (biceps) and lateral (supraspinatus) aspects of the upper arm.

▶ **Explain similarities and differences between golfer's elbow and tennis elbow.**

Golfer's elbow and tennis elbow are similar in that they are characterized by inflammation and irritation of the common tendons that attach at either the medial or lateral epicondyle. These injuries produce localized pain as well as pain with many wrist and hand movements and functions. Golfer's elbow, otherwise known as medial epicondylitis, is a pathology of the common flexor tendons of the wrist and hand located in the anterior–medial forearm. Resisted wrist flexion and forearm pronation, as well as palpation just distal and lateral to the epicondyle over the flexor–pronator muscle group origin, reproduce pain. Passive wrist extension and forearm supination with the elbow extended may also produce pain. In contrast, lateral epicondylitis (or tennis elbow) is a pathology of the common extensor tendons of the wrist and hand located in the posterior–lateral forearm. Signs and symptoms include gradual onset of pain over the anterior aspect of the lateral epicondyle with the majority of tenderness localized to the origin of the extensor carpi radialis brevis tendon. Pain can be reproduced or aggravated with gripping and wrist extensor activities, as well as passive wrist flexion with forearm pronation while the elbow is extended.

▶ **Give details about structures involved, predisposing factors, and signs and symptoms of little league elbow.**

The medial apophysis is a nonarticular growth plate in adolescents that serves as the attachment site for the flexor–pronator muscle group as well as the UCL. In skeletally immature patients, valgus traction forces applied during the late cocking or early acceleration phases of throwing stress the apophyseal plate rather than the tendon or ligament. The resulting injury may start out as an inflammatory response and progress to an avulsion of the apophysis if the repetitive stress continues. Individuals with this condition report a prolonged history of pain with throwing. Signs and symptoms include pain and swelling over the medial epicondyle. In addition, pain and laxity may be present during stress testing of the medial elbow if the apophysitis is irritated.

▸ **Identify the mechanism and structures involved in gamekeeper's thumb.**

Gamekeeper's thumb injuries involve the ulnar (medial) collateral ligament (UCL) of the MCP joint of the thumb. The injury typically results from forced abduction and hyperextension of the thumb, away from the hand, that stretches and tears the UCL. This injury has also been termed skier's thumb because the mechanism often occurs when skiers fall on an outstretched hand while holding on to a ski pole. Signs and symptoms include pain, point tenderness over the medial aspect of the MCP joint of the thumb, swelling, and varying degrees of instability consistent with the degree of ligament injury.

▸ **Detail differences between jersey and mallet finger.**

Jersey finger injuries are flexor tendon avulsion injuries involving the flexor digitorum profundus tendon; they occur when the distal phalanx is forcefully extended while the finger is flexing. Signs and symptoms include immediate pain, swelling, and point tenderness at the attachment of the flexor tendon on the distal phalanx. With complete rupture, the patient is unable to flex the distal phalanx while the proximal joint is held in extension. In contrast, mallet finger occurs when the extended distal phalanx is suddenly and forcefully flexed. Signs and symptoms include pain, point tenderness over the distal attachment, flexion deformity of the distal phalanx, and an inability to actively extend the distal phalanx.

▸ **Identify the location of boxer's fracture.**

Boxer's fracture is typically found in the neck of the fifth metacarpal.

PRACTICE!

For hands-on practice in this area, go to the web resource and complete the following:

Level 2.9, Module J8: Shoulder Injury Assessment and Diagnosis

Level 2.9, Module J10: Wrist and Hand Injury Assessment and Diagnosis

CRITICAL THINKING QUESTIONS

1. A patient walks into your clinic complaining of lateral elbow pain. His chief complaints are pain and stiffness upon waking in the morning, pain while moving the wrist into extension, pain with passive movement into flexion, and weakness and pain while gripping objects. There was no episode of injury per se, but the patient first noticed the signs after a 3 h tennis match with a friend 2 days ago. What injury do you suspect and why?

2. A female swimmer reports to your clinic with complaints of hand numbness following intense swimming during practice. This numbness does not start at the beginning of practice but about halfway through. She feels the numbness in the entire hand and has some aching and weakness along with it. All symptoms resolve within 3 h after practice, only to start up again during the next practice. What injury and pathologies do you suspect and why?

Lower Extremity Injury Recognition

Sandra J. Shultz, PhD, ATC, CSCS, FNATA
Kirk Brumels, PhD, AT, ATC

OBJECTIVES

After reading this chapter, the student should be able to do the following:

- List the most common avulsion fracture sites of the hip and pelvis region.
- Describe the injury mechanism and signs and symptoms of myositis ossificans.
- List the primary functions of menisci.
- Describe the functions of the posterior cruciate ligament and anterior cruciate ligament.
- Identify the contributing factors and signs and symptoms of patellofemoral pain syndrome.
- Describe the mechanism and biomechanics involved in iliotibial band friction syndrome.
- Detail differences between lateral ligament and syndesmotic ankle sprains.
- Describe a Lisfranc fracture.
- Explain the location of a Jones fracture.

This chapter describes various injuries to the hip, pelvis, thigh, knee, lower leg, ankle, and foot and presents information relating to the recognition and examination of these injuries. Familiarity with the injuries that commonly occur to these anatomical structures will facilitate your ability to examine these areas and to interpret your findings accurately. For an overview of general injury mechanisms, classifications, and examination techniques, refer to chapters 7 and 8. Specific tests and techniques are beyond the scope of this text and are not discussed here. For more complete examination strategies for the hip, pelvis, thigh, knee, lower leg, ankle, and foot, refer to Shultz, Houglum, and Perrin (2010).

Hip, Pelvis, and Groin Injury Recognition

Given the structural integrity of the hip and pelvis and the tremendous forces that sport activity can exert on these structures, injuries in this region range from minor strains and irritations to severe joint disruptions. It is important to appreciate the anatomy (figure 10.1, *a* through *c*) and the types of injuries to these structures that you may encounter in physically active people, as well as strategies for proper referral and care.

Considerable forces can be transmitted through the hip and pelvis during weight-bearing activities. Primarily because of the strength and stability of the hip and pelvis, injuries to this region are less common than those to the knee and ankle. However, when injuries do occur, even those that are minor can be painful and debilitating because of the role these structures play in weight bearing and locomotion.

Acute Soft Tissue Injuries

The most common types of acute injury to the hip, pelvis, and groin are contusions, muscle strains, and sprains. Traumatic fractures and dislocations are rare; stress fractures of the femoral neck and avulsion fractures are more common. Because of the relative stability of the hip and sacroiliac joints and the strength of the surrounding ligaments, sprains in this region are less common than in other lower extremity joints. Muscular strains about the hip are relatively common, resulting from

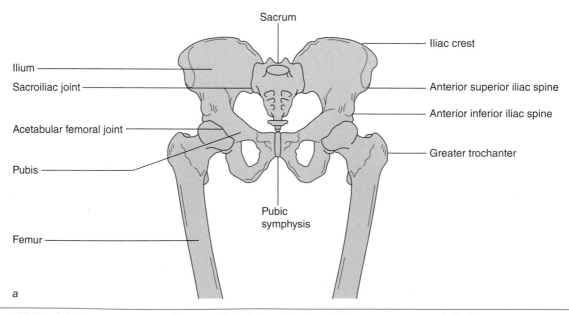

Figure 10.1 *(a)* Bony anatomy and joints of the hip and pelvis. *(b)* Posterior view of the ligamentous support of the hip joint. The pubofemoral ligament can be seen only in the anterior view. *(c)* Ligamentum teres (ligamentum capitis femoris). *(continued)*

overstretching or from a rapid, forceful contraction.

Contusions

Because of their many superficial bony prominences, the hip and pelvis are prone to contusions. Most vulnerable to injury are the lateral hip, iliac crest (**hip pointer**), and coccyx. Contusions to these areas can cause considerable pain and disability. Signs and symptoms include localized pain, swelling, and ecchymosis.

Sprains

Because the hip is a relatively stable joint supported by skeletal anatomy characteristics (deep socket) and numerous ligaments, excessive movement is not common. Due to this decreased movement, sprains in this region are less common than in other lower extremity joints. However, when they do occur, they will most likely limit physical activity.

Sacroiliac Joint

Sacroiliac sprains most often result from jamming mechanisms—for example, when a basketball player comes down from a rebound and lands off balance on a single leg with the leg straight and the back extended. This can transmit sizable forces through the lumbosacral and sacroiliac regions, contusing the joint and possibly disrupting the liga-

ment. Signs and symptoms associated with sacroiliac sprains include pain, swelling, and tenderness over the affected joint and ligaments. Pain may be localized to the involved area but may also be felt as a deep ache or radiating pain into the buttock and thigh.

Hip Joint

Direct and indirect forces that cause excessive rotation or abduction, or that drive the femur posteriorly when the hip is flexed, can stretch or tear the ligaments surrounding the hip joint. Signs and symptoms of a hip joint sprain are pain deep in the joint and difficulty with weight bearing. The patient complains of pain with passive hip movement as the injured ligament becomes taut.

Strains

Muscular strains about the hip are relatively common, resulting from overstretching or from a rapid, forceful contraction. Explosive starts and slipping of the foot during cutting are common mechanisms for strains to the hip flexor and adductor. Abductor strains can result from quick and forceful movements such as cutting away from the side of the plant leg. Improper warm-up, muscle fatigue, and weakness are thought to increase an individual's risk for muscle strain, as

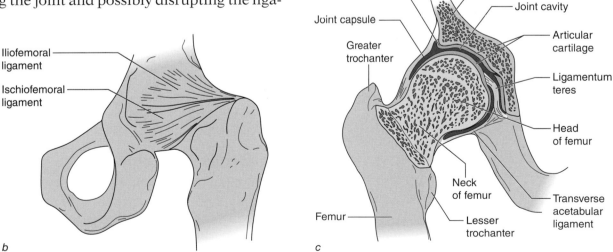

Figure 10.1 *(continued)* *(a)* Bony anatomy and joints of the hip and pelvis. *(b)* Posterior view of the ligamentous support of the hip joint. The pubofemoral ligament can be seen only in the anterior view. *(c)* Ligamentum teres (ligamentum capitis femoris).

these injuries frequently occur during the beginning of practice and preseason training. Signs and symptoms may include pain and a burning or tearing sensation at the time of injury, and the patient may feel or hear a pop. You will note palpable tenderness and spasm in the involved muscle, and you may also palpate a defect with third-degree strains. Swelling, ecchymosis, and pain with passive stretch and active contraction are consistent with the degree of injury.

Chronic or Overuse Soft Tissue Injuries

Because of the repetitive stresses placed on the hip and pelvis during locomotion and cutting and jumping maneuvers, chronic conditions caused by inflammation and muscle tightness are seen more often than acute injuries. Structural and functional abnormalities at the hip can significantly affect the entire lower extremity.

Bursitis and Snapping Hip Syndrome

Bursae are fluid-filled sacs that help reduce friction at various points throughout the body. Although numerous bursae surround the hip and pelvis, chronic bursitis usually involves the trochanteric, iliopsoas, or ischial bursae (figure 10.2).

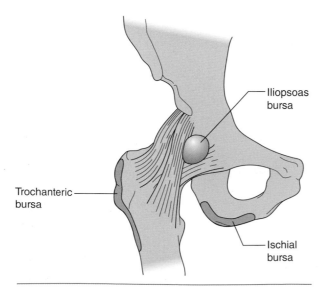

Figure 10.2 Location of the iliopsoas, trochanteric, and ischial bursae.

Bursitis and Snapping Hip Syndrome

The trochanteric bursa sits between the iliotibial (IT) band and the greater trochanter. Tightness in the IT band, repetitive insult to the lateral hip, excessive biomechanical abnormalities, leg length discrepancy (long leg), and running on a slanted street (downhill side) may cause abnormal friction and irritation of the bursa between these structures. The patient complains of pain or deep aching in the lateral hip, has palpable tenderness and crepitus over the greater trochanter, and is unable to lie on the involved side. Swelling and redness occur if the bursa is acutely inflamed.

Iliopsoas Bursitis

Iliopsoas bursitis most often results from overuse activities. The patient complains of pain in the anterior groin with hip flexion. As the bursa is deep to the adductor muscles, it is difficult to examine and palpate for tenderness. Because of the difficulty in palpating the specific structures, iliopsoas bursitis is often mistaken for a muscular strain.

Ischial Bursitis

The ischial bursa, which lies over the ischial tuberosity, may become painful and inflamed with excessive friction. As the ischial tuberosities bear the weight in sitting, repeatedly flexing the hip and extending one leg and then the other (e.g., cycling with an improperly adjusted seat) can irritate the bursa. The patient complains of pain with sitting, has palpable tenderness over the ischial tuberosity, and pain with passive hip flexion and active or resistive hip extension. Ischial bursitis is often difficult to differentiate from proximal hamstring tendinitis.

Piriformis Syndrome

The piriformis muscle is a lateral hip rotator that originates on the sacrum and passes through the greater sciatic notch to its attachment on the posterior superior aspect of the greater trochanter of the femur (figure 10.3). Anatomically, the sciatic nerve usually passes underneath the piriformis as it exits

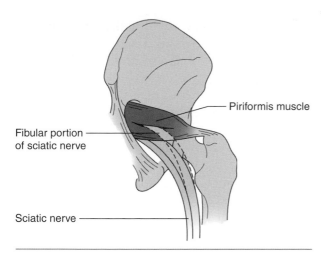

Figure 10.3 In the majority of the population, the sciatic nerve passes underneath the piriformis, but in about 12% of the population it splits, such that its fibular portion passes through the piriformis with the tibial portion still passing underneath.

the greater sciatic foramen. Because of the close proximity of the sciatic nerve to the piriformis muscle, it is prone to irritation in this region.

Traumatic Fractures and Hip Dislocation

Hip fractures, which most frequently occur through the femoral neck, typically result from a direct blow to the lateral hip. Traumatic hip fractures are usually obvious, as the involved leg appears shortened and laterally rotated. While traumatic fractures are often obvious, others, such as stress fractures, are not, as they can mimic the symptoms of a muscle strain. With less obvious fractures, if the patient is able to move the hip and lower extremity at all, she will most certainly be unable or unwilling to bear weight. Pelvic fractures due to crush injuries can be life threatening, as they may cause considerable hemorrhage. Any patient with a suspected traumatic fracture should be examined and continually monitored for shock.

Avulsion Fractures

Avulsion fractures result from a violent contraction producing tremendous tractioning forces through the muscular tendon to the bony attachment. Common sites for avulsion fractures are the anterior superior iliac spine (ASIS, sartorius), anterior inferior iliac spine (AIIS, rectus femoris), lesser trochanter (iliopsoas), and ischial tuberosity (hamstring). Signs and symptoms include immediate pain, swelling, and loss of function.

Hip Dislocation

Hip dislocations are usually easy to identify. Most dislocations occur posteriorly with the hip and knee in a flexed position. A direct blow transmitted up the shaft of the femur, or less commonly an indirect medial (internal) rotational force with the foot firmly planted, can displace the femoral head posteriorly to the acetabulum. Examples of common mechanisms are seen when the knee hits the dashboard during a traffic collision and when someone lands hard on a flexed knee with the full weight directed through the long axis of the femur. In order for the hip to dislocate, significant stretching and tearing of the acetabular labrum and surrounding ligaments must occur. Signs and symptoms include extreme pain, obvious deformity, and inability to move the extremity. The leg appears as shortened and medially rotated (vs. laterally rotated as with a fracture). The patient must be immobilized and immediately transported to emergency medical care via emergency medical services.

Summary

The hip is a very stable joint due to the shape of its bony articulations. Because joint stability is inversely related to joint mobility, hip mobility is sacrificed as a function of stability, and therefore many of the injuries around the hip region are soft tissue injuries. With the exceptions of dislocations, fractures, and acute muscular strains, many hip injuries have an insidious onset that occurs over time. As always, obtain a brief history from the patient as to the mechanism of injury and the location, type, and severity of the symptoms. The patient's responses to questions about the history should allow you to obtain a clear and accurate injury profile and to establish the stage of the injury (acute, postacute, or chronic or overuse)—and, if the injury is chronic, how the pain profile has changed over time. This information is important for determining the structures involved and management protocols.

Knee and Thigh Injury Recognition

Thigh and knee injuries receive much attention in sports medicine, athletics, and society in general, which is perhaps attributable to the numerous pathologies that occur around the thigh and knee. It may also be attributable to the prevalence of these injuries and the debilitating effects of many of them. In any case, recognition and management of thigh and knee injuries have been and will

continue to be in the forefront of sports medicine research and discussion. Pathologies around the thigh and knee quickly affect functional ability and therefore come to the attention of health care professionals relatively quickly after inception. It is important for athletic trainers to understand the various pathologies that can occur in and around the knee joint.

The knee is a complex joint that absorbs and transmits forces through the lower extremity during weight bearing and that provides mobility for locomotion (figure 10.4, a through c). As the link between the

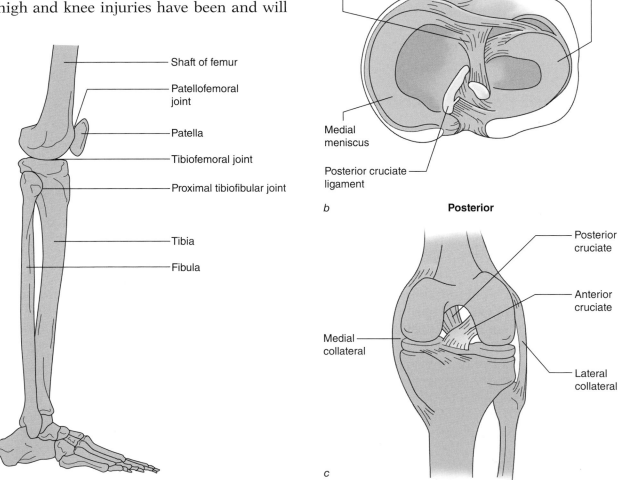

Figure 10.4   (a) Knee bones and joints; (b) medial and lateral menisci at their attachments on the tibial plateau; (c) primary stabilizing ligaments of the knee.

(a) Adapted, by permission, from W.C. Whiting and R.R. Zernicke, 1998, *Biomechanics of musculoskeletal injury* (Champaign, IL: Human Kinetics), 150.

femur and tibia, the knee experiences considerable torque through these long levers during physical activity. These factors make the knee vulnerable to multiple injuries and pathologies.

The knee joint is one of the most frequently injured joints in physically active people. It is particularly susceptible to injury because of its lack of bony stability, its reliance on soft tissue structures for stability, and the large mechanical forces it experiences during sport activity. Compressive, varus and valgus, anterior and posterior shear, and rotational forces are constantly applied to the knee joint during sport activities, particularly those that require running, jumping, cutting, and rapid change of direction. Injury results when either internal or external forces exceed the structural and supportive capabilities of the supporting tissues.

Acute Soft Tissue Injuries

Because the knee relies so heavily on the soft tissue structures for stability and function, injuries to these structures are common. Acute soft tissue injuries can result from both contact and noncontact mechanisms, and with or without the foot in contact with the ground. As with any joint, soft tissue injuries around a joint can affect its function. The loss of function due to injury is exacerbated in the knee joint because of its use in ambulation and activities of daily living.

Contusions

To allow full, unrestricted motion, the knee and thigh are often unprotected during sport activity, leaving the area vulnerable to direct contact with a sport implement, another player, or the ground. Because of the mobility required at the knee, contusions around the joint can be particularly bothersome. Signs and symptoms include pain, swelling, point tenderness, and discoloration. Contusion may also limit range of motion (ROM) and function secondary to pain and swelling.

Quadriceps Contusion

Muscle contusions in the thigh, particularly the quadriceps, can be quite troublesome

and can result in prolonged disability. Quadriceps contusions occur most often when the muscle sustains direct contact while it is contracted rather than relaxed. Significant pain, spasm, and loss of function immediately follow injury. Range of motion into flexion is limited secondary to pain and spasm, but gentle stretching and ice with the knee flexed may afford relief.

Myositis Ossificans

A potential consequence of a quadriceps muscle contusion is myositis ossificans, which occurs when the body's inflammatory response during hematoma absorption causes calcification or forms bony deposits in the muscle. Signs and symptoms of myositis ossificans include a history of severe or repetitive insult to the quadriceps, pain, a palpable mass within the muscle belly, decreased knee flexion range, and decreased quadriceps strength.

Traumatic Bursitis

Direct contact over one of the superficial knee bursae may cause traumatic bursitis. Among the bursae most prone to traumatic injury are the prepatellar, suprapatellar, infrapatellar, and pes anserine (figure 10.5).

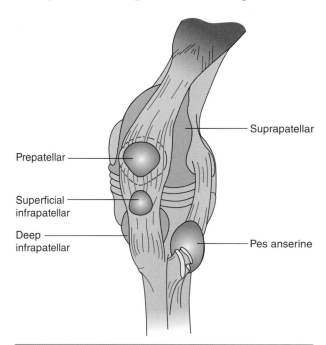

Figure 10.5 Locations of the prepatellar, suprapatellar, infrapatellar, and pes anserine bursae.

Signs and symptoms include immediate observable bursal swelling, redness, and mild pain.

Sprains

The cruciate (anterior, posterior) and collateral (medial, lateral) ligaments act as the primary stabilizers of the knee joint (see figure 10.4c on p. 228). Injury to these ligaments often occurs during athletic activities and may cause considerable instability and activity restriction. Although we discuss each ligament injury separately, injury commonly affects more than one structure, particularly with contact mechanisms. Injuries to more than one ligament, or associated injury of the capsule or meniscus, can result in rotatory or multiplanar instabilities at the knee.

▶ Anterior Cruciate Ligament

The anterior cruciate ligament (ACL) originates from the intercondylar eminence of the tibia and runs in a posterior, lateral, and superior direction to attach on the posterior medial aspect of the lateral epicondyle of the femur. Its primary functions are to limit extension, forward translation (glide), medial rotation, and extreme lateral rotation of the tibia relative to the femur. Both contact and noncontact mechanisms can injure the ACL. Signs and symptoms include immediate pain and unwillingness to move the knee. The patient may also hear a pop at the time of injury. Immediate symptoms usually subside sufficiently within a few minutes to allow a full knee examination. A large joint effusion and loss of motion usually result within 24 h.

▶ Posterior Cruciate Ligament

The posterior cruciate ligament (PCL), which has a wide attachment on the anterior surface of the medial femoral condyle, expands posteriorly under the ACL to attach to the posterolateral tibial plateau. Much shorter than the ACL, it limits extension, posterior translation, and medial rotation of the tibia on the femur. The PCL is most often injured secondary to a direct blow to the anterior tibia that drives it posteriorly on the fixed femur. Common scenarios are making contact with the dashboard during a traffic collision and falling on the anterior tibia with the knee flexed and the foot and ankle plantarflexed. Signs and symptoms include pain, joint effusion, and limited ROM into full flexion and extension. With complete rupture there may be an audible pop at the time of injury.

▶ Medial (Tibial) Collateral Ligament

The medial collateral ligament (MCL) is a broad, fan-shaped ligament that consists of superficial (extra-articular) and deep (intra-articular) fibers. The MCL limits abduction of the tibia on the femur and also assists in limiting extension and lateral rotation of the tibia. Signs and symptoms of MCL injury include pain, mild to moderate swelling, discoloration, and point tenderness in the middle portion of the MCL or near its femoral or tibial attachment. Pain may also occur at the medial joint line if the deep portion of the ligament or its attachment to the medial meniscus is torn. Since the ligament is primarily located outside of the joint capsule, there is usually no joint effusion with an isolated MCL sprain. You will note instability during valgus stress with second- and third-degree injuries.

▶ Lateral (Fibular) Collateral Ligament

The lateral collateral ligament (LCL) runs from the lateral epicondyle of the femur to its attachment on the fibular head. It limits knee extension and adduction of the tibia relative to the femur. The LCL is injured less frequently than the other knee ligaments. The mechanism for LCL injury is a varus force applied to the medial aspect of the knee. Signs and symptoms include pain, lateral knee swelling, ecchymosis, and point tenderness over the fibular collateral ligament. The patient may hear or feel a pop with complete rupture, and you will note varus instability with second- and third-degree injuries. The individual experiences increased pain when the ligament is tensed during full knee flexion and extension and with varus stress. Pain and swelling also limit ROM.

Meniscal Injuries

The menisci are two semilunar cartilages that sit on the tibial plateau, attaching only at their peripheral margins (see figure 10.4*b* on page 228). They are thickest at their peripheral borders and thinner toward the center. They move with the tibia during flexion and extension and with the femur during rotation. They possess no nerves, and their vascular supply is primarily along the periphery. The primary functions of the menisci are to

- help stabilize the joint by deepening the tibial condyles,
- absorb the shock of weight bearing and decrease loading stress,
- lubricate the joint and reduce friction during movement, and
- make joint surfaces more congruent and improve weight distribution by increasing the contact area between the tibia and femur.

Tearing of the medial or lateral meniscus typically occurs from compression and rotation of the femur on the fixed tibia. Cutting and pivoting with the joint in full weight bearing can pinch the meniscus between the femur and tibia and tear it as the femur rotates on the joint surface. Signs and symptoms include pain, swelling, and joint line tenderness. The patient may complain of pain, instability, or the giving way of the knee during cutting or pivoting.

Strains

Muscular strains typically stem from forceful contraction of the muscle during eccentric loading or from overstretching. Inflexibility, fatigue, weakness, muscular imbalance, and inadequate warm-up increase an individual's susceptibility to thigh muscle strains. Recurrent strains are a common problem, as the symptoms often subside and the patient returns to activity before adequate healing has occurred.

▶ Quadriceps Strain

The quadriceps muscle is most often overloaded during sudden acceleration or decel-eration, so injuries most frequently occur during sprinting, kicking, and weightlifting. Injury typically involves the rectus femoris muscle. The patient usually complains of immediate pain, spasm, and loss of function. Pain and weakness with active or resistive extension are consistent with the degree of injury. The individual is palpably tender over the injured area, and a defect may exist with second- and third-degree injuries. Second- and third-degree injuries may also result in observable swelling, ecchymosis, and an altered gait.

▶ Hamstring Strain

Hamstring strains—more common than quadriceps strains—occur most often with sprinting activities. Injury can occur in the midbelly of the muscle, at the distal myotendon junction, or at the proximal insertion on the ischial tuberosity. The patient experiences an immediate sharp or burning pain in the hamstrings at the time of injury. Other signs and symptoms include palpable tenderness and spasm over and around the injured fibers. You will note pain with passive stretching and active or resistive knee flexion, and there may be a palpable defect with second- and third-degree injuries.

▶ Patellar Tendon Rupture

A violent, rapid quadriceps contraction can rupture the midsubstance either of the infrapatellar or suprapatellar tendon. At the time of injury, the patient complains of immediate, severe pain and loss of active knee extension. A pop may also be felt and heard as the tendon ruptures. The patella appears to sit more superiorly with an infrapatellar tendon rupture, and a palpable gap is present between the inferior pole of the patella and tibial tuberosity. Considerable swelling and ecchymosis will likely result within 24 h following the injury.

Chronic or Overuse Soft Tissue Injuries

The soft tissue structures of the knee are also prone to chronic inflammatory conditions caused by repetitive friction and overuse. The soft tissues most often involved are (a) the numerous tendons that cross and attach at the knee joint and (b) the bursae that reduce friction and allow free movement of the tendons. Given the many tendons that cross and attach at the knee, tendinitis resulting from repetitive or overuse mechanisms is a frequent complaint in the physically active. As with most tendinitis conditions, the patient presents with an insidious onset of pain and a history of repetitive activity or a significant increase in training over the past few days or weeks. Initially the patient may feel pain only after activity and cool-down; pain may also occur at the beginning of activity but improve with warm-up. As symptoms worsen, the patient complains of pain during activity as well as throughout the day.

Repetitive kneeling, jumping, and flexing and extending are common mechanisms associated with inflammation of these structures.

Bursitis

Numerous bursae have been identified around the knee; they are typically present between tendons and other joint structures to prevent friction during knee movement. Those most prone to irritation and inflammation are the pes anserine, infrapatellar, prepatellar, and suprapatellar bursae (see figure 10.5 on p. 229). Signs and symptoms of chronic bursitis include pain, redness, and localized swelling. The area is tender to palpation and warm to the touch. Crepitus and bogginess (thickening of the bursal fluid) also occur with chronic bursitis. Flexion of the knee may be painful or limited with patellar bursitis secondary to increased pressure over the bursa as the skin tightens into flexion.

Patellar Tendinitis (Jumper's Knee)

Patellar tendinitis frequently occurs from repetitive jumping (basketball, volleyball, long jump, triple jump), running, or weightlifting (leg extensions, squats, lunges). Overloading the extensor mechanism can cause microtearing and inflammation of either the suprapatellar or infrapatellar tendons. Patellar tendinitis is characterized by symptoms of pain, inflammation, and mild swelling either superior or inferior to the patella. Palpable tenderness and crepitus are often present over the inflamed tendon. The patient complains of pain with passive stretching of the tendon and active or resisted knee extension.

Iliotibial Band Friction Syndrome

Iliotibial band friction syndrome is an overuse injury most typically seen in runners and cyclists. It is caused by excessive friction between the IT band and the lateral femoral epicondyle. At approximately 30° of flexion, the IT band changes from a knee extensor to a knee flexor (figure 10.6). When the knee is flexed less than 30°, the IT band lies anteriorly to the lateral epicondyle and

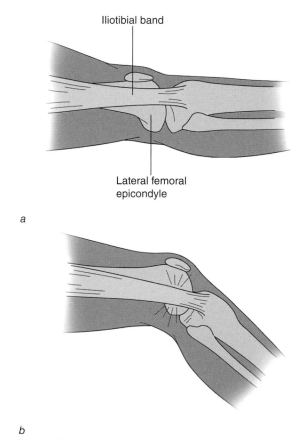

Figure 10.6 *(a)* At less than 30°, the iliotibial band is anterior to the lateral epicondyle and acts as an extensor. *(b)* As the knee flexes to more than 30°, the iliotibial band passes posteriorly to the lateral epicondyle to act as a flexor.

assists with knee extension. As the knee flexes, the IT band rides over the epicondyle at about 25° to 30° of flexion and then sits posteriorly past 30° of flexion, assisting with knee flexion. Irritation occurs with repetitive activity at the transitional range if excessive friction or snapping of the IT band occurs as it passes over the epicondyle.

Signs and symptoms include pain and point tenderness over the lateral femoral condyle just proximal to the lateral joint line. Pain may also radiate up the lateral thigh or down the IT band to its insertion at Gerdy's tubercle. As with other inflammatory conditions, pain is often first noted only after activity and does not restrict activity initially. Pain and snapping may also occur with walking down stairs or squatting, or with flexion and extension movements of the knee around 30° of flexion.

Traumatic Fractures

Traumatic fractures occur less frequently at the knee than at other joints because the ligaments and soft tissues provide most of the stability to the knee joint and thus are more likely to fail. However, as is typical for other body regions, fractures of the knee and thigh are more commonly seen in young, skeletally immature individuals. When you suspect fracture, immobilize the extremity and immediately refer the patient to a physician.

Epiphyseal Fractures

Fractures through the proximal tibial epiphysis, and less often through the distal femoral epiphysis, can result from rotational and shearing forces at the knee joint. Twisting, varus, or valgus forces directed at the knee with the foot firmly planted are the more common fracture mechanisms in the adolescent patient. Signs and symptoms include immediate pain, tenderness along the bone, swelling, loss of function, and possible deformity. The patient may report hearing a pop or snap at the joint. False joint motion, or opening of the epiphyseal joint with varus and valgus testing, may make it difficult

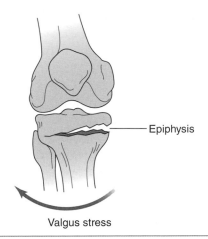

Figure 10.7 Epiphyseal plate injury at the proximal tibia and false joint motion with valgus testing.

to distinguish an epiphyscal fracture from a collateral ligament injury (figure 10.7). You should highly suspect fracture when examining varus and valgus injuries in the adolescent.

Tibial Plateau Fracture

Tibial plateau fractures can result from severe varus, valgus, or rotational forces in combination with axial compression when the foot is firmly planted. The patient complains of severe and immediate pain and is unwilling to move the knee joint. Other signs and symptoms include swelling, tenderness over the proximal tibia, pain with percussion, crepitus, and possible deformity.

Patella Fracture

Fractures of the patella can result from direct contact, as in a fall directly on the patella with the knee flexed, or from indirect forces, such as severe tractioning produced by a forceful quadriceps contraction. The patient complains of sudden and severe pain in the kneecap and is unwilling to contract the quadriceps or extend the knee, or is unable to do so without considerable pain.

Femur Fracture

Femoral shaft fractures resulting from athletic activity are rare because of the relative strength of the femur. When femoral fracture does occur, it usually does so in contact sports such as American football as a result of a severe, direct blow to the midthigh, but such fractures may also occur secondary to severe torsional forces. Femoral shaft fractures are readily apparent; the characteristic deformity is typically a shortened, laterally rotated thigh. Additional signs and symptoms include immediate and severe pain, muscle spasm, and inability to move the extremity. Because of their potential for arterial injury, hemorrhage, and shock, femoral fractures constitute a medical emergency.

Chondral and Osteochondral Fractures

Chondral fractures (fractures of the articular cartilage) and osteochondral fractures (fractures extending through the articular cartilage and into the bone) of the femoral condyle may occur by themselves or concurrently with a ligament injury. Joint compression combined with a varus, valgus, or rotational shearing force can contuse the articular surface and cause a compression or avulsion fracture (figure 10.8), resulting in loose fragments (joint mice) that can produce irritation, locking, and clicking within the joint. Signs and symptoms of chondral or osteochondral fracture include pain, immediate or delayed swelling, locking or clicking,

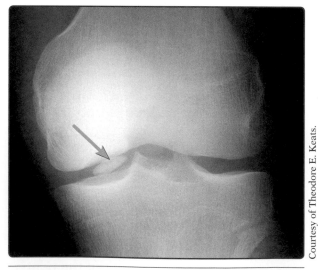

Courtesy of Theodore E. Keats.

Figure 10.8 Osteochondral fracture of the femoral condyle.

and pain with joint compression or weight bearing.

Dislocation and Subluxation

Of the three joints that make up the knee complex, the patellofemoral joint is most prone to subluxation and dislocation. Although dislocation of the tibiofemoral joint is less common, it is a much more serious and potentially limb-threatening injury. Knee dislocations require immediate neurovascular examination and medical referral.

Patellofemoral Subluxation and Dislocation

Patellar dislocations, which can result from either direct or indirect forces, typically occur lateral to the femoral groove secondary to the more lateral angular pull of the quadriceps and the lesser height of the lateral femoral condyle compared to the medial femoral condyle. A direct blow to the medial patella and indirect forces applied by the quadriceps during cutting maneuvers with the tibia laterally rotated can force the patella to displace over the lateral femoral condyle. If the patella remains displaced, the deformity is obvious.

However, often the patella spontaneously reduces, making the injury more difficult to identify. The patient is palpably tender along the medial border of the patella, lateral femoral condyle, and surrounding soft tissue structures. You will note considerable anterior knee swelling, particularly in first-time dislocations, shortly after injury. The patient will be apprehensive when the patella is moved laterally. A physician should examine first-time dislocations or subluxations, especially those resulting from direct trauma, and obtain X rays to rule out any associated chip fractures of the patella or lateral femoral condyle.

Tibiofemoral Dislocation

A total knee dislocation of the tibia and the femur is a very serious, potentially limb-threatening injury that fortunately rarely occurs in sports. Given that the ligaments act as the primary stabilizers of the knee joint, multiple ligaments—including both cruciate ligaments and at least one of the collateral ligaments—must tear in order for the joint to dislocate. In addition to the significant soft tissue damage that occurs, the risk of neurovascular injury is high, particularly with posterior dislocations. Knee dislocations require immediate neurovascular examination and medical referral.

Bony and Articular Defects Secondary to Repetitive Stress

Physical activity subjects the articular surfaces of the tibiofemoral and patellofemoral joints to considerable compressive forces. These forces most often affect the patellofemoral joint, particularly in patients with faulty alignment.

Patellofemoral Pain Syndrome

Patellofemoral pain syndrome (PFPS) is also known as miserable malalignment syndrome or patellofemoral stress syndrome (PFSS). These are vague terms referring to the general condition often called *anterior knee pain*. Anterior knee pain can be caused by a variety of factors that result in patellar malalignment, increased patellofemoral compression, or poor patellofemoral tracking. These include anatomical and biomechanical abnormalities, muscular weaknesses and imbalances, and training errors. An abrupt change in training activity, surface, intensity, or duration that substantially increases the load on the patellofemoral joint may also cause anterior knee pain. Regardless of the cause, the result is the same in each case: pain and irritation consequent to increased patellofemoral compression and pressure. One of the hallmark signs and symptoms of PFPS is poorly localized anterior knee pain that is exacerbated by squatting, climbing stairs, ambulation, or other activity after prolonged sitting (**theater sign**).

Chondromalacia Patella

While chondromalacia patella fits within the general category of PFPS, it is a specific condition characterized by softening, roughening, and eventual degeneration of the lateral articular surface of the patella. Signs and symptoms include general anterior knee pain, crepitus, minor swelling, and increased pain with patellofemoral compression in activities such as deeply bending the knee, extending the knee, or walking up and down stairs.

Apophysitis (Osgood-Schlatter Disease)

In young patients, repetitive tractioning by the patellar tendon can considerably stress the apophysis of the tibial tubercle. During adolescence, the epiphyseal line is weaker than the quadriceps muscle and tendon. Muscle tightness, repetitive jumping, and running during significant growth spurts can excessively traction the apophysis, leading to irritation, inflammation, and partial avulsion. Signs and symptoms include focused anterior knee pain, swelling and tenderness over the tibial tuberosity, and increased prominence of the tibial tuberosity. The patient complains of increased pain with knee extension exercises, squatting, kneeling, and jumping.

Nerve and Vascular Injuries

The nerve and vascular structures are relatively well protected at the knee as they pass through the popliteal space. Only severe joint disruption (dislocation) places these structures at risk. The only exception is the common peroneal nerve, which is vulnerable to injury where it wraps superficially around the head of the fibula.

Peroneal Nerve Palsy

Due to its superficial course around the head of the fibula, the peroneal nerve can be traumatized secondary to a direct blow (contusion), severe cold (ice bag application), or tractioning (varus injury force) (figure 10.9). Signs and symptoms of nerve palsy include pain and tenderness over the distal fibula; numbness, burning, or tingling along the lateral aspect of the leg and into the dorsum of the foot; and motor weakness of

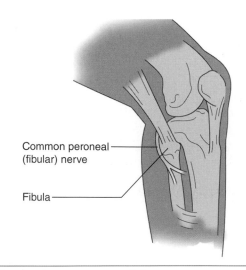

Figure 10.9 Location of the common peroneal nerve where it courses superficially around the head of the fibula.

the dorsiflexors, everters, and toe extensors, causing foot drop.

▶ Popliteal Artery or Nerve Injury

The popliteal vessels and nerves are well protected in the popliteal space. Injury to these structures, although rare, can result from a severe fracture or total knee (tibiofemoral) dislocation. Conduct distal pulse and sensory checks to examine nerve and vessel integrity with any severe knee trauma.

Summary

The knee is not an area in which injury consequences typically threaten life or limb, other than on rare occasions when a knee injury occludes the popliteal artery. However, since this can occur, you must always be alert in your examination of an acute injury to immediate signs and symptoms indicative of a medical emergency. As you approach the patient, note the position of the limb and the individual's response. Often the patient is holding the injured muscle or joint. If the patient is holding a flexed knee, the injury is likely a knee sprain. A position in which the knee is locked straight is more indicative of a fracture, dislocation, or meniscal injury. You will also see many chronic and overuse

injuries in the athletic training facility. These injuries warrant other investigations, including structural and postural examination of the entire lower extremity chain, joint mobility examination, and soft tissue examination, since these are factors that often contribute to these types of injuries.

Lower Leg, Ankle, and Foot Injury Recognition

The primary functions of the leg, ankle, and foot are to provide a rigid lever for propulsion and a stable but adaptable structure to support the body's weight during gait. These functions are fulfilled in part by the skeletal and ligamentous anatomy depicted in figure 10.10, *a* through *c*. Appreciating the balance between mobility and stability at the foot and ankle is essential, as changes in joint function resulting from injury and functional and

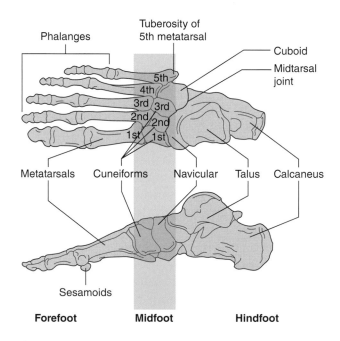

a

Figure 10.10 *(a)* Bony anatomy of the foot, including the hindfoot, midfoot, and forefoot. *(b)* Medial ligaments of the ankle. *(c)* Lateral ligaments of the ankle. *(continued)*

structural abnormalities can tremendously influence this balance and thus influence lower extremity mechanics, stress, and the likelihood of future injury.

Tremendous forces, both compressive and rotational, are transmitted through the weight-bearing structures of the foot, ankle, and leg. Consequently, both traumatic and chronic injuries are frequent in this region. Even seemingly minor injuries can be debilitating given the need for strength and stability of the foot and ankle. While injuries of the leg, foot, and ankle are rarely life threatening, they often result in significant disability due to the weight-bearing demands they must meet. As always, the injury environment, the patient's history, and your observations should guide the breadth and depth of your examination.

Acute Soft Tissue Injuries

Soft tissue injuries commonly occur as a result of direct contact and intrinsic or extrinsic forces acting on the foot, ankle, and leg. The foot and ankle include multiple bones, joints, and ligaments that stabilize the body during weight-bearing activities (figure 10.10, *a* through *c*). Given the tremendous forces exerted on these structures with landing, cutting, and running, the ligaments of the ankle, foot, and toes are prone to injury when activity forces a joint beyond its normal ROM.

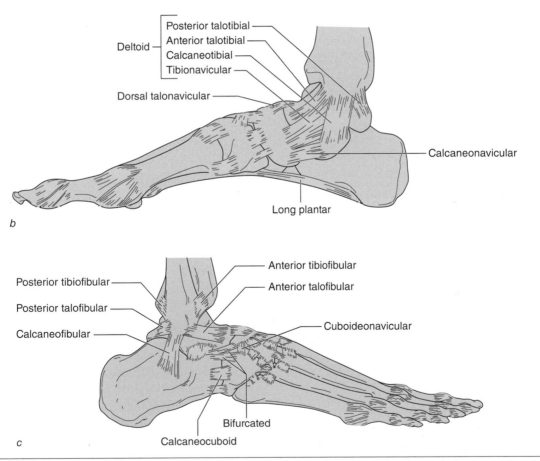

Figure 10.10 *(continued)* *(a)* Bony anatomy of the foot, including the hindfoot, midfoot, and forefoot. *(b)* Medial ligaments of the ankle. *(c)* Lateral ligaments of the ankle.

Contusions

The soft tissue and bony structures of the leg, ankle, and foot are vulnerable to direct trauma in sport activity. Many of the injuries can be quite debilitating due to the intricate functioning of the foot and ankle. Signs and symptoms include pain, swelling, and discoloration. A heel contusion can be particularly problematic. A heel bruise can result from landing hard on the heel during jumping activities or stepping on an uneven surface or a stone at heel strike with little or no footwear protection. A contusion to the fat pad of the heel can cause considerable pain and point tenderness, making it difficult to bear weight or walk with a normal gait. You should closely monitor severe contusions to a muscular compartment for excessive swelling and neurovascular compromise.

Sprains

The multiple bones that make up the foot and ankle are connected via ligaments that must withstand forces during activities of daily living and competition. Specific ligamentous injuries can be the result of acute or traumatic injuries in which the fibers of the ligaments are partially or completely disrupted.

Lateral Ankle Sprains

The most common mechanism of ankle injury involving the lateral ligament complex is inversion with or without plantarflexion (figure 10.11). In a typical scenario, a basketball player comes down on an opponent's foot or lands awkwardly on the outside of his own foot, causing the ankle to turn in (inversion mechanism). The patient complains of immediate pain upon injury and may hear a "pop." Signs and symptoms are consistent with first- through third-degree ligament sprains as detailed for other body parts.

Medial Ankle Sprains

Medial ankle sprains resulting from eversion forces are considerably less common (figure 10.12). This is primarily due to the greater

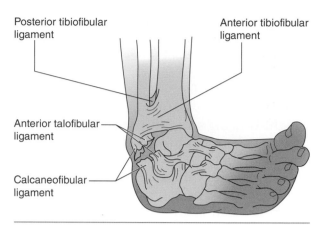

Figure 10.11 Injury to lateral ligaments of the ankle.

stability of the medial ankle, a consequence of the thickness and strength of the deltoid ligament complex as well as the longer lateral malleolus, which prevents excessive eversion.

Syndesmotic Sprains

Syndesmotic, or high ankle sprains, disrupt the tibiofibular ligaments and distal interosseous membrane. Although less frequent than lateral ankle sprains, this injury can result in prolonged disability and recovery when not identified and managed properly. Syndesmotic ankle sprains are typically caused by forced hyperdorsiflexion or lateral rotation of the foot, which forcibly separates the distal tibiofibular joint (figure 10.13). Signs and symptoms include pain and swelling anterior to the ankle joint. Pain in the anterolateral aspect of the ankle with weight bearing, passive lateral rotation of the foot, or forced dorsiflexion also indicates injury to the syndesmosis.

Foot Sprains

Given the number of bony articulations and ligaments in the foot, myriad sprains can result from both direct and indirect forces. Because of the foot's stability, sprains to the mid- and forefoot are less common than sprains to the ankle joint. Sprains to the metatarsal and long arch can result from both chronic overuse and acute traumatic

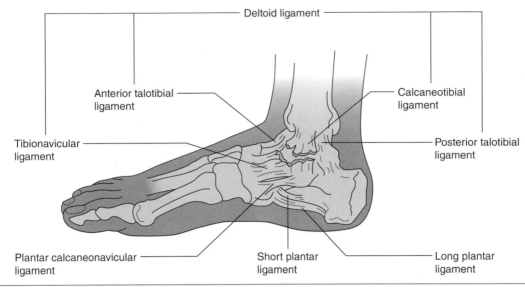

Figure 10.12 Injury to medial ligaments of the ankle. Carefully palpate the distal fibula for possible fracture with all serious eversion injuries.

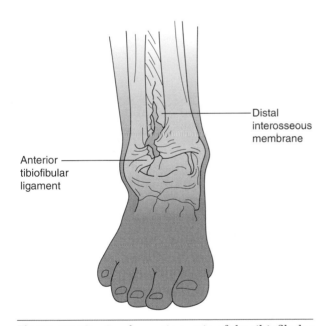

Figure 10.13 Syndesmotic sprain of the tibiofibular joint.

forces that stretch the supporting ligamentous structures, causing midfoot hypermobility and a fallen arch. Signs and symptoms of foot and arch sprains include pain, point tenderness over the involved structure, swelling, discoloration, and difficulty with weight bearing.

Toe Sprains

Toe sprains most often result from direct contact at the end of the toe, such as stubbing or jamming the toe while kicking an unyielding object. However, any direct or indirect mechanism that forces the joint beyond its normal range can result in sprains. Most problematic are sprains to the great toe, also known as **turf toe**. Turf toe can result from extreme dorsiflexion of the first metatarsophalangeal joint during push-off, extreme plantarflexion or axial compression from kicking an unyielding object, or quick stops that slide the foot forward in the shoe. Signs and symptoms of toe sprains include pain, swelling, and ecchymosis.

Strains

Numerous muscles originating from the leg and terminating in the foot and toes are responsible for a variety of ankle and foot motions (figure 10.14). Given the strong mechanical forces associated with running, jumping, and cutting, muscle strains commonly result from overstretch and muscular overload. Signs and symptoms of muscle

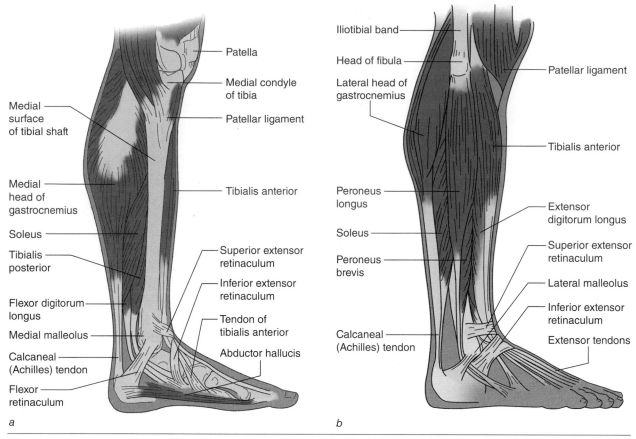

Figure 10.14   Lower leg, ankle, and foot musculature.

and tendon strains include pain with active and resistive movement, pain with passive stretch, muscle spasm, swelling, and point tenderness with possible palpable defect over the injured area.

▶ Rupture of the Achilles (Calcaneal) Tendon

Rupture of the Achilles tendon (figure 10.15) can result from sudden, violent plantarflexion during eccentric loading in full weight-bearing activity. The patient complains of immediate pain and disability and often reports a feeling of being kicked or shot in the calf. Considerable swelling and discoloration also occur, accompanied by an observable defect in the contour of the Achilles tendon. The individual is unable to actively plantarflex the foot.

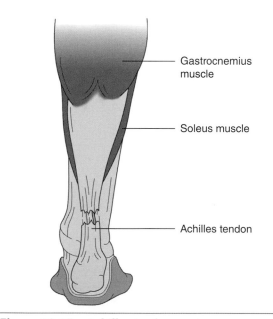

Figure 10.15   Achilles tendon rupture.

Chronic or Overuse Soft Tissue Injuries

Chronic soft tissue injuries in this region are a frequent complaint in physically active people as a consequence of repetitive micro-trauma resulting from abnormal friction, traction, structural mechanics, or some combination of these. Inflammation and swelling of the bursa around the ankle and foot can result from repetitive overuse with running, direct pressure, or friction from poorly fitting footwear.

Retrocalcaneal Bursitis

The retrocalcaneal bursa lies between the calcaneus and the distal insertion of the Achilles tendon (figure 10.16). Inflammation and swelling of this bursa can result from repetitive overuse with running, direct pressure, or friction from poorly fitting footwear. Signs and symptoms include localized swelling, redness, and point tenderness near and around the calcaneal attachment of the Achilles tendon.

Plantar Fasciitis

Inflammation of the plantar fascia is seen most often in patients with abnormal foot alignment and is precipitated by overuse, poor footwear or playing surface, or improper conditioning. The patient's history is your primary evaluative tool. The patient typically complains of a gradual onset of pain and stiffness on the plantar surface of the foot, extending from the heel to the metatarsal heads. Pain is increased upon weight bearing after waking from sleep or after long periods of sitting.

Tendinitis and Tenosynovitis

Tendinitis and chronic strain of the peroneal, posterior tibial, and Achilles tendons are common in the athletic population. In all cases, injury results from repetitive overuse, friction, or tendon traction. Tendinitis may also occur in the toe extensor tendons where they cross superficially on the dorsum of the foot. Signs and symptoms associated with tendinitis include pain, point tenderness, and crepitus over the inflamed tendon; decreased ROM; and swelling. Pain with passive stretch or active or resistive movement of the involved muscle or tendon occurs as well.

Calcaneal Apophysitis (Sever's Disease)

In young, skeletally immature patients, the calcaneal apophysis can become inflamed secondary to repetitive traction stress of the Achilles tendon (figure 10.17). Common signs and symptoms include posterior inferior heel pain, point tenderness, and increased pain with weight bearing, running, or jumping. Decreased dorsiflexion range secondary to tightness of the Achilles tendon during rapid growth phases is likely a predisposing factor.

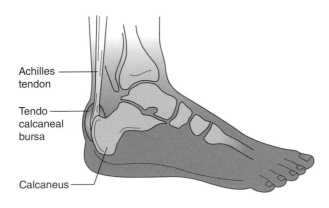

Figure 10.16 Retrocalcaneal bursitis.

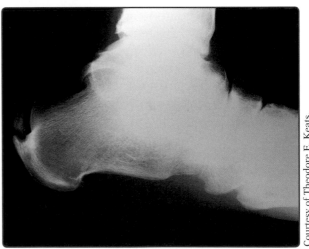

Courtesy of Theodore E. Keats.

Figure 10.17 Calcaneal apophysitis (Sever's disease).

Medial Tibial Stress Syndrome

Medial tibial stress syndrome (MTSS), commonly referred to as shin splints, is usually an inflammation of the periosteum (periostitis) along the posterior medial tibial border at or near the insertion of the long toe or ankle flexors. The condition is typically brought on by abrupt changes in footwear, running surfaces, or training regimen. Medial tibial stress syndrome is characterized by diffuse pain, point tenderness, and inflammation along the medial border of the tibia. The pain is usually diffuse along a broad area of the medial tibial surface.

Traumatic Fractures

Traumatic fractures can result from the same mechanisms that cause ankle and foot sprains. In fact, it is not uncommon for bony fractures to accompany ligamentous injuries as a result of traumatic ankle injury mechanisms.

Tibia and Fibula

Traumatic fractures of the tibia and fibula can result from a direct blow or indirect torsional stress in association with inversion and eversion ankle injuries. Fractures to the fibula shaft can result from a direct blow to the lateral aspect of the leg or from severe eversion or lateral rotation stress. Fractures to the tibial shaft, which are less common, require much greater forces; they can occur in contact sports such as American football with a direct blow to the shin, or in skiing with a severe torsional stress. Signs and symptoms of fracture include immediate pain, swelling, and possible deformity if the fragments are displaced. You will note tenderness over and around the fracture site. Muscle splinting and spasm may also occur. Other signs of fracture include crepitus, pain with bony percussion, or pain with transverse stress such as that produced when the tibia and fibula are squeezed together. You may also note false joint motion or crepitus when manipulating the bone.

Foot

Traumatic fractures in the foot typically involve the metatarsals and phalanges. The mechanisms associated with toe sprains also apply here. Traumatic fractures of the metatarsal shafts most often result from direct trauma, for example when an individual is stepped on by another player or when a weight is dropped on the foot. Pain with longitudinal stress applied to the plantar surface of the foot, axial stress to the bone, or torsional stress applied through twisting the toe often indicates metatarsal fractures. A dislocated fracture of the midfoot characterized by one or more displaced proximal metatarsals is known as a **Lisfranc fracture** (figure 10.18). This fracture is caused in athletics by a direct blow to the Lisfranc joint (between the midfoot and forefoot) or by axial loading along the metatarsals, coupled with either a medially or laterally directed rotational force. Fracture at the base of the fifth metatarsal (**Jones fracture**) is usually caused by indirect loading of the bone with plantarflexion and eversion stress. Avulsion fractures of the proximal fifth metatarsal may also occur at the insertion of the peroneus brevis tendon with inversion stress injuries (figure 10.19). Suspect fracture whenever

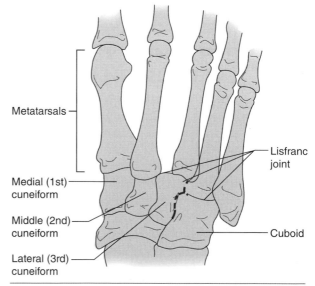

Figure 10.18 Lisfranc fracture.

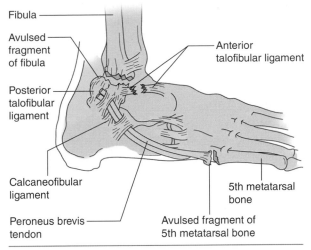

Fibula

Avulsed fragment of fibula

Posterior talofibular ligament

Anterior talofibular ligament

Calcaneofibular ligament

Peroneus brevis tendon

5th metatarsal bone

Avulsed fragment of 5th metatarsal bone

Figure 10.19 Avulsion fractures of both the distal fibula and proximal fifth metatarsal.

there is point tenderness over the base of the fifth metatarsal or pain with resisted eversion. General signs and symptoms of foot fractures are consistent with those previously mentioned.

Stress Fractures

The tibia and metatarsals are the most common sites of leg, ankle, and foot stress fractures, which result from repetitive stress associated with running and jumping activities. Stress fractures of the fifth metatarsal and fibula are also common secondary to repetitive tractioning of the peroneal muscles with eversion and plantarflexion. Tibial stress fractures most often occur in the distal one-third of the tibia, and metatarsal stress fractures most often involve the second or third metatarsal shaft. Symptoms of a developing stress fracture include an insidious onset of pain that initially occurs only during activity and subsides with rest. If the repetitive stress continues, the patient complains of continued pain after activity and into the night. Eventually, if the stressful activity is not curtailed, the patient experiences pain throughout the day. Other signs and symptoms may include localized tenderness over the bone, pain with axial and transverse stress, and swelling.

Exostosis

Excessive calcification, or bone spurs, is identified by radiographic examination and can develop at various locations in the foot and ankle secondary to repetitive stress and contact. A posterior **calcaneal exostosis**, or "pump bump," can result from chronic irritation at the Achilles tendon attachment. Signs and symptoms in addition to the bony prominence include pain, localized swelling, and redness. Inflammation and irritation associated with a calcaneal exostosis may also involve the retrocalcaneal bursa and distal Achilles tendon.

Dislocation and Subluxation

Dislocations of the ankle, hindfoot, and midfoot joints are relatively uncommon. Such injuries require tremendous forces; thus when these dislocations occur, they are almost always associated with fracture. Dislocation of the phalanges commonly results from the same mechanisms that cause sprains and fractures. Dislocations are readily apparent secondary to obvious joint deformity. Immediate pain, swelling, and loss of function also occur.

Nerve and Vascular Injuries

Because of the compartments and tunnels that the nerves and vessels of the lower extremity pass through on their way to the foot, neurovascular compromise is not uncommon. Nerve or vascular compromise or both can result from both acute and chronic compression mechanisms; acute conditions usually represent more serious injury. Immediate recognition and medical referral are imperative.

Morton's Neuroma

Also referred to as metatarsalgia, Morton's neuroma usually occurs at the bifurcation of the lateral plantar nerve as it angles sharply and branches off between the third and fourth metatarsal heads (figure 10.20).

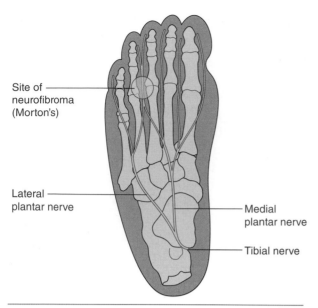

Figure 10.20   Location of Morton's neuroma between the third and fourth metatarsal heads.

This is a prime area of pressure and friction that can cause fibrous tumor formation or tissue buildup around the nerve. Common complaints include pain with weight bearing and tight shoes, burning, numbness, and shooting pain.

▷ Peroneal Nerve Palsy

The peroneal nerve is susceptible to injury with inversion ankle injuries. Since this nerve has a significant sensory branch, the patient complains of sensory changes in the dermatome along the lateral leg and dorsum of the foot. Eversion weakness thought to be due to lateral muscle weakness, as well as pain associated with the ankle sprain, may in fact be the result of superficial peroneal nerve injury. When weakness is prolonged or accompanied by sensory changes, suspect peroneal nerve injury.

▷ Compartment Syndrome

In a **compartment syndrome**, pressure within a muscle compartment increases to the point that it causes neurovascular compromise. There are four muscular compartments in the leg: anterior, lateral, deep posterior, and superficial posterior (figure 10.21). Each is bounded by a thick, elastic fascial sheath that limits compartment expansion

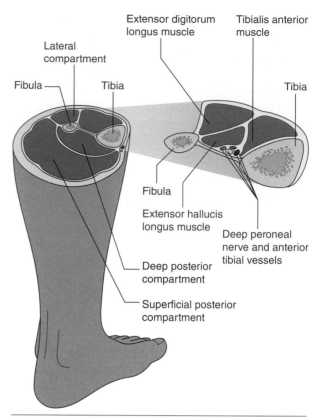

Figure 10.21   Contents of the anterior compartment of the leg.

during significant swelling. A compartment syndrome can be classified as either chronic (exertional) or acute.

• *Chronic (exertional) compartment syndrome.* Chronic or exertional compartment syndrome usually results from excessive muscle hypertrophy during exercise. During activity, tissue pressure remains high during contractions, impeding blood flow and causing muscle ischemia. This transient ischemia causes the patient to stop or slow activity secondary to symptoms of pain, muscular fatigue, a feeling of heaviness within the compartment, and reduced dorsiflexion muscle function. In exertional compartment syndromes, the pressure is usually not high enough to cause vascular collapse and rarely results in a medical emergency. It is common to see fascial defects and muscle herniation through the fascia resulting from increased intracompartmental pressure. Patients who experience exertional compartment syndromes may in severe cases require a surgical fasciotomy to remove the fascial restriction and allow sufficient room for muscle hypertrophy during activity.

• *Acute compartment syndrome.* Acute compartment syndrome represents a medical emergency and typically results from acute trauma such as a fracture, a kick to the leg, or other direct trauma. Intensive exercise can be a causative factor, although this is rarely the case. As a result of the acute trauma, vasodilation and bleeding within the compartment increase pressure and cause venous compromise and eventual collapse. Given the higher pressure of the anterior tibial artery as compared to the veins, blood continues to flow into the compartment even after venous collapse, further contributing to the rising pressure. If the condition is left untreated, muscle ischemia and tissue necrosis occur within 6 to 12 h. Immediate recognition and medical referral are imperative.

Signs and symptoms of an impending acute compartment syndrome include pain out of proportion to the injury that greatly intensifies with plantarflexion of the ankle. The compartment is warm to the touch, and the overlying skin is tense, glossy, and pale. You will observe sensory and motor loss over the distribution of the deep peroneal nerve, with motor deficits ranging from weakness of great toe extension and dorsiflexion to eventual foot drop. (Watch for the five Ps of an impending compartment syndrome: pain, paresthesia, pallor, pulselessness, and paralysis.) If any of these signs are apparent, refer the patient immediately for medical attention. In suspected cases of compartment syndrome, the normal rules of injury management do not apply. Ice should not be applied due to paresthesia and compression is contraindicated as this can create further pressure and vascular compromise. In addition, elevation of the limb is also contraindicated as it further reduces

CASE STUDY

Case Study

Larry is in the middle of his off-season conditioning program. In addition to improving his strength, Larry focuses at this time of year on improving his cardiovascular conditioning. To that end, he has been alternating between running striders and middle distance running. For the past several days, he has noticed a feeling of heaviness and pain in his anterior lower legs. Larry has thought that he might be experiencing an episode of "shin splints" and has been using a home treatment of ice and over-the-counter medication. This seems to help, as the pain subsides substantially and does not bother him until his next workout. However, during his workout today, his sensations were more severe than previously, and Larry complains of "heaviness," pain, tingling, paresthesia, and an inability to dorsiflex his feet. In fact, he tripped several times during his workout and actually had to crawl inside from the stadium and seek the help of Mike, the athletic trainer for the football team.

Think About It

1. What are the possible differential diagnoses for Larry's complaints?

2. What subjective history and evaluative procedures should Mike initiate for Larry's complaints (be specific)?

3. What objective evaluative procedures should Mike conduct for Larry's complaints?

4. When would it be appropriate to refer this case for further diagnostic testing?

5. What further diagnostic testing would be appropriate to confirm or deny the differential diagnoses from question 1?

6. What treatment options are available for the differential diagnoses?

blood flow in an already compromised and ischemic limb.

Summary

Although injuries to the leg, ankle, and foot are rarely life threatening, severe injuries to these areas demand accurate and rapid examination. Obtaining relevant injury history should help you quickly focus on the area of injury. Establish the onset and duration of symptoms to determine the stage of the injury. Identify aggravating and easing factors to determine the level of irritability and also the potential structures involved. Whereas stress fractures are more painful with activity and ease with rest, tendon and muscle injuries may warm up with activity and be more painful at rest. Inflammatory conditions are usually stiff in the morning and loosen as the day progresses, with a return of pain from fatigue and overuse toward the end of the day. With ankle injuries, try to determine whether the injury mechanism resulted in inversion, eversion, or rotation.

Learning Aids

SUMMARY

The bones, joints, ligaments, muscles, tendons, nerves, and vascular structures of the lower extremity are common locations of injuries and pathologies. Injuries to the hip, knee, and ankle can cause varying amounts of disability and affect completion and participation in both activities of daily living and athletic activities. This chapter provides examples of the more frequently seen lower extremity pathologies and also identifies common signs and symptoms to aid in quick recognition. The athletic trainer must be aware of the various pathologies and how to recognize them to facilitate a quick and satisfactory recovery in patients with these injuries and pathologies.

KEY CONCEPTS AND REVIEW

▸ **List the most common avulsion fracture sites of the hip and pelvis region.**

Common sites for avulsion fractures are the anterior superior iliac spine (ASIS, sartorius), anterior inferior iliac spine (AIIS, rectus femoris), lesser trochanter (iliopsoas), and ischial tuberosity (hamstring).

▸ **Describe the injury mechanism and signs and symptoms of myositis ossificans.**

Myositis ossificans occurs when improper or abnormal hematoma absorption causes calcification or the formation of bony deposits in the muscle. The hematoma can occur due to either a direct blow or chronic irritation. Signs and symptoms of myositis ossificans include a history of severe or repetitive insult to the quadriceps, pain, a palpable mass within the muscle belly, decreased knee flexion range, and decreased quadriceps strength.

▸ **List the primary functions of menisci.**

The primary functions of the menisci are to (1) help stabilize the joint by deepening the tibial condyles, (2) absorb the shock of weight bearing and decrease loading stress, (3) lubricate the joint and reduce friction during movement, and (4) make joint surfaces more congruent and improve weight distribution.

▸ **Describe the functions of the posterior cruciate ligament and anterior cruciate ligament.**

The anterior cruciate ligament (ACL) originates from the intercondylar eminence of the tibia and runs in a posterior, lateral, and superior direction to attach on the posterior medial aspect of the lateral epicondyle of the femur. Its primary functions are to limit extension, forward translation (glide), medial rotation, and extreme lateral rotation of the tibia relative to the femur. Both contact and noncontact mechanisms can cause ACL injury.

The posterior cruciate ligament (PCL), which has a wide attachment on the anterior surface of the medial femoral condyle, expands posteriorly under the ACL to attach to the posterolateral tibial plateau. Much shorter than the ACL, it limits extension, posterior translation, and medial rotation of the tibia on the femur. The PCL is most often injured secondary to a direct blow to the anterior tibia that drives it posteriorly on the fixed femur.

▸ **Identify the contributing factors and signs and symptoms of patellofemoral pain syndrome.**

Patellofemoral pain syndrome (PFPS) is a vague term for the general condition often called *anterior knee pain*. Anterior knee pain can be caused by a variety of factors that result in patellar malalignment, increased patellofemoral compression, or poor patellofemoral tracking. These include anatomical and biomechanical abnormalities, muscular weaknesses and imbalances, and training errors. An abrupt change in training activity, surface, intensity, or duration that substantially increases the load on the patellofemoral joint may also cause anterior knee pain. Signs and symptoms of PFPS are poorly localized anterior knee pain that is exacerbated by squatting, climbing stairs, ambulation, or other activity, especially after the person has been sitting or has been still.

▸ **Describe the mechanism and biomechanics involved in iliotibial band friction syndrome.**

Iliotibial band friction syndrome is caused by excessive friction between the IT band and the lateral femoral epicondyle. When the knee is flexed less than 30°, the IT band lies anteriorly to the lateral epicondyle and assists with knee extension. As the knee flexes, the IT band rides over the epicondyle at about 25° to 30° of knee flexion and then sits posteriorly past 30° of flexion, assisting with knee flexion. Irritation occurs with repetitive activity at the transitional range if there is excessive friction or snapping of the IT band as it passes over the epicondyle.

Signs and symptoms include pain and point tenderness over the lateral femoral condyle just proximal to the lateral joint line. Pain may also radiate up the lateral thigh or down the IT band to its insertion at Gerdy's tubercle. As with other inflammatory conditions, pain is often first noted only after activity and does not restrict activity initially. Pain and snapping may also occur with walking down stairs or squatting, or with flexion and extension movements of the knee around 30° of flexion.

▸ **Detail differences between lateral ligament and syndesmotic ankle sprains.**

Syndesmotic, or high ankle sprains disrupt the tibiofibular ligaments and distal interosseous membrane. Syndesmotic ankle sprains are typically caused by forced hyperdorsiflexion or lateral rotation of the foot that forcibly separate the distal tibiofibular joint. Signs and symptoms include pain and swelling anterior to the ankle joint. Pain in the anterolateral aspect of the ankle with weight bearing, passive lateral rotation of the foot, or forced dorsiflexion also indicates injury to the syndesmosis.

The lateral ankle ligament complex is often injured via an inversion mechanism with or without plantarflexion. The patient complains of immediate pain upon injury and may hear a "pop." Signs and symptoms are consistent with first- through third-degree ligament sprains detailed for other body parts but specifically consist of pain over the lateral ligaments distal to the lateral malleolus. Significant swelling and ecchymosis are common with these injuries.

▸ **Describe a Lisfranc fracture.**

A dislocated fracture of the midfoot characterized by one or more displaced proximal metatarsals is known as a Lisfranc fracture. This fracture is caused in athletics by a direct blow to the Lisfranc joint (between the midfoot and forefoot) or by axial loading along the metatarsals, coupled with either a medially or laterally directed rotational force.

▸ **Explain the location of a Jones fracture.**

A Jones fracture occurs at the base of the fifth metatarsal of the foot. It is not to be confused with a fifth metatarsal styloid fracture or a shaft fracture.

PRACTICE!

For hands-on practice in this area, go to the web resource and complete the following:

Level 2.9, Module J2: Ankle Injury
      Assessment and Diagnosis

Level 2.9, Module J4: Knee Injury
      Assessment and Diagnosis

CRITICAL THINKING QUESTIONS

1. A male lacrosse player reports to your clinic for evaluation of a knee injury following practice. He states that he injured his knee yesterday but decided to try to "tough it out" and kept practicing. However, the pain is increasing and is now affecting his function. His mechanism of injury was a twisting during a shot, and he felt a pop and sharp pain in the "inside" and medial aspect of his knee. He complains of tightness, stiffness, pain, locking, and a "loose" feeling. What possible injuries do you need to look for? What injuries do these symptoms occur with?

2. A female soccer player falls to the ground following a lunging motion she made to reach a ball. She complains of very intense upper groin and thigh pain and upon examination has significantly decreased ability to flex her thigh. She states that she heard a "pop" and is extremely tender to palpation near the lesser trochanter. What injuries do you suspect and why?

CHAPTER 11

Head, Spine, and Thorax Injury Recognition

Sandra J. Shultz, PhD, ATC, CSCS, FNATA
Kirk Brumels, PhD, AT, ATC

OBJECTIVES

After reading this chapter, the student should be able to do the following:

- Put in plain words the risks of athletic participation with spinal stenosis.
- Describe the pathology of spondylolysis and spondylolisthesis.
- List concussive signs and symptoms that require immediate referral.
- Explain the differences between disc protrusion, extrusion, and sequestration.
- Detail the differences between pneumothorax and hemothorax.
- Outline signs and symptoms of splenic rupture.

Understanding and recognizing the various injuries and pathologies that can occur in and around the head, spine, and torso are critical for proper examination and management of these injuries. Efficacy and accuracy of diagnostic examinations are severely hampered by insufficient knowledge of the injuries that can occur in these regions. This chapter focuses on injury recognition; specific tests and techniques are not outlined as they are beyond the scope of this text. For more complete examination strategies for the head, spine, and thorax, refer to Shultz, Houglum, and Perrin (2010). For an overview of general injury mechanisms, classifications, and examination techniques, see chapters 7 and 8.

Cervical and Upper Thoracic Spine Injury Recognition

Injuries to the cervical and thoracic spine can range from relatively minor to severe and life threatening. Chronic conditions from faulty posture or mechanics, poor sleeping position, degenerative changes in the spine, athletics-related trauma, and even auto accidents frequently cause a variety of soft tissue pathologies in the physically active. Because of the varied nature and severity of injuries to the cervical spine and the potential for catastrophic consequences, your ability to accurately examine injuries in this area is paramount. Your examination must correctly decipher causes, identify preexisting conditions that potentially led to an injury, and discern the tissue structures involved so you can decide on an appropriate referral or a treatment program. Knowledge of pertinent and basic functional anatomy is critical to appropriate examinations of the cervical spine (figure 11.1).

Your ability to accurately and efficiently determine the nature and extent of the injury could mean the difference between life and death or full recovery and permanent paralysis. In all cases, knowledge of which symptoms and findings dictate immediate medical referral versus conservative care is essential. Cervical and upper thoracic spine injuries can range from minor to catastrophic. The symptoms associated with many of these injuries vary from annoying pain and irritation to life-altering physical changes. Because the cervical spine sacrifices stability for greater mobility, it is more prone to injury than the relatively stable thoracic spine.

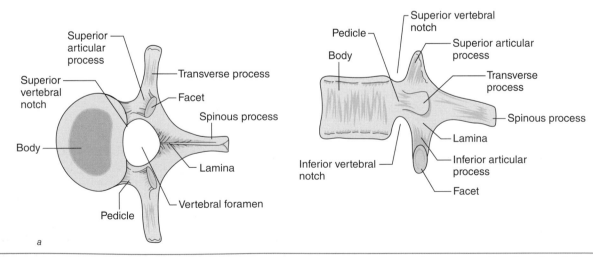

Figure 11.1 Functional anatomy of the cervical and upper thoracic spine. *(a)* Anatomical landmarks of the typical vertebra in superior and lateral views. *(b)* Intravertebral foramen formed by adjacent vertebrae. *(c)* Spinal cord enclosed in the vertebral canal and spinal nerve exiting through intervertebral foramen. *(d)* Disc showing nucleus pulposus and annulus fibrosus. *(e)* Normal curvature of the vertebral column. *(continued)*

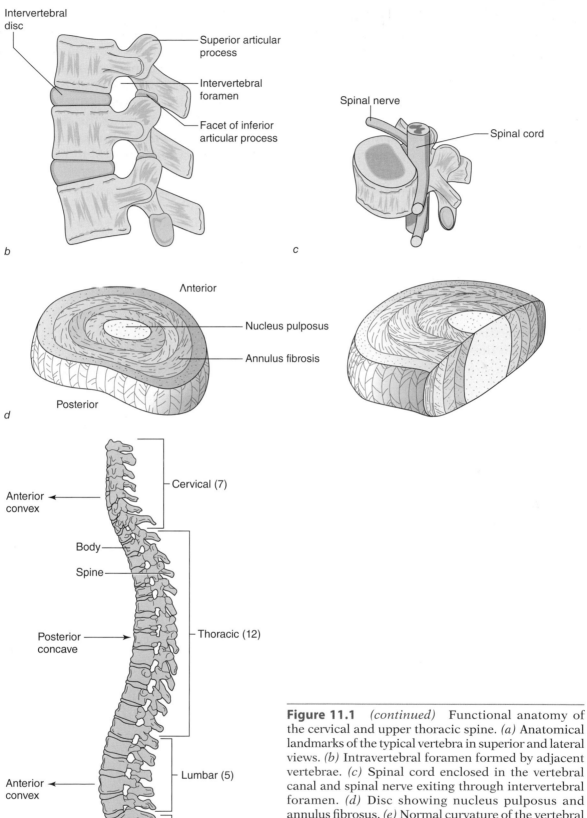

Intervertebral disc

Superior articular process

Intervertebral foramen

Facet of inferior articular process

b

Spinal nerve

Spinal cord

c

Anterior

Nucleus pulposus

Annulus fibrosis

Posterior

d

Cervical (7)

Anterior convex

Body

Spine

Posterior concave

Thoracic (12)

Lumbar (5)

Anterior convex

Sacrum (5)

Posterior concave

Coccyx (4)

e

Figure 11.1 *(continued)* Functional anatomy of the cervical and upper thoracic spine. *(a)* Anatomical landmarks of the typical vertebra in superior and lateral views. *(b)* Intravertebral foramen formed by adjacent vertebrae. *(c)* Spinal cord enclosed in the vertebral canal and spinal nerve exiting through intervertebral foramen. *(d)* Disc showing nucleus pulposus and annulus fibrosus. *(e)* Normal curvature of the vertebral column.

Reprinted, by permission, from J. Watkins, 2010, *Structure and function of the musculoskeletal system,* 2nd ed. (Champaign, IL: Human Kinetics), 32, 33, 122.

Acute Soft Tissue Injuries

Acute soft tissue injuries can result from direct contact, acute overstretch, or mechanical overload mechanisms. Sprains and strains make up the majority of acute soft tissue injuries seen in the cervical and thoracic spine; contusions occur infrequently.

Contusions

Contusions can result from a direct blow to either the soft tissue or the bony prominences of the neck. Although cervical contusions are uncommon, they can cause considerable pain and other symptoms. Signs and symptoms include pain, muscle spasm, and decreased range of motion (ROM). A blow to the base of the neck can also traumatize the brachial plexus, resulting in numbness and weakness in the upper extremity.

Sprains

Cervical and upper thoracic sprains involve the ligamentous and capsular structures that stabilize and connect the vertebrae and their facet joints. Sprains to the cervical and upper thoracic region most often result from compression, or jamming, of the spine into extension. However, cervical sprains may also occur during forceful hyperflexion, hyperextension, or rotational movements. Sudden, forced extension followed by sudden, forced flexion is referred to as **cervical whiplash**. This mechanism can occur in sports and motor vehicle accidents and can result in a combined sprain–strain injury. Typical signs and symptoms include pain, spasm, and restricted ROM.

Strains

Acute strains of the cervical and upper thoracic musculature are common. Isolated muscular strains often result from a single episode of mechanical overload or from violent stretching into flexion, extension, or rotation. Signs and symptoms of cervical and thoracic strain include muscular pain, point tenderness, spasm, and decreased ROM. These symptoms are commonly delayed or gradually worsen up to 24 h following injury as soft tissue swelling and muscle spasm increase. Pain is reproduced with either stretching or contraction of the involved musculature. Depending on the severity of the symptoms, the patient is often seen splinting, or stiffening the neck, rotating or flexing at the trunk rather than at the neck to avoid painful cervical motion.

Chronic or Overuse Soft Tissue Injuries

Many chronic or overuse soft tissue injuries in the cervical and thoracic spine are caused by joint and muscular dysfunction resulting from poor posture and recurrent sprains or strains. The mobile cervical region is particularly susceptible to chronic soft tissue injuries such as spasm, sprains, strains, degenerative disc disease, and facet syndrome.

Degenerative Disc Disease

Degenerative disc changes can occur with recurrent sprains and chronic joint dysfunction. The annulus fibrosis can be weakened or damaged with repetitive injury or stress, reducing disc height and shock-absorbing capability. Signs and symptoms include pain, spasm, motion restriction, and bony changes.

Facet Syndrome

Chronic inflammatory and degenerative changes can affect the facet joints. Chronic inflammation, scarring, and fibrosis of the capsule can result from extension overload, repetitive sprains, and impingement secondary to disc degeneration. Signs and symptoms include pain and decreased motion at the facet joints. Pain is usually exacerbated with extension and rotation to the involved side.

Chronic Cervical Joint Instabilities

As with any joint, a potential complication of cervical sprains is chronic joint instability. Instability of the cervical spine has serious implications in that hypermobility can increase the neurological structures' risk for injury. Instabilities are not easily identifiable during injury examination and typically require radiographic examination in flexion and extension views, so always refer patients who sustain a cervical sprain to a physician to rule out any resulting instabilities.

Bone and Joint Pathologies

Bone and joint pathologies are among the most potentially serious and life-threatening injuries of the cervical spine. These structures are intimately associated with and serve to protect the spinal cord and nerve roots. When forces exerted on the cervical spine are sufficient to displace bone and joint structures, catastrophic injury may result. The primary cause of cervical fractures, dislocations, and subluxations is headfirst contact. Depending on the resulting bending or rotational forces acting on the spinal segment, a variety of fractures or dislocations may occur. Fractures of the vertebral bodies may occur at any level in the cervical spine.

Cervical Spine Fractures, Dislocations, and Subluxations

Headfirst contact, the primary cause of cervical fractures, dislocations, and subluxations, compresses and buckles the cervical spine as it is forced to decelerate the still-moving torso. Immediate recognition of the signs and symptoms associated with cervical fracture or dislocation is paramount to avoiding further injury. Signs and symptoms may include central spine pain, tenderness with palpation of the involved spinous processes, muscle spasm, position deformity, and an unwillingness to move the neck. Neurologic symptoms of associated cord injury such as bilateral sensory deficits (burning hands, paresthesia, numbness, or loss of sensation), motor weakness, and paralysis may be present.

Hyperflexion and Hyperextension Mechanisms

Although impact to the face or the posterior head poses a substantially lower risk to the cervical spine than impact to the top of the head, it can nevertheless cause significant injury. Pure hyperflexion injuries can compress the anterior body and tear the posterior ligaments. Signs and symptoms include pain, point tenderness over cervical musculature, spasm, and restricted movement.

Spinous Process Fractures

Although uncommon, spinous process fractures of the cervical and thoracic spine can result from either hyperflexion or extension mechanisms. Contact or impingement of adjacent spinous processes can cause a push-off fracture with hyperextension mechanisms. Avulsion fractures secondary to traction of attaching ligaments may also occur with hyperflexion injuries. Signs and symptoms associated with spinous process fractures include localized pain, tenderness to palpation, and pain with extreme flexion and extension movements.

Defects and Abnormalities Secondary to Trauma or Repetitive Stress

Although degenerative joint conditions are more commonly seen in older adults, younger people can also exhibit degenerative bony changes due to traumatic injury or repetitive insult. These changes are most commonly seen in patients involved in contact and collision sports such as American football and rugby. Complications associated with degenerative bony changes such as osteophytes and stenosis include structural malalignment, narrowing of the spinal canal or intervertebral foramen resulting in nerve compression, and increased risk of nerve injury.

Osteophytes

Osteophytes, or bone spurs, can arise from the vertebral bodies secondary to degenerative disc changes that increase wear and compression of the joint surfaces. Osteophytes are most commonly found posterolaterally but can also be found anteriorly. Posterolateral osteophytes can narrow the intervertebral foramen, resulting in nerve root compression and increased suscepti-bility to brachial plexus neuropraxia. Signs and symptoms associated with osteophytic changes include decreased ROM, postural changes, neck discomfort that increases with lateral rotation and extension, and neurologi-cal symptoms that increase as intervertebral narrowing progresses.

Spinal Stenosis

Spinal stenosis is more often seen in older adults and is characterized by a developmen-tal or congenital narrowing of the cervical spinal canal. Spinal stenosis can be disabling for anyone, but it is of particular concern in contact sports and may disqualify a patient from participation because of the greater risk of spinal cord injury. The narrowed spinal canal increases the risk for cord compression and injuries resulting from hyperextension or hyperflexion mechanisms. When these factors are coupled with secondary complica-tions such as cervical spine instability or disc herniation, the risk for spinal cord injury is further increased.

Nerve Injuries

Nerve injuries associated with the cervical spine are typically caused by bone or soft tissue encroachment into the spinal canal or intervertebral foramen spaces, causing compression of the nerve structures that run through that space. Spinal cord injury, transient neuropraxia, disc herniation, and brachial plexus injuries are examples of inju-ries caused by external forces acting on the spinal cord or cervical nerve roots. Signs and symptoms of nerve injuries include, but are not limited to, paresthesia, paralysis, numb-ness, burning, tingling, and atrophy.

Transient Neuropraxia

Central cord compression and **transient neuropraxia** can also result secondary to posterior disc herniation, spinal stenosis, congenital fusion, or instability in the cervi-cal spine. Signs and symptoms of transient neuropraxia include sensory changes, such as burning, tingling, or numbness, and motor changes ranging from weakness to tempo-rary paralysis in both the upper and lower extremities (Torg et al. 1996). These symp-toms usually subside within a few minutes but may persist for 1 to 2 days.

Intervertebral Disc Herniation

Cervical disc herniation can result from acute trauma causing compression, flexion, or extension of the cervical spine. More often, it is caused by a gradual weakening or failure of the annulus fibrosis secondary to chronic or repetitive mechanical stress. As a result, the herniated disc material typi-cally protrudes into the intervertebral fora-men, compressing and irritating the exiting nerve root. Signs and symptoms of cervi-cal disc herniation and associated nerve compression include pain and discomfort that improve with cervical distraction and worsen with extension and rotation to the side. The patient exhibits decreased ROM and muscular splinting, tilting the head away from or toward the involved side to avoid compressive and painful positions.

Brachial Plexus Injury

Brachial plexus injury involves mechanical deformation due to compression or stretch-ing of the C5 through T1 nerve roots as they exit the cervical spine. Brachial plexus injuries are often termed stingers or burners because of the classical symptom of imme-diate sharp, burning pain radiating into the arm at the time of injury. The patient also complains of temporary weakness or inability to move the arm. Symptoms may be reproduced with lateral flexion away from the stabilized shoulder or with lateral flexion toward the involved side. Symptoms associated with brachial plexus injury are usually short-lived, and the extremity typi-cally regains full function within minutes. However, neurological symptoms may persist for a few days or even months, depending on the severity of nerve disruption.

Vascular Injuries

Vascular injuries associated with the cervical spine are also caused by bone or soft tissue encroachment that results in compression of various vascular structures in and around the neck. **Thoracic outlet syndrome (TOS)**, probably the most common vascular condition in the cervical region, is due to compression of the subclavian artery as it exits through the thoracic outlet. The thoracic outlet is marked by the anterior scalene muscle anteriorly, the middle scalene posteriorly, and the first rib inferiorly. The brachial plexus complex exits through the thoracic outlet and can also be affected by compressive forces in this area. The vertebral arteries can be compromised in cervical fractures, dislocations, or subluxations.

Summary

Due to the possibility of fatal or catastrophic injuries to the cervical spine, the acute examination strategy centers on eliminating concern about a life-threatening or life-altering cervical spine injury. Decisions regarding movement of the patient and transportation to emergency facilities need to be made during this examination. Clinical examinations usually involve non-life-threatening and nonacute cervical spine injuries.

The most important aspect of the examination strategy for a suspected cervical spine injury is to determine the severity and initiate appropriate emergency transportation procedures. On arriving at the patient's side, do a primary survey to check for consciousness as well as airway, breathing, and circulation and respond accordingly. If the individual is unconscious, assume that he has a spinal cord injury. It is also imperative to stabilize the cervical spine by performing in-line stabilization if you suspect a cervical spine injury. If at any time in your examination a serious neck injury becomes an assumption, no further examination is necessary;

emergency medical services (EMS) should be notified and the patient should be properly stabilized and transported to an emergency care facility.

Thoracic and Lumbar Spine Injury Recognition

Considerable mechanical and muscular forces are exerted on the thoracic and lumbar regions of the spine during the running, jumping, twisting, bending, and lifting activities associated with sport. The lumbar spine provides both mobility and stability for upper extremity and torso movements and effectively absorbs and transmits forces between the upper and lower extremities. Because of its greater mobility and load-bearing function compared to the thoracic and sacral spines, the lumbar spine is particularly susceptible to pain and injury. Back pain, a frequent complaint in the physically active, commonly results from acute traumatic episodes as well as cumulative stress. Although not usual in sport, the most severe consequence of a back injury is paralysis. You must be able to quickly and effectively recognize the signs and symptoms of a serious back injury and manage it accordingly to prevent further injury and neurological insult.

Lumbar and thoracic pain is most often due to acute and chronic strains of the postural muscles supporting the lumbar region. Chronic strain may result from poor posture, poor mechanics, weakness, stiffness, and muscle restrictions. Occasionally, congenital defects or degenerative changes cause low back pain. Traumatic injuries such as fractures may also occur, and you must always consider the potential for spinal cord injury and potential paralysis with severe injuries. Knowledge of pertinent and basic functional anatomy is critical to appropriate examinations of the thoracic and lumbar spine (figure 11.2).

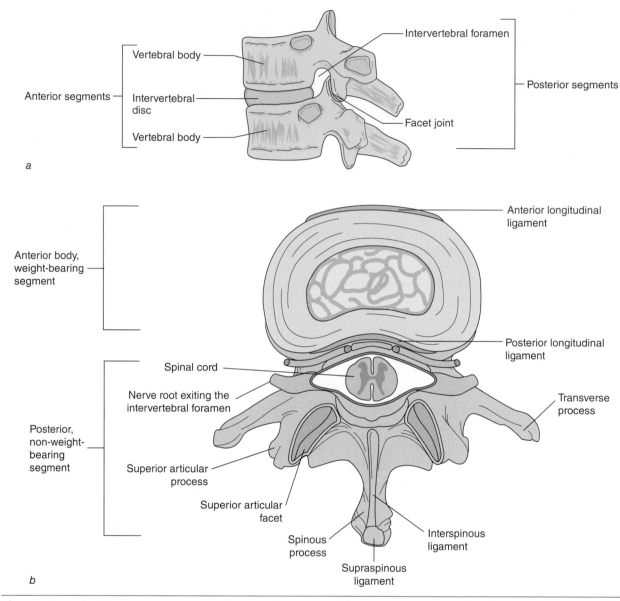

Figure 11.2 *(a)* Functional anatomy of the lumbar spine. *(b)* Transverse section showing the structures of the posterior segment and the relationship of the spinal cord and nerve roots.

(a) Adapted, by permission, from J. Watkins, 2010, *Structure and function of the musculoskeletal system,* 2nd ed. (Champaign, IL: Human Kinetics), 120.

Acute and Chronic Soft Tissue Injuries

Soft tissue injuries make up the majority of injuries encountered in the lumbar spine. The soft tissue injuries that physically active people most commonly experience include contusions, sprains, and strains.

Contusions

The spinal structures vulnerable to direct contact and contusions are the spinous processes and their overlying superficial ligaments. Contusions to these structures may result in point tenderness, localized swelling, and pain with flexion and extension. Contusions to the musculature may cause considerable muscle swelling, stiffness, and spasm resulting in loss of ROM and function. Although these contusions are rarely serious or debilitating, patients who have incurred significant direct trauma to the lower trunk and complain of severe or unrelenting low back pain should be thoroughly examined for possible kidney or other visceral trauma.

Sprains

Sprains in the lumbar and thoracic region typically result from sudden loading or torsion movements. They can also result from direct or indirect trauma that forces the spinal segments beyond their normal ranges of motion, as well as from compressive loading forces.

• *Facet syndrome.* Facet syndrome is an inflammation (**spondylitis**) of the facet joint and its surrounding capsule. Facet syndrome can result from acute trauma or chronic repetitive insult. Extension overload of the facet joint, particularly when combined with rotation, can compress and irritate the joint. Because the facet joint is richly innervated, facet syndrome may be associated with considerable pain. Other signs and symptoms include localized swelling; paraspinal muscle spasm; tenderness upon palpation and movement of the facet joint; and increased pain with extension, compression, and rotation to the involved side. Pain may also be referred down the leg.

• *SI joint dysfunction.* Low back pain can also be referred from a sprain or dysfunction of the sacroiliac (SI) joint. While these conditions and tests are covered in the discussion of the hip and pelvis, they are mentioned here simply to alert you to potential injuries affecting the lumbar spine region.

Strains

The mechanisms for muscular strains are similar to those for sprains, causing sudden contraction or stretching of the involved musculature (figure 11.3). Sudden eccentric loading of an already contracting muscle is also a common cause of muscular strain. Strains can result from a single episode of muscle overload but also frequently result from cumulative stress. Signs and symptoms include pain, point tenderness, muscle spasm, and possible swelling in and around the involved musculature.

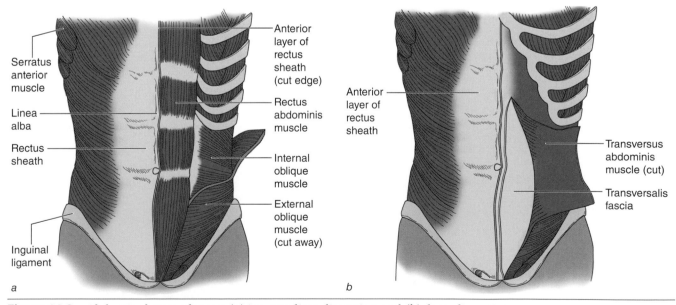

Figure 11.3 Abdominal musculature: *(a)* intermediate dissection and *(b)* deep dissection.

Adapted, by permission, from C.M. Norris, 2008, *Back stability*, 2nd ed. (Champaign, IL: Human Kinetics), 51, 53.

Bone and Joint Pathologies

Bone and joint pathologies are less common than soft tissue injuries in this region. While traumatic fractures may occur in the lumbar and thoracic spine, the vast majority of bone and joint pathologies result from congenital weakening, degenerative processes, or both.

▶ Traumatic Fractures of the Thoracic Spine

Because of the stability of the thoracic spine, fractures and dislocations are rare in sport participants. Thoracic spine fractures typically involve compression of the vertebral body resulting from violent forward flexion or axial loading in a forward flexed position (figure 11.4). Signs and symptoms include localized pain and discomfort, tenderness with palpation over the spinous process of the involved vertebra, muscle spasm and guarding, and increased pain with forward flexion and other movements of the thoracic spine.

▶ Traumatic Fractures of the Lumbar Spine

Traumatic fractures of the lumbar spine are relatively uncommon with sport activities, with the possible exception of high-speed impact sports. The structures most likely to be fractured secondary to acute trauma are the vertebral body, transverse processes, spinous processes, and pars articularis. Fractures of the transverse processes can result from direct trauma, violent torsional movements, or an avulsion of the psoas major muscle following a violent contraction (figure 11.5). Avulsion fractures of the transverse process can cause considerable pain and bleeding. Fractures of the relatively unprotected spinous processes are typically attributable to blunt trauma but may also result from forced hyperflexion of the lumbar spine.

Signs and symptoms associated with fracture include immediate pain, direct tenderness over the vertebral segment, referred pain along nerve distribution, crepitus, decreased ROM, and an unwillingness to move. If the

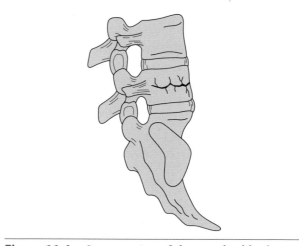

Figure 11.4   Compression of the vertebral body.

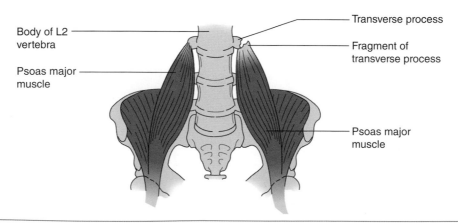

Body of L2 vertebra

Psoas major muscle

Transverse process

Fragment of transverse process

Psoas major muscle

Figure 11.5   Transverse process with psoas avulsion.

fracture encroaches on the spinal cord or nerve root, signs and symptoms of sensory or motor deficits associated with nerve compression or injury may also be present.

Spondylolysis and Spondylolisthesis

A condition that is often attributed to a congenital abnormality but may not manifest itself until the patient is physically active is spondylolysis. **Spondylolysis** involves a fracture of the pars interarticularis, located between the inferior and superior facets. It is typically thought to be a stress fracture secondary to a congenital weakening. **Spondylolisthesis** occurs when the fracture of the pars interarticularis in spondylolysis becomes unstable and forward subluxation of the involved vertebrae occurs. Spondylolisthesis is frequently found in gymnasts, weightlifters, and football lineman secondary to the repetitive flexion and hyperextension common in their sporting activities.

Signs and symptoms associated with spondylolysis and spondylolisthesis are centralized low back pain (possibly radiating into the buttocks and posterior thighs), swelling, muscle spasm, and a straightening of the lordotic curve. Patients with these conditions may exhibit decreased ROM and increased pain with hyperextension. Standing on only the leg of the affected side and extending the spine also increases pain.

Degenerative Pathologies

Degenerative changes of the vertebrae and disc are more frequently the cause of back pain in the physically active adult. Chronic joint inflammatory conditions resulting from cumulative and repetitive stress (e.g., spondylitis, facet syndrome) may also bring about degenerative changes such as osteophytes and capsular fibrosis. Nerve compression injuries of the thoracic and lumbar spine most often involve the nerve roots of the sciatic nerve as they exit the intervertebral foramen of the lumbar vertebrae. Nerve compression can result from an encroaching prolapsed or herniated intervertebral disc (figure 11.6) or from degenerative osteophytes causing stenosis of the intervertebral foramen (figure 11.7).

Intervertebral Disc Herniation

Intervertebral disc prolapse (bulge) or herniation can be caused by both acute trauma and cumulative stress mechanisms. Faulty posture, faulty movement mechanics, weak musculature, and inflexibility can all contribute to repetitive microtrauma that weakens

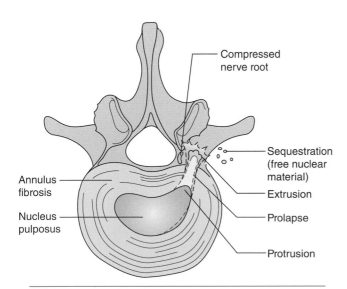

Figure 11.6 Four stages of disc herniation.

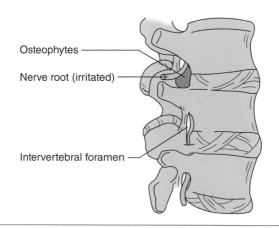

Figure 11.7 Osteophytes and stenosis of intervertebral foramen causing nerve root compression.

the annulus fibrosis and allows protrusion and possible extrusion or sequestration of the disc material (see figure 11.6 on page 259). Twisting and holding a heavy object away from the body while lifting is a frequent mechanism for acute lumbar disc herniation. Signs and symptoms of disc herniation include centralized back pain, point tenderness over the spinal level, muscle spasm, and **sciatica**, or referred pain along the nerve distribution. Signs and symptoms associated with nerve compression are also present; these are covered in the next section.

Nerve Compression Injuries of the Lumbar Spine

Nerve compression can result from an encroaching prolapsed or herniated intervertebral disc (see figure 11.6) or from degenerative osteophytes causing stenosis of the intervertebral foramen (see figure 11.7). When injuries are associated with nerve compression, the patient typically complains of sciatica, or radiating pain down the thigh, lower leg, and foot along the distribution of the sciatic nerve. The specific pain location and pattern depend on the lumbar level at which the nerve is compressed (figure 11.8). Patients exhibiting positive neurological signs require immediate referral. Complaints of bowel or bladder dysfunction with low back pain are considered a medical emergency.

Summary

It is common for patients to report back injuries or back pain some time after their onset. Because the back is complex and has many structures that can be the source of pain, and

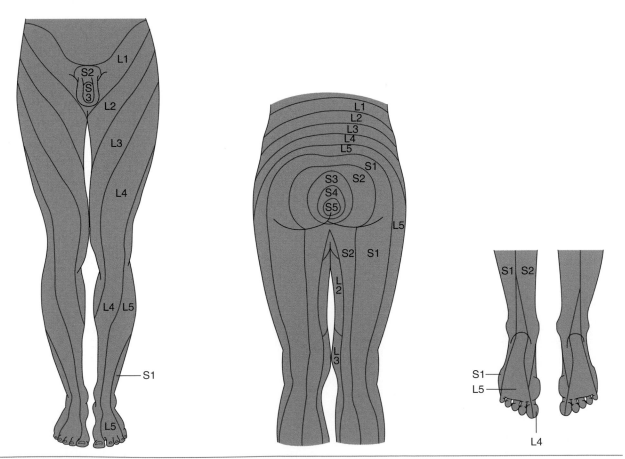

Figure 11.8   Sensory nerve distribution for the lumbar plexus.

because many of those structures can refer pain to the lower extremities, examination of back injuries is a challenging task. It can be difficult to narrow down potential causes of the pain and identify the source of the problem. A systematic approach that uses a thorough history to limit the possibilities, along with a complete objective examination that pinpoints and confirms your suspicions, is critical. Emergency situations resulting from lower back injury include those in which paresthesia, paralysis, radiating pain, or neurovascular symptoms are present.

Head and Face Injury Recognition

This section addresses the recognition of injuries to the head and face and equips you to differentiate signs and symptoms that indicate a life-threatening condition. It is important to realize, though, that head and facial pain can be caused by medical conditions unrelated to sport activity. General medical conditions of the head, eyes, ears, nose, and mouth also cause pain, and it is important to keep those conditions in mind

when a patient complains of head or face pain and symptoms with no known injury mechanism.

The head is a complex anatomical structure that supports the brain and the sensory organs for sight, hearing, taste, and smell. Although patients frequently complain of head and facial pain, the causes can vary widely and may sometimes indicate serious intracranial pathology. For this reason you need to understand the anatomical complexity and function of the structures in the head region in order to adequately examine injury and illness there (figure 11.9).

Even with the use of protective equipment during sport activity, head and facial injuries occur frequently and can range from minor insults to life-threatening conditions. You must be well versed in the etiology and signs and symptoms of each of these conditions and be able to quickly identify symptoms that indicate a medical emergency and immediate medical referral.

Head Injuries

Head injuries are common in athletics, representing the leading cause of death due to

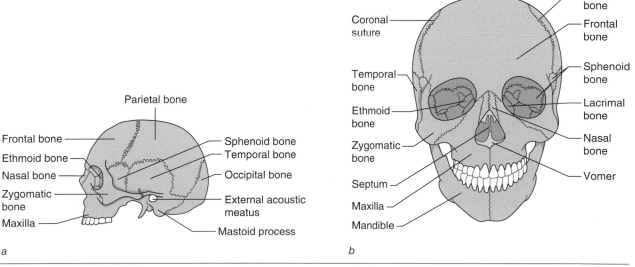

Figure 11.9 (a) Bones of the skull and (b) facial bones. (The palatine bone, which forms the palate that separates the mouth from the nasal cavity, is not visible in this view.)

Reprinted, by permission, from J. Watkins, 2010, *Structure and function of the musculoskeletal system*, 2nd ed. (Champaign, IL: Human Kinetics), 28, 30.

sport activity. A major blow to an individual's head or chin should immediately arouse suspicion of potential head injury. Head injuries are typically classified into three categories:

- Mild head injury or concussion
- Intracranial hemorrhage
- Skull fractures

Concussion

A **concussion**, caused by an agitation or shaking of the brain, is defined as a transient alteration in brain function without structural damage. Clinically, it is defined by the severity of the injury. Multiple grading scales have been developed to classify the degree of mild head injury based on the duration of either unconsciousness or posttraumatic amnesia (see example in table 11.1). While experts do not yet universally agree on the grading and criteria for return to activity following a concussion, they do agree that any patient suffering postconcussion symptoms such as headache, dizziness, nausea, ringing in the ears (**tinnitus**), loss of consciousness, confusion, and amnesia should not participate in contact or collision sports until symptoms clear (Cantu 2001). Signs and symptoms vary considerably from one person to another and according to injury severity. (See the sidebar Signs and Symptoms of Postconcussion Syndrome for more information on the signs and symptoms of concussions.) While it is often fairly easy to recognize second- and third-degree concussions, first-degree concussions may go unnoticed if the patient does not report symptoms.

Intracranial Hemorrhage

When head trauma results in tissue edema or hemorrhage, pressure builds in the intracranial space, ultimately compressing the brain stem, the center for breathing, heart rate, and other life-sustaining functions. Unless pressure is relieved in a timely fashion, death will result. A space-occupying hematoma alters consciousness, vital signs, motor function, and pupillary function. Patients with this injury vary in their level of consciousness from fully awake to drowsy or lethargic,

SIGNS AND SYMPTOMS OF POSTCONCUSSION SYNDROME

- Headache with exertion
- Dizziness
- Tinnitus
- Fatigue
- Irritability
- Frustration
- Difficulty in coping with daily stress
- Impaired memory or concentration
- Eating or sleeping disorders
- Behavioral changes
- Alcohol intolerance
- Decreased academic performance

From NATA 1994.

Table 11.1 Evidence-Based Cantu Grading System for Concussion

Grade	Symptoms
Grade 1 (mild)	No loss of consciousness; posttraumatic amnesia* or postconcussion signs or symptoms lasting less than 30 min.
Grade 2 (moderate)	Loss of consciousness lasting less than 1 min; posttraumatic amnesia* or postconcussion signs or symptoms lasting longer than 30 min but less than 24 h.
Grade 3 (severe)	Loss of consciousness lasting more than 1 min or posttraumatic amnesia* lasting longer than 24 h; postconcussion signs or symptoms lasting longer than 7 days

*Retrograde and anterograde.

Adapted from R.C. Cantu, 2001, "Posttraumatic retrograde and anterograde amnesia: Pathophysiology and implications in grading and safe return to play," *Journal of Athletic Training* 36(3): 246.

to stuporous, to comatose. Symptoms of **intracranial hemorrhage** may not appear immediately following injury but may occur at some delay. However, once symptoms do appear, the patient's condition can deteriorate quickly and result in death if not immediately recognized. Any patient who loses consciousness, even for a brief period of time, should be closely examined and monitored following injury and throughout the next 24 h for signs and symptoms of intracranial hemorrhage. Symptoms of intracranial hemorrhage include, but are not limited to, rapid shallow breathing, hypotension, rapid pulse, pupil irregularities such as inequality and unresponsiveness to light, and varying levels of motor deficits.

Skull Fracture

Skull fractures result from direct impact and are more common in sports using a bat and ball or played on hard surfaces with the patient not wearing a helmet. The fracture may be linear or hairline, resulting from a blunt force, or depressed, resulting from a more focused point of contact. The location of the fracture may be significant, as fractures that transverse a major artery may tear the vessel and cause an epidural hemorrhage. If you palpate a depression or deformity on the skull, be very careful not to apply additional pressure to the area. Signs and symptoms of skull fracture include pain, palpable tenderness, swelling, discoloration, possible bony depression, and loss of consciousness.

Second-Impact Syndrome

A patient who returns to competition and sustains a second minor head trauma soon after an initial head injury may be at risk for second-impact syndrome. **Second-impact syndrome** is characterized by an autoregulatory dysfunction that causes rapid and fatal brain swelling. The individual with a recent history of mild head injury who receives a blow to the head initially exhibits signs and symptoms of a mild concussion. The second impact does not usually result in loss of consciousness, and the patient typically remains upright but may appear dazed (Cantu and

Voy 1995). However, within minutes the patient collapses into a coma and shows signs of cranial nerve and brain stem pressure. The mortality rate of second-impact syndrome is high, so prevention is crucial.

Eye Injuries

Injuries to the eye, which most often result from direct contact, may involve either the corneal surface or internal eye structures. Eye injuries can be quite serious and may result in permanent damage if not recognized immediately or treated appropriately. The following are some of the more common eye injuries seen in athletics.

Periorbital Hematoma

A **periorbital hematoma**, or black eye, is caused by a direct blow and is characterized by discoloration and swelling of the orbital rim and cavity (figure 11.10).

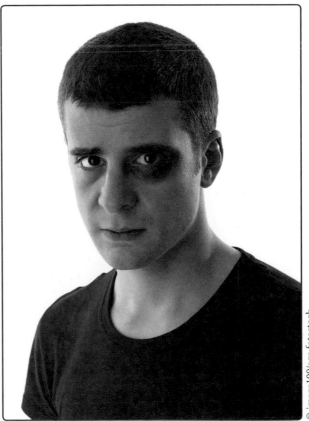

© image100/age fotostock

Figure 11.10 Periorbital hematoma.

Corneal Abrasion

A finger poke to the eye or a foreign body under the eyelid can scratch the outer surface of the cornea, resulting in a corneal abrasion. Abrasions can also occur when an individual attempts to remove a foreign body from the eye or removes a contact lens that has been in place too long.

Corneal Laceration

Lacerations through the full thickness of the cornea are much less common than corneal abrasions but can occur when a sharp object, such as a fingernail, cuts the eye. Immediately refer patients with a corneal laceration to an ophthalmologist for further examination.

Detached Retina

A sudden blow to the head or eye can cause the pigment layer of the retina to tear away or detach from its neural layer on the inner, posterior surface of the eye. A detached retina is not readily observable, but symptoms indicating a possible detached retina include blurred vision, flashes, floating spots, and blind areas in the patient's field of vision. Suspected detached retinas warrant immediate referral.

Hyphema

Direct trauma to the eye can also result in **hyphema**, or an accumulation of blood in the anterior chamber of the eye (figure 11.11).

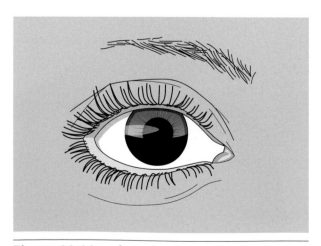

Figure 11.11 Blood in the anterior chamber (hyphema).

Blood in the anterior chamber is readily apparent, as it obscures the iris and pupil. The patient complains of impaired vision, pain, and a feeling of pressure in the eye. Hyphemas indicate a serious eye injury that can cause excessive pressure within the eye or can be associated with further underlying pathology. Keep the patient upright and immediately refer her to an ophthalmologist or emergency room.

Orbital Blow-Out Fracture

A fracture of the orbital floor, also known as a blow-out fracture, occurs from a sudden increase in orbital pressure due to a direct blow to the eye. Blunt trauma such as being struck in the eye with a baseball or racquetball is a common mechanism. The pressure from the blow fractures the thin, inferior wall of the orbit and displaces the wall inferiorly. Signs and symptoms include swelling, discoloration, and point tenderness along the inferior aspect of the eye. The injured eye may appear to sit lower than the uninjured one, and the patient is unable to look up because the inferior eye muscles are trapped at the fracture site (figure 11.12).

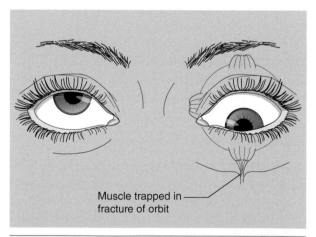

Muscle trapped in fracture of orbit

Figure 11.12 Orbital blow-out fracture with the inability to look upward.

Ear Injuries

Contusions, friction, or repetitive trauma to the external ear can result in bleeding between the skin and cartilage. In some instances, an observable hematoma forms that, if left untreated, causes separation of the cartilage from its nutritional supply. This results in necrosis and degeneration of the cartilage, leading to permanent scarring and deformity, which is known as cauliflower ear (auricular hematoma) (figure 11.13). Lacerations of the ear, though uncommon, can result from a severe direct impact or tension force.

Nasal Injuries

Nasal injuries are the most common facial injury in sport. Nasal fractures are the most common facial fracture, and nosebleeds (**epistaxis**) frequently occur because of the rich blood supply in the nasal mucosa. Direct trauma to the nose is the most common cause of nasal injuries and in severe cases can actually cause a deviation of the septum separating the nasal passageway into two narrow cavities. Minor deviations in the septum to one side or the other are common. However, severe deviations can restrict airflow, and the patient complains of difficulty exchanging air through one side of the nose. In this case, surgery may be necessary to repair the deviation.

Face and Jaw Injuries

Direct contact and glancing blows to the face and chin can result in traumatic injury of other facial bones or the temporomandibular joint (TMJ). Fractures to the mandible, maxilla, or zygomatic arch may result from a direct blow, for example being struck by a ball or another player or contacting the ground in a fall. The most common fracture site is the mandibular angle, near the socket of the third molar (Moore 1992). Often, two fractures occur, one on either side of the jaw.

▶ Facial Fractures

Fractures to the maxillae may also occur concurrently with a nasal fracture, and epistaxis may result. Zygomatic fractures are among the more common facial fractures and usually result from a direct blow to the cheek (figure 11.14). If the fracture is displaced, the cheek appears flattened. Because the zygomatic bone forms part of the orbit, visual acuity and ocular alignment can be affected.

▶ Temporomandibular Joint Dysfunction

Temporomandibular joint dysfunction is characterized by chronic joint pain and crepitus that may also produce headaches

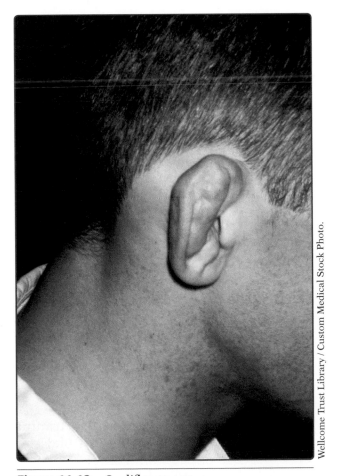

Figure 11.13   Cauliflower ear.

Wellcome Trust Library / Custom Medical Stock Photo.

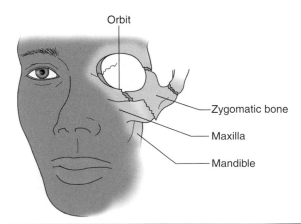

Orbit

Zygomatic bone

Maxilla

Mandible

Figure 11.14   Zygomatic arch fracture.

and neck pain. Causes of TMJ dysfunction are direct trauma, arthritic conditions, poor approximation of the teeth when biting down, muscular tension, and grinding of the teeth at night. Dislocations of the TMJ can also occur.

Dental Injuries

Patients may present with a variety of dental complaints that may or may not be related to sport participation or work activity. They can experience dental pain and injury secondary to either direct trauma to the mouth or tooth and gum disease resulting from poor hygiene. Injuries to the teeth caused by direct trauma to the mouth are classified as fractures, intrusions, luxations, or avulsion (figure 11.15). Tooth fractures may involve a simple chipping of the enamel or may extend into the dentin, pulp, or root. Trau-

matic forces to the mouth can also loosen a tooth in its alveolar process (socket). An axial force applied to the tooth may cause an intrusion, in which the tooth is driven into the socket. If force is applied to the side of the tooth, the tooth may be displaced (luxation) or dislocated. The tooth appears out of alignment or crooked, and the gums may bleed. Dislocated teeth may also be partially extruded, or pulled from the socket. In this case, the tooth may appear longer than the adjacent teeth or may have been removed completely. Completely removed teeth must not be handled roughly or by the root and should be *gently* placed back in the mouth or placed in a tooth-preserving solution immediately. Due to the severity of such injuries, the difficulty of treatment, and the long-term ramifications of improperly managed dental injuries, refer the patient to a dentist for further examination and follow-up.

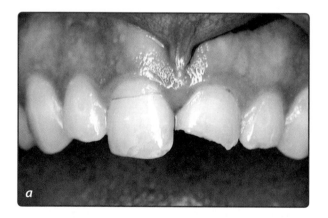
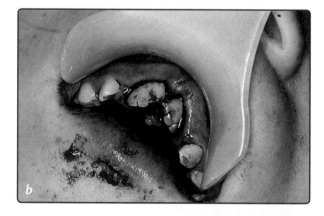
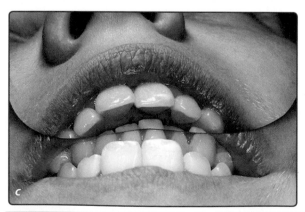
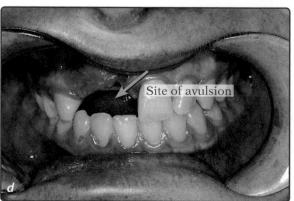

Figure 11.15 *(a)* Fracture, *(b)* intrusion, *(c)* luxation, and *(d)* avulsion of a tooth.

Summary

The goal of recognizing and examining head and facial injuries is to determine the severity of the injuries and whether immediate referral for advanced medical services is warranted. Recognizing life-threatening head trauma or life-altering facial trauma is paramount for proper treatment.

The condition of an individual with a serious brain injury can quickly deteriorate, and death can occur within minutes. It is imperative that you monitor vital signs and level of consciousness every 5 min until you have ruled out serious head trauma or are sure the patient is stabilized or improving. Any one of the following changes is reason for immediate referral:

- Decreasing level of consciousness (decreasing score on Glasgow Coma Scale)
- Increasing blood pressure
- Decreasing or irregular respirations
- Decreasing or irregular pulse
- Unequal, dilated, or unreactive pupil(s)

When examining potential head injuries, your concern is not only whether the patient exhibits any characteristic signs and symptoms, but also whether the signs and symptoms change or worsen over time. Your observation skills must be particularly keen in this examination, as the behavior and response of the patient provide important clues to injury severity. Follow-up examination of mild head trauma during the first 24 to 48 h after injury should include home instructions for the patient and a roommate or family member to watch for signs and symptoms that indicate a worsening condition. It is useful to have a prepared instruction sheet that you can give to the person who will be staying with the patient over the 24 to 48 h following injury. Even in mild cases that appear to warrant little concern about serious brain injury, you should provide this information as a precaution, as signs of intracranial hemorrhage may be delayed or may progress slowly.

Thorax and Abdominal Injury Recognition

You will often be presented with patients complaining of chest and abdominal pain. Although most of these complaints will be associated with minor injuries and illnesses, others may indicate serious underlying pathologies. Examination of the thorax and abdomen is rather complex in that symptoms of underlying pathology may not appear immediately, masking the seriousness of the situation. Injuries to the thorax and abdomen can be described as emergent (on-site) or nonemergent (clinical) depending on whether they are due to acute trauma or underlying or slow-developing pathology, respectively. The ability to recognize the signs and symptoms of internal injury and cardiorespiratory compromise can mean the difference between life and death, and often you will need to repeat examinations over time.

To understand and properly examine chest and abdominal injuries, you must first be familiar with the anatomical orientation and physiological function of the organs and structures of the thorax and abdomen (figure 11.16). Although this chapter presents anatomical orientation where appropriate within the context of various pathologies, you are encouraged to review the general anatomy and physiology of this region before proceeding.

Injuries to the thorax and abdomen can result from a variety of mechanisms. Injury can occur as a consequence of violent muscle contractions and can even occur spontaneously without evidence of direct trauma. Blunt trauma or direct insult is the most common mechanism and the one that presents the greatest concern for serious injury. Although the internal organs of the thorax and abdomen are well protected, they are

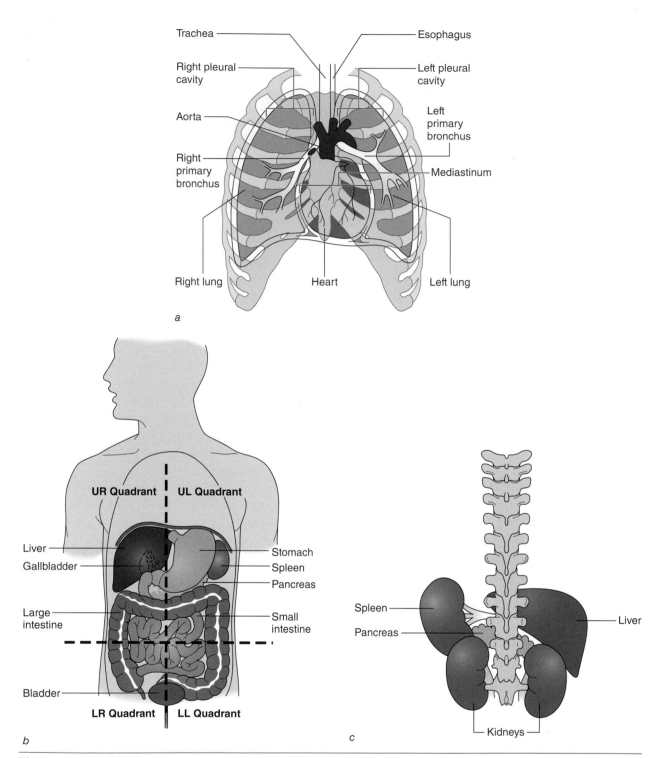

Figure 11.16 *(a)* Thoracic cavity and skeletal rib cage. Note the two pleural cavities and the structures of the mediastinum. *(b)* Anterior view of the organs of the abdominal cavity (note the four quadrants of the abdominal cavity). *(c)* Posterior view of the organs of the abdominal cavity.

vulnerable to injury during sport. Internal injuries often result from a hard fall; a helmet to the chest, lower back, or abdomen; or impact from a baseball, softball, or other sport implement. Because of the potential for life-threatening complications arising from these injuries, you should suspect underlying pathology throughout your examination any time a patient sustains a significant blow to the chest or abdomen.

Thorax (Musculoskeletal)

Injuries to the chest wall and organs of the thoracic cavity can result from direct insult or violent muscle contractions; they also may occur spontaneously as a consequence of intense exercise. The most common injuries resulting from these mechanisms are contusions, strains, sprains, and fractures of the chest wall. The structures most commonly involved are the ribs, sternum, costochondral cartilage, muscles and tendons, and costovertebral joints where the ribs attach to the sternum and vertebral column.

Contusions

Because of the superficial nature of the anterior and lateral chest wall, rib and sternal contusions are common in contact sports with no or inadequate chest protection. Signs and symptoms include localized pain, swelling, discoloration, periosteal irritation, and point tenderness. Deep inspiration may cause pain if the adjacent intercostal muscles or costochondral joints are irritated or injured. Although severe contusions may be difficult to distinguish from fracture, contusions typically do not display signs of bony crepitus or pain with indirect compression of the chest wall.

Sprains

Sprains or separation of the costochondral joint can result secondary to anteriorly directed trauma to the sternum or lateral compression of the chest wall. The patient complains of pain and point tenderness at the costochondral junction. With separation or dislocation, he will also complain of increased pain with deep inspiration, of crepitus or clicking, and of increased prominence of the joint. You may also observe swelling and discoloration.

Costochondritis

Chronic irritation and inflammation of the costochondral junction (**costochondritis**)

can occur following acute, traumatic injury or as a result of chronic stress or repetitive activities such as coughing, rowing, or lifting. The patient may have no history of trauma but complain of a gradual onset of pain in the anterior chest wall and tenderness over the affected joint. Crepitus and mild inflammation may also be present. Rest, ice, and anti-inflammatory medication typically resolve symptoms within a few weeks.

Rib Fracture

While the first through fourth ribs are well protected by the shoulder girdle and the 10th through 12th ribs are more mobile, the rigidly fixed fifth through ninth ribs are prone to fracture. Fractures most commonly occur at the weaker, posterior angle (figure 11.17). Signs and symptoms include localized pain, point tenderness, swelling, discoloration, crepitus, and muscle guarding. Pain increases with indirect chest wall compression, deep inspiration, and coughing, sneezing, laughing, or jarring. Because deep inspiration increases pain, the patient often presents with rapid, shallow breathing to avoid the pain. The patient may also rotate the trunk and lean toward the injured side to prevent muscle tensioning and pain.

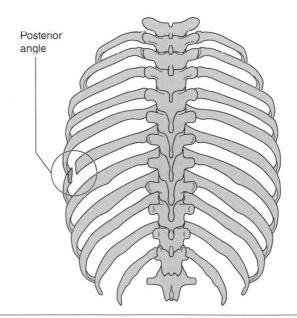

Posterior angle

Figure 11.17 Rib fracture at the posterior angle.

Sternum Fracture

Fractures of the sternum are rare in contact sports. However, sternal fractures can result from a severe, direct blow to the anterior chest (e.g., when another player's helmet or a sport implement, such as a baseball, hits the chest at a high velocity). The patient will likely complain of losing her breath immediately following injury as well as feeling pain with deep inspiration. Examination will reveal localized pain, tenderness, ecchymosis, swelling, and possible deformity. Because of the severity of the blow needed to cause a sternal fracture, always check for underlying pleural (hemothorax, pneumothorax) and cardiac (contusion, tamponade) injury, particularly if the sternum displaces posteriorly.

Thoracic Cavity

The same mechanisms that cause trauma to the musculoskeletal structures of the thorax can also traumatize the heart and lungs or cause internal bleeding—all of which can have life-threatening consequences. Internal injuries in the thoracic region are serious and often life threatening. Lower rib fractures may subsequently lacerate the upper abdominal viscera and result in internal hemorrhage. Although the thoracic cavity is well protected circumferentially by the sternum, ribs, and vertebral column, both blunt and penetrating trauma can injure these vital structures and compromise pulmonary or circulatory function or both. Injuries to the lungs may also occur spontaneously as a consequence of intense exercise.

Pneumothorax

A **pneumothorax** occurs when air enters the pleural cavity located between the lung and the chest wall, thus reducing the volume of the lung (figure 11.18). Severe, life-threatening complications can arise if the air in the pleural cavity continues to increase, progressing to a tension pneumothorax. Increasing pressure caused by the trapped air shifts the mediastinum away from the injured side, compressing the heart and healthy lung and compromising their function (figure 11.19).

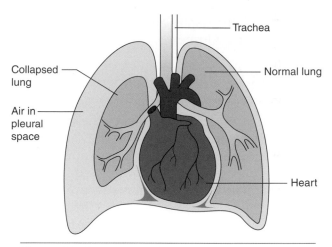

Figure 11.18   Pneumothorax.

A pneumothorax can result from traumatic injury or can occur spontaneously in the absence of trauma. A penetrating injury such as a rib fracture can rupture or lacerate lung tissue and allow inspired air to escape into the pleural space. More common in sport, however, is a spontaneous pneumothorax; this most often occurs in young, healthy patients with no history of trauma and may follow an intense bout of activity that causes small ruptures in the outer surface of the lung tissue. Signs and symptoms associated with a simple pneumothorax include upper chest pain, **dyspnea** (difficulty breathing) or shortness of breath, light-headedness, and decreased breath sounds. Immediately refer patients with a suspected pneumothorax for emergency medical care.

Hemothorax

Traumatic chest injuries, such as laceration of lung tissue or an intercostal artery secondary to a penetrating rib fracture, can result in a **hemothorax**, in which blood, rather than air, fills the pleural space. Signs and symptoms of a hemothorax include lung collapse and reduced or absent breath sounds on the involved side, severe chest pain, dyspnea, cyanosis, hypotension, and the coughing up of frothy blood.

Cardiac Contusion

Blunt trauma to the chest that compresses the heart between the sternum and the spine

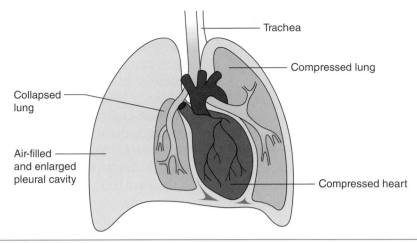

Figure 11.19 Tension pneumothorax and shift of the mediastinum with compression of the heart and healthy lung.

can result in a contusion to the heart muscle. Signs and symptoms of cardiac contusion include chest pain, neck vein distension, possible rhythm disturbance (**arrhythmia**), muffled heart tones, shock, and respiratory or cardiac distress.

Cardiac Tamponade

Blunt trauma to the chest can also cause cardiac tamponade, or hemorrhage within the enclosed, inelastic pericardial cavity surrounding the heart. Cardiac tamponade is characterized by compression of the heart and pulmonary veins, which prevents venous return to the heart. Signs and symptoms include neck vein distension (due to the backup of venous flow), shock, hypotension, cyanosis, severe chest pain, and difficulty breathing. Cardiac tamponade is clearly life threatening and warrants immediate emergency medical care.

Cardiac Concussion (Commotio Cordis)

A condition that has aroused considerable interest in recent years is cardiac concussion. Cardiac concussion, or commotio cordis, is characterized by immediate cardiac arrest and sudden death following a localized blunt, but seemingly inconsequential, blow to the chest. Unfortunately, in most cases, resuscitation attempts have failed and death usually results. When an individual collapses following blunt trauma to the chest, you should immediately exam-

ine for airway, breathing, and circulation and should summon EMS.

Abdomen

Traumatic injuries to the abdominal region include soft tissue injuries of the abdominal muscles, genitalia, and internal organs. While the thoracic cavity is protected by the skeletal rib cage, the abdomen is protected primarily by soft tissue structures; thus contusions and muscular strains are more common injuries in this region. Although these injuries are usually minor, they can cause considerable pain and disability if they are acute. Internal injuries, particularly to the solid organs, are also a concern with mechanisms of blunt trauma and most often involve the spleen and kidney. When a patient presents with a history of severe blunt trauma to the abdomen, you should highly suspect internal injury or hemorrhage. If internal hemorrhage results, the injury becomes life threatening if you do not immediately recognize it and manage it appropriately.

Solar Plexus Contusion

A direct blow to the abdomen over the solar (celiac) plexus can momentarily paralyze the diaphragm and impair breathing. This syndrome, often referred to as getting the wind knocked out of you, commonly results from abdominal impact. Signs and symptoms include abdominal pain, fear, anxiety, and difficulty breathing. The symptoms should dissipate quickly, and normal breathing should resume without the need for medical intervention or treatment.

Testicular Trauma

Testicular trauma or scrotal contusion, which is relatively common among physically active males, results from a direct blow to the external genitalia. This injury can cause considerable pain, spasm, ecchymosis, and swelling. The patient may also complain of nausea and may vomit or faint if pain is severe. Except with severe contusions, the symptoms are usually short-lived and are often relieved when you place the patient in supine and bring his knees toward his chest. The patient is typically able to return to activity after a few minutes.

A potential complication of testicular trauma is torsion of the spermatic cord, in which the trauma rotates the testicle in the scrotum. Signs and symptoms of testicular torsion include immediate or gradual onset of groin pain, heaviness in the scrotum, and change in the normal position or appearance of the testicle. This condition constitutes a medical emergency and requires immediate referral, as blood flow to the testicle is compromised.

Abdominal Muscle Strain

Strain of the abdominal muscles (rectus abdominis, internal and external obliques) can result from a violent muscle contraction or trunk twisting. Chronic or repetitive overuse can also cause muscular strain. Signs and symptoms include pain, muscle spasm, and palpable tenderness. Swelling and discoloration may or may not be present. In essentially all muscle strains, the patient complains of increased pain with muscle contraction or with passive stretching of the involved muscle.

Side Stitch

A side stitch or side ache is characterized by a sharp pain or spasm along the lateral abdominal wall, typically on the right side.

This transient pain occurs most often with intense running activities and more commonly early in the season. Although the exact cause is unknown, the side stitch is typically associated with muscle ischemia and poor conditioning but has also been attributed to intestinal gas or to consumption of a large meal just before activity. The pain often quickly subsides with reducing activity or with deep, steady breathing. Stretching away from the side of pain or raising the arm overhead also relieves symptoms. Once the pain dissipates, the patient is usually able to return to activity without further problems.

Hernia

A **hernia** is characterized by the protrusion of the small intestine through a weakened area in the anterior abdominal wall. The two most common sites of herniation are the femoral ring (figure 11.20a) and the inguinal region (figure 11.20b). Signs and symptoms consist of pain, tenderness, palpable mass, and discomfort with coughing or straining.

Kidney Contusion

In contact sports, kidney contusions can occur secondary to a severe blow to the lower back. The primary signs and symptoms of kidney trauma include deep aching in the lower back and flank region and possible muscle guarding. The pain may also wrap around anteriorly to the lower abdomen. Severe contusions can result in nausea, vomiting, and possible shock. Hematuria is a hallmark of kidney trauma but may not be visible to the naked eye and may require urinalysis for identification. Ask the patient to check the urine for a change in color. Remove players with a suspected kidney contusion from activity and refer them immediately to determine the extent of injury.

Splenic Rupture

Rupture of the spleen can be a rapidly progressive injury that, if not recognized early, can lead to internal hemorrhage and possible death. In fact, splenic rupture is the most common cause of death due to

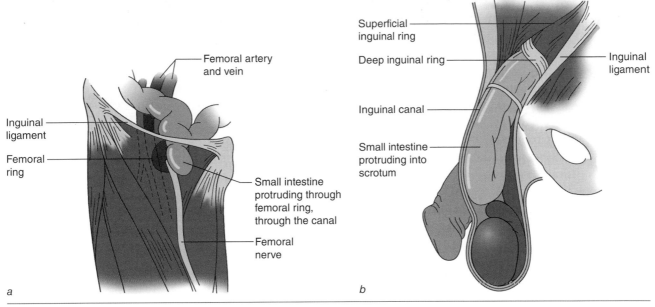

Figure 11.20 *(a)* Femoral hernia and *(b)* inguinal hernia.

abdominal trauma in sport. The spleen sits in the upper left quadrant and is most vulnerable to injury after a systemic illness, such as mononucleosis, that enlarges the organ. Injury to the spleen can result from a direct blow to the left upper abdominal quadrant or a hard fall. Patient complaints typically include left upper quadrant and flank pain, as well as nausea and vomiting. The patient may exhibit signs and symptoms of shock including wet (cold, clammy) skin; pale skin color; and weak, rapid pulse.

Summary

Your first responsibility when recognizing and examining thorax and abdominal pathology is to establish whether the patient is conscious and examine for airway, breathing, and circulation. A rapid, weak pulse indicates internal injury, shock, or both. Also note rhythm for evidence of arrhythmias, which may indicate a cardiac contusion or other cardiac trauma. In cases of abdominal trauma, the victim purposely limits respirations within the upper chest to avoid moving the abdominal region; this limited movement is one reason for rapid and shallow respirations. A blood pressure that falls below 100/60 may indicate shock or internal hemorrhage. Skin that becomes pale, cool, and clammy is an indication of shock and internal hemorrhage. This situation is a medical emergency and warrants immediate referral.

CASE STUDY

Case Study

You are the athletic trainer for your high school soccer team, and Becca is the starting goalkeeper. During the course of a game with your cross-town rival, players collide in front of the goal and Becca is struck on the abdomen. Becca remains down on the field, time is called, and you are summoned to evaluate Becca. When you arrive at her side she is conscious but in obvious pain. When you ask what happened, Becca states that she was kneed in the upper left portion of her abdomen and is in substantial pain. Further examination shows that Becca is not suffering from any other injury, and you are able to remove her from the competitive field with the help of some of her teammates. Sideline evaluation and questioning provide information that Becca has not been feeling well over the past week but did not want to miss the important game and did not report her symptoms, which included fatigue, sore throat, and general malaise. Approximately 5 min have passed since the injury, and Becca's pain has not subsided and in fact has gotten worse. Becca now complains of nausea, and her skin color has gone from flushed to pale. Vital sign examination elicits a weak but rapid pulse and abnormal respirations.

Think About It

1. What do you believe is wrong with Becca? What are your differential diagnoses? What is the worst-case scenario?

2. What history information may either confirm or disconfirm your suspicions?

3. What is the proper management for your suspected diagnosis?

Learning Aids

SUMMARY

Recognition of the causes of injuries to the head, spine, and thorax, as well as of the types of injuries and signs for referral, is critical, as these pathologies can be potentially catastrophic and even fatal. Although these are not among the most common injuries seen in an athletic patient population, understanding the pathology and being able to recognize it are imperative for proper management. Because of the organs and structures involved in injuries to these areas, vital sign examination and evaluation of sensory organs are important components of the assessment and management plans.

KEY CONCEPTS AND REVIEW

▶ **Put in plain words the risks of athletic participation with spinal stenosis.**

The narrowed spinal canal in spinal stenosis increases the risk for spinal cord compression and injuries resulting from hyperextension or hyperflexion mechanisms. When these factors are coupled with secondary complications such as cervical spine instability or disc herniation, the risk for spinal cord injury is further increased. Basically there is not enough room for the spinal cord within the vertebral columns, and normal activities that do not affect someone without spinal stenosis may create problems in someone who does have this condition.

▸ **Describe the pathology of spondylolysis and spondylolisthesis.**

Spondylolysis involves a fracture of the pars interarticularis located between the inferior and superior facets. It is typically thought to be a stress fracture secondary to a congenital weakening. Spondylolisthesis occurs when the fracture of the pars interarticularis in spondylolysis becomes unstable, and forward subluxation of the involved vertebrae occurs. Spondylolisthesis is frequently seen in gymnasts, weightlifters, and football lineman secondary to repetitive flexion and hyperextension associated with their sporting activities.

Signs and symptoms associated with spondylolysis and spondylolisthesis are centralized low back pain (possibly radiating into the buttocks and posterior thighs), swelling, muscle spasm, and a straightening of the lordotic curve. Patients with these conditions may exhibit decreased ROM and increased pain with hyperextension. Standing on only the leg of the affected side and extending the spine also increases pain.

▸ **List concussive signs and symptoms that require immediate referral.**

Unconsciousness or deteriorating levels of awareness

Evidence of lateralizing signs

Abnormal papillary reflexes

Deteriorating vital signs
- Slow and irregular respirations
- Decreased or bounding pulse
- Elevated blood pressure

▸ **Explain the differences between disc protrusion, extrusion, and sequestration.**

The main differences between disc protrusion, extrusion, and sequestration are the type and extent of nucleus pulposus disc material pressing against or through the outer fibrous ring of annulus fibrosis. Disc protrusion occurs when the annulus fibrosis becomes weakened and the nucleus pulposus presses against the weakened wall of the disc, causing a bulge or protrusion. Disc extrusion occurs when the nucleus pulposus is forced through the annulus fibrosis but is still continuous with the material still in the center of the disc. Disc sequestration is a disc extrusion in which the nucleus pulposus involved in the extrusion is separated completely from the rest of the disc material.

▸ **Detail the differences between pneumothorax and hemothorax.**

A pneumothorax occurs when air enters the pleural cavity located between the lung and the chest wall, thus reducing the volume of the lung. A pneumothorax can result from traumatic injury or can occur spontaneously in the absence of trauma. Signs and symptoms associated with a simple pneumothorax include upper chest pain, dyspnea (difficulty breathing) or shortness of breath, lightheadedness, and decreased breath sounds. Immediately refer patients with a suspected pneumothorax for emergency medical care.

A hemothorax occurs when blood, rather than air, fills the pleural space. Signs and symptoms of a hemothorax include lung collapse and reduced or absent breath sounds on the involved side, severe chest pain, dyspnea, cyanosis, hypotension, and the coughing up of frothy blood.

▸ **Outline signs and symptoms of splenic rupture.**

Patients with a ruptured spleen have complaints of left upper quadrant and flank pain, as well as nausea and vomiting. The patient may exhibit signs and symptoms of shock including wet (cold, clammy) skin; pale skin color; and weak, rapid pulse.

PRACTICE!

For hands-on practice in this area, go to the web resource and complete the following:

Level 2.9, Module J6: Thorax and Lumbar Spine Injury Assessment and Diagnosis

Level 2.9, Module J11: Cervical Spine Injury Assessment and Diagnosis

CRITICAL THINKING QUESTIONS

1. You are working as an athletic trainer at a high school football game, and an individual suffers a violent collision and complains of a head injury. You and your team physician have examined the patient and determined that he has suffered a concussion. He has been removed from the game and is sitting on the bench. During your periodic reexaminations you observe that he seems to be becoming more lethargic; he complains of worsening headache, has become nauseous, and has an elevated pulse rate and blood pressure. What pathology should you be concerned about, and what actions would you take?

2. A city employee makes an appointment to see you in your role as an athletic trainer for the town of Maple Grove. This employee complains of significant low back pain that is causing abnormal gait due to discomfort. In addition, she is having problems lifting her toes (dorsiflexion) during walking, which is causing exaggerated hip and knee flexion to swing the leg through. The affected foot lands loudly on the ground during ambulation. In your examination, you note decreased sensation on the dorsal aspect of the foot around the great toe. Discuss the potential pathology and the reasons for the gait abnormalities.

General Medical Conditions

Sandra J. Shultz, PhD, ATC, CSCS, FNATA
Kirk Brumels, PhD, AT, ATC

OBJECTIVES

After reading this chapter, the student should be able to do the following:

- List and briefly describe four general medical conditions that affect the heart.

- List and briefly describe general medical conditions of the respiratory system.

- Identify the two types of eating disorders presented and briefly explain each.

- Explain the female athlete triad.

- Describe the condition called rhabdomyolysis.

- List and briefly describe general medical conditions of the integumentary system.

- Differentiate infections that are viral from those that are bacterial.

- Explain the Epstein-Barr virus and identify the common disorder it often causes.

When caring for the physically active, you may encounter a variety of general medical conditions and disabilities that are not directly related to physical activity but that can affect performance or overall health. The terms "medical condition" and "condition" often refer to abnormalities or deviations within body systems, or specific body parts within a given system, that alter normal function.

Many general medical conditions are preexisting and do not preclude the patient from participation but may result in complications during activity. While patients with preexisting conditions typically understand their condition quite well and take precautionary measures to minimize the risk of complications, it is equally important for you to be aware of these conditions and to recognize signs and symptoms of complications. This chapter addresses general medical conditions that affect the body systems, as well as common ailments that affect the eyes, ears, nose, and throat (EENT).

Cardiovascular Conditions

Athletic trainers need to be familiar with a number of cardiovascular conditions. Some are congenital; some develop over time; and some are acute in nature. Whatever the cause, the athletic trainer needs to be aware of these conditions and be able to recognize them and assist in their management and care.

▶ Coronary Artery Disease

Coronary artery disease (CAD), also known as coronary heart disease, is a chronic cardiovascular condition characterized by hardening and narrowing (atherosclerosis) of the coronary arteries, the vessels supplying blood to the heart. It is the most common form of cardiovascular disease in the United States. Coronary artery disease can reduce blood flow to the heart (cardiac ischemia), during which time the patient may not experience any symptoms (silent ischemia). When symptoms are noted, they include varying degrees of pain (angina), pressure, or discomfort in the chest; shortness of breath; and arrhythmias. In cases of severe or prolonged ischemia, cardiac arrest or heart failure may occur.

▶ Heart Murmurs

Heart murmurs most often occur due to a defective heart valve (American Heart Association 2003). Valves may be stenotic, having an atypically small opening that prevents them from opening completely, while other valves may be unable to close completely. The latter condition leads to regurgitation, or the leaking of blood back through the valve when it should be closed. Murmurs present as an abnormal heart sound upon auscultation, such as a gentle blowing, fluttering, or humming sound. A murmur heard during heart contraction is termed a systolic murmur; diastolic murmurs occur between contractions. Continuous murmurs are heard throughout the cardiac cycle. When you note a murmur, refer the patient to a physician for a medical diagnosis to determine its source and any underlying cardiovascular condition.

▶ Hypertension

High blood pressure is the common term for hypertension, which involves an elevated systolic or diastolic blood pressure and is associated with generalized arteriolar vasoconstriction. Pressure consistently measuring over 140/90 mmHg at rest is considered high. Heredity can play a predisposing role in its onset.

▶ Hypertrophic Cardiomyopathy

Hypertrophic cardiomyopathy is a serious disease of the myocardium (heart muscle), resulting in enlarged muscle cells in the ventricular septum and left ventricular walls. The enlarged left ventricular wall has more stiffness than normal, causing blood to backflow into the atrium and lungs and reducing blood flow to the body.

▶ Hypotension

Hypotension is a subnormal (low) blood pressure. The most common type is orthostatic hypotension, in which the blood pressure drops when the person suddenly stands. Orthostatic hypotension is defined as a decrease of at least 20 mmHg in systolic blood pressure upon movement from a supine to standing position. It can be caused by cardiac pump failure, diminished blood volume available within the vascular system, venous pooling, medication, and **neurogenic** pathologies.

Migraine Headache

Migraines are recurring vascular headaches of sudden onset with associated gastrointestinal and visual disturbances. The exact cause is unknown, but it is believed that migraines may be related to allergies, stress, hormonal imbalance, toxins, or vasomotor disturbances. There is often a family history of migraines. Migraines are divided into the classic and common types:

- Classic migraine attacks are preceded by an aura that occurs 10 to 30 min earlier and produces neurological symptoms. Common symptoms of classic migraines are speech difficulty; tingling of the face or hands; weakness on one side of the body; and intense, throbbing pain that starts on one side of the head around the temple, forehead, eye, ear, and jaw and advances to the other side. Classic migraines last for 1 to 2 days, whereas common migraine symptoms last for 3 to 4 days.
- Common migraines, which are more prevalent, do not have an aura preceding onset. The standard symptom, photophobia, is often accompanied by other symptoms including throbbing around the eye, nausea, vomiting, mood changes, and severe headache.

Mitral Valve Prolapse

The mitral valve, a bicuspid (two-flap) valve that separates the left atrium from the left ventricle, allows blood to flow from the atrium to the ventricle during diastole and prevents backflow into the atrium with ventricular contraction. Due to congenital abnormalities, the mitral valve cusps collapse backward into the left atrium during heart function, allowing blood to leak backward through the valve.

Syncope

Syncope, or fainting, is a sudden, temporary loss of consciousness most commonly resulting from either a physiological or an emotional stress that causes a vasovagal reaction. Syncope most often occurs during standing or with sudden changes in position (sudden sitting or standing). Syncope can also result from reduced blood volume produced by heavy sweating, violent coughing spells that rapidly change blood pressure, heart or lung disorders, side effects of medications, seizures, or any condition that results in inadequate glucose or oxygen supply to the brain.

Respiratory Conditions

Respiratory conditions are common nonorthopedic conditions that affect patients while they prepare for or compete in athletic activities. The athletic trainer needs to be able to recognize these conditions, which range from respiratory difficulties due to various bacterial or viral infections to actual lung disease issues, and assist in their management. Recognizing signs and symptoms of concern and facilitating referral to the appropriate health care professional for further evaluation and treatment are critical in order for patients to continue competition with optimal respiratory function.

Upper Respiratory Conditions

An upper respiratory infection (URI) is any infection that affects any portion of the upper respiratory system (conducting pathway) including the tonsils, nose, throat, sinuses, and neck lymph nodes. Middle ear infections can also be associated with URIs. Upper respiratory infections can be viral or bacterial. The common cold, flu, sinusitis, laryngitis, pharyngitis, and tonsillitis are examples of these conditions.

Common Cold

Common colds are viral infections that affect the upper respiratory system and are sometimes referred to as rhinoviruses. The incubation time is short, 18 to 48 h, with the onset typically heralded by a scratchy throat, sneezing, nasal discharge, and general **malaise**. Fever can sometimes accompany a cold, especially in children. Congestion headache, reduced smell and taste sensations, nasal congestion, cough, and general achiness are frequent complaints. Symptoms usually run their course in 4 to 10 days, but additional factors such as sinusitis, bronchitis, or tonsillitis can extend their duration. Since a cold is caused by a virus, antibiotics are not recommended unless it is apparent that a bacterial infection accompanies the cold.

Influenza

Influenza, or flu, is a viral infection that affects the body in general and the upper respiratory system in particular. Highly contagious, it is spread by infected persons through coughing and sneezing. Symptoms include high fever, chills, general weakness, fatigue, body aches and pains, and inflammation of the upper respiratory system with moderate signs and symptoms of runny nose, sore throat, and dry cough. Mild cases last 2 to 3 days, whereas more severe cases last for 4 to 5 days with residual symptoms of weakness and fatigue persisting for up to a few weeks.

Bronchial and Lung Infections

Infections of the bronchioles and lungs are more serious than URIs. Although bronchitis can be caused by both infections and irritants, pneumonia is a serious lung infection that requires immediate medical referral and treatment.

Bronchitis

Inflammation of the bronchial tree, either acute or chronic, can result from an infection or a reaction to an irritating agent. Acute bronchitis is associated with a URI such as a common cold or other viral infection of the nasopharynx, throat, or upper bronchial tree. It may also be associated with a secondary bacterial infection. While acute bronchitis can affect children or adults, chronic bronchitis occurs commonly in adults and results from chronic diffuse obstructive pulmonary diseases such as emphysema or pulmonary fibrosis.

Pneumonia

Pneumonia is an infection of the alveolar spaces that is usually bacterial but can be viral. A URI frequently precedes pneumonia in a patient. Other factors that influence pneumonia onset in adults include alcoholism, malnutrition, debilitation (being bedridden), aspiration, coma, or bronchial tumor.

Other Respiratory Conditions

Not all respiratory conditions are infectious. Chronic and acute respiratory conditions can be caused or exacerbated by allergens in the environment or can be induced by exercise or stress. These include hay fever, asthma, and hyperventilation.

Hay Fever

Hay fever is an allergic rhinitis that occurs seasonally because of the patient's reaction to airborne pollens. Depending on the allergy, the individual may be most susceptible in the spring, summer, or fall. A profuse watery nasal discharge accompanies itching of the eyes, nose, and mouth. Sneezing is common, along with conjunctivitis, frontal headaches with increased sinus pressure, and irritated nasal mucous membranes.

Asthma

Asthma is a reactive airway disease characterized by paroxysms of dyspnea, coughing, and wheezing that has been seen in increasing frequency over the past few years. True asthma is usually triggered by an environmental irritant, allergen, medication, or exercise that causes a reactive narrowing of the trachea, bronchi, and bronchioles and is accompanied by an inflammatory component. The result is a widespread, reversible narrowing of the airways (bronchospasm).

Signs and symptoms resulting from an acute severe asthma attack include spasmodic coughing, chest pain and tightness, wheezing, high pulse rate, rapid and shallow respirations, retraction of the neck muscles on inhalation, restlessness and agitation, and possible fainting. When the symptoms of reactive airway disease occur only with exercise, the condition is typically referred to as exercise-induced asthma or EIA.

Hyperventilation

Hyperventilation is characterized by a breathing rate or depth exceeding that required to eliminate carbon dioxide (CO_2). Usually transient, it typically results from factors such as metabolic disturbances, panic, or fear and may occur in unconditioned patients during exercise. An individual who is hyperventilating breathes off too much CO_2, which results in respiratory alkalosis. This causes numbness or tingling around the mouth and in the hands and feet, as well as light-headedness. A sharp, stabbing chest pain is also a frequent complaint, causing patients to panic further because they think they may be having a heart attack. The best course of action is to simply calm and reassure the individual in an effort to restore normal respiration rate and depth.

Digestive Conditions

Digestive conditions commonly seen in patients can range from mildly annoying to time-loss pathologies. Some digestive conditions are temporary, often lasting from several hours to several days, whereas others can be chronic in nature with periods of increased symptoms and debilitation. Proper recognition and management are critical, as many digestive disorders affect the nutritional intake and absorption that are important for high-level physical activity.

Appendicitis

Inflammation of the appendix can occur in an individual of any age. You must be aware of signs and symptoms, since immediate referral to a physician is necessary to avoid dangerous and life-threatening situations. Appendicitis can be acute or chronic and is triggered by a bacterial infection lodged within the appendix. Immediate physician referral is necessary for either administration of antibiotic medication or surgical intervention.

Colitis

Inflammation of the colon typically occurs during the second through fourth decades of life as a result of certain food hypersensitivities, bacterial or viral infections, psychogenic disorders, or autoimmune processes. Onset can be sudden but most often is slow and insidious, beginning with bowel urgency, abdominal cramps, or bloody mucus in the stools before progressing to looser stools, frequent bowel movements, and severe cramps. Physician referral is recommended. Treatment often includes bed rest; fluid intake; change in diet; intravenous medication and supplements; medications such as anticholinergics (to reduce intestinal motility), antibacterial agents, and glucocorticoids; and stress management techniques.

Constipation

Constipation can result from a variety of factors, including poor hydration, stress, poor diet, medications, and neurogenic disorders. Constipation is frequently asymptomatic but can cause cramps and general abdominal discomfort. Prevention of constipation includes adequate hydration, dietary reduction in simple carbohydrates, an increase in complex carbohydrates and fresh fruits and vegetables, and a balanced diet.

Diarrhea

Diarrhea is characterized by loose, liquid, or frequent bowel movements. Diarrhea is usually short-term, but if it lasts for more than 2 weeks it is considered persistent or chronic. It is a symptom of many conditions, including ulcerative colitis, parasitic infections, bacterial infections, diverticulitis, irritable bowel syndrome, malabsorption syndrome, and gastroenteritis. Diarrhea can also be caused by medication reactions, food additives such as sorbitol or fructose, food allergies, travel with exposure to contaminated water or food, excessive use of laxatives, or stress and anxiety.

Esophageal Reflux

Esophageal reflux occurs when the esophageal sphincter between the esophagus and stomach does not close completely. Acid from the stomach can enter the esophagus and cause what is commonly termed heartburn. The condition is aggravated when the patient is recumbent, so patients should be encouraged to sleep in a semirecumbent position.

Gastritis

Gastritis is an acute or chronic condition in which the mucous membrane of the stomach becomes irritated or inflamed. Acute gastritis can result from ingestion of abrasive substances such as alcohol, salicylates (e.g., aspirin), antibiotics, sulfur products, excessively acidic or spicy food, or allergenic foods. Acute gastritis is usually of short duration, subsiding within 24 to 48 h, and presents with symptoms of nausea, vomiting, headache, vertigo, sensation of fullness, malaise, and possible fever. Treatment includes abstaining from solid foods and ingesting only clear liquids.

Gastroenteritis

Gastroenteritis is an inflammation of the stomach and intestine mucous membrane—acute conditions that people commonly refer to as food poisoning. The cause is ingestion of virus or bacteria or excessive intake of irritating substances such as alcohol, salicylates, cathartics, or heavy metals. The severity of the symptoms directly relates to the nature and dose of the irritant ingested. The person experiences a sudden onset of nausea, as well as vomiting, malaise, abdominal cramps, and diarrhea. A fever usually occurs if the condition is infection based.

Indigestion

Indigestion is a nonspecific term that refers to either improper digestion or deficient absorption of food in the digestive tract. Also known as digestive upset, or dyspepsia, it can result from irregular eating, ingestion of foods to which the person is unaccustomed or allergic, and anxiety or stress.

Irritable Bowel Syndrome

Irritable bowel syndrome is a noninflammatory, nonserious disorder that affects the large bowel. The accompanying symptoms reflect the failure of the large bowel to function smoothly. The cause is unknown, but the syndrome occurs more often in women than in men; symptoms are seen more often during menstruation and times of stress and are aggravated with ingestion of fats, chocolate, milk products, alcohol, and caffeine. A significant number of people with irritable bowel syndrome demonstrate depression, anxiety, or other psychological problems. Symptoms include abdominal cramps with painful constipation or diarrhea.

Ulcers

Ulcers involve a more severe form of gastritis and include an erosion of the mucous membrane of the stomach, duodenum, or lower esophagus. Ulcers can take the form of duodenal or gastric ulcers and are also referred to as peptic ulcer disease. They are thought to be caused primarily by bacteria. Physician referral for antibiotic medication, accompanied by medication to reduce stomach acid, is the usual approach to treatment.

Eating Disorders

Abnormal eating habits can affect physical and athletic performance due to poor nutritional absorption, storage, and use. Disordered eating patterns such as anorexia nervosa and bulimia can be life threatening. Due to the combination of physical and psychological components of eating disorders, a multifaceted approach to management often proves to be most effective.

Anorexia Nervosa

Anorexia is a severe psychological disorder characterized by a self-induced food aversion and extreme weight loss. Although the condition can affect males, females are 10 times more often affected and usually experience amenorrhea as a side effect. Anorexia typically begins either in the preteen years or early in the teen years but may not manifest until the 30s or 40s.

Anorexia may appear initially as normal dieting and concern about weight loss but then becomes an obsession to be thin. Patients with anorexia do not see themselves as thin even when their appearance is emaciated and they are grossly underweight. Food and caloric intake and expenditure become their central focus; they often limit food intake to 300 to 600 calories daily. Signs and symptoms include weight loss greater than 25% of body weight, behavior directed toward weight loss, peculiar patterns of handling food, intense fear of gaining weight, disturbances in body image, and amenorrhea in women.

Bulimia Nervosa

Patients who have bulimia are of normal weight but use techniques such as vomiting and ingestion of diuretics and laxatives to prevent weight gain. Patients suffering from bulimia tend to be slightly older than those with anorexia. Like people with anorexia, they have an exaggerated fear of getting fat; but they do not attempt to lose weight, only to maintain it. Episodes of uncontrolled binge eating followed by vomiting are frequent. Patients with bulimia are often outgoing perfectionists who enjoy pleasing others. Because of frequent vomiting episodes, symptoms such as enlarged salivary glands around the throat become evident, and tooth enamel is dissolved by stomach acids. Calluses on the knuckles and sores at the corners of the mouth may also be present. Irregular heart rate, muscle weakness, kidney damage, and epileptic seizures are additional symptoms that can result from frequent vomiting and electrolyte disturbances. Because outward signs are minimal and subtle, bulimia is more difficult to detect than anorexia. However, at times these conditions are found in tandem, and weight loss is evident (bulimarexia).

Obesity

Although prevalent in the general population, obesity is not normally seen in the athletic population. Weight over 40% to 50% of the desired weight is considered morbidly obese and can be life threatening.

Reproductive and Genitourinary Conditions

Conditions that affect the reproductive and genitourinary systems in athletic patients can originate from both nonathletic and athletic events. While some conditions occur in athletes and nonathletes alike, others are caused directly by competition in athletics. Recognition, education, and confidentiality are very important in treating these conditions properly.

Kidney Stones

Kidney stones is the common term for urinary calculi. Found anywhere in the urinary system, including the kidney, ureter, bladder, or urethra, kidney stones are composed of precipitated urinary salts. If a stone moves from the kidney and obstructs the ureter, severe renal colic ensues as the smooth muscle of the ureter forcefully contracts to relieve the obstruction. The pain, which is extreme, may start in the back or the flank and radiate across the abdomen into the groin, genitalia, and inner thigh. Small stones eventually pass through the ureter and are discharged. Larger stones may require surgical intervention to relieve the obstruction.

Urethritis

Urethritis, or inflammation of the urethra, is also known as a urinary tract infection (UTI) that is isolated to the urethra. This type of infection occurs more frequently in women than in men and is a poorly understood phenomenon. Symptoms, although not always present, may include urinary frequency and urgency, painful or burning urination, cloudy or even reddish urine if **hematuria** is present, general malaise, and lower abdominal pain. Antibacterial medications usually resolve the problem within a couple of days, but antibiotics are taken for up to 2 weeks to ensure a cure.

Urinary Tract Infection

As just discussed, urethritis is a form of UTI. A UTI also occurs if the bacterial infection spreads to other segments of the urinary system. In advanced cases, the infection spreads to the bladder and ureter. When kidneys are affected, symptoms of urethritis as well as other symptoms such as back pain, fever, nausea, and vomiting can be present.

Spermatic Cord Torsion

Spermatic cord torsion, or testicular torsion, occurs when the testicle twists on the spermatic cord, leading to venous occlusion and engorgement followed by arterial ischemia and possible testicular infarction (figure 12.1). Occurrence can either be traumatic or based on predisposing factors. This condition constitutes a medical emergency and requires immediate referral, as blood flow to the testicle is compromised.

Epididymitis

Epididymitis is an inflammation of the epididymis, one of a pair of ducts that carry sperm from the seminiferous tubule of the testicles to the vas deferens. Epididymitis can result from UTI, venereal disease, tuberculo-sis, mumps, or inflammation of the prostate gland or urethra.

Hydrocele

A hydrocele is an accumulation of fluid around the testicle. Hydroceles are most common at birth and usually resolve without assistance by 18 months of age with the closure of the processus vaginalis. Adult hydroceles result from direct trauma, infections, or radiotherapy. There is commonly no pain. Physician referral is necessary with any changes in the size, shape, or consistency of the testicle.

Varicocele

A varicocele is an enlargement of the internal spermatic veins that develops because of defective valves in the veins, allowing backflow into the testicle (figure 12.2). This can result in sterility. Pain or a significant size difference in the testicles is an indication for surgical repair. Surgery is usually successful, and sperm count is restored in up to 70% of patients.

Testicular Cancer

Testicular cancer is a highly treatable and curable cancer that occurs predominantly in males 20 to 35 years of age. While trauma is not considered a cause of testicular cancer, the tumor may be first detected during an injury examination, as a lump on the testicle is commonly the first sign.

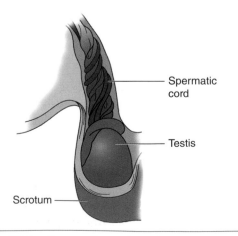

Figure 12.1　Spermatic cord torsion.

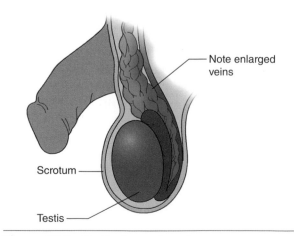

Figure 12.2　Testicular varicocele.

Gynecological Conditions

Gynecological conditions can occur in female athletic patients due to normal life stage issues or as a result of excessive or intense exercise. Menstrual dysfunctions, painful menses, and vaginal infections, for example, are conditions that can cause discomfort and affect athletic performance. Proper recognition, management, education, counseling, and confidentiality are important aspects of care for these patients.

Menstrual Dysfunction

Female patients may complain of a variety of menstrual dysfunctions, including pain, menstrual irregularity, and loss of menses.

Amenorrhea

Amenorrhea is the absence of a menstrual cycle. The three types of amenorrhea are primary, secondary, and irregular. Primary amenorrhea is present when menstruation has not started by age 16. Secondary amenorrhea occurs when menstruation stops in a woman who has previously menstruated. Factors that can produce secondary amenorrhea include pregnancy, menopause, stress, weight change, breast-feeding, anemia, excessive exercise, ovarian cysts, and medications. The incidence of osteoporosis (bone loss) and of stress fractures is higher in amenorrheic women than in others. Physician referral is necessary to determine the cause of amenorrhea and appropriate treatment.

Female Athlete Triad

The female athlete triad is considered a serious yet preventable syndrome composed of three interrelated conditions: disordered eating, amenorrhea, and osteoporosis. While each component of the triad represents a medical problem in itself, experts agree that the combination of the three conditions can significantly affect the health of the young female patient.

Oligomenorrhea

Oligomenorrhea is defined as an irregular menses, characterized by infrequent or light periods or both. Causes can include rapid weight loss, anorexia or bulimia, high levels of or significant changes in exercise, and some medications and illicit drug use. Refer the patient to a physician, who will determine the cause of the oligomenorrhea before selecting the most appropriate treatment.

Dysmenorrhea

Dysmenorrhea, also known as menstrual cramps, includes pain during menstruation that is severe enough to interfere with normal activity. Additional symptoms can include nausea, vomiting, and severe abdominal pain. Over-the-counter analgesics and anti-inflammatories may adequately relieve pain. Hot baths and massage may also encourage muscle relaxation and increase circulation.

Pregnancy and Exercise Considerations

Occasionally you may encounter and work with a physically active female who is pregnant. The following sections discuss the physiological changes that occur with pregnancy and some precautions you should be aware of with the physically active female. Pregnancy does not preclude physical activity; but pregnant patients should follow certain precautions, and their physician should always closely monitor them. Once you are aware that a patient is pregnant, consult a physician before letting her embark on an exercise program. Exercise levels will depend on the patient's overall health, current physical conditioning, exercise goals, and exercise tolerance. Generally, women who have achieved a level of fitness prior to pregnancy should be able to maintain that level throughout pregnancy. However, as physiological changes occur, they may need to modify the types of activities they engage in.

Pelvic Conditions

Pain or symptoms in the pelvic and vaginal regions are usually caused by yeast and bacterial infections. These conditions include vaginitis, candidiasis, and pelvic inflammatory disease.

Vaginitis

Vaginitis is the medical term for vaginal infections. Of the number of organisms that can cause vaginitis, the most common are bacteria, yeast, and parasites. Untreated conditions can lead to pelvic inflammatory disease, endometritis, cervicitis, and other obstetric complications. Treatment includes antibiotic medication.

Candidiasis

Candidiasis, or yeast infection, is actually caused by a fungus. Small numbers of this fungus are present normally in the vagina, but when the number increases, symptoms can occur. Causes include tight clothing; warm weather; stress; diabetes; pregnancy; obesity; and medications such as antibiotics, steroids, and birth control pills. Symptoms can include pain during sex, vaginal itching and burning, and a curd-like white discharge. Treatment includes over-the-counter antifungal medication inserted as vaginal suppositories, creams, or tablets.

Pelvic Inflammatory Disease

Pelvic inflammatory disease (PID), also called salpingitis, is a serious complication of sexually transmitted diseases. It is a bacterial infection that attacks the female reproductive system, spreading from the vagina to the womb, fallopian tubes, and ovaries. It occurs as a result of an untreated bacterial infection of the vagina. Gonorrhea is a common preceding infection. Symptoms may not always be present but may include painful stomach cramps, bleeding, fever, chills, an upset stomach, and an odorous discharge. If left untreated, the condition can lead to sterility and is in fact the major cause of sterility in young women.

Breast Conditions

It is not uncommon for the breasts to feel tender before menstruation. Normal changes in the breast affect both breasts simultaneously and symmetrically. However, there may be times that a patient comes to you out of concern about changes in the appearance or feel of the tissue in one of the breasts. In the majority of these cases the changes are benign, but they should be examined and malignancy (cancer) ruled out.

Benign Conditions

Benign (noncancerous) conditions can be caused by **fibrocystic changes** and **fibroadenomas**. Because it is often difficult to differentiate between benign and malignant changes in breast tissue without diagnostic tests, refer all patients (whether male or female) who note breast tissue changes to a physician for proper diagnosis.

Cancer

Breast changes such as lumps, dimpling, or puckering of the skin and thickening or swelling that do not go away may be warning signs of breast cancer, warranting immediate referral to a physician for examination. Other signs and symptoms to be concerned about include skin irritation, distortion, retraction, scaliness, and changes or tenderness in or secretion from the nipple. While breast cancer cannot be prevented, it can be effectively treated and cured if recognized early. Educating your patients and encouraging breast self-examination in women 20 years and older may ultimately save a life.

Sexually Transmitted Diseases and Diseases Transmitted by Body Fluid

Various diseases that are prevalent in society are transmitted through sexual contact or other transfer of bodily fluids. These diseases can be transferred from one individual through the exchange of seminal or vaginal fluid, oral or fecal contact, or blood contact. Many of these diseases can be prevented with proper precautions such as abstinence or protected sex, proper wound care, and appropriate food preparation. Although these conditions may involve dangers of transmission to other patients, confidentiality and education are of utmost importance.

Human Immunodeficiency Virus and Acquired Immunodeficiency Syndrome

The human immunodeficiency virus (HIV) weakens the immune system by destroying lymphocytes (T-cells), impairing the body's ability to defend itself against potentially deadly infections and malignancies. Human immunodeficiency virus advances through a progression of stages, beginning with transient infections, continuing to complex diseases related to acquired immunodeficiency syndrome (AIDS), and ending in AIDS itself. Approximately 70% of those infected with HIV develop AIDS within 10 years. Acquired immunodeficiency syndrome is actually a collection of life-threatening diseases that occur as the patient's immune system becomes progressively weaker and less resistant to infection and malignancies.

Hepatitis

Hepatitis is an inflammation of the liver caused by either infectious or toxic substances. It is one of the most frequently reported infectious diseases in the United States, surpassed only by gonorrhea and chicken pox. The five known types of hepatitis are A, B, C, D, and E. They are defined by the manner of transmission and the length of time the patient can remain a carrier. Hepatitis A and E are communicated through fecal–oral transmission following food handling without proper hand washing and can evolve into epidemic situations. Hepatitis B, C, and D are transmitted through blood, semen, and other bodily fluids. Refer patients suspected of having hepatitis to a physician. Care of patients with hepatitis requires using sterile technique with open wounds and properly disposing of contaminated items.

Chlamydia

Chlamydia is the most common bacterial sexually transmitted disease in the United States. Teenage girls and young women under the age of 25 have the highest incidence rate. Signs and symptoms include painful urination (dysuria) and a pus discharge in males and vaginal discharge, pelvic pain, and dys-

uria in females. Antibiotic therapy under the guidance of a physician is the standard of care for those infected with the disease.

Genital Warts

Genital warts, or condylomata acuminata, are located in the perineum and perianal region. They are caused by the human papilloma virus (HPV). Genital warts are contracted through sexual contact, and the patient typically has a history of unprotected sexual contact with an infected person or with multiple partners.

Gonorrhea

Gonorrhea is a bacterial infection, and the infection rate is climbing rapidly. Females aged 15 to 19 have the highest rate of gonorrhea. Sexual intercourse is the chief means of transmission.

Syphilis

Syphilis is an acute venereal bacterial condition. The syphilis bacterium is transmitted during vaginal, rectal, or oral sex; it can also be transmitted through open wounds or through direct contact with bodily fluids or blood. If symptoms occur, they are usually seen as genital or anal lesions in the form of a **chancre** that starts as a papule and then ulcerates. Although prevention and education are viewed as effective approaches to eliminating the disease, antibiotic therapy is the standard treatment for patients who have contracted syphilis. One dose of penicillin usually cures syphilis.

Endocrine Conditions

Endocrine complications can occur in patients, and good disease management involves a multimember approach. Athletic trainers must be aware of these conditions and may be called upon to be an active participant in treatment protocols. Many endocrine disorder conditions require daily medication and continual monitoring but do not often prevent an individual from participating in competition or exercise.

Diabetes Mellitus

Diabetes mellitus is an autoimmune disorder that causes a deficiency in glucose metabolism. Insulin, a peptide hormone responsible for glucose utilization, is either not secreted or is prevented from being used in the body. Diabetes mellitus occurs as one of two types: insulin-dependent diabetes mellitus (IDDM), or type 1 diabetes, and non-insulin-dependent diabetes mellitus (NIDDM), or type 2 diabetes. IDDM usually occurs in nonobese children and adults, whereas NIDDM most often occurs in obese adults and children. IDDM results from insufficient insulin production in the pancreas. Patients with NIDDM have an insulin-producing pancreas, but their body's sensitivity to the insulin hormone is significantly diminished.

Glycemic Reactions

If a patient with diabetes has too much insulin in the body, the blood glucose levels drop below normal and a hypoglycemic reaction occurs. If the insulin level is too low, glucose levels are elevated above normal levels and the body becomes hyperglycemic. You must be aware of the differences in the signs and symptoms between these two conditions, since the treatments are opposite (table 12.1).

• *Hypoglycemia (insulin shock).* Hypoglycemia, or insulin shock, can be life threat-

ening. The symptoms, which are nonspecific, include sweating, trembling, fatigue and weakness, light-headedness, irritability, headache, intoxicated behavior, apprehension, mental confusion, and—in advanced stages—convulsions and coma. Memory loss, lack of coordination, and slurred speech may also be noted. If the patient in insulin shock is unable to swallow, do not attempt to force liquids or foods; instead, arrange for immediate transportation to an emergency care facility for intravenous glucose administration to avoid possible brain damage or death. Since activity lowers blood glucose levels, you should closely monitor individuals with diabetes during times of unexpected increased activity and during early-season workouts when diet, insulin, and activity balances may not yet be established.

• *Hyperglycemia (diabetic coma).* In its advanced stages, hyperglycemia is referred to as hyperglycemic shock, or diabetic coma. This condition develops over a period of days as the patient's blood glucose levels rise. Failure to take insulin, severe illness or infection, physical or emotional stress, or poor dietary control can disrupt glucose levels and lead to this condition.

If you are unsure whether the patient suffers from hypoglycemia versus hyperglycemia, administer sugar. If the patient does

Table 12.1 Comparison of Hypoglycemia and Hyperglycemia

Signs and symptoms	Hypoglycemia	Hyperglycemia
Onset	Rapid onset, occurring within minutes	Slow onset, occurring over hours and even days
Neurological changes	Irritability, mental confusion, dizziness, bizarre behavior, slurred speech, memory loss, headache, dilated pupils; in severe cases, seizures and coma	Lethargy, mental confusion, listlessness
Skin	Cold, clammy; profuse sweating	Warm and dry
Muscular changes	Weakness, fatigue, muscle tremors, incoordination, ataxic gait	Weakness and fatigue
Cardiorespiratory changes	Weak, rapid pulse; no breath odor	Rapid pulse (tachycardia); deep, rapid breathing (Kussmaul respirations); characteristic odor of acetones on breath
Genitourinary and gastrointestinal changes	None	Nausea and vomiting; excessive urination, thirst, or eating

not start to respond within 2 or 3 min after receiving sugar, candy, or sweetened beverages, you should suspect hyperglycemia.

Hyperthyroidism

Hyperthyroidism can develop during times of emotional or physical stress. It is an autoimmune condition in which an excessive amount of thyroid hormone is present in the body. This increases the body's metabolic activity and causes weight loss regardless of increased food intake. With an increase in metabolic activity comes a concomitant increase in body temperature, so the patient does not tolerate hot environments, suffers from excessive sweating, and must significantly increase fluid intake. Increased sympathetic activity results in an increased heart rate, tremors, and protruding eyeballs. Treatment is ablation of the thyroid tissue with surgery or radiation, or control of thyroid levels with medication.

Hypothyroidism

Hypothyroidism may result from an iodine deficiency but can also occur following radiation exposure or from hypothalamic or pituitary damage. Many of the symptoms are the opposite of those seen with hyperthyroidism. Since thyroid hormones regulate the rate at which the body uses calories for energy expenditure, hypothyroidism reduces body metabolism and causes weight gain even without any change in caloric intake. Additional effects are loss of appetite, intolerance to cold, decreased sweating, reduced heart rate, constipation, coarse and dry hair, premature graying in young adults, thick and dry skin, swollen eyelids, numbness and tingling in the hands, lethargy, slowness of movement, and sleepiness. Hypothyroidism is treated with regular administration of synthetic thyroid hormone medication to deliver normal thyroxin levels throughout the body.

Pancreatitis

Pancreatitis, an inflammation of the pancreas, can be either acute or chronic. The most common cause is a partial obstruction of the pancreatic duct because of a penetrating duodenal ulcer, edema following surgery or abdominal trauma, peritonitis, or systemic disease. Symptoms include nausea, vomiting, and severe pain that can be cramping and dull or poorly defined. Refer people with suspected pancreatitis to the physician for diagnosis and treatment with antibiotics, analgesics, or surgery.

Musculoskeletal Conditions

Muscle, bone, and joint disorders can be very disabling to the physically active. As athletic trainers increasingly care for physically active adults and mature adults, they more frequently encounter general complaints of muscle and joint pain. While joint-specific pathologies are discussed in separate chapters of this text, the following sections deal with more generalized muscle, bone, and joint disorders.

Arthritis

Arthritis is a disease characterized by pain and inflammation of one or more joints. Arthritis occurs when these conditions result in long-term pain, inflammation, and joint deformity. Other signs and symptoms include early morning stiffness, increased warmth around the affected joint, and reduced joint mobility. Patients suffering from arthritic symptoms should consult their physician before beginning or continuing their exercise program.

Osteoarthritis

Osteoarthritis is characterized by degeneration of the cartilaginous surface of the joint, which results in joint pain, stiffness, swelling, and decreased range of motion. Osteoarthritis can result from genetic predisposition, injury that disrupts the cartilaginous surface or joint mechanics, overuse, and obesity. The joints most often affected include those in the cervical and lumbar regions, fingers, hips, knees, and great toes. Treatment includes activity modification; anti-inflammatory medications; weight loss; and with severe degeneration, joint replacement.

Gout

Increased levels of uric acid in the blood (uricemia) can lead to gout, an acute arthritis marked by joint inflammation due to the deposition of urate crystals in the joints. Gout can affect any joint but is most common in the great toe, foot, and knee. Pain and swelling of the joint accompanied by chills and fever are the hallmarks of gout. You may also note hypertension and back pain. Symptoms are recurrent and more prolonged with subsequent episodes. Treatment for gout attacks typically includes non-steroidal anti-inflammatory drugs (NSAIDs) and may include corticosteroid drugs for severe attacks.

Fibromyalgia

Fibromyalgia (fibrositis) is a chronic myofascial disorder characterized by chronic musculoskeletal pain, fatigue, and localized tenderness. Pain is most often experienced around the neck, shoulders, upper back, elbows, and lower back. The cause of the condition is unknown. The presence of fibromyalgia is determined by exclusionary diagnosis–based negative blood tests, X rays, and prolonged muscular tenderness for 3 months or more. There is no known cure for fibromyalgia at this time.

Rhabdomyolysis

Rhabdomyolysis is an acute, sometimes fatal disease caused by severe destruction of skeletal muscle that results in injury to the kidney. Any time skeletal muscle is damaged, myoglobin is released into the bloodstream, which is ultimately filtered by the kidneys. When severe skeletal damage releases extremely large amounts of myoglobin, kidney failure may occur when the myoglobin occludes the kidney structures or breaks down, releasing metabolic by-products that can be toxic to the kidneys. Severe skeletal muscle damage may also cause fluid to shift from the bloodstream into the muscle, leading to hypovolemic shock and reduced blood flow to the kidneys, creating a medical emergency.

Neurological Conditions

Neurological disorders represent a wide range of conditions of varying etiologies that ultimately affect some aspect of the nervous system. As with musculoskeletal injuries, the neurological conditions discussed here can be either acute or chronic in nature. However, due to the structure and function of the nervous system, any nervous system condition has the potential to be extremely debilitating, disabling, or both.

Tetanus

Tetanus is commonly called lockjaw. Caused by the tetanus bacillus, it enters the body through an open wound that has been in contact with dirt or soil. The bacillus attaches to the local nerve, moves to the spinal cord, and becomes anchored to the motor nerves. It prevents normal synaptic inhibition so that a tetanic contraction of the muscles occurs. Most commonly, it produces stiffness of the jaw and neck, with stiffness of the extremities occurring less often.

Epilepsy

Epilepsy is a chronic condition characterized by recurring seizures. Seizures are a spontaneous and involuntary neurological aberration caused by unregulated and abnormal electrical brain activity; they can last from a few seconds to a few minutes. The many causes of epilepsy include head trauma, infectious diseases, metabolic disorders, tumors, congenital abnormalities, and drugs.

Seizures are classified as partial, or focal, and generalized. Partial or focal seizures affect only certain parts of the brain and usually involve only one part of the body, such as the face or arm, in a **tonic–clonic** activity. Generalized seizures are of various types, but the most common are petit mal and grand mal seizures. Petit mal seizures are brief episodes of consciousness impairment that occur in childhood and are usually outgrown by the age of 20. A grand mal seizure, also called a tonic–clonic seizure, occurs with a sudden loss of consciousness; the person falls to the ground as the body's muscles enter a state of total tonic contraction.

Reflex Sympathetic Dystrophy

Reflex sympathetic dystrophy (RSD) is a multisystem, multisymptom disorder. Its effect on the sympathetic nervous system results in a multitude of symptoms and problems. It usually follows an injury and most frequently affects the hand in upper extremity injuries or the foot in lower extremity injuries. The etiology is unknown. The primary symptom of RSD is severe, constant pain, usually a burning sensation that occurs in the involved extremity, especially distally. It is accompanied by pitting or nonpitting edema, bluish skin, coolness of the distal extremity, and reduced motor function.

Meningitis

Meningitis is an infection of the cerebral spinal fluid that can be either bacterial or viral. It is sometimes referred to as spinal meningitis. Bacterial meningitis is usually more severe and can result in brain damage, hearing loss, or death. Viral meningitis is rarely as serious, with recovery occurring in about 7 to 10 days. Establishing whether the cause of meningitis is bacterial or viral is crucial to effective treatment.

Symptoms are similar for all meningitis and occur over several hours to a couple of days. They include headache, stiff neck, and high fever. Nausea, vomiting, confusion, photophobia, and drowsiness can also occur.

Integumentary Conditions

Skin conditions can arise from various sources such as bacteria, fungi, viruses, parasites, and other external agents like chemicals and poisons. Many of these conditions can be treated with over-the-counter medications, but some need referral to physicians for prescription medication. Concern for the individual patient with a skin infection is warranted, but concern must also be given to others if the condition has contagious properties. The best approach for many skin conditions is prevention through cleanliness, personal hygiene, and hand washing.

Bacterial Infections

Bacterial infections are typically of staphylococcal origin and are usually characterized by pustules. In many cases the site of bacterial infections is in hair follicles.

Abscess

An abscess, which can occur in many different sites and can be either acute or chronic, is a localized bacterial infection that appears as a collection of pus. Common signs and symptoms include local tissue destruction and edema. Acute abscesses usually present as a localized area of pain and increased warmth, demonstrating typical signs of inflammation.

Acne Vulgaris

Although acne vulgaris is commonly seen in adolescents, it can also occur as an adult-onset condition. It is the result of a hereditary disorder of the hair follicles and oil glands that causes blackheads, cysts, and pustules of varying depths on the face, neck, chest, shoulders, and back.

Carbuncle

A carbuncle is a painful, localized staphylococcus-based infection that affects the skin and subcutaneous tissue. Carbuncles occur most frequently in men and are commonly located on the back of the neck. Signs include fever, a pus-filled lesion, and local pain. Refer carbuncles to a dermatologist, who can debride the area and prescribe antibiotics.

Cellulitis

Cellulitis is an inflammation of soft or connective tissue. It usually involves skin and subcutaneous tissue and has a tendency to spread. Any infecting organism can cause cellulitis, but the most frequent cause is streptococci or staphylococci bacteria that affect an area of reduced resistance following injury or other trauma. Cellulitis is characterized by a general redness of the skin, swelling, pain, and warmth that vary directly in proportion to the severity of the condition. Cellulitis requires physician referral so that proper antibiotic therapy can be instituted.

Folliculitis

Folliculitis, usually staphylococcal in origin, is an inflammation of the hair follicle. The inflammatory site becomes a pustule and displays signs of inflammation: redness, localized swelling, and tenderness (figure 12.3). The treatment is to dry the pustule with astringents or other agents used with acne vulgaris, or even oral antibiotics when the folliculitis is prominent.

Furuncle and Furunculosis

The common name for a furuncle is a boil—a localized infection of a hair follicle (figure 12.4). The common source of infection is staphylococcus bacteria, and a boil is most often found on the neck, axillae, face, buttocks, and breasts. The local area is red, edematous, and tender. Since staphylococcal infections are highly contagious, the patient must refrain from sport participation until the infection has healed. Should the boil rupture, the infection can spread to surrounding tissues. Treatment includes moist hot packs and 10% topical benzoyl peroxide; the physician may order oral antibiotics.

Impetigo

Impetigo, a contagious bacterial infection caused by either staphylococci or streptococci, is highly contagious in young children. It begins as pustules that go on to rupture and crust over (figure 12.5). These most commonly occur on the face and head but can spread to other areas. Treatment includes referral to a physician for antibiotic medication.

Viral Infections

Some integumentary conditions have a virus as their source. It is important that proper

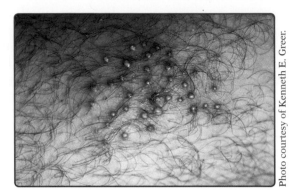

Photo courtesy of Kenneth E. Greer.

Figure 12.3 Folliculitis.

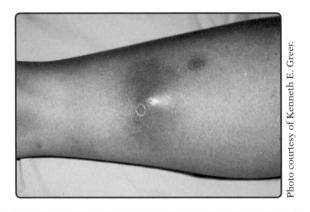

Photo courtesy of Kenneth E. Greer.

Figure 12.4 Furuncle (boil).

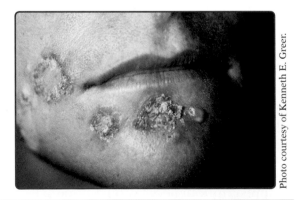

Photo courtesy of Kenneth E. Greer.

Figure 12.5 Impetigo.

identification and recognition occur quickly in these conditions to facilitate treatment and limit the incidence of transfer to other parts of the body and other individuals.

Molluscum Contagiosum

Molluscum contagiosum, a viral contagious infection of the skin, is characterized by small, round, flesh-colored papular lesions that occur most commonly on the face, trunk, axilla, perineum, and thigh (figure 12.6). You may see many or only a few papules. Participants in contact sports frequently transmit this disease. Physician referral is necessary for treatment with prescribed medications.

Herpes Simplex

Herpes simplex infections are contagious viral infections caused by herpes virus I and II. They are characterized by an eruption of groups of vesicles (figure 12.7) and have a tendency to reactivate and reappear with stress or fever. Herpes virus I that occurs on the lips or around the nose is also called a fever blister or cold sore. Herpes virus II occurs on the genitalia.

Herpes Zoster

Herpes zoster is associated with two diseases; one occurs in childhood and the other in adulthood. The childhood version is known as chicken pox (varicella) and the adulthood version as shingles (zoster). Physician referral is recommended; however, there is no known treatment for herpes zoster. Symptomatic relief can occur with application of topical lotions or powders. Analgesics can relieve pain.

Verruca Plantaris

Verruca plantaris is commonly referred to as a plantar wart (figure 12.8). Caused by a virus, it results in hypertrophy and thickening of the epidermis layers. It occurs on the bottom of the foot and is flattened because of the pressure of bearing weight. The thickening can cause pressure and discomfort.

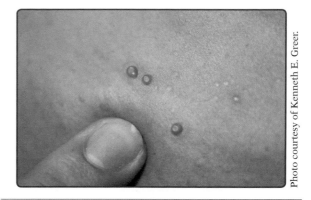

Photo courtesy of Kenneth E. Greer.

Figure 12.6   Molluscum contagiosum.

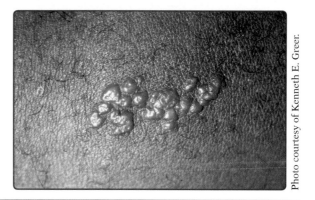

Photo courtesy of Kenneth E. Greer.

Figure 12.7   Herpes simplex I.

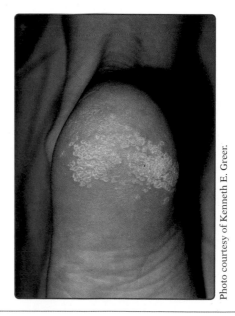

Photo courtesy of Kenneth E. Greer.

Figure 12.8   Verruca plantaris (plantar wart).

Verruca Vulgaris

Verruca vulgaris is a common wart caused by a papilloma virus (figure 12.9). These warts occur in areas of frequent trauma or infection such as the hands, elbows, knees, face, and scalp.

Fungal Infections

Fungal infections are common among sport participants. Most fungal infections are referred to as tinea or ringworm infections. The specific names of most fungal infections reflect their location on the body.

Ringworm

Although ringworm is one of many fungal diseases of the skin (tinea infection), the term is commonly used for a fungus that affects the scalp, trunk, and upper extremities. It is also known as tinea corporis. The lesion is a well-defined ringed eruption that has red or brown plaques with a raised border and may itch or burn (figure 12.10).

Tinea Capitis

This highly contagious ringworm infection, typically seen in children, affects the scalp (figure 12.11). The lesions are scaly, grayish patches in which the hair becomes dull, broken, and thin. The affected area can include either small ringed patches or much of the scalp. You must refer to a physician for necessary topical medication, since tinea capitis does not spontaneously resolve.

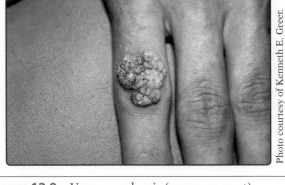

Figure 12.9　Verruca vulgaris (common wart).

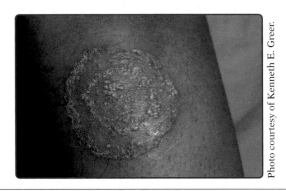

Figure 12.10　Tinea corporis (ringworm).

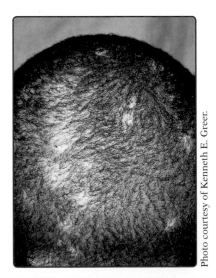

Figure 12.11　Tinea capitis (ringworm of the scalp).

Tinea Cruris

Tinea cruris (jock itch) is a fungal infection that affects the groin (figure 12.12). It has the characteristic ringworm appearance and can cause itching, redness, scaling, and cracking. Antifungal medications for treating tinea cruris are available in over-the-counter and prescription doses. Not sharing towels and clothing are good prevention habits that limit spread of the fungus.

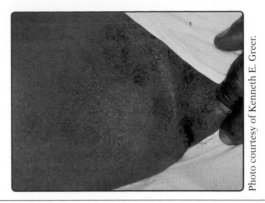

Figure 12.12 Tinea cruris (jock itch).

Tinea Pedis

Tinea pedis (athlete's foot) is a fungal infection that affects the feet (figure 12.13). The skin can appear red, scaly, and cracking and is often itchy. Prevention and treatment for tinea pedis are the same as for other ringworm infections. Cleansing and drying the feet properly, wearing clean socks, and avoiding walking barefoot are appropriate prevention steps.

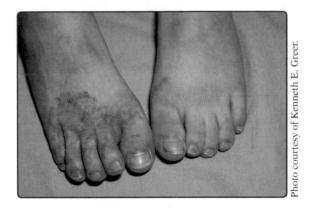

Figure 12.13 Tinea pedis (athlete's foot).

Tinea Versicolor

Tinea versicolor is a noncontagious ringworm infection that affects the horny layers of the skin and hair follicles (figure 12.14). A yeast fungal infection, it appears first as a salmon-colored, then as a scaly, patch of skin that does not pigment. Usually found on the trunk, it appears as either a white or a brown patch of skin.

Parasitic Infestations

Parasitic infestations of lice and itch mites can infect and irritate the skin. Many of these infections are found in the hair of the scalp and pubic regions. Proper treatment includes prescription medication and personal hygiene measures.

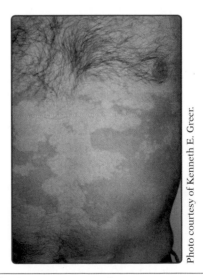

Figure 12.14 Tinea versicolor.

▶Pediculosis

Pediculosis is an infection of the skin caused by lice (figure 12.15). The affected body region is indicated by the name: pediculosis capitis is caused by the head louse, pediculosis corporis by the body louse, and pediculosis pubis by the crab louse. Lice of this third type infest hairs of the genital region; infestation is commonly referred to as crabs. The most prevalent symptom is severe itching. Pediculosis is transmitted through direct contact with infected patients. Treatment includes physician referral for medication to eradicate the parasite. Thorough laundering of clothing and bed linens is also necessary.

▶Scabies

Scabies is caused by the itch mite. The impregnated female mite burrows into the skin and deposits her eggs in the tunnel. The larvae hatch and accumulate around hair follicles. Typical signs and symptoms include the appearance of elevated burrows on the skin and itching. The most common sites are the interdigital spaces of the hands and the axilla, trunk, and genital regions (figure 12.16).

Inflammatory Conditions

Inflammatory conditions are integumentary conditions that cause localized and regional inflammation of the skin. These conditions are often characterized by redness, soreness, itching, burning, and swelling.

▶Dermatitis

Dermatitis is simply defined as an inflammation of the skin. Contact dermatitis, the most common dermatitis condition, is a delayed reaction to direct contact with an allergen (figure 12.17). It is characterized by erythema, edema, itching, and vesiculations of varying degrees. The first step in treatment is to remove the offending substance.

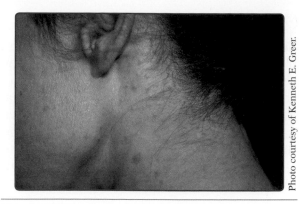

Figure 12.15 Pediculosis capitis.

Photo courtesy of Kenneth E. Greer.

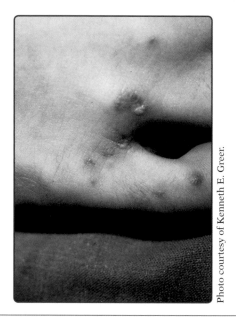

Figure 12.16 Scabies.

Photo courtesy of Kenneth E. Greer.

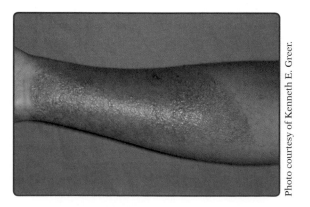

Figure 12.17 Contact dermatitis.

Photo courtesy of Kenneth E. Greer.

Eczema

Eczema is the generic term used to describe chronic dermatitis. It is characterized by scaling, erythematous, edematous, papular, vesicular, crusty skin and is often accompanied by itching and burning (figure 12.18). As with other forms of dermatitis, removing the irritant is key to treatment.

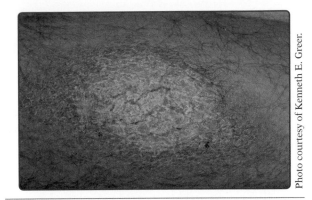

Figure 12.18 Eczema.

Psoriasis

Psoriasis is a usually chronic condition of unknown etiology that exhibits characteristic eruptions on the extensor surfaces of the extremities, especially the elbows, knees, back, and scalp (figure 12.19). The eruptions are circumscribed, erythematous papules covered with silvery scales.

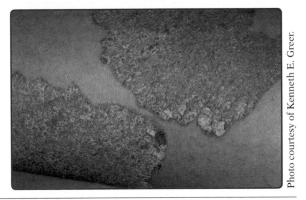

Figure 12.19 Psoriasis.

Environmental Exposures

Other skin conditions occur due to environmental factors such as allergens and exposure to heat or cold, chemicals, and poisons. Signs and symptoms of these conditions differ according to source of irritant.

Hives

Hives, or urticaria, is a dermal hypersensitivity reaction to an allergen. Common allergens include any substance that causes an abnormal reaction upon exposure, such as insect bites, foods, dust, mold, or certain medications. A **wheal** formation that occurs on the skin can range from small red dots to large, raised, reddened areas (figure 12.20).

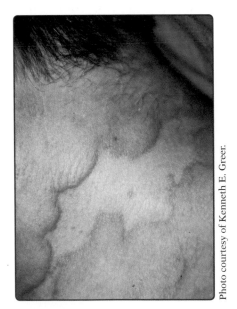

Figure 12.20 Hives in a wheal formation.

Frostbite

Frostbite is a potentially serious condition of local tissue destruction consequent to exposure to cold that freezes the superficial and possibly deeper tissue layers. It can range from mild to severe. Mild cases display erythema, itching, numbness, and mild pain. If exposure to cold continues, the skin can become pale, waxy, and firm to the touch. Severe cases are characterized initially by paresthesia and painless blisters and ultimately lead to tissue destruction and gangrene (figure 12.21).

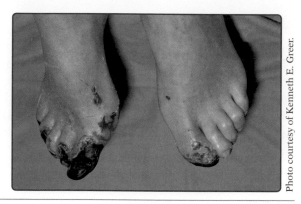

Figure 12.21   Severe frostbite.

Photo courtesy of Kenneth E. Greer.

Sunburn

Redness, pain or burning, itching, and increased skin heat characterize sunburn, a common skin condition caused by overexposure to the sun's ultraviolet rays. Blisters may also be present with more severe sunburns, causing the damaged skin layer to peel off a few days later. When the sunburn is severe and occurs over a large portion of the body, there may also be fever and general malaise.

Other Lesions

Other lesions involving the dermis can result in tissue or fluid buildup due to mechanical friction or glandular occlusion. These conditions include, but are not limited to, blisters, calluses, and sebaceous cysts.

Blisters

A blister is a separation of the skin's dermal and epidermal layers caused by a heat buildup from friction. Fluid, either serous or blood, fills the area (figure 12.22). The preferred treatment is to protect the area with a sterile bandage. If the blister breaks, cleanse the area using sterile technique; apply an antiseptic ointment and secure with a sterile dressing.

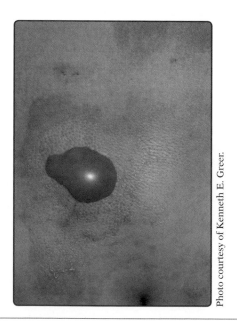

Photo courtesy of Kenneth E. Greer.

Figure 12.22   Blister.

Calluses

Calluses are the result of excessive friction. Skin builds up in an area of high friction as a means of self-protection (figure 12.23). Calluses typically form on the feet and hands over areas of high friction, stress, and bony prominences. As the callus forms, the skin becomes thicker and less flexible and elastic, moving as an abnormally large unit and becoming more susceptible to tears. Calluses should be kept trimmed and manageable, though not completely removed so as to leave sufficient protection of more sensitive skin layers.

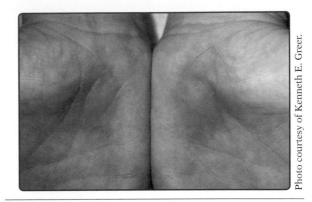

Figure 12.23 Callus.

Photo courtesy of Kenneth E. Greer.

Sebaceous Cysts

A sebaceous cyst is a benign cystic skin tumor that develops because of occlusion of a sebaceous gland in the dermis. It is a firm, round, movable, and nontender mass that most commonly develops on the scalp, face, back, or scrotum (figure 12.24). An infected cyst causes discomfort. Treatment includes physician referral for excision of the cyst sac.

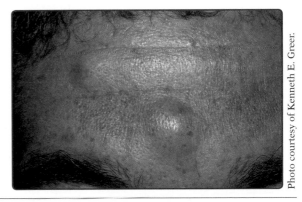

Figure 12.24 Sebaceous cyst.

Photo courtesy of Kenneth E. Greer.

Eye, Ear, Mouth, Nose, and Throat Conditions

Injuries and pathology associated with the eyes, ears, mouth, nose, and throat are very common and pervasive both in athletics and among the general population. In fact, there are so many conditions that affect these areas that a physician specialty is dedicated to their treatment. Continuation of athletic competition or exercise depends on the location and the condition itself.

Eye Conditions

Injuries to the eye most often result from direct contact and typically involve the cornea or internal eye structures. Eye injuries can be quite serious and may result in permanent damage if not recognized early or treated properly.

Conjunctivitis

Conjunctivitis, or pinkeye, is irritation and inflammation of the outer surface of the eye or inner eyelid. It can be caused by allergies, infection (viral or bacterial), or direct contact. Viral conjunctivitis, which frequently accompanies an upper respiratory infection, is quite contagious and can easily spread to the unaffected eye or to teammates. It is imperative that the patient avoid touching the eye when possible and immediately washes her hands after having done so to avoid spreading the infection.

Sties

The glands and hair follicles of the eyelid can become irritated and swollen as a consequence of infection or obstruction. A sty is an infection or obstruction of a ciliary gland of the eyelid.

Ear Conditions

Injuries to the ear include lacerations and hematoma caused by blunt trauma to the side of the head. In addition to ear injuries caused by sport participation, many ear conditions caused by infection and illness can affect sport participation. Early recognition and treatment of these pathologies help limit the time lost from activity.

▶ Impacted Cerumen

Excessive wax buildup in the external auditory canal can lead to hearing loss, tinnitus, and feelings of pressure or pain within the ear. On observation, the wax accumulation is visible in the ear canal.

▶ Otitis Externa (Swimmer's Ear)

Otitis externa, or bacterial infections from water accumulation in the swimmer's ear, are a common cause of inflammation in the external ear canal. Signs and symptoms of otitis externa include pain, itching or burning, and possible drainage from the ear. The external ear may be tender to palpation, and pulling on the earlobe increases pain.

▶ Otitis Media

Otitis media is characterized by inflammation or infection of the tympanic cavity or middle ear. Within this cavity are the auditory ossicles (malleus, incus, and stapes) as well as tympanic muscles and nerves. Infections of the middle ear and tympanic membrane (eardrum) can be extremely painful. Signs and symptoms include severe earache, swollen and red eardrum, fever, dizziness (vertigo), tinnitus, and possible hearing loss.

Mouth

Injuries to the mouth and related structures may or may not be related to sport participation. Dental pain and injury can be secondary to either direct trauma to the mouth or to tooth and gum disease resulting from poor hygiene. Injuries to the teeth caused by direct trauma are classified as fractures, intrusions, luxations, or extrusions.

▶ Gingivitis

Gingivitis is an inflammation of the gum that results from bacteria in and around the gums caused by food deposits and inadequate brushing or flossing. Brushing the teeth too aggressively or in a lateral versus up-and-down motion can also irritate the gums. The gums appear red and swollen, and the patient complains of pain and bleeding when brushing the teeth.

▶ Periodontitis

Periodontitis, a more serious condition caused by bacteria, results in loss of alveolar bone and recession of the gum line. Signs and symptoms include pain and bleeding with brushing, tooth sensitivity to cold and hot drinks or foods, red and swollen gums, breath odor, and possible loosening of the teeth.

▶ Dental Cavities

Tooth pain may result from dental caries (cavities) or abscess. Decay and degeneration of the tooth enamel, allowing exposure, irritation, and infection of the tooth's pulp, cause dental caries. If the infection passes through the root of the tooth into the periodontal tissues, an abscess may form in the adjacent gum.

Nose

Nasal conditions other than direct trauma injuries often are a result of viral or bacterial infections or allergic irritants. Many of these conditions are considered nuisances, but in severe cases they can affect and limit athletic participation.

▶ Rhinitis

Acute inflammation or infection of the nasal passageways, usually virus or allergy based, results in annoying nasal mucosa discharge. Obstructed breathing (congestion) can occur with excessive mucosal discharge and swelling of the nasal passages. A runny nose and sneezing are often the first signs of an upper respiratory infection. Medications are used to control mucosal discharge and decrease congestion.

Sinusitis

Inflammation of the nasal and facial sinuses can result from either viral or bacterial exposure but is also commonly associated with predisposing conditions such as chronic rhinitis, obstructive drainage, allergy exposure, general debilitation, dental abscess, or exposure to extreme temperature and humidity.

Throat

Throat conditions other than direct trauma injuries often are a result of viral or bacterial infections or allergic irritants. Discomfort from throat conditions can vary from being slightly annoying to limiting one's ability to breathe and swallow. Limitation of physical activity will be based on the patient's symptoms and how they affect his ability to participate.

Pharyngitis

Inflammation of the pharynx can result from either a viral or a bacterial infection and is often an extension of sinusitis, tonsillitis, or adenoid infection. Chills, fever, hoarseness, and **dysphagia** commonly accompany a burning or dry throat. Treatment includes rest, fluid intake, and medication for symptomatic relief. Antibiotics are used for bacterial infections.

Laryngitis

Acute inflammation of the larynx usually results secondary to a common cold, sinusitis, pharyngitis, or tonsillitis. A tickling sensation or rawness in the throat with a frequent need to clear the throat is often accompanied by hoarseness or a change or loss of voice. Treatment includes bed rest, fluid ingestion, and resting the voice; bacterial conditions indicate antibiotic medication.

Tonsillitis

Although acute inflammation of the tonsils often results from a bacterial infection, chronic tonsillitis is frequently related to predisposing factors such as a common cold or adenoiditis. Acute tonsillitis presents with signs and symptoms of chills, fever, malaise, headaches, body aches, and severe pain in the throat with difficulty swallowing. Symptoms of chronic tonsillitis, on the other hand, include a sore throat, mild fever, and nasal discharge.

Viral Syndromes

Viral syndromes are systemic conditions caused by viral infections. They are often highly contagious and may have prolonged symptoms. Complications such as enlarged visceral organs and sterility may result from one or more of these conditions.

Epstein-Barr Virus

The Epstein-Barr virus (EBV) is a member of the herpes virus family (Venes 2010). The virus is spread via saliva and is the cause of infectious mononucleosis. But while the symptoms of mononucleosis typically resolve in 1 or 2 months, EBV remains latent in cells of the throat and blood for the rest of the person's life. The virus can periodically reactivate in infected persons, usually without symptoms of illness.

Infectious Mononucleosis

The EBV causes most cases of infectious mononucleosis, or mono. This condition can affect any age group, but most cases are seen in patients aged 15 to 30. The disease is transmitted through direct contact with the saliva of an infected patient. A common means of transmission is sharing beverage containers or food utensils.

Incubation is 2 to 7 weeks after contact, and symptoms can last a few days or several months. Most commonly, they disappear in 1 to 3 weeks. Symptoms are vague and include general malaise, headache, fatigue, chilliness, appetite loss, and puffy eyelids.

As the disease progresses, additional symptoms—swollen and tender lymph glands, sore throat, and fever—emerge. Tenderness and enlargement of the spleen, difficulty swallowing, and bleeding gums can also occur. If an individual of any age competes while the spleen is enlarged, there is a chance of rupture; thus an enlarged spleen contraindicates physical activities requiring contact or jostling. Refer suspected cases to the physician for a diagnosis.

Measles

Measles is a highly contagious viral infection (rubeola) transmitted through the air; a patient can contract measles by breathing the same air as an infected person. Because of the ease of transmission, epidemics—usually occurring in the spring in a cycle of 2 or 3 years—are common. The incubation period is about 9 to 11 days, with about 2 weeks passing between exposure and the appearance of the measles rash. The rash, which begins about 3 or 4 days after the other symptoms, takes the form of irregular papules around the hairline of the face and neck and rapidly spreads to the trunk and extremities. The disease takes 10 to 14 days to run its course.

Mumps

Mumps is a highly contagious viral infection that affects the salivary glands, especially the parotid glands. It is spread through droplet infection or direct contact with saliva.

Systemic Conditions

Systemic conditions are typically multisymptomatic and affect entire organ systems. Many systemic conditions are caused by bacterial infections, but they also can occur due to viral infections, vitamin or mineral deficiencies, or congenital traits.

Bacteremia

Bacteremia (also known as bacterial sepsis or septicemia) is characterized by the presence of bacteria in the blood. It occurs when an infection overwhelms the local defenses at the original infection site (e.g., skin, respiratory, genitourinary, gastrointestinal) and enters the bloodstream, initiating a systemic response that adversely affects blood flow to vital organs.

Lymphangitis

Acute streptococcal infections in the extremities can lead to lymphangitis, an inflammation of the lymphatic vessels. Signs and symptoms include red streaks extending from the infected area to the axilla or groin, fever, chills, headache, and general malaise.

Lymphadenitis

Lymphadenitis is inflammation of the lymph nodes, which can be caused by a variety of conditions resulting from bacterial infection or other inflammatory conditions that drain bacteria or toxins into the lymph. It is commonly associated with lymphangitis.

Iron Deficiency Anemia

Anemia is characterized by a deficiency of red blood cells, hemoglobin, or total blood volume. Although there are various causes of anemia, iron deficiency anemia occurs the most frequently. A deficiency of iron in the blood decreases the quantity of red blood cells. Since red blood cells contain hemoglobin, the oxygen carrier of the blood, anemia reduces the body's ability to deliver oxygen to cells throughout the body.

Sickle Cell Anemia

Sickle cell anemia is a genetic mutation of the red blood cells. Normal red blood cells are round, but sickle cells are sickle shaped. The condition occurs most predominantly in African Americans. Signs and symptoms include pain in the chest, joints, back, and abdomen that can range from mild to severe; swelling in the feet and hands; jaundice; kidney failure; repetitive infections; or gallstones or stroke at an early age.

CASE STUDY

Case Study

Maria is the athletic trainer for the men's basketball team at a local community college. The team is participating in an all-day basketball tournament, with games at 10 a.m., 12:30 p.m., and 3 p.m. During the third game of the day, Terry, who is diabetic, begins to feel unwell. Because of the game schedule, the players, including Terry, were not able to spend much time eating and had only granola bars and some juice at around 11:30 a.m. Terry had a good breakfast and his glucose levels were appropriate prior to the first game; but after a quick recheck during the third game, he and Maria notice that his levels are lower than recommended by his physician.

Think About It

1. What do you think Terry is suffering from? What symptoms are commonly associated with Terry's condition?

2. What two factors have caused the low glucose levels, and what could happen if this goes untreated? What is happening at a cellular level in this situation?

3. What should Maria do to help Terry? What should she do if he loses consciousness?

4. In the future, what should Maria and Terry do when the activity schedule is similar to prevent these symptoms?

Learning Aids

SUMMARY

While many of the conditions discussed in this chapter are general medical conditions that may arise during normal activities and over the course of life, they can certainly have an impact on physical performance. In addition, many can be directly caused by or linked to participation in athletics and physical activity and need to be recognized and managed by the athletic trainer. Therefore, it is important for athletic trainers to understand these conditions and their implications for referral and continued participation.

KEY CONCEPTS AND REVIEW

▸ List and briefly describe four general medical conditions that affect the heart.

- Coronary artery disease (CAD), also known as coronary heart disease, is a chronic cardiovascular condition characterized by hardening and narrowing (atherosclerosis) of the coronary arteries, the vessels supplying blood to the heart.

- Heart murmurs most often occur due to a defective heart valve. Valves may be stenotic, having an atypically small opening that prevents them from opening completely, while other valves may be unable to close completely.

- Mitral valve prolapse: Due to congenital abnormalities, the mitral valve cusps collapse backward into the left atrium during heart function, allowing blood to leak backward through the valve.

- High blood pressure is the common term for hypertension, which involves an elevated systolic or diastolic blood pressure and is associated with generalized arteriolar vasoconstriction.

- Hypertrophic cardiomyopathy is a serious disease of the myocardium (heart muscle), resulting in enlarged muscle cells in the ventricular septum and left ventricular walls.
- Hypotension is a subnormal (low) blood pressure. The most common type is orthostatic hypotension, in which the blood pressure drops when the person suddenly stands.
- Syncope, or fainting, is a sudden, temporary loss of consciousness most commonly resulting from either a physiological or an emotional stress that causes a vasovagal reaction.

▸ **List and briefly describe general medical conditions of the respiratory system.**

- An upper respiratory infection (URI) is any infection that affects any portion of the upper respiratory system (conducting pathway) including the tonsils, nose, throat, sinuses, and neck lymph nodes.
- Bronchial and lung infections can both cause infections of the bronchioles and lungs; pneumonia is a serious lung infection that requires immediate medical referral and treatment.
- Bronchitis, or inflammation of the bronchial tree, either acute or chronic, can result from an infection or a reaction to an irritating agent.
- Pneumonia is an infection of the alveolar spaces that is usually bacterial but can be viral.
- Common colds are viral infections that affect the upper respiratory system and are sometimes referred to as rhinoviruses.
- Influenza, or flu, is a viral infection that affects the body in general and the upper respiratory system in particular. It is highly contagious and is spread by infected persons through coughing and sneezing.

- Hay fever is an allergic rhinitis that occurs seasonally because of the patient's reaction to airborne pollens.
- Asthma is a reactive airway disease characterized by paroxysms of dyspnea, coughing, and wheezing.
- Hyperventilation is characterized by a breathing rate or depth exceeding that required to eliminate carbon dioxide (CO_2).

▸ **Identify the two types of eating disorders presented and briefly explain each.**

- Anorexia nervosa: Anorexia is a severe psychological disorder characterized by a self-induced food aversion and extreme weight loss. Although the condition can affect males, females are 10 times more often affected and usually experience amenorrhea as a side effect. Food and caloric intake and expenditure become their central focus; they often limit food intake to 300 to 600 calories daily. Signs and symptoms include weight loss greater than 25% of body weight, behavior directed toward weight loss, peculiar patterns of handling food, intense fear of gaining weight, disturbances in body image, and amenorrhea in women.
- Bulimia nervosa: Patients who have bulimia are of normal weight but use techniques such as vomiting and ingestion of diuretics and laxatives to prevent weight gain. Episodes of uncontrolled binge eating followed by vomiting are frequent.

▸ **Explain the female athlete triad.**

The female athlete triad, considered a serious yet preventable syndrome, is composed of three interrelated conditions: disordered eating, amenorrhea, and osteoporosis. While each component of the triad represents a medical problem in itself, experts agree that the combination of the three conditions can significantly affect the health of the young female patient.

▸ **Describe the condition called rhabdo-myolysis.**

Rhabdomyolysis is an acute, sometimes fatal disease caused by severe destruction of skeletal muscle that results in injury to the kidney. Any time skeletal muscle is damaged, myoglobin is released into the bloodstream, which is ultimately filtered by the kidneys. When severe skeletal damage releases extremely large amounts of myoglobin, kidney failure may occur when the myoglobin occludes the kidney structures or breaks down, releasing metabolic by-products that can be toxic to the kidneys. Severe skeletal muscle damage may also cause fluid to shift from the bloodstream into the muscle, leading to hypovolemic shock and reduced blood flow to the kidneys, creating a medical emergency.

▸ **List and briefly describe general medical conditions of the integumentary system.**

General medical conditions of the integumentary system occur due to bacterial, viral, fungal, or parasitic conditions. Most of these conditions are not life threatening, but they can be annoying and highly contagious. Proper management is critical to alleviate the spreading of the infection from person to person.

▸ **Differentiate infections that are viral from those that are bacterial.**

Bacterial infections are typically of staphylococcal origin and are usually characterized by pustules. In many cases the site of bacterial infections is in hair follicles and is generally localized to a single body part or region. Viral infections are caused by a virus and can be systemic in nature. Symptoms of viral infections may involve larger areas and other body systems and are resistant to antibacterial treatments.

▸ **Explain the Epstein-Barr virus and identify the common disorder it often causes.**

The Epstein-Barr virus (EBV) is a member of the herpes virus family. The virus is spread via saliva and is the cause of infectious mononucleosis. But while the symptoms of mononucleosis typically resolve in 1 or 2 months, EBV remains latent in cells of the throat and blood for the rest of the person's life.

PRACTICE!

For hands-on practice in this area, go to the web resource and complete the following:

Level 2.10, Module K2: Common Syndromes and Diseases

Level 2.10, Module K6: Sudden Illnesses and Communicable Diseases

CRITICAL THINKING QUESTIONS

1. You are the newly hired athletic trainer for the Yellow Tree school district. You have been asked by school administrators to produce a lecture on illness prevention for the student-athletes and parents of the district. Produce a PowerPoint presentation outlining, very specifically and memorably, ways to best avoid common bacterial, viral, and environmental illness pathologies.

2. One of your wrestlers has been recently diagnosed with a severe case of molluscum contagiosum. Outline a treatment and management plan consistent with the National Athletic Trainers' Association's position statement on skin diseases.

Acute
and Emergency Care

The NATA BOC (2011) identifies acute care of injuries and illnesses (AC) as a specific domain. They state that, "Athletic trainers are often present when injuries or other acute conditions occur or are the first healthcare professionals to evaluate a patient. For this reason, athletic trainers must be knowledgeable and skilled in the evaluation and immediate management of acute injuries and illnesses." Competencies in this domain are the focus of part III.

Chapter 13 discusses the immediate or acute care of an athletic injury. The chapter covers the gamut, from the emergency situation, in which you may only monitor vital signs and prepare the victim for transfer to the emergency medical services, to the situation of the walk-in patient seeking evaluation and care of an illness or injury.

Chapter 14 covers immediate and emergency care procedures used to prevent the exacerbation of life-threatening and non-life-threatening conditions to reduce the risk of morbidity and mortality. In reading this chapter, you will review the ABCs and immediate steps for preventing a serious or potentially serious injury from getting worse. The chapter discusses the permissions you will need before rendering any emergency treatment and how to gain that permission in advance; the emergency medical services (EMS) team; and the development of the emergency action plan for your setting.

COMPETENCIES

Prevention and Health Promotion (PHP): PHP-17-b, c, g, and h

Clinical Examination and Diagnosis (CE): CE-16, 20h, and 21j

Acute Care of Injuries and Illnesses (AC): AC-2-7, 9, 10, 12-14, 19-28, 30, 34, 36-b, d, j, 39, and 40-42

Acute Care

Susan Kay Hillman, ATC, PT

OBJECTIVES

After reading this chapter, the student should be able to do the following:

- Explain the eight steps in developing an emergency action plan.

- Identify the elements of "vitals," or vital signs, and explain each.

- Explain the American College of Surgeons' ranking of trauma hospitals.

- Explain the numbers given as the blood pressure reading—what they are and what they represent.

- Explain methods used in controlling bleeding.

- Explain the sterile technique and compare and contrast it to Universal Precautions.

- Explain the difference between the head-squeeze and the trapezius-squeeze techniques of manual stabilization of the cervical spine.

- Explain the two techniques for moving the patient onto a spine board from a supine position.

Handling emergencies is not a day-to-day function of the athletic trainer, but athletic trainers do often need to deal with an injury that just happened, that is, to render acute care. In medical specializations, the acute care physician or **physician's assistant** focuses on patients with acute illness or injury that will be cared for in emergency departments, trauma units, intensive care units, or specialty practices. The athletic trainer's role in acute care is to provide immediate life-supporting care and to activate emergency medical services (EMS).

Planning Foundations for Acute Care Situations

As you recall from chapter 1, various individuals are a part of the sports medicine team and may be the ones you call upon in an acute care situation. Whoever you are, wherever you are, you need to have thought about what to do in the case of a serious injury or other emergency. Forming that emergency action plan is a critical step in making any emergency a very manageable one.

The Emergency Care Plan

One can never be too prepared for an emergency situation. Just as in the case of doing CPR, if and when we need to use the emergency procedures, our minds will be flooded with information—and the more automatic the response, the better. Creating an emergency plan is a good way to ensure all members of the coaching and medical staff are well prepared to handle an emergency situation (see the sidebar Items to Consider When Creating an Emergency Care Plan, and also see chapter 14 for a thorough discussion of each of the sidebar items). It also is wise to practice the steps of the emergency plan several times throughout the school year or sport season. Having every member of the coaching and medical staff familiar with the emergency care plan is a great asset if

an emergency ever arises. As an example, consider a situation that actually occurred during a college football practice. During tackling drills in the early phase of the practice, a linebacker made a hit, lowering his head and striking the ball carrier. The linebacker collapsed suddenly and then lay motionless on the field. Because this was a practice day, the only staff on the field was the supervising ATC, three student volunteers, several coaches, and one equipment person. The player could not move; his level of consciousness was diminished, and he was calling people by the wrong name and making strange requests.

This player had a concussion, and in view of the type of drill that had led to the concussion, one could suspect that his neck may also have been injured. The athletic trainer, coaches, and equipment man safely and quickly immobilized the individual's spine on a spine board as one of the volunteers was instructed to call 911. Preplanning with the entire athletic department staff allowed smooth teamwork in helping this player.

Every member of the sport staff has a responsibility in the total athletic injury emergency care plan. In an emergency situation, anyone may be called upon, and everyone must be knowledgeable and ready to help. Every team should develop an emergency care plan that outlines game and practice coverage; emergency procedure steps; and other elements of emergency care such as communication, transportation, and record keeping. See figure 13.1 for a sample emergency plan from National Youth Sports Safety Foundation, Inc.

Role of the Athletic Trainer

The athletic trainer is usually present at the time of an injury and must understand how to provide acute or immediate care. Acute care can be thought of as the immediate care or "first aid" for the injured patient. As the athletic trainer and the first on the scene, you will be the professional best prepared to render first aid and cardiopulmonary resus-

ITEMS TO CONSIDER WHEN CREATING AN EMERGENCY CARE PLAN

- Game and practice coverage: Outline the duties of those regularly in attendance. Anticipate the personnel who might be available, delineate duties, and discuss contingency plans.
- Procedure steps: Know what will be done. Outline the steps to be taken in various emergency situations.
- Communication systems: Know how to contact emergency medical services. Ensure that there is a working telephone near all practice and game facilities. On or next to each telephone, have appropriate emergency numbers and directions for calling for an ambulance.
- Equipment: Appropriate emergency care equipment and supplies must be available and in proper condition for use. Include emergency equipment in annual inventory and ordering.

- Emergency care facilities: Contact local emergency care facilities to establish protocol for registration of injured participants. Preregister the entire team if possible. Discuss procedures to be followed when emergency medical needs arise.
- Transportation: Arrange for an ambulance crew to be in attendance during events or notify a local ambulance company of event location, time, and preferred access routes.
- Personnel training: Training and retraining of all personnel need to be accomplished periodically.
- Record keeping: Review commonly used and accepted abbreviations for medical terms as well as methods of recording medical information. Always make a record of the injuries and treatment provided.

citation (CPR) if needed. But how would you feel if you *thought* you were providing the best care of an ill or injured but were told later that what you did delayed the needed emergency care and that the individual's condition suffered seriously? What if death resulted? It is very important not only to understand the scope of practice (what your state laws say) regarding the ability of the athletic trainer to provide emergency and acute care, but also to learn and practice the skills and techniques involved. The athletic trainer should be skilled in the acute management of sprains, strains, **lacerations**, **contusions**, fractures, and dislocations as well as in CPR and rescue breathing. Chapter 14 provides instruction on CPR and rescue breathing. Chapters 9, 10, and 11 of this text present detailed discussion on the recognition of various musculoskeletal conditions (sprains, strains, dislocations, contusions).

Care and treatment of these conditions is quite uniform and is discussed later in this chapter.

Role of the EMS Team

As you learned in the first chapter of this book, the EMS team involves a number of levels of emergency care providers. The basic EMT (emergency medical technician) seldom provides any more care than the certified athletic trainer, yet the EMT may be the only person on the ambulance that arrives to take the patient to the hospital. The EMT-P (paramedic) has specialized training that allows advanced monitoring and care involving intravenous (IV) care and delivery of medicines via injection. The larger the community, the more likely it is that a paramedic will be on the ambulance you call. If not, realize that the ambulance crew may not

The emergency care plan addresses immediate needs for medical assistance in the instance of traumatic injury or illness. The emergency care plan assigns specific duties for effective evaluation, transport, and follow-up of the situation. It affects coaches, spectators, practice, and game personnel as well as participants. The emergency care plan must address situations that may occur from the first practice through the last team meeting; it covers weekdays as well as weekends.

A checklist is attached for duties assigned to specific individuals or information pertinent to the specific team or sport.

This plan may be used for any sport, for any site where the team practices or competes. It must be available at all times. The plan should include information regarding vehicular access that changes for game days; or changed access when the sideline is set up for the game. The National Federation of State High School Associations (NFHS) recommends placing the plan in a plastic "sleeve" and posting it at each specific athletic venue.

Should an injury occur that requires medical assistance; the following are critical items that need to be addressed by a coach, ATC, designated first aid responder, athletic administrator, or some combination of these personnel.

- Primary evaluation
- ABCs
- Accessing EMS immediate primary care
- Notification of athletic trainer or designated first aid responder by radio or telephone, if not on-site
- Notification of parent
- Report all injuries to coach or team administrators within 24 h

(The following are recommended but shall not supersede procedures adopted by your school's athletic department.)

Emergency care cards, first aid kit, and quick access to ice shall be the standard for each practice and event.

In case of a catastrophic injury, no information should be given to any party other than EMS. The ATC or coach or both shall notify the athletic administrator. The athletic administrator shall be responsible for contacting the principal of the school. The athletic administrator or principal will release appropriate information to the media. Other strategies can be developed by individual schools.

The following is a template for use at individual schools by individual teams. Other emergency plan templates are available from a variety of groups. The National Federation of State High School Associations' *NFHS Sports Medicine Handbook* offers such a form.

Emergency Care Plan

Date: _____ School: _____

Coach: _____ Contact Number: _____ Sport: _____

Game site street address: _____

Specific directions to game site from nearest major intersection: _____

_____

_____

Practice site street address: _____

Specific directions to practice site from nearest major intersection: _____

_____

_____

Figure 13.1 Sample emergency plan. *(continued)*

Instructions. Please complete and distribute a copy to all members of your coaching staff, the athletic administrator, designated first aid responder, and athletic trainer. Discuss this plan with your coaching staff. Proper preparation can lead to quick, appropriate action.

Where should EMS come to have quick access to the injured athlete? _____

_____

Who will give primary care to the athlete? _____

Where is the first aid kit? Where are the emergency care cards? _____

_____

Who calls EMS? _____

From which cell phone or telephone will the call to EMS be made? _____

Who will notify the parents that the athlete is being transported to an emergency care facility? _____

To which emergency care facility will athletes be transported? _____

Who will notify the athletic administrator or athletic trainer? _____

Who will manage the rest of the team while care is given to the injured athlete? _____

Who will open any gates or doors for EMS? _____

Who will meet EMS and direct them to the injured athlete? _____

Who will travel with the injured athlete to the emergency care facility? _____

Who will follow up with the parents? _____

Who will document the injury? _____

Who will speak to a parent in the instance of catastrophic injury? _____

Emergency Telephone Numbers

EMS: _____   Athletic Trainer: _____

Emergency Care Facility: _____   Athletic Administrator: _____

Figure 13.1 *(continued)*   Sample emergency plan.

ATC for Virginia High School League prepared by Nancy Burke. Used by permission.

be able to extend the care you can provide but can help you prevent further trauma and expedite the trip to the hospital.

Role of Hospitals

Knowledge of the types of hospitals in your area is very important in the management of acute injuries and emergencies. The American College of Surgeons (ACS) ranks hospitals according to the level of care they provide; Level I trauma centers are the highest-ranking hospitals for emergency situations (see the sidebar Trauma Level Designations). As an athletic trainer, you should be aware of the local hospitals and what each is equipped to handle. Your knowledge in this area can help ensure that an injured person receives the care needed. Imagine this: You are at the spring football game, complete with officials. During a play from scrimmage, a linebacker breaks through the offensive line and sacks the quarterback. That is all expected, but the referee is caught behind the line of scrimmage and gets knocked down during the play. He is in serious pain with a fractured **humeral head** (shoulder). You and the team doctor send him by ambulance to the closest hospital. Unfortunately, the extent of the injury is not conveyed to the ambulance driver, and the level of care needed is not available at the hospital closest to the field. The referee has to be transferred to a hospital prepared to care for a fracture of this type, which further delays his treatment. If you had known which hospitals in the area were equipped to handle the level of care needed, you could have informed the ambulance driver and helped the referee receive more immediate care.

Essentials of the Acute Examination

Any time you approach a patient who is not moving and talking, you must take caution not to move her until you know the type and degree of injury. This evaluation is rapid and is accomplished in a systematic fashion to allow care to be rendered as soon as possible.

This systematic evaluation of the patient comprises the *primary survey* and *secondary survey*.

Primary Survey

As noted in chapter 8, a primary survey determines the status of life-threatening or limb-threatening conditions using the ABCs of emergency medical care: examination of Airway, Breathing, and Circulation. Your first goal is to tend to life-threatening conditions by examining the patient's airway, breathing, and circulation for respirations and pulse. You should also evaluate other vital signs and check for severe bleeding at this time. When you come upon an injured patient, you usually start talking to him to find out what he felt and where he hurts. If the individual is able to talk, you can safely assume that he is breathing and has a pulse. If he fails to respond, your job is to discover what is not working and provide rescue breathing and perhaps CPR. You will learn more about primary surveys in chapter 14.

TRAUMA LEVEL DESIGNATIONS

- Level I trauma centers are equipped to provide the highest level of trauma care. The most severely injured patients are taken to these facilities. A full range of specialists and equipment is available in-house 24 h a day.

- Level II trauma centers work with Level I centers to provide comprehensive trauma care. They provide 24-h availability of essential specialties and equipment, but those specialists may not be in-house at all hours.

- Level III trauma centers do not have all specialists available, but they do have resources to provide emergency resuscitation and intensive care for trauma patients. Usually these hospitals are in rural areas or smaller communities. In the case of exceptionally severe injuries, Level III hospitals have special transfer arrangements with Level I or II trauma centers.

- Level IV centers exist in some states where there are insufficient resources for a Level III center. Level IV centers provide the initial evaluation, stabilization, and diagnosis and the access to a Level III or higher trauma center. These hospitals may provide surgery and critical-care services as well. A trauma-trained nurse is available on-site, but physicians are on call. If the hospital is not open 24 h, it is required to have an after-hours trauma response protocol.

Secondary Survey

Once you know that the individual is breathing and his heart is pumping, you can perform an examination to determine the presence of other injuries. A secondary survey is a rapid examination of the seriousness of the injury, and the conclusions you formulate determine how you should remove the patient from the site. Usually, the athlete is able to tell you what happened, what he felt, and how bad the pain is currently. If he is in severe pain, you may not be able to gain much information about what happened. Teammates may be able to describe the incident. In your survey of the limbs and spine, you should palpate and question the individual about his discomfort. Discovering the extent of the injury is the purpose of the secondary survey and is covered in chapter 8 of this text.

Vital Signs

This chapter does not discuss the emergency care of sport participants, only the initial evaluation prior to referral. If the patient reports to the treatment center with complaints of illness, it is wise to measure and record vital signs, or "vitals." Likewise, emergencies that affect the patient's **systemic** function (spinal cord injury, concussion, cardiac trauma, heat exhaustion, and so on) necessitate evaluation of vital signs and treatment until EMS arrives and takes over the care.

Vital signs are measures of bodily functions and vary depending on the age and condition of the individual. An elderly patient on supplemental oxygen may need more extensive vital signs taken than a young, fit individual. Generally, if you refer the patient to emergency care, the staff will ask for vitals; the ones evaluated for an athletic individual are pulse, blood pressure, respiratory rate, and temperature. Not all acute care presentations require vitals, but it is good to know how to take these measures so you can use them when needed. The normal levels and levels of concern for each vital sign are listed in table 13.1.

Pulse

The pulse is an indication of the rate and quality of the heartbeat. A rate higher than normal is called **tachycardia**; a rate lower than normal is called **bradycardia**. In tachycardia, the heart chambers don't have enough time to fully fill, so each beat sends less blood (oxygen) to the body and to the heart itself. In bradycardia, the heart is not pumping fast enough to supply the body and the heart itself with sufficient blood (oxygen), and in time the heart may stop. If the pulse is weak and your technique is good, it may be that the heart muscle is not working at its full capacity. Any of these findings should alert you to the fact that things are not normal and that EMS is needed. Continue to monitor the pulse and be ready to render cardiac compression if the heart stops beating.

Taking the pulse may be second nature to you at this point in your education, but did you know that taking the pulse at the carotid artery in the neck (figure 13.2a) could lower the heart rate? This would only happen if you unintentionally rubbed in the area of the carotid, over the area called the **carotid sinus**. The carotid sinus is the point at which the common carotid artery branches into two: the internal carotid and the external carotid. Rubbing of the carotid sinus can

Table 13.1 Vital Sign Values

Vital sign	Normal resting value	Level that creates concern
Pulse	60-100 beats per minute	>100 beats per minute (tachycardia) or <60 beats per minute (bradycardia)
Blood pressure	90/60 to 120/80 mmHg	140/90 mmHg
Respiratory rate	12-20 breaths per minute	Over 20 breaths per minute at rest
Temperature (oral)	98.6° F +/−1°	>100° F

stimulate nerves in the arterial wall and decrease the heart rate. If you have learned to take a pulse, you likely also learned not to use your thumb but to use your fingertips. The reason is that you might feel a larger artery in the tip of your thumb while trying to palpate, and the presence of the two pulses would be confusing. To accurately measure heart rate, place the tips of your index and long fingers on the thumb-side, **palmar** (palm side) crease of the wrist; this pulse is called the radial pulse (figure 13.2b). You should be able to detect a beat. If you are unable to find the pulse there, shift your fingers, lighten the touch, and try again. Once you find the pulse, count the number of beats you feel during a 30-s period. You can calculate the number of heartbeats per minute just by simple multiplication using 30, 15, or even 10 s of beats. The longer the time period used (up to 1 min) to count the beats, the more accurate your readings.

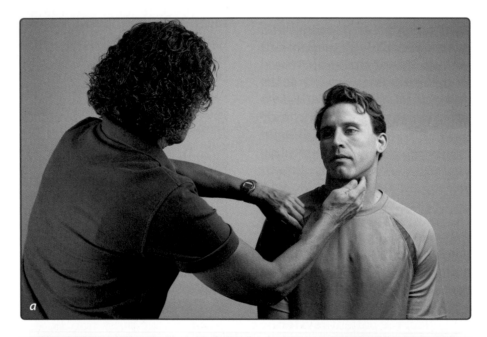

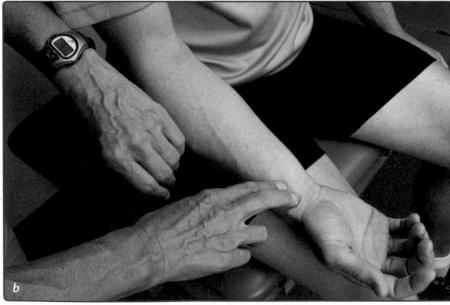

Figure 13.2   Locations for taking the *(a)* carotid and *(b)* radial pulse.

Blood Pressure

Blood pressure (BP) is the measure of pressure in the **peripheral** vessels during the function of the heart. It is the combination of the amount of blood (cardiac output) and the resistance in the peripheral vessels. An abnormal BP (higher BP = **hypertension**; lower BP = **hypotension**) is an indication of a change in **cardiac output**, a change in peripheral resistance, or both. In hypertension, high enough pressure in the vessels could cause a vessel to rupture. Rupture of a vessel in the brain is called a stroke; rupture of a vessel of the heart is called a heart attack. In hypotension, the pressure in the vessels is low, and the brain, heart, and other tissues may not receive enough blood. If the brain doesn't get enough blood (or oxygen carried in the blood), the person will faint.

Many brands of small machines are available for patients to use to measure their own blood pressure. Clinicians, however, should learn to take blood pressure using a **sphygmomanometer** and **stethoscope**. The sphygmomanometer is a blood pressure cuff, a rubber bladder covered with nylon that has Velcro closures. A long tube connected to the cuff has a bulb and controller at its end. The cuff is placed around the patient's arm just above the elbow, wrapped around the arm, and secured with the Velcro. Using the blub at the end of the tube, the cuff is inflated to a pressure between 130 and 150 mmHg; then, using the controller, the cuff is slowly deflated while the examiner listens for a heart sound with the stethoscope. As the pressure in the cuff decreases, the examiner listens for the heart sounds and pays attention to the readings on the dial.

The stethoscope must be placed over the **brachial artery** at the elbow. You can easily find the brachial artery by flexing your elbow using your biceps. As you flex the elbow, notice the tendon that appears as the biceps contracts. This is the tendon of the **biceps brachii**. Just medial (toward the midline of the body) is the brachial artery. Light fingertip pressure there allows you to palpate the brachial artery, the spot where you should place the stethoscope in taking blood pressure (BP). Figure 13.3 demonstrates how to take blood pressure following these steps.

There are two numbers on the dial to pay attention to while the pressure in the cuff is

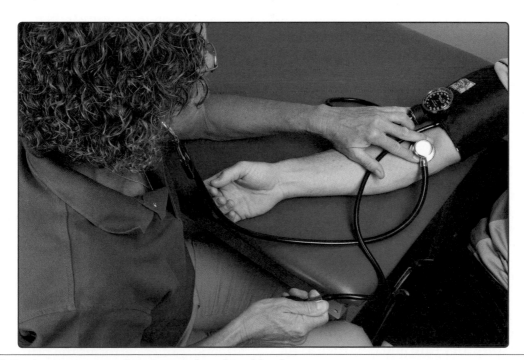

Figure 13.3 Accurate setup of equipment for taking blood pressure.

decreasing. The first number, the top number in the BP reading, is the **systolic** pressure and is arrived at when the first sound is heard. The second number, the bottom number in the reading, is the **diastolic** pressure and is arrived at when the sound disappears. The systolic pressure is the pressure during the pumping phase of the heart, and the diastolic pressure is the pressure during the refilling of the heart chambers. Together, these two numbers comprise the blood pressure reading, expressed as 120/80 or 143/92, for example.

Unfortunately, errors can occur in the process of taking BP. The stethoscope may be in the wrong position; the cuff may be too small for a large patient's arm; or the clinician's hearing may be compromised by extraneous noises or other hearing difficulties. Those factors would play a role in the accuracy of the BP reading. If the reading is inaccurate, it lacks **validity**: It is not a valid measure of the actual BP. Additionally, having multiple technicians taking a BP can lead to inaccuracies. For example, if a patient's BP is being tracked and each time she comes to the clinic to have her BP measured a different technician performs the evaluation, there could be inaccuracies given that not all technicians would use exactly the same technique. However, if only one clinician takes the BP and uses the same technique every time, the repeat measures would be consistent, indicating **reliability** of the measurement. Your goal should be to be as accurate as possible (achieve validity) and to obtain measurements that are consistent (achieve reliability).

Respiratory Rate

Determining the rate and quality of the patient's breathing is the objective of measuring respiratory rate. If the patient is not breathing satisfactorily (is breathing too fast or too slow), the amount of oxygen in the blood will be insufficient (**hypoxia**) and tissues will be damaged. If the brain does not get enough oxygen, fainting will result.

The number of breaths per minute is termed **respiratory rate** and is written as the number of breaths per minute. Watching the patient for 30 s or for 1 min usually provides a good measure of respirations. The quality of the breath should be noted as well. Patients with asthma or other forms of chronic obstructive pulmonary disease (**COPD**) have distinct qualities to their breathing that you should note in your reporting of vitals.

Temperature

A patient's temperature indicates the body's internal heat. Too much internal heat can be damaging to body organs and must be reduced. Body temperature, a vital sign to obtain if the patient complains of illness, is assessed using an oral thermometer. Depending on the time of day, a resting person with an oral temperature over 99° to 99.5° F is considered to have a fever. The best way to measure core temperature is to use a rectal thermometer, since cold (or hot) drinks and mouth breathing affect oral temperature readings. The rectal thermometer is more invasive than the oral thermometer, so researchers opt for small **thermistors** in capsule form to record internal (gut) temperature. The capsule is ingested, and for the next day or two the thermistor works its way out of the digestive tract, sending core temperature information wirelessly. The average oral temperature is 98.6° F; the rectal temperature is often about 1° F higher.

Immediate Care for Emergency Problems

The very first thing you must do when approaching an injured patient is determine her ability to breathe and ascertain that her heart is working (circulation). You can make certain assumptions regarding airway and breathing based simply on calling to the victim and asking questions. A verbal response indicates that the airway is open and the victim is breathing. If the heart is not beating, the body will not sustain brain activity and the victim will become **unconscious**. Rather than wait for that to occur, the athletic trainer performs the primary survey and renders proper care for airway, breathing, and circulation (ABCs), as you will learn about in detail in chapter 14.

When the primary survey shows no difficulties but the secondary survey uncovers a fracture or dislocation, emergency splinting of the limb is needed. A later section of this chapter covers splinting, but at this point it is important to remember that your objective is to do no harm. Splinting the injury in the position in which it is found is highly recommended. If a joint dislocation compromises blood flow, reduction may be an urgent need. Unless you are specifically trained in doing the reduction, you should not attempt it and must quickly get the patient to a qualified practitioner. Always realize that when trauma is perceived as severe, the likelihood exists that the patient will go into **shock**. Monitor the patient and be sure to provide complete care.

Shock

When oxygen supplied to the brain by circulating blood is insufficient, fainting results. But fainting is just one of the signs that a patient may be going into shock. Shock is a typical manifestation of heavy internal or external bleeding, spinal cord injury, heart conditions, dehydration, or severe allergic reactions. Signs and symptoms of shock include the following:

- Low blood pressure (key sign)
- Rapid and shallow respiration
- Cold, clammy skin
- Rapid and weak pulse
- Dizziness or fainting

Shock requires immediate medical attention. Call 911 and summon an ambulance that can provide an IV with fluids. The sooner you get the patient to medical help, the greater the chance of avoiding damage to internal organs.

Severe Bleeding

Hemorrhage is another word for bleeding and can refer to visible bleeding or internal

bleeding. Management of internal bleeding in the thorax, abdomen, or cranium is outside the scope of practice of the athletic trainer but must be recognized during evaluation of injuries as a potential pathology so that proper medical attention can be obtained. Usually, internal bleeding results in a drop in the blood pressure and possible fainting, which indicates more trauma than may meet the eye. When the blood is contained within a joint or in the muscle tissue, visible signs like swelling may be present. The athletic trainer can manage internal bleeding of this type through use of compression and elevation of the injured area to a level above the heart. Elevation of the limb often requires lowering the level of the heart, thus putting the patient in a supine position during the application of the ice and compression. If the bleeding is visible, the athletic trainer should be well prepared to manage the situation using Universal Precautions.

Universal Precautions

Our first impulse in seeing blood is often to grab a tissue or cloth and put it on the wound. This may be acceptable in the case of your own wound; but if you are treating another person, you need to use Universal Precautions.

In an effort to limit the risk of infection to health care providers via **bloodborne pathogens**, the Centers for Disease Control and Prevention (CDC) recommends that blood and certain body fluids of all patients be considered potentially infectious. This assumption encourages individuals to follow **Universal Precautions**, meaning that they should routinely take care to prevent skin and mucous membranes from coming into contact with a patient's blood or with certain body fluids.

Blood and body fluids containing visible blood, as well as semen, vaginal secretions, tissues, and bodily fluids such as synovial fluid, are potentially infectious. Tears, nasal secretions, saliva, sputum, sweat, urine, feces, or vomit are not unless they contain visible blood. Appropriate barriers include gloves, a mask, a gown, and eye protection.

However, the CDC also recognizes the appropriateness of something as simple as a thick gauze pad, which may be used to cover a small spot of blood as long as the gauze is thick enough to prevent blood from soaking through and contacting the health care provider's skin.

Other precautions include frequent, regular hand washing during work with patients and the disposal of any used sharp instruments into **impervious** ("sharps") containers. Those working with needles must remember that a needle should not be recapped by hand but immediately disposed of into the sharps container. Sharps containers should be located throughout the health care facility to allow immediate access wherever wounds are treated. Additionally, soiled cloth or gauze should be disposed of into clearly marked red biohazard bags. Gloves worn during the care of a patient must be removed, and the outside of the glove should not be allowed to touch the provider's skin (see figure 13.4). The gloves, once they are removed and are inside out, should also be disposed of into the biohazard bag, and these bags must be closed and disposed of according to strict guidelines. The Occupational Safety and Health Association (**OSHA**) publishes guidelines for preventing occupational hazards, and the National Athletic Trainers' Association also has guidelines for preventing transmission of bloodborne pathogens. According to the CDC, "pathogens of primary concern are the human immunodeficiency virus (HIV), hepatitis B virus (HBV), and hepatitis C virus (HCV)" (Centers for Disease Control and Prevention 2010).

If a provider comes into contact with potentially infected blood or body fluids, the proper reports should be filed. Figure 13.5 presents a sample exposure report form. Once the report is submitted to the medical director, follow-up tests for infection are performed on the provider.

Controlling Visible Bleeding

Visible blood should warn the rescuer to take steps to control the bleeding. In some accidents the victim is bleeding badly and may be in need of immediate help. Remember that controlling bleeding is not your first concern; the biggest concern is to keep the patient breathing. Once the airway is established and breathing is spontaneous or assisted, bleeding can be managed. There are four ways to control bleeding. The first three are the most practical and useful; the last method can be used only as a last resort and if the rescuer has the equipment and training.

- *Direct pressure.* Applying pressure with a soft, sterile cloth or bandage often slows the flow of blood enough to allow natural clot formation to occur. Preventing contamination may be the first thought when one encounters a bleeding patient. Sterile cloths are often not readily available on the athletic field unless they are in the athletic trainer's medical kit. If sterile cloth is not available, a clean, dry cloth can be used. Profuse bleeding needs to be controlled; if it is not, the patient could die. It is less likely that a person will die because you applied a clean but not sterile cloth to the wound to control the flow of blood. The cloth should be clean and free of any known bacteria, dirt, grease, or other soil.

- *Splinting.* The rationale for use of a splint to control bleeding is that in the case of broken bones, the bleeding occurs because the ends of the bones are injuring adjacent tissues. As long as the bones are free to move, they can continue to damage vessels and dislodge clots that are beginning to form. Immobilization of the fracture may be sufficient in itself to stop bleeding. Think about an individual with a severely broken leg, such as a compound fracture—a fracture in which the end of the bone has pierced through the skin. The wound should be padded with sterile cloth; the leg should then be held in the position in which it was found; and one or more objects made of firm material, like a board, should be used to stabilize the bones. The wound should be padded with sterile cloth if possible—clean cloth if not—and bandaged to the immobilization device.

- *Pressure over the major artery.* When direct pressure over the wound does not

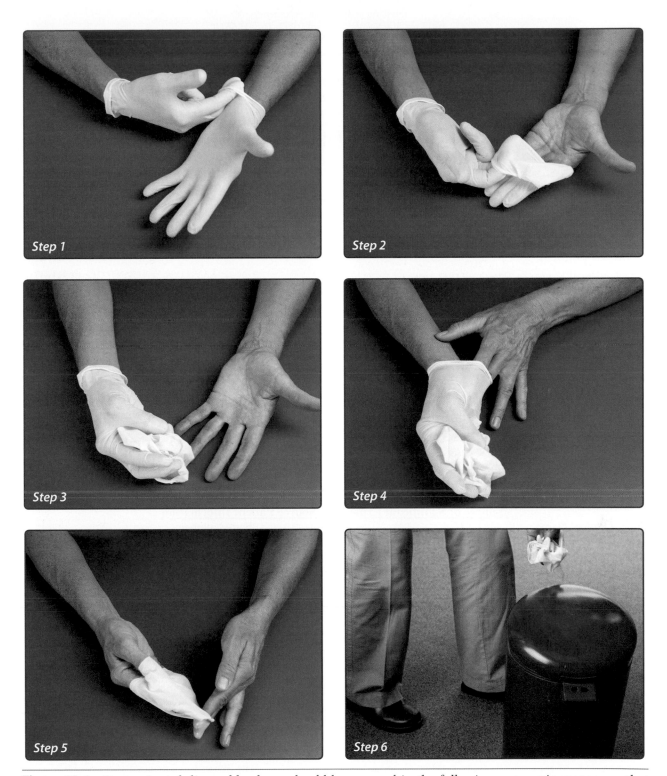

Figure 13.4 Contaminated disposable gloves should be removed in the following systematic manner so that they do not contaminate the skin. Step 1: Use your dominant hand to grasp your nondominant hand at the palm. Step 2: Carefully pull off the glove of the nondominant hand. Step 3: Hold it in your dominant hand. Step 4: Work your nondominant hand under the palm side of the glove on the dominant hand. Step 5: Once the fingers of your nondominant hand are to the glove finger holes, slowly push the glove over the fingers of your dominant hand. Carefully pull the glove off. Step 6: Dispose of gloves in proper container.

Form 350 9/05

State of Utah – Labor Commission
Division of Industrial Accidents
160 East 300 South, 3rd Floor - P.O. Box 146610
Salt Lake City, UT 84114-6610
(801) 530-6800 – (800) 530-5090 – Fax (801) 530-6804

Emergency Medical Service Provider Exposure Report Form

Complete this form to document exposure to blood and/or other body fluids. Most unprotected exposures do not result in an infection, however, some people can be exposed to a disease and not have any symptoms of illness. It is important that you document any significant exposure incident.

Significant Exposure – EMS Provider Information

Exposed Provider, use your last initial, first initial, last 4 digits of Social Security number for ID # ex.(ab1234) ID # _____

Employee Name _____ DOB ___/___/___ Sex _____
            (Last)   (First)   (M)   M or F
Home Phone _____ Work Phone _____ Employer/Agency _____
Contact Person at Employment / Agency _____ Contact Phone _____
Date _____ Incident # _____

Mechanism of Exposure (check all that apply)

Body Fluid Exposure		Other Body Fluid w/Blood		How Were You Exposed?	
	Blood		Saliva		Splash in Eye
	Birth Fluids		Urine		Splash in Mouth or Nose
	Pericardial Fluids		Feces		Bite
	Pleural Fluid		Pus		Puncture w/Hollow-bore Needle
	Synovial Fluid		Sputum		Puncture Cut w/Other Sharp Implement
	Cerebrospinal Fluid		Other		Open Wound
	Semen				Rash / Dermatitis
	Vaginal Secretions				Abrasion

What protective equipment were you using at the time of exposure? (check all that apply)

	Bag-Valve-Mask		One Way Resuscitation Mouthpiece		Paper Gown
	Gloves		N-95 Mask		Other
	Eye Protection		Surgical Mask (Less than N-95 rating)		

Source of Significant Exposure – Source Patient Information

Source Patient Name _____ Phone Number _____
Source Patient Address _____ (Street Address) DOB ___/___/___
_____ (City, State, Zip) Sex M___ F___

☐ I hereby give my permission to the facility named below to draw and test my blood for any or all of the following: ☐HIV Antibody, ☐HBV/Surface Antigen and, ☐HCV Antibody. I understand that the results of this testing are private information and will be confidential.

☐ I refuse to have my blood drawn and tested. I understand that a court order may be pursued to require me to have blood testing done.

Source Patient (or responsible) Signature _____ Date ___/___/___

Receiving Facility/Testing Laboratory

Receiving Facility _____ Date Specimen(s) were obtained ___/___/___
Testing Laboratory _____ Date Specimen(s) were submitted ___/___/___
Did patient expire? ☐Yes ☐ No   Was the patient under the jurisdiction of the State Department of Corrections (Prisoner or Parolee)? ☐Yes ☐ No
Name of Person submitting report _____
Title _____ Phone Number _____ Date Report was submitted ___/___/___

If onsite post exposure counseling is not available contact any of the following. http://www.ucsf.edu/hivcntr/Hotlines/PEPline.html 24/7
Or call (800) 537-1046. (801) 538-6096 or (800) FON-AIDS 8-5 M-F (hospital clinicians may receive 24/7 help with PEP counseling by calling 1-888-448-4911)
The Laboratory must report the test results of the source patient testing to the EMS Agency/Employer Contact person listed above.
* The EMS Agency/Employer must submit the Employer's First Report of Injury/Illness (Form 122) when this form is completed by an EMS Provider.

Figure 13.5 Exposure report form.

Reprinted from State of Utah: Labor Commission.

control the bleeding, or if the bleeding is from a large surface area so that direct pressure is not possible, pressure over a major artery can slow the blood flow. Your knowledge of the arterial system of the human body is important for identifying the location of the most proximal major vessel; generally, the major vessel is in the **axilla**, the groin, the back of the knee, or the front of the elbow. Direct pressure to the major artery can compress it. If this does not seem to slow the blood flow, reapply the pressure and attempt to sandwich the artery between your fingers and a firm part of the victim's anatomy, such as a bone or bony prominence. It is not necessary to follow Universal Precautions when applying direct pressure over a major artery unless the area is covered with blood.

• *Tourniquet.* A **tourniquet** is the last thing to try in order to control bleeding and is a method to avoid unless you are a trained paramedical professional. A tourniquet should not be applied unless bleeding is copious and cannot be controlled by direct pressure. Vigorous attempts to control with direct pressure should be continued. Once a tourniquet is placed, it should not be removed or loosened by anyone but a doctor. A tourniquet should be used only when a decision has been made to save the patient's life by sacrificing the limb. This is a decision that only the trained emergency care provider should make.

Sterile Technique

When one is bandaging an open, bleeding wound on the field, the use of proper sterile technique is seldom possible. The objective in this case is to keep the wound as clean as possible and usually to pad and protect it so that the individual can return to play. Once the player is in a controlled environment, the wound can be properly cleaned and dressed. Providers working in a treatment center or clinic can take care to follow sterile technique. Whenever providers are treating an open wound, they should make every effort to prevent **contamination** of the wound by practicing sterile technique. Remember, we

cannot actually provide a sterile environment, but we can take measures to minimize contact with nonsterile surfaces. Generally, lacerations and abrasions are treated using Universal Precautions to prevent the transfer of bloodborne pathogens between the patient and the clinician, but true sterile technique is not followed. On the other hand, if you are treating a postsurgical site, or cleaning the pin holes on an external fixator after a bone fracture, for example, you should follow the sterile technique.

If you have had the opportunity to observe surgery, you have witnessed sterile technique. You may have noticed that the patient is draped with a sterile covering and that only the operative site is exposed. The use of a sterile work surface is the first step in preparing the work area. The sterile cloth is often prepared as part of a special packet of materials commonly used in wound cleaning (**debridement**). The instruments (scissors, forceps, and so on) are wrapped with the cloth, and the entire package is sterilized in an **autoclave**. After autoclaving, the inside of the cloth is sterile, but the outside is considered contaminated. Once the cloth is unfolded, the sterile side faces upward and makes an ideal barrier upon which to perform the wound debridement. All instruments and gauze used to treat the wound must be sterile and can be placed on the sterile cloth.

The person who will do the wound care puts on a scrub cap to cover his hair, a mask for the nose and mouth, and shoe covers. Washing the hands down to the elbows is called the "scrub" and requires repetitive circular motions on each surface of each appendage. Hospitals have specific requirements on the number of scrub strokes for each area. During scrubbing for the sterile technique, scrubbing your hands 25 to 30 strokes on each surface of each finger, followed by scrubbing (25 times) each surface of the arm in small sections, sends the germs off the hands and arms to drain off the elbow. This is repeated for the other side; care is taken not to touch the washbasin or anything nonsterile, and then the hands are allowed to air dry. If a sterile towel is available, it may be used to dry the hands. A sterile gown is donned with the help of an assistant who holds the nonsterile inside surface of the autoclaved gown and lays it over the shoulders of the clinician. The assistant ties the gown using the inside ties. Next, the sterile gloves are put on. Now the provider is "sterile," but only from the chest to the waist and from the elbows to the fingertips. Care must be taken to separate the sterile items from nonsterile items and to keep them apart throughout the procedure. Only autoclaved items or items commercially packaged as sterile can be considered sterile. If a sterile gauze pad or bandage is needed, an assistant will tear the package open and allow the pad to drop onto the sterile surface without touching the pad or the sterile field.

Nonserious Acute Injuries

When your secondary survey indicates a sprain, strain, or contusion, the problem is typically not as serious as a fracture, dislocation, or hemorrhage. These conditions, however, may seem like a very serious injury to the patient. These patients can be helped from the field and taken to the sideline or the clinic setting and rested from activity and for further evaluation. Treatment of these injuries is with ice, compression, and elevation. The acronym for the treatment is RICE: rest, ice, compression, and elevation.

- **R**est means resting from any use of the injured area rather than general sleep-type rest. If an injured joint is difficult to rest, the application of a sling or brace may be warranted.
- **I**ce is applied to constrict blood vessels and reduce swelling. Ice can be provided as crushed ice, cubed ice, ice bucket, or whirlpool. The type of ice application you choose will be based on the availability of alternate forms of ice, the body area treated, and the ability to apply the ice and also elevate the extremity.

- **C**ompression can be applied by means of an elastic bandage wrapped around the injured area, a compression sleeve, or a pneumatic compression unit. Compression should be applied during the ice application but is continued or reapplied following icing.
- **E**levation of the injured area above the level of the heart. Elevating the extremity, or lowering the level of the heart, may be necessary. Joints and body areas close to the trunk are more difficult to elevate. In such cases, if it is possible to position the patient with the injured area a little higher than the heart, this is satisfactory.

Spinal Fractures

When the mechanism of injury or the secondary survey suggests the potential of spinal injury, precautions should be taken to stabilize the patient prior to transporting. Relying on injury mechanisms alone is not sufficient in anticipating spinal injury; in fact, in a position paper for the National Association of EMS Physicians, Domeier states, "Currently, spinal immobilization is often performed based only on the mechanism of injury without consideration of the patient's symptoms and physical findings" (Domeier 1999). If the patient is unable to move an extremity or feel your pinch or touch, a spinal fracture should be suspected and spinal stabilization rendered. Stabilization is critical in that if a vertebra is fractured or displaced, the spinal cord may be injured. The state of the spinal cord at the time of the injury should be protected during stabilization and transport.

Whenever an individual suffers an injury to the head, a cervical spine injury should be suspected. In stabilization of the cervical spine, the neck should be immobilized as well as the space between the shoulders, and the skull must be firmly packed to avoid movement. The first responder on the scene will provide the initial stabilization manually using either a head-squeeze or a trapezius-squeeze technique (figure 13.6).

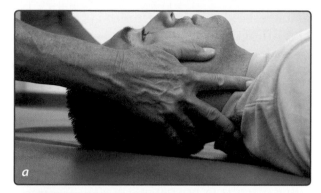

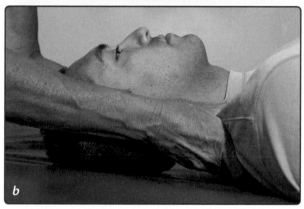

Figure 13.6 Cervical spine stabilization using the *(a)* head-squeeze technique and the *(b)* trapezius-squeeze technique.

the jaw thrust is necessary. In the preceding description, the second and third fingers appear to refer to the index and long fingers, respectively. Boissy and colleagues (2011) studied movement occurring with each of the two cervical spine manual immobilization techniques and found "little overall difference between the HS and TS when a patient is cooperative." They noted, however, that "when a patient is confused and trying to move, the HS is much worse at controlling movement compared with the TS" (p. 80).

Once the medical staff arrives with the emergency equipment, manual stabilization of the cervical spine is transferred to a special immobilization collar. The most widely accepted cervical immobilization is via a commercial cervical **extraction collar** (figure 13.7) that can be sized for the length as well as the girth of the neck.

Following stabilization of the cervical spine in the collar, the patient is transferred to a rigid board called a **spine board**. Then the patient's head is stabilized with foam or other soft materials that hold the patient's head snugly and securely on both sides, from

• ***Head squeeze (HS):*** The lead rescuer lets the patient's head rest in the palms, with the hands on both sides of the head and fingers placed so that the **ulnar** fingers can grab the mastoid process below and the second and third fingers can apply a jaw thrust if necessary (Boissy et al. 2011).

• ***Trapezius squeeze (TS):*** The rescuer grabs the patient's trapezius muscles on either side of the head with the hands (thumbs anterior to the trapezius muscle) and firmly squeezes the head between the forearms, with the forearms placed approximately at the level of the ears (Boissy et al. 2011).

In application of the head squeeze, the little finger is usually at the mastoid, and the ring finger touches the sides of the neck. The long and index fingers also stabilize the neck in relation to the head but can be moved if

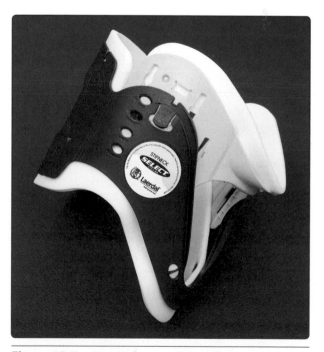

Figure 13.7 Cervical extraction collar.

the shoulders to the skull. This combination of splint and padding, fixed to a rigid spine board using adhesive tape, special straps, or both, provides excellent stabilization of the spine. In an extensive review of literature, the Spine Section of the American Association of Neurological Surgeons and the Congress of Neurological Surgeons concluded, "It appears that a combination of rigid cervical collar with supportive blocks on a rigid backboard with straps is effective at achieving safe, effective spinal immobilization for transport. The longstanding practice of attempted cervical immobilization using sandbags and tape alone is not recommended" (Spine Section of AANS and CNS 2001, p. 1).

Heat Illness

Core temperature is the temperature at which the body functions. This temperature is maintained within a very narrow range that allows body functions to occur. A core temperature above that range is called hyperthermia, and a core temperature below the range is called hypothermia.

As you learned in chapter 4, heat illness can take many forms. Heat exhaustion should be treated as soon as it is detected, and heatstroke is a true medical emergency. If you suspect that a patient is suffering from heatstroke, the best thing you can do is to call for emergency transport and cool the patient down immediately. Remove heavy clothing and submerge the patient in a cold bath; if that is not available, pack the patient in cold towels and ice packs at the axilla and groin areas especially. Call 911 as soon as possible. Put the listener on speaker phone on your cell while you continue treating the patient. Don't waste time!

Asthma and Other Forms of Bronchospasm

Air enters the lungs through the bronchial tree, a branching passageway that turns into smaller and smaller **bronchioles** until its termination deep within the lungs at the **alveoli**. The alveoli are small pouches or sacs that provide air to the capillary bed surrounding them. If parts of the bronchial tree become blocked, breathing becomes more difficult and less air is available to the circulating blood. Irritants or allergens can cause constriction of the bronchioles (the last segment of the bronchial tree prior to the alveoli), or bronchospasm. Several factors can cause bronchospasm:

- Medical conditions: Conditions such as asthma, hay fever, or upper respiratory infections may produce secretions that enter the bronchial tree.
- Environmental factors: Airborne allergens or pollutants, or chemicals like chlorine in the pool, pesticides, fertilizers, and even caulk or paint, can cause bronchiole constriction.
- Medications: Some people experience bronchial spasm when taking aspirin or anti-inflammatory medicines.

The decreased airflow into the lungs is in part due to the **constriction** of the air passageways but can also be due to inflammation in the bronchial tree.

Asthma is a form of bronchial spasm and is usually a combination of spasm and inflammation. A patient previously diagnosed with asthma usually has a prescription for an inhaler. Undiagnosed patients who begin complaining of shortness of breath and wheezing may be suffering from acute **bronchitis** or may be showing signs of asthma. When breathing difficulty begins to cause hypoxia, the patient's lips may appear a bluish color; the pulse rate increases, and the patient becomes more and more panicked. This patient requires immediate medical attention at a hospital or special care clinic. One treatment for acute, severe bronchospasm uses mechanical **ventilators**, which are machines that breathe for the patient. The ventilation may be combined with inhaled bronchodilators to open the airways and intravenous **corticosteroids** to help control the inflammatory condition.

Signs of increased respiratory stress include sudden shortness of breath, use of **intercostal** (rib) **muscles** and neck muscles to assist with breathing, and difficulty blowing the air out of the lungs. A patient demonstrating these signs should be treated with a rescue **inhaler** if it has been prescribed, **pursed-lip breathing**, and removal from the activity and the cold air if she is outdoors in cold weather. Things that often make asthma worse include exercise, exposure to cold air, and increased air density (early mornings and evenings). If rest and a controlled environment do not ease the symptoms, medical care should be sought before acute respiratory distress results.

A patient with **exercise-induced asthma (EIA)** is different from a patient with asthma. With EIA, patients have no trigger other than exercise and do not experience asthma under any other circumstances. Exercise-induced asthma is treated with the use of prescription inhalers and by modification of activity.

Posttraumatic Head Injury

Some sports, as well as some leisure activities, involve a risk of injury to the head. The risk of some severe injuries (e.g., skull fracture) can be reduced if individuals wear well-designed and well-fitted protective helmets and mouth guards (see chapter 5). However, it has not been shown that protective equipment reduces the risk of other head injuries, such as concussion. A blow to the head is a common mechanism for both brain injury and cervical spine injury. The astute clinician always checks the cervical spine when attending to a patient with an acute head injury. The greatest concern with trauma to the head is injury to the brain, **traumatic brain injury** (TBI).

The occurrence of concussions certainly cannot be prevented, yet there are many things that should be done to prevent complications from the injury. According to the Consensus Statement on Concussion in Sport (McCrory et al. 2009), a suspected concussion can involve one or more of the following clinical domains:

- Symptoms: somatic (e.g., headache), cognitive (e.g., feeling as though one is in a fog), or emotional (e.g., lability)
- Physical signs (e.g., loss of consciousness, amnesia)
- Behavioral changes (e.g., irritability)
- Cognitive impairment (e.g., slowed reaction times)
- Sleep disturbance (e.g., drowsiness)

A concussion should be suspected if any one of these components is present. An appropriate management strategy should be put into place (McCrory et al. 2009). The authors of the Consensus Statement on Concussion further recommend the following steps when a player shows any symptoms of a concussion:

- The player should be medically evaluated on-site using standard emergency management principles, and particular attention should be given to excluding a cervical spine injury.
- The appropriate disposition of the player must be determined by the treating health care provider in a timely manner. If no health care provider is available, the player should be safely removed from practice or play and urgent referral to a physician arranged.
- Once the first aid issues are addressed, an assessment of the concussive injury should be made using the SCAT2 or other similar tool.
- The player should not be left alone following the injury, and serial monitoring for deterioration is essential over the initial few hours after injury.
- A player with diagnosed concussion should not be allowed to return to play on the day of the injury.

During the sideline evaluation, the patient's cognitive function should be tested using a battery of tests that evaluate attention and memory. The Maddocks score and the Standardized Assessment of Concussion (SAC) are excellent tests to use in the sideline evaluation of cognitive function. These quick sideline tests are only the initial screening; further **neuropsychological** evaluation must be conducted off the field to help detect subtle **cognitive** changes. See the SCAT2 form (figure 13.8 on p. 329) for these evaluative tests.

Clinical Evaluation of Concussion

The SCAT2 (figure 13.8) battery of tests has been developed for both the preparticipation baseline evaluation and the postconcussion evaluation. The SCAT2 is a standardized way of evaluating a concussion and can be used with patients from 10 years of age upward. **Neuroimaging** studies and sophisticated balance testing are sometimes used when symptoms point to an **intracranial** lesion or **brain stem** pathology, respectively. Neuropsychological assessment is the assessment with the highest clinical value in concussion evaluation. **Neuropsychologists** or other highly trained individuals should review the neuropsychological (NP) tests. The NP test is performed before the patient is released to return to activity and will be an asset to making that determination.

Return-to-Play Parameters

The majority of concussions resolve over a period of a few days, with the scores on the SCAT2 test returning to the preinjury baseline in many instances. During the recovery, it is important to minimize offensive lights, sounds, and activity and to allow the brain a rest period. This cognitive rest includes limiting or eliminating mental activities such as schoolwork, texting, or playing computer or video games. Once the symptoms (headache, brain fog, and so on) disappear, a gradual return to activity should commence.

The return to sport or exercise should be gradual, with frequent monitoring of symp-toms. Realize that the patient might want to return to sport, so asking him to report any headaches, brain fog, or other symptoms may not be effective. As new physical challenges are introduced, the patient should be questioned regarding his symptoms. If the symptoms do not increase within 24 h of the change in activity level, the patient may move on to the next step upward in the activity ladder (see table 13.2; McCrory et al. 2009).

Clinicians should also be aware of specific **statutes** and policies that may affect the return-to-play decision. Several states have passed sport concussion **legislation**, which specifically defines who may clear an individual to return, how the return-to-play progression should proceed, or both. Additionally, the National Collegiate Athletic Association (NCAA), the National Federation of State High Schools (NFHS), and many state interscholastic athletic associations have developed policies that include participant, coach, and parent education; signed acknowledgement of risk forms; criteria for removal from play; and criteria for return to play. It is important to understand and follow any laws or policies that affect concussion management in your specific work setting.

Anaphylaxis

Anaphylaxis is a severe and rapidly developing reaction affecting multiple body systems at once. An anaphylactic reaction occurs when an allergen is ingested or injected into the body and thus arrives in the bloodstream for rapid distribution throughout the body. Thus the anaphylactic response is very widespread and affects a variety of body systems. Many allergic responses are mild, with itching or hives, but the severe, systemic reaction that can become life threatening is allergic anaphylaxis.

Most people with allergies know the possible triggers and early warning signs of trouble. They also are usually aware of, and in possession of, emergency anaphylaxis treatment kits. Bee stings may be the most common type of allergic anaphylaxis. People

SCAT2

 FIFA®

Sport Concussion Assessment Tool 2

Name _____

Sport/team _____

Date/time of injury _____

Date/time of assessment _____

Age _____ Gender ☐ M ☐ F

Years of education completed _____

Examiner _____

What is the SCAT2?[1]

This tool represents a standardized method of evaluating injured athletes for concussion and can be used in athletes aged from 10 years and older. It supersedes the original SCAT published in 2005[7]. This tool also enables the calculation of the Standardized Assessment of Concussion (SAC)[3,4] score and the Maddocks questions[5] for sideline concussion assessment.

Instructions for using the SCAT2

The SCAT2 is designed for the use of medical and health professionals. Preseason baseline testing with the SCAT2 can be helpful for interpreting post-injury test scores. Words in italics throughout the SCAT2 are the instructions given to the athlete by the tester.

This tool may be freely copied for distribtion to individuals, teams, groups, and organizations.

What is a concussion?

A concussion is a disturbance in brain function caused by a direct or indirect force to the head. It results in a variety of non-specific symptoms (like those listed below) and often does not involve loss of consciousness. Concussion should be suspected in the presence of **any one or more** of the following:

- Symptoms (such as headache), or
- Physical signs (such as unsteadiness), or
- Impaired brain function (e.g., confusion) or
- Abnormal behavior.

Any athlete with a suspected concussion should be REMOVED FROM PLAY, medically assessed, monitored for deterioration (i.e., should not be left alone) and should not drive a motor vehicle.

Symptom Evaluation

How do you feel?
You should score yourself on the following symptoms, based on how you feel now.

	none	mild		moderate		severe	
Headache	0	1	2	3	4	5	6
"Pressure in head"	0	1	2	3	4	5	6
Neck Pain	0	1	2	3	4	5	6
Nausea or vomiting	0	1	2	3	4	5	6
Dizziness	0	1	2	3	4	5	6
Blurred vision	0	1	2	3	4	5	6
Balance problems	0	1	2	3	4	5	6
Sensitivity to light	0	1	2	3	4	5	6
Sensitivity to noise	0	1	2	3	4	5	6
Feeling slowed down	0	1	2	3	4	5	6
Feeling like "in a fog"	0	1	2	3	4	5	6
"Don't feel right"	0	1	2	3	4	5	6
Difficulty concentrating	0	1	2	3	4	5	6
Difficulty remembering	0	1	2	3	4	5	6
Fatigue or low energy	0	1	2	3	4	5	6
Confusion	0	1	2	3	4	5	6
Drowsiness	0	1	2	3	4	5	6
Trouble falling asleep (if applicable)	0	1	2	3	4	5	6
More emotional	0	1	2	3	4	5	6
Irritability	0	1	2	3	4	5	6
Sadness	0	1	2	3	4	5	6
Nervous or Anxious	0	1	2	3	4	5	6

Total number of symptoms (Maximum possible 22) ▭

Symptom severity score
(Add all scores in table, maximum possible: 22 x 6 = 132) ▭

Do the symptoms get worse with physical activity? ☐ Y ☐ N
Do the symptoms get worse with mental activity? ☐ Y ☐ N

Overall rating
If you know the athlete well prior to the injury, how different is the athlete acting compared to his/her usual self? Please circle one response.

no different	very different	unsure

Figure 13.8 The SCAT2. *(continued)*

Cognitive & Physical Evaluation

1 Symptom score (from page 1)

22 **minus** number of symptoms | of 22

2 Physical signs score

Was there loss of consciousness or unresponsiveness? | Y | N
If yes, how long? _____ minutes
Was there a balance problem/unsteadiness? | Y | N

Physical signs score (1 point for each negative response) | of 2

3 Glasgow coma scale (GCS)

Best eye response (E)

No eye opening	1
Eye opening in response to pain	2
Eye opening to speech	3
Eyes opening spontaneously	4

Best verbal response (V)

No verbal response	1
Incomprehensible sounds	2
Inappropriate words	3
Confused	4
Oriented	5

Best motor response (M)

No motor response	1
Extension to pain	2
Abnormal flexion to pain	3
Flexion/Withdrawal to pain	4
Localizes to pain	5
Obeys commands	6

Glasgow Coma score (E + V + M) | of 15

GCS should be recorded for all athletes in case of subsequent deterioration.

4 Sideline Assessment – Maddocks Score

"I am going to ask you a few questions, please listen carefully and give your best effort."

Modified Maddocks questions (1 point for each correct answer)

At what venue are we at today?	0	1
Which half is it now?	0	1
Who scored last in this match?	0	1
What team did you play last week/game?	0	1
Did your team win the last game?	0	1

Maddocks score | of 5

Maddocks score is validated for sideline diagnosis of concussion only and is not included in SCAT2 summary score for serial testing.

5 Cognitive assessment
Standardized Assessment of Concussion (SAC)

Orientation (1 point for each correct answer)

What month is it?	0	1
What is the date today?	0	1
What is the day of the week?	0	1
What year is it?	0	1
What time is it right now? (within 1 hour)	0	1

Orientation score | of 5

Immediate memory

"I am going to test your memory. I will read you a list of words and when I am done, repeat back as many words as you can remember, in any order."

Trials 2 & 3:
"I am going to repeat the same list again. Repeat back as many words as you can remember in any order, even if you said the word before."

Complete all 3 trials regardless of score on trials 1 & 2. Read the words at a rate of one per second. Score 1 pt. for each correct response. Total score equals sum across all 3 trials. Do not inform the athlete that delayed recall will be tested.

List	Trial 1	Trial 2	Trial 3	Alternative word list		
elbow	0 1	0 1	0 1	candle	baby	finger
apple	0 1	0 1	0 1	paper	monkey	penny
carpet	0 1	0 1	0 1	sugar	perfume	blanket
saddle	0 1	0 1	0 1	sandwich	sunset	lemon
bubble	0 1	0 1	0 1	wagon	iron	insect
Total						

Immediate memory score | of 15

Concentration
Digits Backward:
"I am going to read you a string of numbers and when I am done, you repeat them back to me backwards, in reverse order of how I read them to you. For example, if I say 7-1-9, you would say 9-1-7."

If correct, go to next string length. If incorrect, read trial 2. One point possible for each string length. Stop after incorrect on both trials. The digits should be read at the rate of one per second.

Alternative digit lists

4-9-3	0 1	6-2-9	5-2-6	4-1-5
3-8-1-4	0 1	3-2-7-9	1-7-9-5	4-9-6-8
6-2-9-7-1	0 1	1-5-2-8-6	3-8-5-2-7	6-1-8-4-3
7-1-8-4-6-2	0 1	5-3-9-1-4-8	8-3-1-9-6-4	7-2-4-8-5-6

Months in Reverse Order:
"Now tell me the months of the year in reverse order. Start with the last month and go backward. So you'll say December, November ... Go ahead"

1 pt. for entire sequence correct

Dec-Nov-Oct-Sept-Aug-Jul-Jun-May-Apr-Mar-Feb-Jan | 0 | 1

Concentration score | of 5

---

[1] This tool has been developed by a group of international experts at the 3rd International Consensus meeting on Concussion in Sport held in Zurich, Switzerland in November 2008. The full details of the conference outcomes and the authors of the tool are published in British Journal of Sports Medicine, 2009, volume 43, supplement 1.

The outcome paper will also be simultaneously co-published in the May 2009 issues of Clinical Journal of Sports Medicine, Physical Medicine & Rehabilitation, Journal of Athletic Training, Journal of Clinical Neuroscience, Journal of Science & Medicine in Sport, Neurosurgery, Scandinavian Journal of Science & Medicine in Sport and the Journal of Clinical Sports Medicine.

[2] McCrory, P., et al. Summary and agreement statement of the 2nd International Conference on Concussion in Sport, Prague 2004. *British Journal of Sports Medicine*. 2005; 39: 196-204.

[3] McCrea M. Standardized mental status testing of acute concussion. *Clinical Journal of Sports Medicine*. 2001; 11: 176-181.

[4] McCrea M., Randolph C., Kelly, J. Standardized Assessment of Concussion: Manual for administration, scoring and interpretation. Waukesha, Wisconsin, USA.

[5] Maddocks, D.L., Dicker, G.D., Saling, M.M. (1995) The assessment of orientation following concussion in athletes. *Clin J Sport Med*. 5(1): 32–3.

[6] Guskiewicz K.M. Assessment of postural stability following sport-related concussion. *Current Sports Medicine Reports*. 2003; 2: 24-30.

Figure 13.8 *(continued)* The SCAT2. *(continued)*

6 Balance examination

This balance testing is based on a modified version of the Balance Error Scoring System (BESS)[6]. A stopwatch or watch with a second hand is required for this testing.

Balance testing
"I am now going to test your balance. Please take your shoes off, roll up your pant legs above the ankle (if applicable), and remove any ankle taping (if applicable). This test will consist of three twenty-second tests with different stances."

(a) Double-leg stance:
"The first stance is standing with your feet together with your hands on your hips and with your eyes closed. You should try to maintain stability in that position for 20 seconds. I will be counting the number of times you move out of this position. I will start timing when you are set and have closed your eyes."

(b) Single-leg stance:
"If you were to kick a ball, which foot would you use? [This will be the dominant foot] Now stand on your non-dominant foot. The dominant leg should be held in approximately 30 degrees of hip flexion and 45 degrees of knee flexion. Again, you should try to maintain stability for 20 seconds with your hands on your hips and your eyes closed. I will be counting the number of times you move out of this position. If you stumble out of this position, open your eyes and return to the start position and continue balancing. I will start timing when you are set and have closed your eyes."

(c) Tandem stance:
"Now stand heel-to-toe with your **non-dominant foot** in back. Your weight should be evenly distributed across both feet. Again, you should try to maintain stability for 20 seconds with your hands on your hips and your eyes closed. I will be counting the number of times you move out of this position. If you stumble out of this position, open your eyes and return to the start position and continue balancing. I will start timing when you are set and have closed your eyes."

Balance testing – types of errors
1. Hands lifted off iliac crest
2. Opening eyes
3. Step, stumble, or fall
4. Moving hip into > 30 degrees abduction
5. Lifting forefoot or heel
6. Remaining out of test position > 5 sec

Each of the 20-second trials is scored by counting the errors, or deviations from the proper stance, accumulated by the athlete. The examiner will begin counting errors only after the individual has assumed the proper start position. **The modified BESS is calculated by adding one error point for each error during the three 20-second tests. The maximum total number of errors for any single condition is 10.** If an athlete commits multiple errors simultaneously, only one error is recorded but the athlete should quickly return to the testing position, and counting should resume once subject is set. Subjects that are unable to maintain the testing procedure for a minimum of **five seconds** at the start are assigned the highest possible score, ten, for that testing condition.

Which foot was tested?　　☐ Left　　☐ Right
(i.e., which is the **non-dominant** foot)

Condition	Total errors
Double-Leg Stance (feet together)	of 10
Single-leg stance (non-dominant foot)	of 10
Tandem stance (non-dominant foot at back)	of 10
Balance examination score (30 **minus** total errors)	of 30

7 Coordination examination

Upper limb coordination
Finger-to-nose (FTN) task: "I am going to test your coordination now. Please sit comfortably on the chair with your eyes open and your arm (either right or left) outstretched (shoulder flexed to 90 degrees and elbow and fingers extended). When I give a start signal, I would like you to perform five successive finger-to-nose repetitions using your index finger to touch the tip of the nose as quickly and as accurately as possible."

Which arm was tested?　　☐ Left　　☐ Right

Scoring:　　5 correct repetitions in < 4 seconds = 1

Note for testers: Athletes fail the test if they do not touch their nose, do not fully extend their elbow or do not perform five repetitions. Failure should be scored as 0.

Coordination score ⟶ of 1

8 Cognitive assessment

Standardized Assessment of Concussion (SAC)

Delayed recall
"Do you remember that list of words I read a few times earlier? Tell me as many words from the list as you can remember in any order."

Circle each word correctly recalled. Total score equals number of words recalled.

List	Alternative word list		
elbow	candle	baby	finger
apple	paper	monkey	penny
carpet	sugar	perfume	blanket
saddle	sandwich	sunset	lemon
bubble	wagon	iron	insect

Delayed recall score ⟶ of 5

Overall score

Test domain	Score
Symptom score	of 22
Physical signs score	of 2
Glasgow Coma score (E + V + M)	of 15
Balance examination score	of 30
Coordination score	of 1
Subtotal	**of 70**
Orientation score	of 5
Immediate memory score	of 5
Concentration score	of 15
Delayed recall score	of 5
SAC subtotal	**of 30**
SCAT2 total	**of 100**
Maddocks Score	**of 5**

Definitive normative data for a SCAT2 "cut-off" score is not available at this time and will be developed in prospective studies. Embedded within the SCAT2 is the SAC score that can be utilized separately in concussion management. The scoring system also takes on particular clinical significance during serial assessment where it can be used to document either a decline or an improvement in neurological functioning.

Scoring data from the SCAT2 or SAC should not be used as a stand alone method to diagnose concussion, measure recovery, or make decisions about an athlete's readiness to return to competition after concussion.

Figure 13.8 (continued) The SCAT2. (continued)

Athlete Information

Any athlete suspected of having a concussion should be removed from play and then seek medical evaluation.

Signs to watch for

Problems could arise over the first 24-48 hours. You should not be left alone and must go to a hospital at once if you:

- Have a headache that gets worse
- Are very drowsy or can't be awakened (woken up)
- Can't recognize people or places
- Have repeated vomiting
- Behave unusually or seem confused; are very irritable
- Have seizures (arms and legs jerk uncontrollably)
- Have weak or numb arms or legs
- Are unsteady on your feet; have slurred speech

Remember, it is better to be safe.
Consult your doctor after a suspected concussion.

Return to play

Athletes should not be returned to play the same day of injury. When returning athletes to play, they should follow a stepwise symptom-limited program, with stages of progression. For example:

1. rest until asymptomatic (physical and mental rest)
2. light aerobic exercise (e.g., stationary cycle)
3. sport-specific exercise
4. non-contact training drills (start light resistance training)
5. full contact training after medical clearance
6. return to competition (game play)

There should be approximately 24 hours (or longer) for each stage and the athlete should return to stage 1 if symptoms recur. Resistance training should only be added in the later stages.
Medical clearance should be given before return to play.

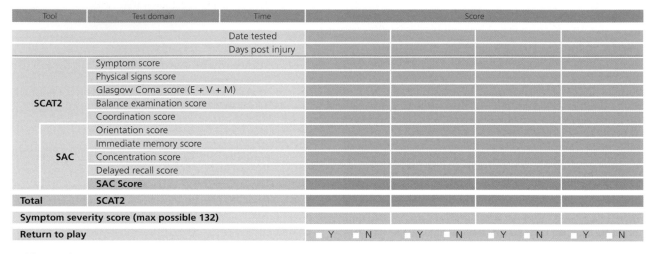

Tool	Test domain	Time	Score			
		Date tested				
		Days post injury				
SCAT2	Symptom score					
	Physical signs score					
	Glasgow Coma score (E + V + M)					
	Balance examination score					
	Coordination score					
SAC	Orientation score					
	Immediate memory score					
	Concentration score					
	Delayed recall score					
	SAC Score					
Total	SCAT2					
Symptom severity score (max possible 132)						
Return to play			☐ Y ☐ N	☐ Y ☐ N	☐ Y ☐ N	☐ Y ☐ N

Additional comments

_____

_____

✂ -

Concussion injury advice (To be given to concussed athlete)

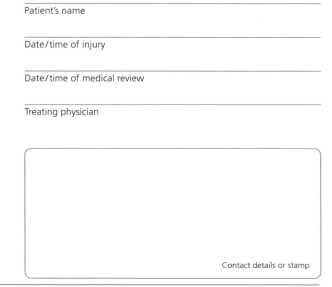

This patient has received an injury to the head. A careful medical examination has been carried out and no sign of any serious complications has been found. It is expected that recovery will be rapid, but the patient will need monitoring for a further period by a responsible adult. Your treating physician will provide guidance as to this time frame.

If you notice any change in behavior, vomiting, dizziness, worsening headache, double vision, or excessive drowsiness, please telephone the clinic or the nearest hospital emergency department immediately.

Other important points:

- **Rest and avoid strenuous activity for at least 24 hours**
- **No alcohol**
- **No sleeping tablets**
- **Use paracetamol or codeine for headache. Do not use aspirin or anti-inflammatory medication**
- **Do not drive until medically cleared**
- **Do not train or play sport until medically cleared**

Clinic phone number _____

Patient's name

Date/time of injury

Date/time of medical review

Treating physician

Contact details or stamp

Figure 13.8 *(continued)* The SCAT2.

Reprinted from McCrory et al. 2009.

Table 13.2	Graduated Return-to-Play Protocol	
Rehabilitation stage	Functional exercise at each stage of rehabilitation	Objective at each stage
1. No activity	Complete physical and cognitive rest	Recovery
2. Light aerobic exercise	Walking, swimming, or stationary cycling, keeping intensity <70% MPHR (maximal personal heart rate); no resistance training	Increasing HR (heart rate)
3. Sport-specific exercise	Skating drills in ice hockey, running drills in soccer; no head impact activities	Addition of movement
4. Noncontact training drills	Progression to more complex training drills, for example, passing drills in football and ice hockey; may start progressive resistance training	Exercise, coordination, and cognitive load
5. Full contact practice	Following medical clearance, participation in normal training activities	Restoring confidence and assessment of functional skills by coaching staff
6. Return to play	Normal game play	

who are prone to allergic anaphylaxis to bee stings often carry an epinephrine auto-injector with them when the risk of bee stings is high.

If a patient is unaware of an allergy and shows signs of anaphylaxis, call 911 immediately. If the patient is aware of the allergy and has an epinephrine auto-injector, inject the **epinephrine** immediately and rub the injection point to distribute the medicine. If the patient is conscious, elevate the feet to bring more oxygenated blood to the brain. Stay with the patient until the ambulance arrives. If the patient stops breathing, begin rescue breathing; if the heart stops, begin cardiac compressions.

Exercise-induced anaphylaxis has been described in the literature and is reported to be a "rare disorder in which anaphylaxis occurs after physical activity. The symptoms may include **pruritus**, hives, **flushing**, wheezing, and GI involvement, including nausea, abdominal cramping and diarrhea. If physical activity continues, patients may progress to more severe symptoms, including **angioedema**, **laryngeal edema**, hypotension and ultimately, **cardiovascular collapse**. Cessation of physical activity usually results in immediate improvement of symptoms" (Huynh 2011).

Care Principles for Musculoskeletal Injuries

The greatest majority of injuries seen in physically active individuals are injuries to the musculoskeletal system: bone, joints, muscles, and the tissue connecting them. Acute care of an injury to a patient in the midst of a game may differ slightly from the acute care of an injury presented by the patient in the clinic. On the field, the primary and secondary surveys provide information regarding the need for immediate on-the-field care and answer questions on the method to be used to move the individual from the field. A patient who reports to the treatment clinic may have an acute injury that surfaced overnight, or may have an issue that arose during sport participation but did not require immediate medical attention. In this acute situation, the primary survey is skipped since the patient is ambulatory and able to talk. Whatever the presentation, the immediate (acute) care of the musculoskeletal injury will involve the RICE treatment described earlier. Asking the individual to rest does not mean asking her to become sedentary; rest is for the injured joint or extremity. When picturing how to rest a shoulder or elbow, you might think of using a sling. That would be a good choice. In addition to a sling, some injuries may benefit from a splint, and lower extremity injuries may require ambulatory assistance, for example, with crutches.

Splinting

Splinting is a commonly used technique in the acute care of orthopedic injuries. The primary purpose of splinting is to immobilize above and below the fracture, spanning past the adjacent joints if possible. When one is splinting a joint injury, the splint should cover the bone proximal and distal to the injured area.

Splints can be made of various materials; the important thing is the length parameter. Hikers have been known to use branches from trees to immobilize a fracture while they were in a remote location. In the clinic and on the field, splinting materials are usually available. Splints can be wooden, aluminum, hard plastic, or **pneumatic**. Care must be taken to avoid pressure over nerves and to allow easy access to a distal pulse point. Pressure on a nerve that is close to the surface (ulnar nerve at the medial **epicondyle** of the humerus or **common fibular nerve** at the lateral aspect of the **fibular head**) can lead to compression on the nerve, further complicating the orthopedic injury under treatment. The pulse should be taken before splinting, again after the splint is applied, and occasionally thereafter until the splint can be removed. A diminishing pulse indicates increased pressure on the artery and must be reported to emergency personnel.

Splinting of an injury on the playing field is done to allow the participant to be safely moved from the play area. Once the individual is to the sideline or has been moved into a clinic room, the splint is usually removed for further evaluation. In the event of a fracture, however, once applied, the splint is not removed until the **radiology** staff or physicians deem this appropriate. Many of the materials that splints are made with are **radiolucent**, meaning they need not be removed for a **radiograph**.

Crutches

Crutches are often needed to fully rest a lower extremity injury. Several types of crutches are available, but two types are most commonly used: underarm and forearm crutches. The underarm crutch is best for someone unaccustomed to crutches who will have to use the **ambulatory** device for only a short period of time (less than a month). Underarm crutches require some upper body strength but not as much as the forearm crutches do. Forearm crutches were designed by Lofstrand and are often referred to as Lofstrand crutches; they are also sometimes called Canadian crutches. Regardless of the name, these crutches put the weight on the forearms rather than the axillae. A cuff fits around the forearm, and the hand rests on a handle. These crutches are more often used for people who need to use crutches for an extended period of time. The forearm crutch allows more use of the hands, making long-term crutch walking less of an inconvenience.

The axillary crutch (figure 13.9*a*) is fitted with the patient standing if possible. The crutch tip is situated about 6 to 8 in. away from the patient's foot during upright standing. In this position, the axillary pad of the crutch should be about two or three finger widths (about 1 in.) from the patient's axilla. If the patient is unable to stand, the approximate height of the axillary pad is usually 16 in. less than the patient's height. The hand should be positioned on the hand rest, and the elbow should be bent approximately 30°. Axillary crutches can be adjusted for overall height and hand pad position. The forearm crutch (figure 13.9*b*) handle should position the elbow at around 15° to 20° of flexion, and the crutch length should be sufficient to place the crutch tip about 6 in. in front of the foot and about 2 to 3 in. to the side. The forearm cuff should be about 1 to 1/2 in. from the elbow.

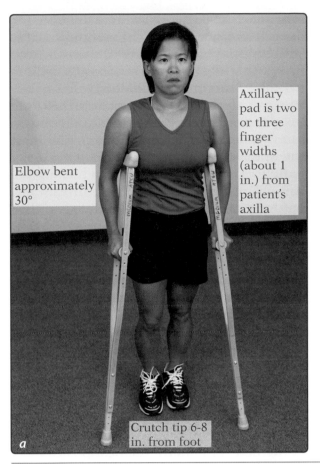

Elbow bent approximately 30°

Axillary pad is two or three finger widths (about 1 in.) from patient's axilla

Crutch tip 6-8 in. from foot

a

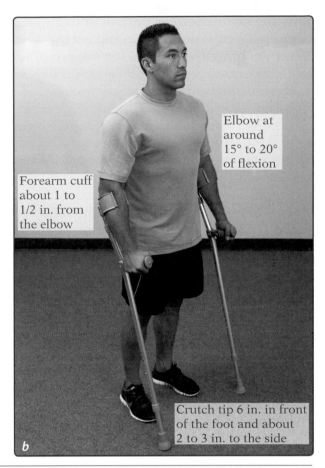

Elbow at around 15° to 20° of flexion

Forearm cuff about 1 to 1/2 in. from the elbow

Crutch tip 6 in. in front of the foot and about 2 to 3 in. to the side

b

Figure 13.9 Fitting *(a)* an underarm crutch and *(b)* a forearm crutch.

Moving and Transporting Injured Patients

Patients may require assistance in moving from the location where they were injured to a medical facility. If the injury does not involve a weight-bearing bone or joint and there is no reason to suspect spinal injury, the patient may be assisted with walking. When you decide to walk patients from the place of injury, monitor their pulse rate and cognitive level as you move them from lying to sitting and then to standing. **Syncope** (fainting) could result if the patient is moved from the ground to standing too quickly. Hypotension in this situation is termed **orthostatic hypotension** and results because of a sudden drop in the blood pressure as the patient stands up.

Moving the Injured Patient Onto a Spine Board

If a spinal injury is suspected, care must be taken to stabilize the spine both during the transfer onto the spine board and while the patient is on the spine board. Stabilizing the entire spine and moving the head and body as a unit help to minimize further damage. The Spine Section of the American Association of Neurological Surgeons and the Congress of Neurological Surgeons reported that "3%-25% of spinal cord injuries occur after the initial traumatic insult, either during transit or early in the course of management" (Spine Section of AANS and CNS 2001, p. 1). Extreme care must be taken in moving a patient with a suspected spine injury. Often the patient is not in a supine position and must be positioned on the board in supine. Although four individuals could act together to move an injured person, it is wise to practice and repractice the skills and techniques with your medical team.

Moving the Patient From a Prone Position

If the patient is lying facedown (prone) or semiprone, he should be rolled onto his back using the log-roll method (figure 13.10). Before he is moved, a cervical immobilization collar should be applied. The immobilizer is slid under the patient's neck, with care taken to keep the neck in the position in which it was found. Once the collar is applied, the log roll can commence. At least four individuals are required to roll the patient onto the spine board: Three are needed to complete the roll, and one is needed to position the board.

The lead rescuer positions her hands to stabilize the cervical spine, taking care to anticipate the end position if she's turning the patient from prone to a supine position so that her arms do not become crossed. This rescuer remains at the patient's head and instructs the other rescuers in the operation. Rescuer 2 is positioned at the shoulders, rescuer 3 at the patient's hips. Rescuers 2 and 3 reach across the patient to take a firm grasp of his body. These two rescuers share in the responsibility of rolling the body and should overlap their arms in grasping the patient. Rescuer 4 obtains the spine board and positions it near the patient. The board will need to be between the patient and the rescuers so that the patient can be rolled onto his side and then down onto supine on the spine board. The lead rescuer instructs the other rescuers in any adjustments that should be made as well as communicating what the team will be doing. On the command of the lead rescuer, the rolling begins. The rescuers roll the patient toward his side and continue rolling into a supine position on the waiting board. Once the person is on the board, small adjustments in position may be made using a slide method. Rescuers positioned around the patient, on the command of the lead rescuer, slide the patient on the surface of the board to obtain the best position.

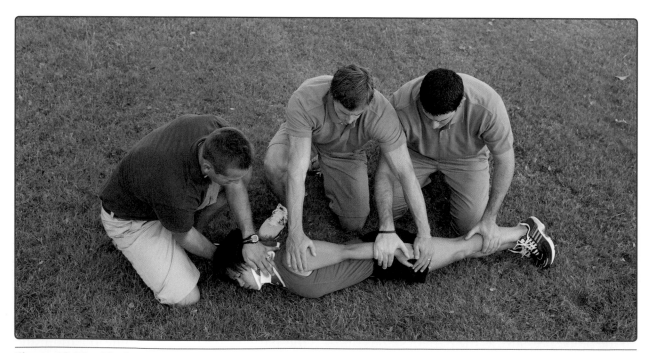

Figure 13.10 The log-roll method.

Moving the Patient From a Supine Position

Once the cervical immobilization collar has been applied, there are two methods of lifting the patient onto a spine board from a supine position: the log-roll method and the lift and slide method. In a study of head motion during the two lifting techniques, Boissy and colleagues (2009) found the lift and slide method superior to the log-roll method. The log-roll method just described is the same if the patient is found in a supine position, with the exception of the amount of movement required. In this technique, the rescuers are on one side of the patient, and the spine board is positioned on the patient's opposite side. The lead rescuer instructs the team how much to roll, when to stop, and when to begin the gradual roll back onto the spine board. It is important to move patients only a minimum distance to position them safely on the board. While the rescuers have the patient rolled upward, rescuer 4 gently slides the board between the patient and the surface.

In the lift and slide method, once the cervical immobilizer collar is applied and the lead rescuer is still in control of the head and the team, the rescuers position themselves straddling the patient at the shoulders, hips, and legs (see figure 13.11). The lead rescuer stabilizes the head and neck as she orders the team to lift the patient in unison. The lift is only high enough to slide the spine board under the patient, and guiding the lift is the responsibility of the lead rescuer. The rescuers must have a stance wide enough to allow the board to slide between their feet. The lead rescuer determines the stop point for the sliding board so that the patient is well positioned; "Slide the board until you hit my shoe" is an adequate command. When the board is in position, the lead rescuer gives the command to lower the patient on a specified count (usually a count of 3). Once the patient is on the board, minor adjustments can be made using a slight lift and slide technique.

When the patient is in the proper position, head padding and straps are applied in a crossing fashion to stabilize the patient on

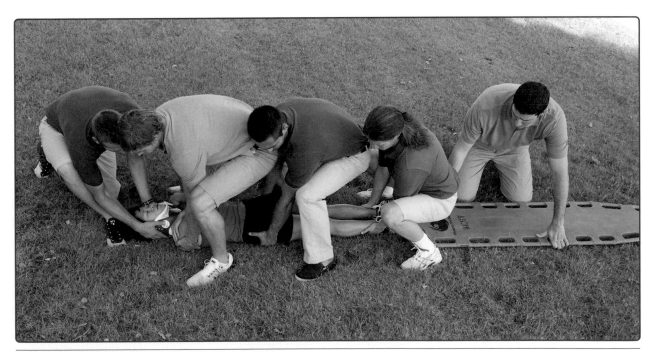

Figure 13.11   The lift and slide technique.

the board. When the straps are secure and the head is well padded and strapped, the spine board may be lifted. The lead rescuer gives the instructions, for example, "We will lift on 3 and bring the board to the level of the gurney." The team lifts the board and places it gently on the waiting gurney. Monitoring of the patient's condition (level of consciousness, vital signs) should continue until he is transferred to the next level of care.

Moving the Injured Patient Off the Field

If the injury involves a weight-bearing bone or joint, that extremity should be stabilized before the patient is moved. The injury must be splinted so that the bones or joints above and below the injury are immobilized. Once the bone or joint is stabilized, the patient may need to be transferred onto a stretcher and moved on a rolling gurney or transported by a manual carry or a **wheeled transporter** (wheelchair or motorized or nonmotorized transporter).

Manual Carry Techniques

When individuals have an injury to the upper extremity, it is usually very simple to help them off the playing surface. When the injury involves the weight-bearing lower extremity, the patient will require help getting off the field. The help may be assistive, or the individual may need to be picked up and carried. The condition of the patient, patient size, and the rescuers' sizes all factor into the decision of how to help. When the rescuers are as tall as or taller than the patient, the patient can place one arm over the two rescuers' shoulders as they assist him to the sideline (see figure 13.12). Often, the other participants on the court or field are the same size as the injured individual and can be used to help him to the sideline. If it is deemed best to pick the patient up and carry him, the technique is similar to the assist; but the rescuers interlock their arms to form a seat and backrest. The interlocked arms are situated under the

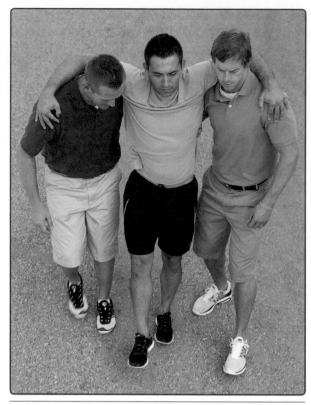

Figure 13.12 Assist method of helping an injured patient off the playing surface.

patient's thighs and behind him to support his back (see figure 13.13). This technique works well if the individual is smaller than the rescuers.

Transporting the Injured Patient From an Unstable Surface

In athletics, it is not uncommon to have an unstable surface from which to work to stabilize the spine of a participant. Two settings in which the surface is unstable are the swimming or diving pool and the gymnastics pit, a foam-filled pit for vaulting and tumbling. In each of these settings, the rescue team must practice repeatedly to ensure that they can respond to an emergency should one occur.

Swimming Pool

In the swimming pool, the spine board is **buoyant**, giving the task unique challenges.

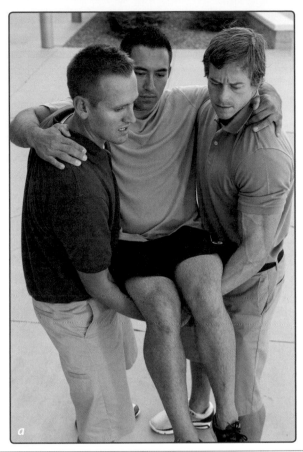
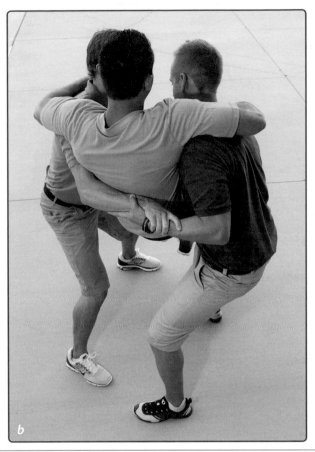

Figure 13.13   Carrying an injured patient off the playing surface. *(a)* Front view and *(b)* rear view showing the rescuers' interlocked arms.

(figure 13.14). Once the lead rescuer stabilizes the cervical spine, the spine board may be brought into the pool. With continuous immobilization of the cervical spine, the other rescuers **submerge** the board enough that it can be brought under the body of the injured swimmer. Once the board is parallel to the floor of the pool, the board is allowed to rise up and bring the swimmer to the surface. If it is too difficult to submerge the board, the patient may need to be gently floated to the pool edge where additional leverage can be obtained.

Care is taken throughout the procedure to keep the neck and spine in an immobile position. Once strapped onto the board, the patient can be extricated from the pool, with several individuals assisting in the lift. Rescue breathing may be needed and is difficult to perform when the rescuer is in the water unsupported. As the rescuer rises to give the rescue breaths, the board and patient will submerge. This makes it necessary to move the patient to the side of the pool and to use the wall for support or quickly move the patient out of the pool to begin needed steps of CPR. The situation calling for CPR in the pool necessitates a more rapid extrication from the water to enable correct performance of chest compressions.

Gymnastics Foam Pit

When a gymnast appears to have injured the spine and is lying in the foam pit, the rescuers must take extreme care as they enter the pit so that they do not cause movement of the foam supporting the patient (figure 13.15). If the position of the injured patient is such that a rescuer can lie on the edge of the pit and effectively stabilize the cervical spine,

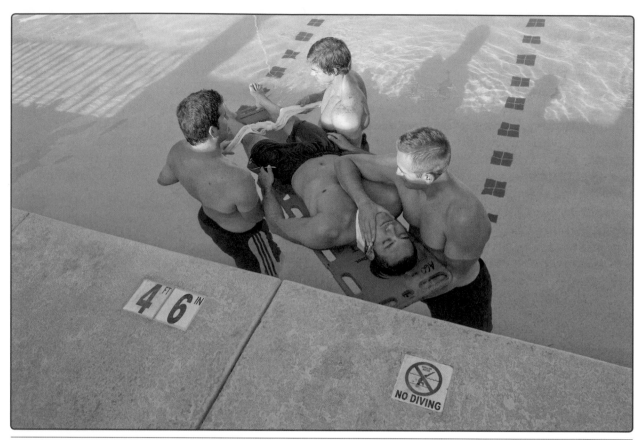

Figure 13.14 Preparing for extrication from a swimming pool.

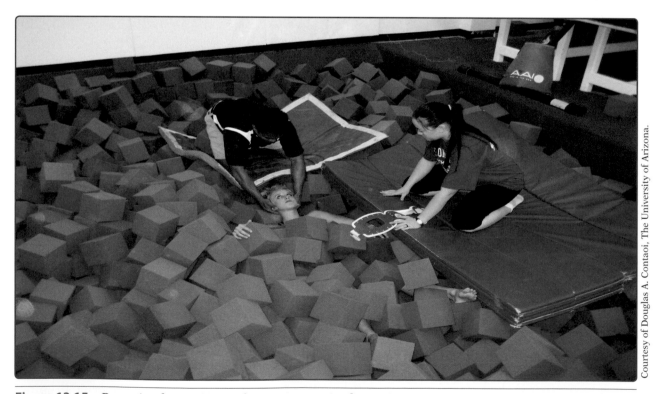

Figure 13.15 Preparing for extrication from a gymnastics foam pit.

this should occur before anyone enters the pit. When possible, place mats on the foam blocks to provide a more stable surface from which to work. Once the rescuers are situated next to the patient, they should stabilize her using manual immobilization and then apply the neck immobilization. The spine board is then handed to one of the rescuers. Using the best lifting technique possible, the rescuers move the patient onto the spine board and stabilize her as in any spine boarding situation. Lifting the patient from the pit is possible once she is stabilized on the spine board.

Transporting the Injured Patient to a Campus Health Center

College campuses usually have a student health center where radiographs can be obtained and other medical professionals are available. To transport a patient with a non-life-threatening condition, call your campus police department. These personnel are often able to provide car transportation for the patient. Using a personal car for transport is not recommended because of the liability involved. Should you wish to transport the patient to the athletic department's medical care center, you could use a golf cart set up for transport or a simple wheelchair. If the injury is not severe and does not involve weight-bearing bones or joints, the athlete may be allowed to walk to the athletic department or student health center if accompanied by two assistants. If the patient is walking, two assistants must be ready to do a two-person carry should he have difficulties.

Transporting the Injured Athlete to a Hospital

When an injured individual's condition warrants hospital care, 911 should be called. Once the ambulance arrives, the care of the patient is transferred to the emergency personnel on the ambulance. Be sure to relay any and all of the patient's pertinent medical information to the emergency providers. Some ambulance companies permit a rider to accompany the patient. Should that be possible, be sure to respect the need to follow ambulance and hospital **protocol** and not interfere with the providers' duties.

Should the patient need to go to the hospital in a nonemergency situation, you may elect to use a school vehicle for the transport. Be aware that if you use a school employee and vehicle to transport an injured patient, liability for further injury is upon the driver and the school. Use of a personal vehicle for transporting an injured patient is not recommended because of the increased personal risk involved.

Learning Aids

SUMMARY

Acute care in athletics differs from the acute care of minor injuries. This chapter provides details on the acute care of serious illness and injury in athletics. Injuries to the spine pose the greatest concern with respect to skilled stabilization and transport. It is important to understand the use of the spine board to stabilize the spine, as well as the use of splints to cover the joints above and below an injured bone in the stabilization of an upper extremity fracture.

Transporting an injured player from the field or court can be done in a variety of ways once the injury is identified and stabilization provided. The rescuer must understand the techniques and then practice them. It is only through practice that the skills can be refined to the point that one is able to help in a real emergency. Thought and practice must occur in all venues: outdoor fields, tracks, indoor courts, vast areas like a golf course, aquatic venues, and even the gymnastics foam pit. Practice of spine stabilization and transport must occur in those settings with the people who will most often be present. This is all part of the well-designed emergency care plan: Think, discuss, map it out, and practice.

Severe bleeding should usually abate with immobilization of the injured area and direct pressure over the wound. If the hemorrhage continues, other techniques can be used to stop the bleeding. Whenever blood is present, care must be taken to avoid direct contact between the patient and the provider through the application of Universal Precautions. If a wound is susceptible to infection, the sterile technique may need to be employed.

Musculoskeletal injuries are often acute yet not serious. The general treatment of those injuries is rest, ice, compression, and elevation (RICE). Rest is provided through splinting and sometimes the use of crutches. Application of splints and fitting of crutches present other practice opportunities that will enable the provider to act efficiently and quickly.

Acute care is not limited to injuries to structures of the musculoskeletal system; it also includes conditions that could compromise bodily function. When sufficient oxygen does not reach the tissues, tissue will incur damage. The most important tissue is the brain. Lack of oxygen to the brain results first in fainting but could escalate to death. Oxygen is provided to the bloodstream, but this depends on a good working environment between the lungs and the heart. Low oxygen levels can occur with asthma and bronchitis; and if not enough oxygen is provided to the bloodstream, the brain does not receive sufficient oxygen and fainting will occur. Likewise, if the heart is not working effectively, the brain is the organ at highest risk. Many acute care conditions affect the interaction between the cardiovascular and respiratory systems, resulting in fainting, shock, or both.

Acute care is a complex and multifaceted subject area. Through the reading of this chapter you should realize the depth and breadth of injuries and illnesses that are or could become serious and that require astuteness, skill, and efficiency on the part of the health care provider.

KEY CONCEPTS AND REVIEW

▶ **Explain the eight steps in developing an emergency action plan.**

(1) Game and practice coverage, (2) procedural steps, (3) communication systems, (4) equipment, (5) emergency care facilities, (6) transportation, (7) personnel training, and (8) record keeping.

▶ **Identify the elements of "vitals," or vital signs, and explain each.**

The elements of vitals are pulse, blood pressure, respiratory rate, and temperature. Pulse indicates the function of the heart. The pulse rate indicates how fast the heart is working; the faster the rate, the less time for the chambers to fill. A very slow rate may indicate that the heart is going to stop. Blood pressure indicates the cardiac output and the peripheral resistance in the vessels. Blood pressure that is too high is a risk for vessel rupture; blood pressure that is too low will cause fainting. Respiratory rate indicates the rate and quality of the patient's breathing. If it is not enough, fainting may occur. Body temperature indicates the presence or absence of a fever, or the person may be suffering from heat illness if the internal temperature cannot be dissipated.

▶ **Explain the American College of Surgeons' ranking of trauma hospitals.**

The ACS ranks hospitals according to the level of care they can provide. Level I trauma centers have a full range of specialists in-house 24 h a day and are the best centers for the handling of severe trauma. The other levels, II through IV, have progressively fewer services available.

▶ **Explain the numbers given as the blood pressure reading—what they are and what they represent.**

The top number is the first thump sound heard when blood pressure is taken and is the systolic reading, the pressure during the pumping phase of the heart. The bottom number, the last thump sound heard when blood pressure is taken, is the diastolic reading, the pressure during the refilling phase of the heart.

▶ **Explain methods used in controlling bleeding.**

Means of controlling bleeding include direct pressure on the wound; splinting of a fracture to stop movement and allow clotting; pressure over a major artery proximal to the injury site; or, as a last resort, a tourniquet.

▶ **Explain the sterile technique and compare and contrast it to Universal Precautions.**

Sterile technique is a system of cleaning, gowning, and working so that anything that comes into contact with the patient's open wound is sterile. It is similar to Universal Precautions in that both methods require clinicians to cover themselves. However, with sterile technique the reason for gowning and gloving is to prevent contamination of a wound, while Universal Precautions are used to prevent transferral of bloodborne pathogens between the patient and the clinician.

▶ **Explain the difference between the head-squeeze and the trapezius-squeeze techniques of manual stabilization of the cervical spine.**

In the head squeeze, the rescuer cradles the patient's head in the palms of his hands, with the little fingers at the mastoid process of the skull, the ring finger touching the skull and neck, and the index and long fingers stabilizing but ready to apply the jaw thrust if needed. In the trapezius-squeeze technique, the rescuer's hands are on the patient's trapezius, and the patient's head is sandwiched between the rescuer's forearms. The two methods were found to be equally effective if the patient was cooperative, but the trapezius squeeze was more effective if the patient was confused and trying to move.

▶ **Explain the two techniques for moving the patient onto a spine board from a supine position.**

The two techniques are the log roll and the lift and slide method. In the log roll, the patient is rolled onto her side; the board is moved into position opposite the rescuers; the patient is rolled onto the tilted spine board; and then the patient and board are returned to the horizontal position as a unit. In the lift and slide, the rescuers stand over the patient and on command lift the patient in unison while the board is slid under the patient. On command, the rescuers lower the patient's body in unison to the surface of the board. If minor adjustments are needed, the rescuers slide the patient at the lead rescuer's commands.

PRACTICE!

For hands-on practice in this area, go to the web resource and complete the following:

Level 1.4, Module C3: Emergency Action Plans

Level 1.4, Module C8: Rest, Ice, Compression, Elevation, and Support (RICES)

Level 1.4, Module C9: Open Wounds

CRITICAL THINKING QUESTIONS

1. You are working a soccer game when you see two players collide as they both attempt to head a ball. The visiting player seems to have dropped to the ground limp, while your player has bounced back up immediately. As you approach the downed player, you notice that he is not moving, but you

can see the rise and fall of his chest. Explain your steps in this acute care situation.

2. You are having dinner at a hotel with your cross country team when suddenly one of the girls quickly stands up and grabs her throat. You immediately go to her side and ask her what is wrong. She can barely breathe and is pointing down her throat. As you look inside her mouth you can see the uvula swelling and almost closing the airway. What can you do?

3. You are the senior student trainer working with the football team. Your duties include on-the-field care of any "early outs." The early outs generally are the kickers and players in any skill position with whom the coach wants some extra time. This day, the linebacker coach has brought six linebackers out early to practice some drills. You are watching the drills when two players collide and one really gets his "bell rung." You begin to question him and notice immediately that he is talking strangely. He asks you for a Popsicle! Then when a female offers him water, he calls her "Mom." What should you tell the coach about letting the player continue to practice? What is your plan for care of this patient?

CHAPTER 14.

Emergency Care

Susan Kay Hillman, ATC, PT

OBJECTIVES

After reading this chapter, the student should be able to do the following:

- Identify the appropriate first aid procedures for a variety of injuries and illnesses.

- Explain the ABCs of emergency care.

- Explain methods of obtaining consent for various levels and situations of treatment.

- Identify the members of the emergency medical services team and their role in helping an injured patient.

Emergency care skills are skills that should be practiced over and over, and the steps in care should be rehearsed and reviewed often. Your athletic training supervisors will be able to tell you about situations they were involved in, perhaps making you think of things you wouldn't have had they not shared their experience. We all begin our athletic training or coaching exposure by listening and watching as more experienced people go about their jobs. Soon we are allowed to practice the skills and eventually take over, to lead the drill, exercise, or conditioning; but we're so intent on doing the job correctly that sometimes we fail to understand exactly why we are doing what we're doing. As we become more and more comfortable with the process of performing the skill or the job, we can step back and question ourselves why a particular technique was chosen, what other techniques could have been used, and, perhaps most importantly, whether the technique works— and if it does, why it does. This evidence for the practice is the basis of "evidence-based practice," the goal for everything we do in athletic medicine (see chapter 23).

Understanding the why, what, how, and when of injury management is our ultimate goal. This allows us to become thinkers rather than just robots. If you already know some of the injury management skills from previous chapters and courses, this chapter will assist you in the application of that knowledge. In this chapter we discuss the emergency situation and what you might do, the emergency care plan, and the emergency care team members and duties.

First Aid, Emergency Care, and Cardiopulmonary Resuscitation

If someone asked you what to do for a patient needing CPR (**cardiopulmonary** resuscitation), you would probably respond "ABCs." To those who have been trained in the area of first aid, ABCs is a mnemonic that stands for

- A = airway: Is the victim's airway open so he can breathe?
- B = breathing: Is the breathing smooth, or does it sound obstructed or noisy in some way?
- C = circulation: Is the heart beating to provide circulation to the rest of the body?

We all know that many other questions are answered, almost subconsciously, before the initiation of CPR. If you were not present when the person collapsed, you survey the scene. If you come upon a car wreck with gasoline spilled over the road, you might decide that the scene is unsafe for evaluation of the victim and that it is necessary to immediately relocate the victim. On the game field, if you see an individual "go down," you might evaluate the scene subconsciously and already be at the next question—"What happened?" All of these steps are important in the overall care of an injured person.

Two major organizations instruct and credential people in the performance of CPR: the American Heart Association and the American Red Cross. The differences are minor; the important thing is to be trained and then to be retrained at regular intervals. We might think that once we know CPR we could perform it at any time. The fact is that when we first learn the skills we are concentrating on the tasks at hand, and the procedures are quite rehearsed. If we encounter an actual emergency, we may not have time to think— we have to react quickly and automatically.

If you have not yet been instructed in CPR, you may want to plan to attend a course. Often local agencies offer training, or you may have a first aid course on your campus that includes training, testing, and certification in CPR. The essential aspects of CPR include chest compressions and rescue breathing. The American Heart Association changed the standard procedure for CPR so that it starts with the chest compressions rather than the rescue breaths. The rationale is that the rescue breaths delay the performance of the chest compressions, the essential task to keep the blood circulating.

Chest compressions are administered through use of the heels of the hands over the body of the sternum (avoiding contact with the zyphoid process). The depth of compression and the rate of compressions are important and vary depending on the size of the victim. The sidebar Steps of CPR provides a summary of the steps of CPR.

Every emergency situation necessitates two evaluations, or surveys. Even though athletic trainers are often present at athletic practices and events, they cannot see everything that occurs. Unless the entire injury is seen, the medical provider should perform both the primary and secondary survey. If the injury is seen, often the astute athletic trainer has an idea of just what joint or body part was involved in the injury and can skip some of the steps along the way. He always will check the joint above and below the injury, but may not do a complete survey of all body parts. However, when you have no knowledge of what happened you will need to learn as much as you can about the injury.

The primary survey, the ABCs, is the first step in the evaluation of the injured person. Obviously, if you come to the aid of an injured person who is alert and speaking to you, you will not need to render CPR, but taking the pulse and monitoring respiration rate are still important. Once the ABCs have been established, the spine and extremities must be evaluated. This second evaluation, of the spine and extremities, is called the **secondary survey**. Since there is no immediate indication that life is at risk, the secondary survey is not a part of the emergency unless there are significant findings like bleeding or orthopedic deformities. Chapter 8 provides details about the secondary survey and all aspects of the physical examination.

Bleeding

At this point you should quickly review the discussion in chapter 13 of the care of severe bleeding. Remember that when you encounter blood, the first step is to institute Universal Precautions. The habit of handing a sterile cloth to the individual while you put on gloves is a good one to develop. Once gloves are on (and mask if necessary), control the bleeding by direct pressure. If a fracture is causing the bleeding, splinting the fracture

STEPS OF CPR

1. Ask someone to call 911. If nobody is available, you should quickly make the call.

2. Try to get the victim to respond. If she doesn't respond, roll her onto her back.

3. Start chest compressions. Place the heel of your hand on the center of the victim's chest. Put your other hand on top of the first with your fingers interlaced.

4. Press down so that you compress the chest at least 2 in. in adults and children and 1.5 in. in infants. The rate should be at least 100 compressions per minute.

5. If you've been trained in CPR, you can now open the airway with a head tilt and chin lift unless a neck injury is suspected.

6. Pinch the victim's nose closed. Take a normal breath, cover the victim's mouth with yours to create an airtight seal, and then give two 1 s breaths as you watch for the chest to rise.

7. Continue compressions and breaths— 30 compressions, two breaths—until help arrives.

may help control the blood flow. If control is not possible with those two methods, use direct pressure over a major artery; and if that fails to slow the bleeding, use a tourniquet only as a last resort.

Obvious Orthopedic Deformity

In addition to checking for bleeding, you will need to know whether there is something torn or broken that may be causing bleeding you can't see. If patients are alert, you must tell them you are going to check for broken bones. As you feel along the contours of each of the limbs, the hips and pelvis, and the trunk, you should continue to talk to the patient. Ask questions like "Can you feel me touching you?"; "Do you have any pain here?"; "Can you wiggle your toes? Your fingers?" Questions such as these will apprise you of the patient's level of consciousness as well as tell you more about where the injury may be. This scenario is more like the typical situation you might encounter on the athletic field—the individual is injured, but you may not know the exact nature of the injury. Bleeding is suspected whenever there is significant trauma. Internal structures may be bleeding if torn, and this bleeding must be controlled just as the bleeding from an open wound must be controlled. Remembering the flowchart shown in figure 14.1 as you progress through your evaluation of the injured person will enable you to prioritize these steps much more quickly.

First Aid for Sudden Illnesses

Individuals are not often overcome with sudden illness, but that emergency certainly may occur. When people become ill suddenly, they often exhibit some warning signs before an emergency situation develops. Signs that there may be some problem include changes in skin color (the skin becomes pale or flushed); unusually heavy perspiration; complaints of feeling dizzy, light-headed, or weak; and vomiting or **diarrhea**. The prob-

lem has become much worse if the patient exhibits changes in level of consciousness or an inability to move, demonstrates slurred speech, complains of severe headache, or has difficulty breathing. Sometimes the patient or the situation can give you a good idea of what is wrong. For example, if the temperature and humidity are quite high, the person may be experiencing heat illness; or, if you know someone has diabetes, you may reason that the problem is a diabetic coma or an insulin reaction. When you know the cause of the problem, you can provide better care.

When there is no clue to the reason for a sudden illness, the best measures are to care for any life-threatening conditions first and then, if the person's life is not in danger, to treat the symptoms. Help get the individual comfortable, prevent overchilling or overheating, watch for signs of decreased level of consciousness, and seek medical assistance or call emergency medical services (EMS). Always remain with the patient to monitor her condition and to provide any emergency care needed. Don't leave the scene until the ambulance personnel or the physician has taken over the patient's care and you have provided all the vital information you have gained.

The Emergency Care Plan

As you discovered in chapter 13, establishing a plan for emergency situations is very important. If you have ever been in a situation where your mind just went blank, imagine that feeling when the stress of the emergency is upon you. That would not be a good place to be, so preparation is critical. Walk each and every practice venue with an eye on what would need to happen should an emergency occur. Where is the closest phone? Will a cell phone work in the area? How close can an ambulance come to that location? What is the easiest access to the court or field? Will someone need to control the fans or crowd? All these and more questions need to be asked and answered in the emergency care plan for each location where people will

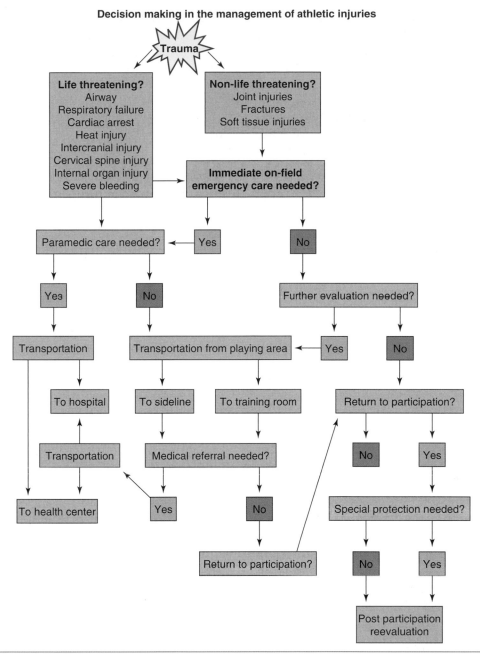

Figure 14.1 Decision making in the management of athletic injuries.

be practicing and competing. Adequate staff must be on site and trained for any situation that may arise.

Game and Practice Coverage

Regardless of the setting, sports with a high potential of serious injury should have medical coverage during practices and games. The list of sports with a high potential of serious injury may vary from school to school. If the staff is trained and the emergency guidelines allow the staff to place an injured patient on a spine board, the necessary equipment should be at hand. Each individual athletic trainer responsible for a sport team should know which patients have conditions that might predispose them to sudden illness. Knowledge of patients with diabetes, sickle cell anemia, epilepsy, or heart conditions allows the sports medicine specialist to prepare for any potential problems. The emergency plan should be discussed and practiced with all members of the support and coaching staffs so that any person available at the time of an emergency can be of significant assistance.

Emergency care to be provided for game coverage should be established each year (Ray and Konin 2011). Sometimes schools contract with local emergency providers. Ambulance staff on hand for the game should be dedicated to emergencies on the playing field or court, and a separate ambulance should be available for emergencies in the stands. In the event that one ambulance is taken from the site, a replacement ambulance should be sent for immediately. These services should be arranged for before the season begins, and members of the ambulance company should meet with the team coaches, medical staff, or both, prior to the first game.

Emergency Procedure Steps

When an emergency situation arises, we want to be prepared. The best way to prepare for an emergency is to plan. If you were not very familiar with the team, facility, or community, it would be wise to involve the athletic administrator, coach, team physician, and community **EMS** personnel in formulating your plan for emergency care at specific events, as well as to involve them in issues concerning team and crowd control, immobilization, transportation preferences, and communication protocols. All questions should be addressed prior to the start of the sport season.

The following steps should be taken in any emergency situation:

- First responder assesses the situation for severity and nature of the injury and calls for help if needed.
- Provision of needed injury management begins with the first on the scene.
- Second responder assists in managing injury, in directing functions of various personnel available to help, or both.

- Team (first responder, second responder, and other personnel) stabilizes the injury to allow for transportation.

The activation of the EMS system depends on the nature and severity of the injury and the level of knowledge and skill of the responders.

Communication Systems

The medical staff should have at least one cellular telephone at each athletic venue. If the practice or game area is indoors and cellular phone reception is hampered by the architecture of the building, it is essential to have a regular phone with a dedicated line. Access to this phone must be very convenient—not through dark hallways and locked doors. Immediate access to EMS may make all the difference in the well-being of a patient.

At some schools where athletic fields are spread out over the campus, communication may occur through a central dispatcher, often by walkie-talkie radio transmission. Although this system involves an additional step for contacting EMS, it can function quite well in some situations. It is very important that the line stay clear of idle chitchat so that the response to an emergency call can occur without delay.

Wherever a land-line telephone is located, written instructions for contacting EMS should be on or near it (see the sidebar Sample of Emergency Procedures for Posting at Telephone). This information should include the telephone number to call, the words to say, and the exact directions to the location of the injured player. As soon as EMS has been contacted, someone should be sent to whatever entrance or other specific location the ambulance has been instructed to go to. That person should direct the ambulance to the appropriate building or field. If these procedures are not planned for and followed, help can be delayed. As an example, an athletic trainer was leaving a busy campus building and noticed a group gathered around a student who appeared unresponsive. The athletic trainer felt that the situation was under control since medical people were attending to the student. On the way to the parking area, the athletic trainer saw an ambulance. It became obvious that the ambulance driver did not recognize the location and would need assistance. The athletic trainer signaled for the driver to park in a fire lane and waited for the paramedics to disembark. She directed them to the location of the group she had noticed earlier. The paramedics shouted "Thanks! We had no idea!" as they hurried to the aid of the victim. Precious time can be lost if proper procedures are not followed.

In addition to the communication that might occur before the telephone call (internal communication) and the call to the emergency care service (external communication), on-site communication is critical in the total care of the patient. The **first responder** (the first medical person to render attention to the victim) is often the athletic trainer. It becomes that first responder's duty to give the **EMT** or **paramedic** (or both) any medical information known about this patient. By passing on bits of information pertaining to etiology (cause) and any pathology

(physical problems) relating to the patient, one gives the emergency personnel a better understanding of what is occurring.

Once the members of the ambulance crew determine that the patient needs to be taken to the hospital, they will notify the emergency care facility. If the condition of the patient is not a threat to life or limb, it is permissible to call upon a parent or other authorized person for transportation. In this case it is necessary to call the hospital or health care provider to alert the medical staff of the patient's problem, the method of transportation, and the estimated time of arrival. When possible, it is best to speak directly to the person who will be caring for the patient upon arrival.

One final form of communication, which may be among the most important, is notification of the patient's parents and the school administrators. Certainly the parents need to know what has happened, and in general it is best to have the team athletic trainer or team physician make this notification. If the patient is under the age of consent, or a minor, the hospital will want to contact the parent or guardian for permission to treat. Of course there are situations, such as a

SAMPLE OF EMERGENCY PROCEDURES FOR POSTING AT TELEPHONE

EMERGENCY PROCEDURES, BASKETBALL FLOOR

1. Call 9-911 from this phone.
2. Identify yourself: name, position. "This is Joe White, head athletic trainer at State University."
3. Explain the emergency: "A player on the men's basketball team fell and is unconscious."
4. Be ready to answer any questions: Is there a pulse, is he breathing?
5. Explain how to enter the basketball arena: "Enter from University Drive, going west off State Street. Turn right at the entrance to the loading dock (just before the parking garage). Come down the ramp. The rolling door will be open."
6. Stay connected until THE OTHER PERSON HANGS UP.
7. Go open the rolling door (use the #91 key in the desk drawer). Get someone to stand at the top of the ramp to signal the ambulance and direct the driver down the ramp.

true emergency, in which consent to treat the minor is implied, allowing care to be rendered immediately. Notification of the school administrators may be thought of as a courtesy, yet these are usually the people who receive requests from parents and the press for information about the incident. The administrator need have only sufficient information to understand what happened (e.g., Joe Black collided with the goalpost and was unconscious) and where the patient is being taken for further care (e.g., he is being taken by ambulance to St. Vincent's Hospital). Other information may be helpful to the administrator (and the coach) and, with the exception of confidential medical information, may be provided.

Equipment

Emergency equipment is important to have at hand when it is needed. Many companies manufacture storage bags that can be used to organize and transport stretchers, spine boards, cervical immobilization devices, and other equipment that may be needed on the athletic field or court. This equipment should be the same equipment that is used in emergency situation practice sessions. Some schools may not have sufficient personnel to provide emergency care to an injured patient, relying instead on local emergency services. There are no known regulations that require schools to have emergency equipment on hand, yet it may be very wise to be sure that life support could be provided in the case of an emergency.

Emergency Care Facilities

Most communities have an emergency care facility nearby. In some small, rural towns, the only emergency service may be through the volunteer fire department. Most firefighters are trained as EMTs, and this care is certainly helpful during an athletic crisis or other emergency. In large metropolitan areas, where emergency care facilities are available locally, there may be many hospitals within a short distance of the athletic facility.

Knowing the locations of the hospitals and the best routes to get to them is important if you ever plan to transport ill or injured patients yourself or to have a family member transport them. Additionally, it is helpful to know where the closest fire station is in the event an ambulance is needed.

Visiting the local fire station and discussing the potential emergency needs of the team or school may be of help in the future. Familiarizing fire station personnel with your practice facilities may be beneficial if an ambulance is needed at a practice site. Information about how to enter the restricted grounds of some schools can be especially critical.

Transportation

An injured or ill patient must be transported with extreme care. If the problem could become worse, medical attention during transport could be required. This is a situation that calls for use of an ambulance. In some situations in athletics, the injury is significant but life or limb would not be at risk during transport to the emergency room or physician's office via a school or personal car. However, you should be familiar with the liability involved should you elect to use your own car for such purposes.

If one decides that transport of the patient is safe, it is prudent to document as much of the case as possible. Aspects such as peripheral circulation (distal to the injury) and neurological status should be noted and recorded. Additionally, before the person is moved, injured joints or bones must be properly immobilized. If there is any doubt about the safety of personal transportation of the individual, professional services (EMS) should be employed for that purpose.

Obviously if the injury necessitates CPR, EMS should be activated immediately. Whether summoned for life support or for transportation of a spinal injury or other orthopedic or medical reasons, once EMS personnel arrive, care of the patient becomes the job of the ambulance personnel, and transportation as well as medical care will be provided by the EMS team. The responsibilities of the on-site medical team are transferred to the EMS personnel at that time.

Personnel Training

Whenever a number of people will be on hand for an athletic event, everyone associated with medical services should be familiar with the emergency procedures to be conducted. When only a few medical and athletic training personnel are present, coaches and sometimes other support staff may be called upon to provide help.

Yearly completion of CPR training should be a requirement for all students and staff members expected to help in a cardiac emergency. Training of all teachers and administrators in CPR is beneficial, not only for the sake of the patients and students, but also to better prepare each person to handle an emergency at school or home.

If the emergency policy includes preparing injured patients for transport by ambulance, those who will be involved should receive instruction and should also have practice—before the season begins—in the preferred techniques for lifting and turning the victim. The physicians responsible at the games should play an active role in establishing the procedure the emergency team is to follow. Involving the ambulance staff with the medical staff is critical to ensuring good understanding and open communication between the groups. Schedule a meeting in which all members of the emergency response team will plan, review, and rehearse the procedures to follow in the event of an emergency on the playing field. Be sure to discuss the specific duties of each individual who will be present at each type of event.

Record Keeping

Just as with any injury, emergency care rendered must be documented for the patient's medical records. The record should include all treatments performed by the school personnel, as well as the times of the EMS call and ambulance arrival. The ambulance crew,

according to regulations set forth by their governing parties, will monitor the condition of the patient. The ambulance crew may be required to perform particular tests regardless of what information the first responders have provided. This should not pose a problem, especially if lines of communication are well developed and active.

Careful documentation of the emergency situation is very important in the event that the patient or family later files a lawsuit against the medical care providers. This is likely to happen in the situation in which a patient suffers loss of limb or life. Naturally, the family will want to know exactly what happened and what was done, and the court may call for this information. Relying on memory is not good enough; you must have carefully written records (see figure 14.2).

Consent to Treat

The health care provider must receive "permission" to treat the patient; this is termed *consent*. Consent for treatment, by law, is required prior to any medical treatment to a patient. Consent is often assumed because of the relationship of the participant to the coach or athletic trainer. Usually that assumption is correct because of prior planning and documentation by the school administration. Legally, consent must be obtained from every participant before the first day of practice. If the participant is under the legal age of consent, the parents or guardian should sign consent-for-treatment forms that will allow medical aid in the event it is ever necessary during athletic participation on the team(s) with which you are working. Some states have laws that permit minors to give their own binding consent for medical attention. As to medical care, your state may have a law that permits minors to be treated as adults if they are self-supporting, married, or pregnant. If you are the person in charge of medical care of the participants, you may want to contact the legal department (your athletic director can refer you to the appropriate person) to obtain help in designing

---

Name of injured person: _____

Time of injury: _____　Date of injury: _____

Place injury occurred: _____

_____

Nature of emergency: _____

_____

Immediate steps taken: _____

_____

Primary Survey

Vital signs: _____　Pulse: _____

Blood pressure: _____　Respiration rate: _____

Secondary Survey

Bone or joint injury: _____

Soft tissue injury: _____

First respondent: _____

Secondary respondent(s): _____

Immediate management: _____

_____

EMS notification time: _____　EMS arrival time: _____

Emergency care facility: _____ Attending physician: _____

Notification of parent/guardian: _____ Time and date of notification: _____

Person contacted: _____

Name of person completing report: _____ Date: _____

Figure 14.2　Sample emergency report form.

Reprinted by permission of Nancy Burke.

medical consent-for-care forms. Figure 14.3 is an example of a consent form.

Community–Based Emergency Medical Services

Anyone working in athletics will have occasion to call on or work with the community-based EMS. A visit to the nearby fire station to introduce yourself will go a long way in establishing lines of communication between your athletic team or school and the ambulance and paramedic team. Often, if you devote the time and energy to meeting those responsible for emergency transport, they will work with you in establishing preferred methods of transport, open lines for communication, and other details of your emergency care needs.

In the 1990s, demand for EMS became greater than the supply of EMTs, so the U.S. Department of Transportation developed

In presenting my son/daughter for diagnosis and treatment

Name: _____ for _____

☐ Mother   ☐ Father   ☐ Legal Guardian   ☐ Son   ☐ Daughter

of _____ years of age, hereby voluntarily consent to the rendering of such care, including diagnostic procedures, surgical and medical treatment, and blood transfusions, by authorized members of the hospital staff or their designees, as may in their professional judgment be necessary.

I hereby acknowledge that no guarantees have been made to me as to the effect of such examinations or treatment on my child's condition.

I have read this form and certify that I understand its contents.

We/I hereby give our (my) consent to

_____

(Name of Person/Agency)

who will be caring for our (my) child

_____

(Name of Child)

for the period _____ to _____ to arrange for routine or emergency medical/dental care and treatment necessary to preserve the health of our (my) child.

We/I acknowledge that we are (I am) responsible for all reasonable charges in connection with care and treatment rendered during this period.

Name: _____   Family physician: _____

Address: _____   Pediatrician: _____

_____   Surgeon: _____

Telephone no.: _____   Orthopedist: _____

Name of health insurance carrier: _____   Child's allergies, if any: _____

_____

_____

_____

_____   Date of last tetanus booster: _____

Group no.: _____   Medicines child is taking: _____

Agreement no.: _____

Signature: _____   Date: _____
          Mother, Father, or Legal Guardian

Witness: _____   Date: _____

In case of emergency I can be reached at:

_____

_____

Figure 14.3 Emergency medical authorization form.

the EMT-Basic National Standard Certification. The addition of the EMT-B personnel to the EMS team increased the number of trained individuals available for prehospital emergency services. Today, EMS involves a number of professionals who all work to provide emergency care in the shortest time possible. The members of the EMS network are listed in table 14.1.

Accessing the Emergency Network

In the United States, the emergency network is usually activated by dialing 911 on any telephone. Although many think of this number merely as a way to call police, fire, and ambulance, it has other important functions. A 911 call coming in to the dispatch desk automatically generates certain information. Even if someone were only to dial 911 and hang up, the dispatcher would know the telephone number from which the call had originated. This system is the same as the systems people purchase for their homes that let them call a special number to find out where missed calls originated. The same system operates in caller-ID devices. Knowledge of the caller's telephone number enables the dispatcher to return an interrupted 911 call to attempt to find out whether there actually is some kind of trouble.

You should not assume that 911 for emergency is the number to dial when visiting another country. Whenever you are traveling outside the United States, especially with sport teams, it is important to know the local emergency access numbers. For example, in the United Kingdom, the number for emergencies is 999, and in Australia it is 000. Take the time to check with local health care providers to establish the protocol for obtaining emergency medical assistance.

As mentioned earlier, a visit to the local provider of ambulance service is extremely valuable. Usually this is the nearest fire department; most firefighters are also trained as EMTs. When you contact or visit the EMTs, it is helpful to discuss all aspects of your emergency plan—from the preferred gate for entering the practice or game area to the techniques for placing an individual on a spine board for immobilization and transport.

In addition to establishing the lines of communication and discussing the emergency care plan, it is advisable to schedule a training session. During this session, all members of the medical/emergency care team work together to perform actual techniques to be used in the event of head injury, spinal injury, or cardiac emergency. This cooperation between the athletic training staff, the ambulance crew, and the attending physicians allows all members of the emergency response team to understand the concerns and skills of the others.

Table 14.1	Members of the Emergency Medical Services Network
Personnel	**Individuals involved and job duties relating to EMS network**
Dispatchers	The 911 dispatcher calls to appropriate DPS (Department of Public Safety) team
Emergency medical technicians, emergency medical technicians-paramedic	Emergency care on the scene rendered by the EMT, EMT-P personnel, ambulance transportation to medical facility
Hospital personnel	Admissions personnel, nurses, and technicians who prepare the patient for medical care
Poison control centers	Phone consultant provides name and process of administering antidotes for ingested poisons
Physicians	Hospital- or community-based physicians who care for the injured
Other allied health personnel	Radiologists, anesthesiologists, and medical specialists who provide special care

Transportation Systems

Because of the cross-training of many public safety personnel, transportation may be provided by groups other than ambulance crews. Depending on the local policies and the level of trauma, police or fire departments may dispatch officers to provide assistance in transporting the injured subject to the emergency facility or to the hospital.

Regardless of the means by which your patient arrives at the hospital, if a DPS (Department of Public Safety) agency provides the transportation from your location, agency protocols and orders must be followed. When working with a medical/emergency care team that has its own physician, you must realize that your physician's orders will become secondary to the orders given by the medical director responsible for that team. Be sure to discuss this issue with your team physician to avoid misunderstandings that can arise in emergency situations when the EMS chain of command is not understood in advance.

Roles and Responsibilities of EMS Professionals

The EMS system is made up of several professionals working together to provide the best and fastest emergency care. Each member of the emergency team has specific roles and responsibilities set forth by federal, state, and local agencies. Each state may have some rules of its own; if interested, you could check with the local professionals to obtain complete information about the roles and restrictions for each of the emergency response team members.

First Responders

Although not a specifically trained person in all states, the first responder is the first medically trained individual to arrive at the scene of an injury or sudden illness. This person may be a firefighter, police officer, school nurse, coach, athletic trainer, lifeguard, teacher, or one among many other professionals with some level of emergency training. The first responder, at the least, has successfully completed a first aid course. This person's duty is to provide the specific care that she has been trained to provide. If the first responder is a lifeguard and the injury is a diabetic coma, the lifeguard may only treat for shock or may call 911 and monitor the vital signs. If you are the first person on the scene of an injury, you are the first responder. You are obligated to provide whatever care a person with your training and experience level would afford the injured person; this is your duty.

Emergency Medical Technician

The EMT is the allied health professional most commonly associated with ambulance calls. One should realize, however, that there are two levels of EMTs: basic (EMT-B) and intermediate (EMT-I). There are greater differences than one might think between the "B" and the "I," in that the EMT-I is nearer to the level of the paramedic. The EMT-B (commonly called the EMT) is often the first member of the EMS team to arrive at the scene of an accident or to respond to an emergency call. The EMT typically attempts to care for the patient after having learned what preliminary care was given by the first responder, the first non-EMS person on the scene.

Paramedic

The paramedic (EMT-P), as well as the EMT-I, has had advanced training in prehospital care. The paramedic is the team member who has the most advanced training in Advanced Life Support (**ALS**), including skills in intravenous (IV) therapy, advanced pharmacology, cardiac monitoring, defibrillation, advanced airway maintenance, and intubation as well as other advanced assessment and treatment skills. This person can provide further immediate treatment before the patient is transported to the hospital.

Emergency Room Physician

The physician on duty in the emergency room is often the medical director of the EMS team. Through an understanding of the situation that has caused the injury (etiology of the injury), the physician can continue the care initiated by the EMTs and EMT-P. Physicians often assist the EMTs and paramedics in developing skills of assessment and treatment, allowing the physicians to "extend their arms" through the EMS team. This is done through continued training in various situations. Like athletic trainers who come to know the team physician so well that they can predict with high confidence what the doctor will do, the EMS personnel out in the field often have to act on behalf of the doctor. They need to know the tests the doctor is going to want and what treatment he would want to try first, second, and third. The paramedics and EMTs working closely with the emergency physician often build a trusting relationship that allows the physician additional insight into the patient's exact condition at the remote location.

Emergency Care Equipment

Not only is it wise to understand what to do in the case of a broken leg or "blown-out" knee; it is critical to understand what to do in the case of a life-threatening emergency. It is the life-threatening injury that will remain in your memory for years to come. Let's try to make that memory a pleasant one! Having the proper equipment available in the event of an injury is not the only step in being prepared; having the proper training to allow use of that equipment is essential. It is not wise to purchase equipment that you are not trained or skilled enough to use. Purchase and provide only equipment that will be useful to the majority of the staff members providing medical coverage for the contest or event.

• *Airway management.* Management of airway conditions, although infrequently required in sport, is essential; and all medical, allied medical, and coaching staff members should possess the skills involved. Remember, the "A" of the ABCs is Airway and is a critical step in emergency care. Every athletic trainer should possess certain supplies for managing airways, and some can provide supplemental oxygen. Minimally, the athletic trainer should have a pocket mask at hand. A pocket mask provides a physical barrier between the patient and the provider for use in giving rescue breaths. This mask serves to decrease the potential of transmission of bloodborne pathogens through Universal Precautions. Various airway management devices and supplies for delivery of supplemental oxygen are usually available on the ambulance.

• *Cardiac equipment.* Today, many athletic trainers, coaches, and others (such as airline attendants) who may be involved in a potential cardiac emergency are able to provide cardiac monitoring and defibrillation using the **AED**, a portable monitor and defibrillator. These devices have verbal and visual step-by-step instructions for analysis of the heart's rhythm, application of the electrodes, and delivery of cardiac conversion techniques. Large companies are beginning to train employees in AED use and CPR and to provide AEDs throughout the workplace.

• *Maintenance of equipment.* All equipment used for emergency care of the injured patient must be available and in proper condition for use when the need arises. Checking the equipment on a regular basis is essential to ensure its working order. Any time a piece of equipment is used, a designated staff member should check all supplies associated with it and make sure that all items are returned to their proper locations. It is wise to inspect all emergency care equipment prior to each season, regardless of how often it was used during the previous season. Electrical equipment, such as semiautomatic defibrillators, should be professionally checked for power output, circuitry, and other functions. Equipment that is expendable (single use) should be discarded once it has been used and should be replaced immediately. Products such as vacuum splints should be tested to ensure against leaks or malfunctions of the pump apparatus.

Learning Aids

SUMMARY

Emergencies are not frequent in athletics; but when they occur, you must be prepared. Not infrequently, an athletic trainer is called upon during team travel when an emergency arises. Understanding the ABCs of emergency care is just the beginning. Understanding the importance of the primary and secondary surveys is essential for thorough and complete care of the injured individual. Once a full understanding of emergency care is achieved, an action plan for handling emergencies can be devised for your particular sport situations. At the time of an actual emergency, the more reminders available, the more clear the provider's thinking can be. Having written instructions next to any landline phone in the treatment area will help if you ever need to send someone to that phone to call 911. Athletic trainers are often the first on the scene when an athletic emergency occurs, but they should never feel they are alone in the care of this potentially serious situation. The EMS team should be at ready access. Having cultivated a good working relationship with the local EMS providers is a great asset if an emergency occurs.

KEY CONCEPTS AND REVIEW

▶ **Identify the appropriate first aid procedures for a variety of injuries and illnesses.**

The first step (primary survey) is to determine the extent of emergency care needed. Once the primary survey shows that the injured person has a good airway and strong heartbeat, the secondary survey can begin. The purpose of the secondary survey is to look for any signs of injury that need atten-

tion. Always treat the most serious condition first before moving on to less serious ones.

▶ **Explain the ABCs of emergency care.**

The ABCs are the order of actions one performs when the condition of a victim appears serious and the person may need CPR.

- A stands for Airway. Make sure that the airway is open and there are no obstructions.
- B stands for Breathing. Look, listen, and feel: Check for breathing by looking for chest rise and fall; listen for sounds of respiration and note the quality of the sounds, and feel the sensation of breath on your cheek as you watch for chest rise and fall.
- C stands for Circulation. Check the pulse to determine if blood is being pumped through the body. Since blood to the brain is most important, checking the carotid pulse is appropriate.

▶ **Explain methods of obtaining consent for various levels and situations of treatment.**

Legally, consent must be obtained from every participant before the first day of practice. If the participant is under the legal age of consent, the parents or guardians must sign consent-for-treatment forms that will allow medical aid in the event it is ever necessary during athletic participation. Some states have laws that permit minors to give their own binding consent for medical attention. As to medical care, your state may have a law that permits minors to be treated as adults if they are self-supporting, married, or pregnant. If you are the person in charge of medical care for the participants, you may want to contact the legal department (your athletic director can refer you to the appropriate person) to obtain help in designing medical consent-for-care forms.

▶ Identify the members of the emergency medical services team and their role in helping an injured patient.

- The first responder is the first person on the scene. This may be the athletic trainer.

- The EMT is often the first access to the hospital. The EMT will stabilize the patient and prepare to transport him to the closest facility to care for his injury or condition.

- The EMT-P may arrive with the ambulance crew. This professional will be able to provide intravenous medication and other needed injections to further stabilize the patient.

- The emergency room physician(s) will be the emergency care providers at the hospital. They will provide the medical care for the condition.

PRACTICE!

For hands-on practice in this area, go to the web resource and complete the following:

Level 1.4, Module C4: Cardiopulmonary Resuscitation

Level 3.3, Module N3: Emergency and Acute Care

CRITICAL THINKING QUESTIONS

1. You are the coach and athletic trainer for a small high school. No physician is available to the team, and the school nurse is in only on Thursdays. One of your wrestlers reports to you on Tuesday saying that he has been feeling "hot and cold" since yesterday. Overall he admits he is not feeling very well, but his biggest complaint is the chills and fever. Discuss the steps you would take in evaluating this individual for participation. Explain why the patient may be complaining of "chills."

2. You are traveling with your volleyball team to a rural high school to play in a tournament. On the drive you have to take a less traveled county road. The coach is driving along when he spots something lying in the middle of the road. As the van nears the "object," it becomes clear that it is a man. The man appears to be breathing and is surrounded by a pool of blood. The coach shouts to you to grab your medical bag and come with him to aid the victim. As you approach the man, you see that his pants are torn and that the femur is protruding through his skin. What do you do?

The therapeutic interventions (TI) section of the NATA BOC (2011) competencies states that, "Athletic trainers assess the patient's status using clinician- and patient-oriented outcome measures. Based on this assessment and with consideration of the stage of healing and goals, a therapeutic intervention is designed to maximize the patient's participation and health-related quality of life." The four chapters in this part of the book present information on many facets of this task.

Chapter 15 provides concepts of rehabilitation and healing through its discussion of the principles of rehabilitation and healing, the formulation of rehabilitation goals, parameters of therapeutic exercise, and the process of helping the patient recover from the grief over loss following an injury.

Chapter 16 introduces the therapeutic treatment modalities used in athletics. The various forms of heat and cold are presented, as well as the indications and contraindications for their use. Various specialized modalities are discussed, including their uses, application techniques, and indications and contraindications.

Chapter 17 provides information on therapeutic exercise parameters and techniques. This discussion provides information on stretching and strengthening techniques and the differences between the two types of techniques. The concepts of proprioception, plyometrics, and open and closed chain are presented.

Chapter 18 covers pharmacology in athletic training. The classification system of drugs is presented to help readers understand "controlled substances" versus over-the-counter medications, for example. Readers will learn how to find more information on specific prescription medications as well the regulations on use of prescription drugs in settings such as the Olympics or other international athletics. Other topics include medicinals used for inflammation, pain, infection, colds, and other conditions.

COMPETENCIES

Prevention and Health Promotion (PHP): PHP-46, 47, and 49

Clinical Examination and Diagnosis (CE): CE-14, 17, 19, 20f-j, 21a, c, d, j, m, and n

Therapeutic Interventions (TI): TI-7-10, 11a-f, 13-15, 19-27, 29, and 30

Concepts of Rehabilitation and Healing

Peggy A. Houglum, PhD, ATC, PT
Kirk Brumels, PhD, AT, ATC

OBJECTIVES

After reading this chapter, the student should be able to do the following:

- List the seven principles of rehabilitation.
- Explain what "prevent deconditioning" means if a patient has an injured knee.
- Discuss how to formulate objective and measurable goals in a rehabilitation program.
- Define the essential parameters of therapeutic exercise in sequential order.
- Compare strength and muscle endurance and give examples of each.
- Define functional activities as used in a therex program.
- List the stages of grief as described by Kubler-Ross and relate each stage to an event in a patient's coping process.
- Discuss the three healing phases of tissue.
- Explain the term *chronic inflammation*.
- List treatment modalities used to affect healing.
- Identify factors that could affect the patient's healing over which the clinician has no control.

This chapter introduces you to many of the concepts relating to rehabilitation and healing. No matter how much we concentrate on injury prevention, injuries will always occur and need to be managed. The injury healing and rehabilitation process begins immediately following an injury, and understanding the principles underlying the process is essential for helping patients to recover. Rehabilitation and wound healing principles go hand in hand; therefore the athletic trainer must be aware of and address both during each patient interaction.

Components of a Rehabilitation Program

This section deals with the general principles, objectives, and goals of a musculoskeletal rehabilitation program. We present an overview of the components of a rehabilitation program with emphasis on examination and assessment and rehabilitation progression procedures. It is critical for athletic trainers to understand general principles and progressions relating to rehabilitation in order to enable a timely return to activity.

Rehabilitation Principles

There are seven principles of rehabilitation; principles are the foundation upon which rehabilitation is based. This mnemonic may help you remember the principles of rehabilitation: ATC IS IT.

> **A**void aggravation
> **T**iming
> **C**ompliance
> **I**ndividualization
> **S**pecific sequencing
> **I**ntensity
> **T**otal patient

• *A: Avoid aggravation.* It is important not to aggravate the injury during the rehabilitation process. Therapeutic exercise, if administered incorrectly or without good judgment, has the potential to exacerbate the

injury, that is, make it worse. The primary concern of the therapeutic exercise program is to advance the injured individual gradually and steadily and to keep setbacks to a minimum.

• *T: Timing.* The therapeutic exercise portion of the rehabilitation program should begin as soon as possible—that is, as soon as it can occur without causing aggravation. The sooner patients can begin the exercise portion of the rehabilitation program, the sooner they can return to full activity. Following injury, rest is sometimes necessary, but too much rest can actually be detrimental to recovery.

• *C: Compliance.* Without a compliant patient, the rehabilitation program will not be successful. To ensure compliance, it is important to inform the patient of the content of the program and the expected course of rehabilitation. Patients are more compliant when they are better aware of the program they will be following, the work they will have to do, and the components of the rehabilitation process.

• *I: Individualization.* Each person responds differently to an injury and to the subsequent rehabilitation program. Expecting a patient to progress in the same way as the last patient you had with a similar injury will be frustrating for both you and the patient. It is first necessary to recognize that each person is different. It is also important to realize that even though an injury may seem the same in type and severity as another, undetectable differences can change an individual's response to it. Individual physiological and chemical differences profoundly affect a patient's specific responses to an injury.

• *S: Specific sequencing.* A therapeutic exercise program should follow a specific sequence of events. This specific sequence is determined by the body's physiological healing response and is briefly addressed in the next section of this chapter.

• *I: Intensity.* The intensity level of the therapeutic exercise program must challenge the patient and the injured area but at the same time must not cause aggravation. Knowing when to increase intensity without overtaxing the injury requires observation of the patient's response and consideration of the healing process.

• **T: Total patient.** You must consider the total patient in the rehabilitation process. It is important for the unaffected areas of the body to stay finely tuned. This means keeping the cardiovascular system at a preinjury level and maintaining range of motion, strength, coordination, and muscle endurance of the uninjured limbs and joints. The whole body must be the focus of the rehabilitation program, not just the injured area. Remember that the total patient must be ready for return to normal activity or competition; providing the patient with a program to keep the uninvolved areas in peak condition, rather than just rehabilitating the injured area, will help you better prepare the patient physically and psychologically for when the injured area is completely rehabilitated.

Rehabilitation Team Members

Rehabilitation includes health care professionals working as a team. Some team members are primary in that they are the health care professionals who are routinely involved in rehabilitation of the patient. Secondary rehabilitation team members are individuals within the health care umbrella who may be called upon to offer services or consultation when unusual or specific needs are required for a successful rehabilitation outcome. The sidebar Primary and Secondary Rehabilitation Team Members outlines the various team members.

Rehabilitation Objectives

Any therapeutic exercise program has two basic objectives. The first directly relates to

PRIMARY AND SECONDARY REHABILITATION TEAM MEMBERS

Primary Team Members
- Athletic trainer
- Physician
- Patient
- Orthopedist
- Podiatrist
- Ophthalmologist
- Psychologist or counselor
- Physical therapist

Additional Primary Team Members for Athletes
- Athletic training student (athletic therapy student in Canada) or other health care student
- Parents or spouse
- Coach
- School nurse

Secondary Team Members
- Emergency medical technicians
- Orthotist
- Pharmacist
- Kinesiologist
- Exercise physiologist
- Nutritionist
- Attorney
- Supervisor
- Peers

Additional Secondary Team Members for Athletes
- Sport team members
- Equipment manager
- Teachers
- Athletic administrator

the principle just discussed, treating the total patient. This objective is to prevent deconditioning of uninjured areas. The second objective is to rehabilitate the injured part safely, efficiently, and effectively.

Prevent Deconditioning

Preventing deconditioning includes providing exercises for the cardiovascular system, the uninvolved areas of the injured extremity or segment, and the uninvolved extremities. The patient can also maintain good strength and range of motion of the trunk, upper body, and uninvolved lower extremity by using weights and performing other exercises. For example, exercises for the involved-side hip and ankle can be used to prevent deconditioning of those areas without applying undue stress to the injured knee.

Because of the nature of the injury or the medical restrictions involved, you may need to use your imagination to develop exercises that challenge the uninjured parts but do not harm the injured area; but it is important to design programs with the objective of maintaining current conditioning levels as much as possible.

Rehabilitate the Injured Part

Good knowledge of the injury, the healing process, and methods of rehabilitation is paramount to achieving the objective of rehabilitating the injured part. You must use good judgment along with this knowledge to enable the patient to progress safely and effectively through the therapeutic exercise program.

Therapeutic exercise can be used to enhance and promote recovery, but it can also be harmful and ineffective if used incorrectly. It is your responsibility as a health care professional to know the appropriate use of this highly effective yet potentially dangerous therapy.

Rehabilitation Goals

Goals are results one strives to achieve. In therapeutic exercise, the ultimate goal is the return of patients to their former activity. That return should be quick yet safe and should be pursued aggressively but carefully. This means that you must work diligently with the appropriate tools to enhance healing of the injury, restore the parameters that have become deficient, and help patients regain confidence in their ability to return to at least the same level of competence as before the injury. The program should stress the patient just enough to provide appropriate gains using a regular progression of adequate challenges to make continual progress.

Objective and Measurable Goals

Goals should be objective and measurable whenever possible. Goals are occasionally subjective; an example is the goal of decreasing the patient's perceived pain. However, you can achieve some objectivity in measuring pain by asking patients to rate their pain on a 10-point scale. Other parameters such as girth, range of motion, and strength can be objectively measured and provide more concrete goals.

It is necessary to assess and record these measurements at various stages in the therapeutic exercise program, most obviously at the beginning and at the conclusion but also routinely throughout the program. Changes in measurements will help you and the patient identify positive gains and areas still in need of improvement. This record also enables you to more easily notice when changes do not occur as frequently as expected and decide what specific modifications are needed.

Short- and Long-Term Goals

When an injury is severe enough to restrict sport participation or normal activity for at least a month, both long-term and short-term goals should be set. A long-term goal is the final desired outcome of a therapeutic exercise program. For example, returning the patient to a former level of athletic competition is a long-term goal. Specifically, this involves returning the patient to normal levels of all parameters that allow full return to sport participation, including flexibility, strength, endurance, coordination, and skill execution. Definitive levels of these parameters are different for each patient and depend on the patient's sport, specific position, age, skill level, and level of participation. **Short-term goals** provide both you and the patient with objective aims on the way toward the long-term goals. Both short-term and long-term goals are expressed in terms of objective measures of what the patient is to accomplish within the given time frame and under what conditions. Short-term goals, established weekly or biweekly, depend on the patient's response to the injury and ability to progress, the stage of the rehabilitation process, and the severity of the injury.

Short-term goals are important because they give the patient something concrete to work toward and a psychological boost toward achievement. Looking at long-term goals can be overwhelming, but focusing on short-term goals gives the patient direction and establishes a logical progression for the rehabilitation process.

Examination and Assessment

To evaluate goal attainment, clinicians continually examine and assess the injury and its healing process. These assessments should occur from the time the injury happens to the time the patient is ready to return to sport participation or normal activity. Therapeutic exercise programs are one area in which clinicians make frequent assessments.

The only way to establish goals is to examine the patient and assess her current condition on the first day of rehabilitation. For each deficiency you find, you decide what realistic short-term goals the patient can achieve toward correcting that deficiency within a specific amount of time. You also reassess the patient's deficiencies regularly throughout the rehabilitation to decide on new and appropriate short-term goals once the previous goals have been met.

Rehabilitation Progression

The progression of a good therapeutic exercise program is challenging yet safe. Accurate examination and assessment of the patient's response to the exercises and treatment are necessary for achieving such a progression. The progression should accord with the severity and type of injury and the response to the injury and treatment. A good progression challenges the patient without causing deleterious effects such as increased pain, swelling, or decreased ability to perform.

- *Exercise progression.* One aspect of progression is the type of exercise. For example, a strength progression may advance from isometrics to isotonics to isokinetics to plyometrics. The patient begins with a level that is challenging but not irritating to the injury, which is determined, in part, by the severity of the injury and the clinician's assessment of the patient's current ability.

- *Program progression.* Another level of progression involves the program itself: A program should be designed to emphasize different types of goals as it progresses. Keep in mind that you cannot expect a patient to perform advanced skill drills before flexibility and strength have been achieved, and that full strength cannot be achieved until flexibility is restored.

Basic Components of Therapeutic Exercise

The total rehabilitation program includes two basic elements, therapeutic modalities and therapeutic exercise. Modalities are used to treat and resolve the effects first seen in injury: spasm, pain, and edema. Therapeutic exercise (therex) is an essential and critical factor in returning the patient to sport participation or normal activity. Modalities are used prior to therex, since spasm, pain, and edema must be resolved before the patient is able to tolerate exercise. If the therapeutic exercise program is to be effective, however, specific parameters must be addressed sequentially. Each parameter must be restored to at least preinjury levels if the patient is to safely resume normal activity or full sport participation. These parameters in their proper sequence are

1. flexibility and range of motion;
2. muscle strength and endurance; and
3. proprioception, coordination, and agility.

Therapeutic exercise must address these parameters in proper order: first, flexibility and range of motion; next, muscular strength and endurance; and finally, proprioception, coordination, and agility. Each of these parameters is based on the previous ones—much as in the building of a pyramid, in which stones are placed one on the other, layer by layer, until the structure is complete. This concept will become clearer as we discuss each parameter.

Flexibility and Range of Motion

There is a technical difference between flexibility and range of motion, but in functional terms the difference is nominal. The term **flexibility** is often used to refer to the mobility of muscles and the length to which they can extend. If a muscle is immobilized for a period of time, it tends to lose its flexibility, or degree of mobility. If stretching exercises are incorporated into a routine conditioning program, the muscle tends to maintain its flexibility or length. Inflexibility usually means that a muscle, not a joint, has limited mobility.

Range of motion refers to the amount of movement possible at a joint. Range of motion is affected by the flexibility of the muscles and muscle groups surrounding the joint. If a muscle lacks flexibility, the joint may not have full range of motion. Range of motion is also affected by factors such as mobility of the joint capsule and ligaments, fascial restraints, regional scar tissue, and strength. Because of the close clinical relationship between range of motion and flexibility, the terms are often used interchangeably; but keep in mind that technical differences do exist between them.

A properly designed therapeutic exercise portion of a rehabilitation program places a priority on regaining lost range of motion and flexibility first. Achieving flexibility early is necessary for two important reasons. First, the other parameters are based on the flexibility of the affected area. The second reason for emphasizing range of motion first has to do with the impact of the healing process. As injured tissue heals, scar tissue is laid down. As scar tissue matures, it contracts. This contraction process is important in eventually minimizing the size of the scar; but it also can be detrimental because as the tissue contracts, it pulls on surrounding tissue, causing loss of motion, especially if the scar crosses a joint.

During healing, a window of opportunity exists during which scar tissue mobility can be optimally influenced. Once that time frame has passed, the likelihood of successfully achieving full range of motion is diminished considerably.

Strength and Muscular Endurance

As the patient's flexibility progresses, achieving normal strength and muscular endurance becomes the priority. With any injury, some strength is lost. The amount of strength and muscular endurance lost depends on the area injured, the extent of the injury, and the amount of time the patient has been disabled by the injury.

Muscular strength is the maximum force a muscle or a muscle group can exert. The most common way to measure it is to determine the amount of weight the muscle or muscle group can lift in one repetition. Muscular endurance is the muscle's ability to sustain a submaximal force in either a static activity or a repetitive activity over a period of time.

Of all the parameters achieved during therapeutic exercise, strength is probably most obvious and most frequently sought following an injury. Muscular strength and endurance are two dimensions within a continuum of muscle resistance. They also affect each other: When strength improves, endurance increases, and vice versa.

Proprioception, Coordination, and Agility

Proprioception, **coordination**, and **agility** are often omitted in a therex program. It is too often assumed that because range of motion and strength are restored, the patient is ready to resume normal activity or full sport participation. This is not the case at all. Impaired balance, proprioception, or coordination—either from injury to the structures controlling these parameters or from lack of practice in a specific skill—increases risk of injury.

A variety of factors affect a patient's proprioception, coordination, and agility. A number of factors in turn are affected by these capabilities, including muscular power, skill execution, and performance. To develop optimal proprioception and coordination, one must first achieve enough flexibility and strength. Coordination and agility are based on the patient's having enough flexibility to perform the skill through an appropriate range of motion and enough strength, endurance, and power to perform it repeatedly, rapidly, and correctly. This is why proprioception, coordination, and agility are the last parameters to focus on—optimal levels require the foundations of good flexibility, strength, and endurance.

The final stage addressing coordination and proprioception evolves into the execution of normal drills that mimic the patient's actual activities. **Functional and activity-specific exercises**, the final step before the return to competition, involve execution of these activities. Functional activities are exercises that precede activity-specific exercises in a rehabilitation program. They commonly involve multiplanar movements and provide greater stresses and demands than single-plane strength exercises. They may include precursor activities to sport-specific exercises like walking prior to running or easy (soft) tossing prior to throwing. They prepare the patient for the more advanced skill demands she will experience in sport-specific activities. Sport-specific activities are exercises that include drills used within a specific sport. They differ from functional activities in that they are specific to sport performance. In this final stage, patients regain the confidence necessary to perform at their prior activity level. When a patient can perform well and with confidence, the clinician can be assured that the goal of fully rehabilitating the patient has been achieved. At that time a return-to-play decision is made by the physician, who ultimately determines when a patient is ready to return to competition based on the information provided by the clinician about the patient's status and function.

Psychological Considerations in Rehabilitation

Many psychological factors have a direct and sometimes profound influence on the overall results of a rehabilitation program. The clinician must be aware of these factors to be able not only to promote optimal results but also to encourage and provide needed support to the patient.

Stages of Grief

Kubler-Ross (1969) outlined stages of grief that people go through when confronted by the prospect of their own death or that of a loved one. Some authors (Peterson 1986; Rotella 1985) have suggested that patients with an injury that keeps them out of competition also go through the process, although this has never been measured or conclusively proven. Since anecdotal reports indicate that injured patients go through the process, we discuss it here. Kubler-Ross's stages of grief are denial, anger, bargaining, depression, and acceptance.

1. *Denial.* At first, the patient does not believe the injury is severe and feels that he will return to competition in a day or two.

2. *Anger.* As the reality of the severity and consequences of the injury sets in and the patient is forced to see the difficulty he is

having in recovery, he expresses anger as a release of genuine feelings of frustration and helplessness. The anger is often directed at whomever is present. It is helpful to remember that during this phase the patient is angry because of the injury and the situation he is in, not because of any actions or words of the people around him. Attempts to calm, rationalize with, or help the patient see what is really happening are often futile at this point.

3. *Bargaining.* In this stage, the patient attempts to bargain with his health care provider over management recommendations. The bargaining process typically involves negotiating to defer anticipated long-term consequences for immediate gratification. For example, an athlete might ask to postpone surgery in order to play in the upcoming game or say things like "If you let me play in one more game, I will work very hard in my rehabilitation."

4. *Depression.* As the patient more fully recognizes the reality of the situation, he enters the next stage, depression. His sense of self-worth declines, and he feels he has no physical or emotional control. Not participating with the team can cause feelings of isolation, further adding to self-doubt and low self-esteem. It is during this phase that rehabilitation becomes the most difficult for both the athletic trainer and the patient. The patient has difficulty complying with the rehabilitation program and may not attend scheduled treatment sessions or may not fully participate in them.

5. *Acceptance.* In this final phase the patient begins to fight the battle against the physical limitations and psychological downswing experienced during the previous stages.

Progression Through the Stages

Changes throughout the grieving process are not abrupt; rather, the patient goes through gradual transitions and can fluctuate between stages. For example, a patient who has entered the depression phase may swing back into the anger phase but later return to the depression phase. As patients progress through depression, they display less and less anger. In the acceptance phase, they may regress to depression before acceptance is complete.

You must be aware that these swings occur and are natural. Seeing that the stages form a continuum, with denial and acceptance on the extremes and adjacent phases overlapping, may help you deal with patients as they go through the grieving stages.

The Clinician's Role in Psychological Recovery

Supporting the patient in psychological recovery is vital to achieving the goals of therapeutic exercise and rehabilitation programs. Clinicians are crucial to this process because of the role they play in affecting the patient's response to injury and commitment to the rehabilitation program. A patient who suffers a time-loss injury may go through emotions similar to those of the five stages of grieving: denial, anger, bargaining, depression, and acceptance. To ensure compliance with the therapeutic exercise program, the clinician must recognize the importance of the patient's psychological state, communicate effectively, educate, provide support, set goals cooperatively, establish rapport, and make the program interesting. Whether you work with physically active patients or other populations prone to musculoskeletal injuries, they will exhibit better compliance if you educate them about the type and extent of the injury; inform them about the rehabilitation process; and communicate in a respectful, open, and honest manner.

Communication

Using good communication skills throughout the rehabilitation process is important. Being a good and active listener is a communication skill that every clinician should develop. Repeating what the patient says about uncertainties, worries, and goals is an active listening skill that demonstrates your interest and concern. Making good eye contact is a simple yet important part of communication. Being aware of the environment and realizing whether it is conducive to good listening and communication are also necessary. Simply being at the same eye level, instead of standing and looking down at the patient, encourages communication.

Offering encouragement about patients' physical efforts throughout the therapeutic exercise program positively affects their psychological response. Encouragement also improves compliance. When someone with authority and expertise whom the patient respects offers support and encouragement, performance and compliance are both enhanced.

Goal Setting With the Patient

Goal setting is important in facilitating patient compliance and enhancing attitude. The patient's assistance in setting goals offers two benefits: The patient feels she has some control over the situation and sees that working together to establish goals ensures mutual understanding of and agreement on those goals. It is natural for an injured patient to feel a loss of power or control, so regaining control is important.

You and the patient should have the same goals. If you have a goal that conflicts with the patient's goals, failure is certain. You and the patient should understand each other's goals, agree on them, and work together to achieve them.

Monitoring the patient's progress, using goals, recording objective changes, and setting new and more challenging goals are all methods of providing patients additional incentives to adhere to the therapeutic exercise program. Patients may be able to discern some benefits from the program; but providing them with more objective, concrete measurements enhances their willingness and motivation to continue.

Supporting the Patient

The members of the patient's support system vary depending on the environment. The clinician is central to the support system and acts as the support system coordina-tor to help the patient achieve a successful outcome. Support team members can assist the patient with home exercises, provide encouragement, and share with the clinician observations or concerns noted outside the treatment environment.

Establishing Rapport With the Patient

Treating a patient on a frequent, if not daily, basis, the clinician develops a rapport with him. The rapport results from the interaction between the two people, their mutual respect, and their desire to achieve the same goals. Establishing rapport can be a challenge with difficult personalities. In these cases it is the clinician's responsibility to put aside her own feelings and act in a professional manner.

Making the Program Interesting

Personalizing the program, making goals challenging yet achievable, and using your imagination to make the program interesting are important to overall success and the patient's compliance. The therapeutic exercise program can be boring and laborious or can be stimulating for both you and the patient. It is up to you to ensure that it is stimulating if your common goals are to be achieved.

Return-to-Competition Criteria

If you work with physically active patients, returning to competition is nearly always the goal of the therapeutic exercise program. By the time the patient is ready to return to full sport participation, you have fully examined and assessed the injured area, the patient's ability to withstand the demands of the sport, and the patient's readiness to return to competition. Full readiness to resume sport participation means that the injured area has no pain or swelling and has full range of motion, flexibility, strength, and endurance. The patient must also be able to perform the sport skills and coordination tasks at an appropriate functional level.

You and the patient must remember that the physician has the final word on when the patient is able to return to competition. It is through your communication with the physician regarding the patient's response to treatment, his ability to perform activities required in the sport, and the status of the injured area that the physician can make that determination.

Concepts of Healing

Knowing as much as you can about the healing process is important for developing a safe and effective therapeutic exercise program. Performing an exercise before the injured area is ready to tolerate that level of stress can impede healing and cause additional injury. As a professional who rehabilitates musculoskeletal injuries, you have a duty to understand healing and realize the impact of the therex techniques you apply. Many aspects of healing are still not completely understood, even among experts. This section presents the most current information we have on the body's response to injury and the process that it undergoes in an effort to return to normal.

It is common knowledge that an injury produces a scar during healing. Although sometimes the body actually replaces damaged tissue with normal tissue, with musculoskeletal injuries it is more frequently the case that the end result of the healing process is scar tissue.

When an injury occurs, the healing process that follows depends on the extent of the injury and the approximation of the wound site's stump ends. If the separation of tissue is small, a bridge of cells binds the ends together. This is called healing by **primary intention**. This type of healing commonly occurs with minor wounds. It is also seen in surgical incisions in which the stump ends are sutured together. In more severe wounds where the stump ends are farther apart and cannot be bridged, the wound heals by producing tissue from the bottom and sides of the wound to fill in the space created by the wound. This is called healing by **secondary intention**. This type of healing may occur in second-degree sprains in which ligament tissue is torn and not surgically repaired. Healing by secondary intention usually takes longer and results in a larger scar.

Healing Phases

Whether the body heals by secondary or primary intention, the process is consistent and predictable in normal situations. We do not entirely understand the process, but we can determine the outcomes of each phase. Healing is a continuum of changing events. To understand and clarify this process, researchers and clinicians divide the events into three different phases. Keep in mind, however, that as far as the body is concerned, the process is continuous, without clear-cut delineations (figure 15.1). The body merely continues the process until the end is reached. The three phases designated by researchers and clinicians are

1. the inflammation phase;
2. proliferation, or the fibroblastic phase; and
3. remodeling, or the maturation phase.

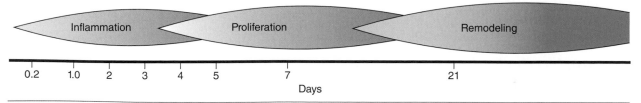

Figure 15.1   Tissue healing process. Note the overlap of these phases.

During inflammation, the injury is contained and stabilized and debris is removed. During proliferation, fibroblasts, myofibroblasts, and collagen peak to begin granulation tissue formation and angiogenesis. During remodeling, wound contraction is well under way, and type III collagen is converted to type I collagen to stabilize and restore the injury site. Each phase has a different duration, different characteristics, and different goals, as outlined in table 15.1.

Inflammation Phase

When an injury occurs, the body attempts to stabilize the injured site by rushing chemicals and cells into the area (Hildebrand et al. 2005). Completion of these extremely complex processes takes 3 to 5 days. A simplified account of these processes is presented in figure 15.2.

The body is extremely busy during this phase in its attempt to protect the site and begin the return to status quo. Inflammation often has negative connotations, but it is an important and necessary step in the healing process. Without inflammation, the body would be unable to heal completely. If inflammation did not occur, proliferation, maturation, and final resolution would not take place; the wound would remain unhealed. Inflammation becomes deleterious when it is prolonged, extending beyond the normal healing time. To make appropriate decisions about when to employ modalities and therapeutic exercise techniques, the clinician must first understand the events that occur in the healing process. Let us examine the series of events involved in this first phase of healing.

Vasoconstriction and Vasodilation

When an injury occurs, blood and lymph vessel walls suffer damage. The immediate local **vasoconstriction** that occurs in the small vessels is followed quickly by **vasodilation**. You may have observed this reaction if you ever suffered a laceration. At first there is no bleeding, but within a few seconds the wound starts to bleed.

Cellular Reactions

It is at this moment of injury that the inflammation phase begins. The vasodilation causes the release of blood and blood products into the injured site, including blood platelets and serum proteins. As these products accumulate in the injury, chemicals are released and other cells are attracted into the area, making an effective tissue "glue," a fibrin plug. In addition to blood vessels, the more fragile lymph vessels are also damaged at the time of injury. Leakage from these vessels is also halted by the formation of the fibrin plug. Once fluid accumulates in the extracellular spaces as it does during an injury, the only way it can be removed is through the lymph system. Unfortunately, because the lymph vessels are plugged by the fibrin plug to stop leakage, their ability to remove the extra fluid from the area is compromised.

Table 15.1 Phases of Healing

Phase	Duration	Characteristics	Goal
Inflammation	Up to about 5 days	At onset of injury, area is warm, red, swollen, and tender.	Stabilize and contain area of injury
Proliferation	Up to about 21 days	Scar tissue is red and larger than normal because of edema.	Dispose of dead tissue, mobilize fibroblasts, and restore circulation
Remodeling	Up to 1 year or more	Water content of the scar is reduced; vascularity and redness are reduced; scar tissue density increases.	Stabilize and reestablish the area

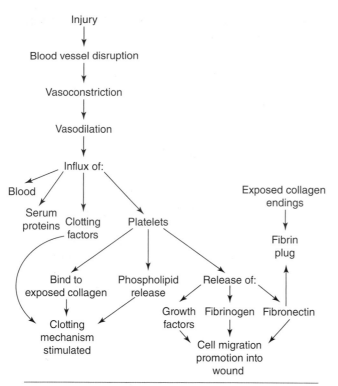

Figure 15.2 Immediate injury response.

Chemical Reactions

There is an intimate interaction between cells and chemicals throughout healing. Some cells stimulate the production of chemicals, and certain chemicals at the injury site stimulate the arrival to or the production of specific cells in the area. This process of attraction or stimulation is called **chemotaxis**. A good example of chemotaxis is the series of events that causes vascular permeability. Vascular permeability is a crucial event in the early inflammation phase. It allows cells and chemicals that normally remain in the bloodstream to enter the injury site and perform their functions to ultimately heal the injured tissue and return the area to as close to normal as possible.

Signs of Inflammation

Many complex events occur during the inflammation phase. The injured area undergoes intense activity. We see evidence of the degree of activity as common signs of inflammation, including localized redness, edema, pain, increased temperature, and loss of normal function. To understand these cardinal signs, we need to examine the histological reasons behind them and recognize what is actually happening. The increase in local cellular and chemical activity increases local temperature, making the skin warm to the touch. Histamine and other released hormones and vasodilation cause redness. Edema or swelling is the result of increased substances in the area and the blockage of lymph vessels whose normal responsibility of drainage is restricted by the newly formed fibrin plug. Finally, pain results from the chemical substances that are released at the site and the pressure from edema on nerve endings.

Proliferation Phase

Although many cells and chemicals are involved during the inflammation phase, the **macrophages** are most responsible for removing debris from the area. Once this task is accomplished, the next step in the healing process is the development and growth of new blood vessels and granulation tissue. This transition from debridement to angiogenesis and granulation tissue formation marks the beginning of the **proliferation phase**. Angiogenesis occurs at a rapid rate during this phase. This is important since scar tissue formation requires vascular production and supply if subsequent events of healing are to occur.

Remodeling Phase

Some of the activities that begin during the proliferation phase continue during the **remodeling phase**. One example is wound contraction. **Myofibroblasts** are responsible for this activity. Some of the fibroblasts convert to myofibroblasts to contract the wound's size. The entire mechanism is very complex and yet to be fully understood. Wound contraction makes the scar smaller. This is advantageous, but it can be detrimental in situations in which joints are affected.

If an injury occurs at or near a joint, scar tissue contraction and adhesions can cause a loss of motion at that joint. Normal tensile strength does not return until a year or more after the injury (and in fact seldom returns to its preinjury level), but the additional support provided by surrounding tissues and the strength of those surrounding tissues may permit a return to sport participation or normal activity sooner than that.

Chronic Inflammation

Normal healing of tissue occurs in the sequence just described. Occasionally, the injury does not progress along this process as it should. It gets stuck in the inflammation phase and is unable to proceed with healing. This condition is referred to as **chronic inflammation**. Recall that in acute inflam-mation, injured cells produce chemicals that work at the local injury site to initiate healing and to debride the area. As the area is cleared of waste and foreign matter, these cells diminish in number, but in chronic inflammations they remain at the site.

Factors That Affect Healing

A number of outside influences can profoundly or subtly affect the healing process. To assist the healing process, clinicians can apply some of these influences. Other factors can be controlled by the patient, parents, or physician. Still others, such as age and systemic diseases, cannot be controlled. Figure 15.3 outlines the injury and healing process and the difference an effective rehabilitation program can make in tissue healing and its

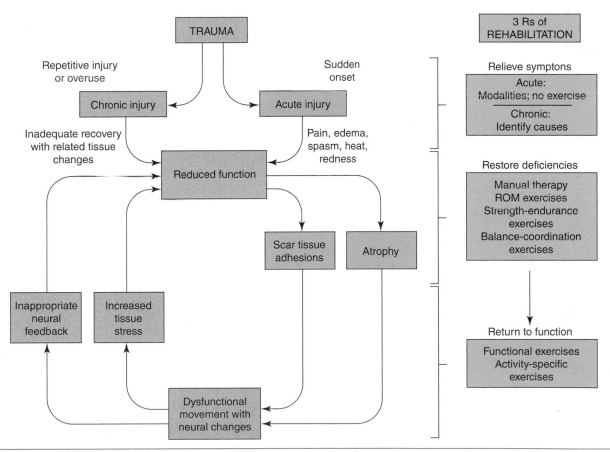

Figure 15.3   The injury process and appropriate types of rehabilitation techniques.

outcome. It is important for a clinician to know appropriate techniques that positively influence the healing process.

Treatment Modalities

Among the treatment modalities most frequently used to enhance healing are electrical stimulation and thermal modalities such as ice, superficial heat, and deep heat. Chapter 16 of this text profiles modalities and their effects on tissue healing and provides more specific information on how modalities can affect inflammation.

- *Ice.* Ice is used during rehabilitation to reduce inflammation caused by therapeutic exercise. After therapeutic exercise such as vigorous stretching or strengthening, signs of new inflammation, such as increased edema, occasionally appear. Although ice does not affect existing edema, it can reduce new edema that results from overstretching or strengthening exercises that are too vigorous.

- *Electrical stimulation.* Electrical stimulation during the first week after injury has been shown to enhance protein synthesis to help promote healing. Protein synthesis is seen in tendons, but because the structure of tendons and ligaments is similar, the treatment may also have the same effects when applied to ligaments. Electrical stimulation can also be applied to muscles to relax muscle spasm, facilitate muscle contraction, and encourage reactivation and recruitment of dormant muscle fibers. When facilitating muscle contraction, electrical stimulation may also assist in relieving local edema by pumping fluid into the lymph system, which reduces pain. With less pain, the patient may be more willing to exercise.

- *Heat.* Heat can be advantageous after the inflammatory phase when applied before exercise. It can increase circulation, which encourages healing and better exchange of nutrients and waste products; relax muscles to allow better exercise execution with less pain; and reduce tissue viscosity to make an area more pliable for stretching.

- *Ultrasound.* Ultrasound has the benefit of producing thermal as well as mechanical effects. A contraindication to continuous ultrasound is in the acute inflammatory phase, when heat is deleterious. Pulsed ultrasound is indicated at that time. It is believed that ultrasound promotes collagen, neovascular, and myofibroblast production. As a source of deep heat, it may be a useful prestretch application for tendon and capsular adhesions at depths that cannot be effectively reached by superficial heat.

It is important for the clinician to know the desired results and choose a modality that will best facilitate those results. As the patient progresses in the rehabilitation program, fewer modalities are required because the injury is more closely approaching normal function and metabolism.

Drugs

Injured individuals often consult with a clinician for information about the drugs that have been prescribed after an injury. Therefore clinicians should have a basic understanding of medications, should be aware of their own limited knowledge, and should readily refer the patient to either the physician or the pharmacist for additional information.

Anti-inflammatory medications are often used in the musculoskeletal injury recovery process. The most frequently used are the nonsteroidal anti-inflammatory drugs (**NSAIDs**). Although research does not demonstrate a significant advantage of NSAIDs for injuries, there is enough evidence to warrant their use. The NSAIDs are used to reduce pain and promote healing by minimizing inflammation in both acute and chronic injuries. Refer to chapter 18 for information on types of drugs and how they work.

Other Modifying Factors

A number of other factors affect healing. Factors over which the clinician has no control include quality of surgical repair, patient's age, systemic diseases, and wound size. Other factors, such as infection, spasm, and swelling, can be reduced by appropriate and timely treatment.

- **Surgical repair.** The physician's surgical and sterile techniques have a direct effect on the healing of surgically repaired injuries. Infection complicates and delays the healing process. The quality of the surgeon's repair technique and follow-up care directly influences when rehabilitation can begin.

- **Age.** Age can be a factor that alters healing. Blood supply is often impaired with age, and a good blood supply is crucial for any injury to heal properly. A poor blood supply delays healing or prevents an injury from healing properly. Diseases associated with age such as osteoporosis also can affect healing.

- **Disease.** Certain systemic diseases can impede healing. If a patient has diabetes, human immunodeficiency virus, arthritis, endocrine disease, connective tissue disease, carcinoma, or other systemic diseases, extra care should be taken with healing wounds. Other conditions that can delay healing include renal, hepatic, cardiovascular, and autoimmune diseases. These conditions are not often seen in younger patients, but the clinician who encounters any of them is wise to be especially cautious.

- **Wound size.** As a rule of thumb regarding wound size, the greater the injury, the more time necessary for healing. The larger the destruction of tissue and separation of tissue ends, the longer it will take for the body to debride the area and connect the stump ends. According to another rule, the greater the injury, the greater the amount of scar tissue needed in the healing process. As we noted previously, scar tissue can impede rehabilitation especially if it occurs around a joint. If the joint is immobilized for a lengthy period of time, scar tissue is more apt to contract and limit range of motion.

- **Infection.** Infection is a possibility any time an open wound occurs, whether it is an abrasion, a surgical wound, or a needle stick from an injection or aspiration. Precautions should always be taken to prevent infection, regardless of the source or size of the wound. Infection always delays healing. When an infection occurs, the wound site will have more scar tissue than it would have had otherwise.

- **Nutrition.** Nutrition plays an important part in healing. The clinician should encourage good nutrition through well-balanced meals to enhance healing. Diets lacking in protein, vitamins (especially A and C), or minerals (especially the trace minerals zinc and copper) make healing more difficult. See chapter 3 for more detailed information on nutrition.

- **Muscle spasm.** **Spasm** is a reflex that occurs with injury as the body attempts to minimize and protect the injury by immobilizing the area. Spasms result in ischemia by restricting blood flow. Applying immediate first aid to the area is important in reducing spasm and ultimately improving the rate of tissue healing and the function of the injured part.

- **Swelling.** The amount of swelling for similar injuries varies from one person to another. As a general rule, the more severe the injury, the greater the swelling. Swelling is caused by fluid in the interstitial spaces, which can include blood, watery fluid from damaged cells, and plasma fluids. Edema puts pressure on sensitive nerve endings, causes reflex muscular inhibition, and negatively affects nutrient exchange at the site of injury. These factors ultimately increase pain, reduce function, and slow healing. The greater the amount of accumulated extravascular blood and fluid, the greater the symptoms of inflammation and the longer it will take the body to progress from inflammation to proliferation. It therefore is crucial for the clinician to apply immediate treatment to minimize the edema and promote healing. Minimizing edema also reduces inflammation, pain, and loss of function.

The Role of Therapeutic Exercise in Healing

Now that you have an understanding of the healing process, it is time to consider how this knowledge can help you design therapeutic exercise programs for injured individuals. Your knowledge of the events and timing of the healing cycle should help you know what to do and when to do it to promote the patient's safe and timely return to competition or normal activity.

The clinician can influence healing positively or negatively, depending on the treatment and when it is applied. Knowledge plays a vital part in the delivery of treatment, but knowing how to apply a treatment is the easy part. Knowing when to apply treatment and the consequences or benefits of applying it is more difficult.

Although immediate treatment after an injury is considered first aid, it is really the first step in rehabilitation. Rehabilitation involves two aspects of treatment beyond on-site evaluation and immediate care. Therapeutic modalities are often first applied to reduce spasm and pain, promote healing, and allow the next phase of rehabilitation—therapeutic exercise—to begin. Therapeutic exercise allows the patient to resume normal activity or full sport participation. Various aspects of therapeutic exercise are discussed in chapter 17 of this text.

CASE STUDY

You are the athletic trainer at Lucas Hills High School, where Hunter is a junior basketball player. Hunter and his team just finished a successful basketball season in which the team lost in the state semifinals. Hunter had a great year and was selected to the all-conference team as a point guard. He has had some college scouts at his games and is looking forward to a great summer league season in which he hopes to improve his skills and his stock among the college coaches. Hunter would love the opportunity to play basketball on scholarship at one of several schools that have programs in his area of academic interest.

After the semifinals, several teammates invited Hunter to join them for a weekend of skiing and snowboarding at the local ski resort. Unfortunately, Hunter had an accident while skiing and injured his knee. He has just returned to your athletic training clinic at the high school following an appointment with the local orthopedic surgeon, Dr. McElroy. Hunter is quite upset about the news he has received, as Dr. McElroy diagnosed him with an anterior cruciate ligament rupture and medial meniscus tear and recommended surgery.

Think About It

1. As you work with Hunter, what are the emotions that you can expect in him over the next few days, weeks, or months?

2. Hunter has a lot of questions regarding time frames and how long it takes for tissue to heal. How would you explain the healing process to Hunter in terms that he can understand?

3. Outline the goals for Hunter's rehabilitation and the principles that you will adhere to as you work with him to reach these goals.

SUMMARY

Decisions on which rehabilitation activities to use in patient care are often specific to the patient, the injury, and the patient's long-term goals. In addition, all athletic trainers should be familiar and comfortable with the individual exercises and activities that prove effective in their work setting. However, the timing of implementation of rehabilitation exercises should always take into account the principles of tissue healing. In addition, rehabilitation progression should always follow a sequential program of increasing demands and functional activities. Being familiar with the concepts of rehabilitation and healing and implementing interventions according to this knowledge are of paramount importance for effective recovery.

KEY CONCEPTS AND REVIEW

▶ **List the seven principles of rehabilitation.**

Avoid aggravation, timing, compliance, individualization, specific sequencing, intensity, and total patient

▶ **Explain what "prevent deconditioning" means if a patient has an injured knee.**

Preventing deconditioning includes providing exercises for the cardiovascular system, the hip and ankle of the injured extremity, and the uninvolved leg and both arms. The patient can also maintain good strength and range of motion of the trunk, upper body, and uninvolved lower extremity by using weights and performing other exercises.

▶ **Discuss how to formulate objective and measurable goals in a rehabilitation program.**

Objective goals and measurements should be formulated through the use of a feedback scale to track changes in pain perception, tape measurements to evaluate girth and muscle hypertrophy, goniometers to evaluate range of motion, and various strength measurement techniques and devices. All this information can be compared to norms or to the opposite limb to help set parameters for short-term and long-term goals.

▶ **Define the essential parameters of therapeutic exercise in sequential order.**

Improve flexibility and range of motion; muscle strength and endurance; and proprioception, coordination, and agility

▶ **Compare strength and muscle endurance and give examples of each.**

Muscular strength is the maximum force a muscle or a muscle group can exert. The most common way to measure it is by determining the amount of weight the muscle or muscle group can lift in one repetition. Muscular endurance is the muscle's ability to sustain a submaximal force in either a static activity or a repetitive activity over a period of time—the number of times a particular exercise or lift can be accomplished in one exercise session.

▶ **Define functional activities as used in a therex program.**

Functional activities are exercises that precede sport-specific activities in a rehabilitation program. They commonly involve multiplanar movements and provide greater stresses and demands than strength exercises. They may include precursor activities to sport-specific exercises such as walking prior to running or easy (soft) tossing prior to throwing. Functional activities prepare the patient for the more advanced skill demands they will experience in sport-specific activities.

▶ **List the stages of grief as described by Kubler-Ross and relate each stage to an event in a patient's coping process.**

- Denial: The patient doesn't believe that the injury is severe and feels that she will return to competition in a day or two.

- Anger: As the reality of the severity and consequences of the injury sets in and the patient is forced to see the difficulty she is having in recovery, she expresses anger as a release of her genuine feelings of frustration and helplessness.

- Bargaining: In this stage the patient attempts to bargain with her health care provider over management recommendations. The bargaining process typically involves negotiating to defer anticipated long-term consequences for immediate gratification.

- Depression: As the patient more fully recognizes the reality of the situation, she enters the next stage, depression. Her sense of self-worth declines and she feels she has no physical or emotional control. Not participating with the team can cause feelings of isolation, further adding to self-doubt and low self-esteem.

- Acceptance: In this final phase the patient begins the battle with physical limitations and the psychological downswing experienced during the previous stages.

▸ **Discuss the three healing phases of tissue.**

- Inflammation phase: When an injury occurs, the body attempts to stabilize the injured site by rushing chemicals and cells into the area. Completion of these extremely complex processes takes 3 to 5 days.

- Proliferation, or fibroblastic phase: Although many cells and chemicals are involved during the inflammation phase, the macrophages are most responsible for removing debris from the area. Once this task is accomplished, the next step in the healing process is the development and growth of new blood vessels and granulation tissue. This transition from debridement to angiogenesis and granulation tissue formation marks the beginning of the proliferation phase.

- Remodeling, or maturation phase: Some of the activities that begin during the proliferation phase continue during the remodeling phase. One example is wound contraction, which myofibroblasts are responsible for. Some of the fibroblasts convert to myofibroblasts to contract the wound's size. The entire mechanism is very complex and yet to be fully understood.

▸ **Explain the term** *chronic inflammation.*

This occurs when the injury does not progress along the usual healing process but gets stuck in the inflammation phase and is unable to proceed in healing.

▸ **List treatment modalities used to affect healing.**

Treatment modalities most frequently used to enhance healing include electrical stimulation and thermal modalities such as ice, superficial heat, and deep heat.

▸ **Identify factors that could affect the patient's healing over which the clinician has no control.**

Factors over which the clinician has no control include quality of surgical repair, patient's age, systemic diseases, and wound size.

PRACTICE!

For hands-on practice in this area, go to the web resource and complete the following:

Level 2.4, Module E2: Injury and Illness Pathology

CRITICAL THINKING QUESTIONS

1. A freshman basketball player injured her knee in a jump stop on the second day of practice. She had never been injured before and is now having a hard time with the rehabilitation. She fails to show up for treatment, is often late when she does make it, and rarely smiles. Discuss her stage of coping from the standpoint of the Kubler-Ross theory and suggest ways you can help her become an active and engaged participant in her own rehabilitation program.

2. You have been doing the rehab for a senior defensive lineman on the college football team who underwent shoulder reconstruction during the off-season. He is now able to do all the exercises you ask him to, and he is quite strong and has good range of motion. You are considering adding some functional exercises to his program on Monday and give him Friday off. Monday he reports in for treatment and rehab and tells you he "tested it just a little" over the weekend. You ask how he feels, and he tells you the only thing that bothered him was doing the "swim move." He admits that he is nervous about getting his arm hit while it is in the air on the "swim." Use your imagination and design some functional exercises to stress his shoulder in the range where he feels vulnerable.

Therapeutic Modalities

Craig R. Denegar, PhD, ATC, PT, FNATA

OBJECTIVES

After reading this chapter, the student should be able to do the following:

- Identify the most common indications for therapeutic modality application.

- Describe the common forms of heat and cold, the main treatment goal, and general precautions and contraindications for each.

- Identify the parameters that need to be considered when TENS is applied to relieve pain or recruit muscle contraction.

- Describe the parameters, precautions, and contraindications for ultrasound.

- Identify two FDA-approved uses of LASER.

- Describe the advantages and disadvantages of manual versus mechanical cervical traction.

- Identify the uses, setup, precautions, and contraindications for lumbar traction.

- Identify two of the many forms of manual therapy.

- Describe how EMG biofeedback can be applied in rehabilitation.

Rehabilitation specialists have used therapeutic modalities since the ancient Greeks (Hippocrates). A **therapeutic modality** can be defined as a device or apparatus having curative powers. Heating lamps and pads, cold packs, ultrasound, laser, and diathermy are among the devices that have been used by athletic trainers and other rehabilitation specialists over the years. Times and technologies have changed. The once common heating lamp has been replaced with hydrocollator packs, while low-power laser therapy has been approved for use in the United States only since 2002. Advances in the understanding of human physiology have also changed how therapeutic modalities are viewed and used.

The definition in the preceding paragraph, specifically the term "curative powers," requires explanation. To cure literally means to rid of disease. In fact, the therapeutic modalities applied by athletic trainers do not rid of disease. Moreover, most applications of modalities likely have little effect on the rate of tissue repair. Therapeutic modalities, however, when used appropriately in the context of a comprehensive plan of care, can reduce pain and facilitate the recovery of function. Thus, the therapeutic modalities discussed in this chapter might be better classified as **physical agents**, treatments that cause a change to the body. The scientific basis for the use of therapeutic modalities has grown, providing a greater understanding of how modality applications affect nerve, muscle, and connective tissues. Thus whether we label the devices and treatments therapeutic modalities or physical agents, we are really discussing devices and treatments used to help injured patients achieve treatment goals and return to normal activity including work and sport.

Technology and the expanding knowledge about how the human body functions and responds to injury are not the only changes that are affecting the use of therapeutic modalities. Evidence-based medicine represents a new paradigm in the practice of medicine and health care. Today clinicians are expected to integrate the best available research into their plans of care and treatment recommendations. Such evidence is derived from studying the response of patients to the treatments in question. Thus, it is not sufficient to rely on proposed physiological responses in selecting treatments when evidence from clinical trials is available. In some cases there is evidence that a modality is effective in achieving a particular treatment goal in patients with a particular condition, and in others, evidence that a treatment is ineffective. The body of evidence from which clinical decisions are made grows daily, requiring today's clinicians to continue to keep abreast of new findings. These efforts and the evolution of evidence-based practice are made possible by the advancements in information technology. The Internet, very familiar to today's student, did not exist when most of the authors contributing to this book were in college. Today's technology permits clinicians greater and more rapid access to research findings from around the world than ever before possible. The application of such research is reshaping how health care, including the use of therapeutic modalities, is practiced.

Regardless of the modality and the available evidence, it is also essential that the treatments be administered safely. Burns, cold-induced nerve injuries, and other adverse events can occur when appropriate patient screening and use of devices do not occur. "Do no harm" is the first rule in medicine and health care. The safe and effective use of therapeutic modalities requires knowledge, vigilance, and a commitment to continuing education. This chapter was developed to provide a foundation for and overview of the use of therapeutic modalities in athletic training.

Applications

As mentioned earlier, rather than providing a cure, therapeutic modalities are applied to facilitate the recovery of function. The ability to move and perform athletic and work-related tasks can be lost following injury or surgery and because of medical conditions such as osteoarthritis. In addition, therapeutic modalities are applied in the context of a comprehensive plan of care. What effects can therapeutic modalities have that facilitate recovery, and how does modality application fit into a plan of care? To answer this question we have to consider what limits function. The first consideration is pain. Pain identifies that something is wrong and causes us to seek medical attention. While essential and productive, pain makes us miserable and results in muscle spasm, loss of joint mobility, and loss of neuromuscular control. One of the primary goals in the plans of care for many patients is pain control. Cold, superficial heat, and electrotherapy can reduce pain. Furthermore, the relief of pain often allows patients to progress to therapeutic exercises aimed at restoring function. By taking a comprehensive view of the patient's needs, the athletic trainer can identify treatment goals and determine when one or more modalities can facilitate the achievement of those goals.

Swelling is also associated with injury and joint disease and can cause pressure that results in pain, can limit joint motion, and can inhibit neuromuscular control. Following injury, RICE is often recommended. RICE is an acronym for Rest, Ice, Compression, and Elevation. While the role of ice in curbing swelling is debatable, protecting injured tissues, elevating the injured limb, and applying ice are still sound recommendations.

As just noted, pain and swelling affect how the body controls muscle activity. For example, following knee injury or surgery, many patients have difficulty recruiting strong contractions of the quadriceps muscles. It has also been found that patients with low back pain exhibit impaired control over some abdominal and low back stabilizer muscles. Neuromuscular electrical nerve stimulation and **electromyograhic (EMG)** biofeedback are modalities that can be applied to facilitate restoration of normal neuromuscular control.

Scar tissue can cause adhesions and restrict motion following injury or surgery.

Modalities can be used to heat tissue prior to stretching and joint mobilizations to facilitate the restoration of joint motion. Seiger and Draper (2010) reported substantial success in patients with long-standing loss of ankle motion, despite treatments to restore motion, when diathermy was used to heat tissues before mobilization. It is important to note that vigorous heating of deeper tissues cannot be accomplished with heat packs, warm whirlpools, or other forms of topical heat because of the insulating effects of adipose. This is just one example that points to the clinician's need to understand the pathology and the treatment goal, understand the effects of various modalities on the body, and have the specific knowledge to apply diathermy safely and effectively in combination with manual therapy.

Lastly, while the application of therapeutic modalities does not provide a cure, there is a limited but growing body of research suggesting that modalities can accelerate repair in some circumstances. Modalities including ultrasound, electrotherapy, and laser have been applied in efforts to promote healing in slow-to-heal and nonhealing wounds for many years. Similarly, pulsed electromagnetic fields and ultrasound have been shown to promote healing in some nonunion fractures (Walker, Denegar, and Preische 2007). These applications are not universally effective, and investigation into the optimal treatment parameters continues. There is now evidence that in some cases it is possible to accelerate fracture healing with pulsed ultrasound delivered by devices specifically designed to affect bone repair (Walker et al. 2007). Laser in combination with a regimen of eccentric exercise has also been shown to speed recovery from Achilles tendinopathy (Bjordal et al. 2008) and to speed healing of skin abrasions (Hopkins et al. 2004). Certainly there is much to be learned about the extent to which tissue repair can be accelerated, including the conditions and patients most likely to respond. Through research, however, new technologies will emerge to assist athletic trainers in rendering optimal care to patients.

Cold and Superficial Heat Treatments

Cold and superficial heat are probably the most commonly applied therapeutic modalities. These modalities conduct heat away from or to the body. The application of cold decreases the temperature of the skin and deeper tissues. The application of heat also increases tissue temperature; however, clinically meaningful increases occur only in the superficial tissues and joints. Heating in deeper tissues including muscle is limited and of little clinical consequence. Heating of deeper tissues including muscle and tendon can be accomplished with ultrasound and diathermy, which are discussed later in this in chapter.

Cold Applications

Cold can be applied with an ice pack, a commercial cold pack, a commercial cold water circulating unit, cold water immersion or whirlpool, or by ice massage. In the simplest application, an ice pack—crushed ice in a waterproof bag—is placed or wrapped on the skin to cool tissues. This is an inexpensive treatment that also allows for compression and elevation of the injured part. Commercial cold packs are another option; however, crushed ice applied directly to the skin is inexpensive, safe, and effective in reducing tissue temperatures and thus is generally preferred.

Cold water circulating units (figure 16.1), also called cryocuffs (a term derived from the trade name Cryo/Cuff), are similar to ice packs in that a cold surface is placed on or near the skin. Cold water is pumped into a cuff, which is then placed on or near the skin to withdraw heat from the tissue. Use of a cuff filled with cold water results in less tissue cooling than the direct application of an ice pack but can provide hours of mild cooling without the need to remove braces and wraps and without the mess of ice packs.

Cold water immersion and cold whirlpools are also used to administer cryotherapy (figure 16.2). Immersion in 40° to 50° F (4-10° C) water or a 50° to 60° F (10-15° C) whirlpool cools tissue as well as an ice pack does. Warmer water is used in a whirlpool because the movement of the water continually breaks down the thermopane, the boundary layer of water around the body part that is warmer than the cold bath (figure 16.3).

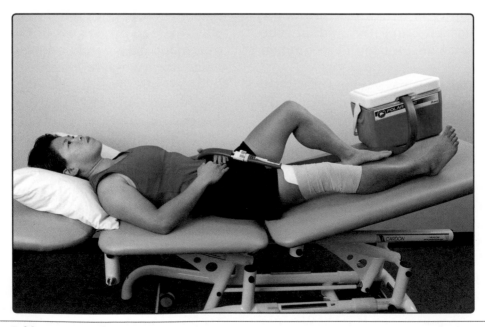

Figure 16.1 Cold water circulation unit.

Loss of the thermopane allows tissues to cool more rapidly. These application methods offer a couple of advantages: The entire limb or joint can be cooled, and active exercise can be performed during the cooling process. However, cold water immersion is not ideal for first aid or during the acute inflammatory response because the injured limb cannot be elevated.

In ice massage, another inexpensive form of cryotherapy (figure 16.4), water frozen in a paper or Styrofoam cup is used to cool and massage the skin. Ice massage should not be applied as a first aid treatment or during the acute inflammatory response because it is incompatible with compression. However, ice massage reduces pain prior to therapeutic exercise and relieves postexercise discomfort. Ice massage can also reduce the sensitivity of tender or trigger points in individuals who have **myofascial pain syndrome** and is readily available for home-based treatment.

One more method of cold application warrants brief mention. Vapocoolant sprays result in very superficial, rapid cooling through evaporation (figure 16.5). There is virtually no temperature change below the epidermis; however, vapocoolant sprays numb an area briefly and may be effective in the management of tender trigger points associated with myofascial pain syndrome (Travel and Simons 1983).

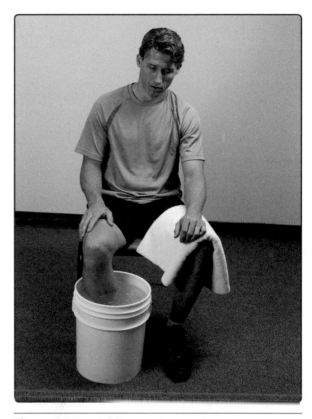

Figure 16.2   Cold water immersion.

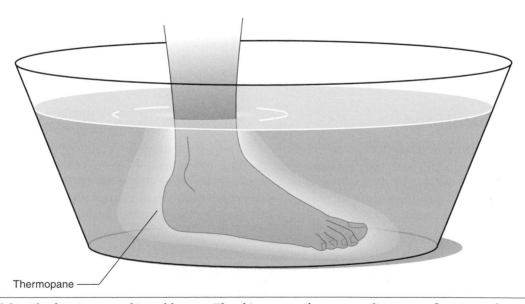

Thermopane

Figure 16.3   The foot immersed in cold water. The skin warms the surrounding water, forming a thermopane on the boundary layer, which is warmer than the cold bath.

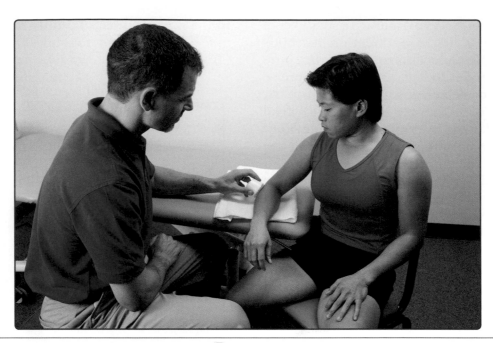

Figure 16.4   Ice massage.

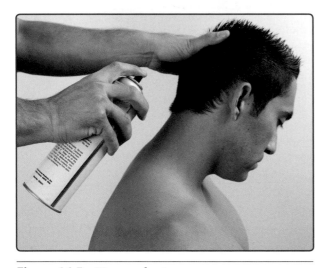

Figure 16.5   Vapocoolant spray.

Heat Applications

The most common form of superficial heat is the moist heat pack, usually a hydrocollator pack. Hot water tanks called hydrocollator units are found in most athletic training rooms and sports medicine clinics. The heat packs are filled with a gel that retains heat. By placing the pack into a hydrocollator tank (170° F, or 76.6° C), you have ready access to superficial heat. At that temperature, direct contact would burn the skin, so the packs must be wrapped in terry cloth covers and towels for protection. When using heat packs with individuals who are at risk for skin injury (i.e., those with circulatory compromise), and in circumstances in which the person lies on the hot pack, be certain to provide sufficient insulation.

Warm water whirlpools are another common form of superficial heat. Whirlpools permit heating around an entire limb or joint. The motion of the water also massages the tissue, which may add to the analgesic and antispasmotic effects of superficial heating. Whirlpools also allow for active or passive motion during heating. The temperature of the water must be maintained within a safe range. Water that is too hot can scald the skin, and whirlpool temperatures should never exceed 115° F (46° C). Because treatment in a whirlpool also stresses the body's ability to dissipate heat, whirlpool treatment can result in hyperthermia and heat illness. The larger the portion of the body immersed in the whirlpool, the greater the heat stress. Table 16.1 provides reasonable guidelines for maximum whirlpool temperatures for various areas of the body.

Moist heat packs and warm whirlpools are the most commonly applied superficial heating modalities. However, paraffin baths, heat lamps, and fluidotherapy are also classified as superficial heating devices. Paraffin baths are filled with seven parts paraffin wax and one part mineral oil heated to 125° to 127° F (51.6-52.7° C). Because of the lower specific heat of the wax compared to water, higher temperatures are used than with whirlpool baths. Paraffin is most commonly used in treating the hand and wrist. The hand is washed and then dipped into the paraffin (figure 16.6). The hand is then removed until the wax hardens. This procedure is repeated four or five times until there is a thick layer of

Table 16.1 Maximum Whirlpool Temperature by Body Part*

Body part	Degrees F	Degrees C
Wrist and hand	112	44.4
Foot and ankle	110	43.3
Elbow	108	42.2
Knee	106	41.1
Thigh	104	40.0

*Assuming well-ventilated whirlpool area and absence of medical conditions that require precaution in warm, humid environments.

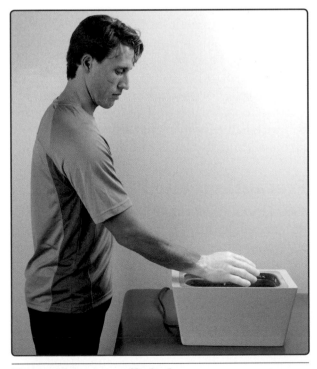

Figure 16.6 A paraffin bath.

warm wax around the treated area. The hand is placed in a plastic bag or an oven mitt; the plastic bag allows you to remove the wax at the end of treatment without making a mess, but the oven mitt holds heat longer. Paraffin cannot be applied if there are open wounds, as the wax will contaminate the wound.

Heat lamps were once commonly used to provide superficial heat. For cost and convenience reasons, heat lamps have been replaced by moist heat packs. Fluidotherapy has been referred to as a dry whirlpool (figure 16.7). A fluidotherapy unit contains ground cellulose material that can be heated to 120° to 125° F (48.8-51.6° C) and then blown around the chamber with forced air. The result is heating through convection and a massage. Fluidotherapy allows passive or active movement during treatment. It is also possible to position patients so that the affected limb is not held in a gravity-dependent position as occurs with use of a whirlpool. Individuals with properly dressed open wounds can be treated with fluidotherapy without the risk of contamination.

Treatment Goals With Cold and Superficial Heat

The goal of most applications of cold and superficial heat is to relieve pain. Pain is associated with muscle guarding and muscle spasm, and cold and heat can also reduce the tone and tension in muscle. The mechanisms through which cold and superficial heat relieve pain are complex and to some extent dependent on the methods of application. Ice packs, commonly applied initially after injury for 20 to 30 min, reduce tissue temperature and slow nerve conduction velocity. As a result of the decreased nerve conduction velocity, fewer pain signals reach the spinal cord and ultimately the higher brain centers. Cold applied for 20 to 30 min also directly affects muscle temperature and therefore tension.

The mechanisms by which superficial heating reduces pain are more complex and less well understood. Heat likely increases activity in neural pathways in the spinal cord

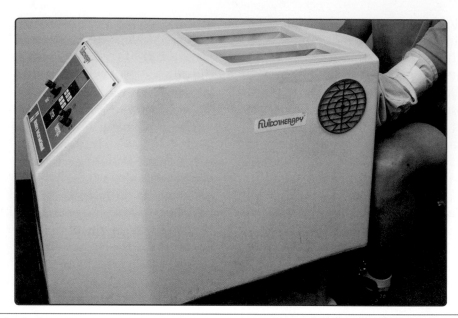

Figure 16.7   Fluidotherapy.

and brain that ultimately trigger the release of pain transmission–inhibiting neuropeptides (**enkephalin**) that block the transmission of pain signals at the dorsal horn of the spinal cord. The mechanisms by which superficial heating relieves muscle tension are also complex and not fully understood. Unlike cold, which has a substantial effect on muscle tissue temperature when applied for 20 or more minutes, hydrocollator packs and other forms of superficial heat have a minimal effect (<1 °C) on muscle tissue temperature. Thus, decreases in muscle tension and muscle spasm following the application of superficial heat result from alterations in neural signals to muscle rather than reduced activity due to changes in tissue temperature.

Cooling of tissues also reduces metabolic activity and the demand for oxygen and nutrients. Following the initial trauma in injury, some cells die in a process known as secondary cell death. Cold application has been hypothesized to reduce secondary cell death. The extent to which cold affects this process is not known, and recent evidence suggests that some secondary cell death is necessary to the injury repair process. At this time neither the optimal parameters (length of application, frequency of application, and time over which treatments should continue)

nor the full effect of cold application on the secondary cell death process is fully understood. It is certainly reasonable to continue to use cold following injury to relieve pain, as no harmful effects have been identified when cold is applied appropriately; however, the effect of cold on reducing secondary injury and facilitating recovery requires additional research.

Although superficial heat has little effect on muscle tissue temperature, synovial fluid temperature can be increased when heat is applied around a joint. Such heating can provide relief of pain and stiffness associated with osteoarthritis and may allow patients to more fully engage in exercises to improve strength and decrease stiffness.

Precautions and Parameters

The safe use of therapeutic modalities depends on appropriate patient screening, parameter selection, and treatment monitoring. Cold application is contraindicated in individuals with somewhat rare conditions, including **cold urticaria** (an allergic reaction to cold exposure) and Raynaud's phenomenon (characterized by constriction of arteries and arterioles in an extremity with cold exposure), and rare conditions including cold-induced hemoglobinuria (paroxymal cold hemoglobinuria) and cryoglobulinemia. Hemoglobinuria occurs when the rate of red blood cell breakdown exceeds the rate at which hemoglobin combines with other proteins. Cryoglobulinemia is a condition in which an abnormal clumping of plasma proteins (cryoglobulins) is stimulated by cold application. It is also possible to injure peripheral nerves lying just below the skin with cold. The ulnar nerve at the elbow, the common peroneal nerve at the posterior lateral aspect of the knee, and the lateral femoral cutaneous nerve at the proximal anterior thigh are most vulnerable.

Thermal burns are the greatest risk posed by superficial heat. The athletic trainer must not exceed recommended levels of heating, must be certain to sufficiently insulate hot packs, and must be certain that the patient has normal sensation and vascular supply to the area to be heated. But injury is not the only concern associated with superficial heat. Bacteria thrive in warm, moist environments. Whirlpools should be thoroughly cleaned and disinfected after each use. Clean covers and toweling are needed to cover hot packs. Special caution must be taken in patients with open wounds.

Cold and superficial heat are typically applied for 20 to 30 min. Cooling of the skin occurs rapidly, while deeper tissues cool more slowly. A 20-min application of cold will result in prolonged reductions in muscle tissue temperature after the cold is removed when the patient remains at rest. The typical treatment time for superficial heat application appears to be based on clinical observation and the collective experiences of clinicians. Short treatments do not result in relief of pain and muscle spasm; and most people, left to their own discretion, apply heat for 20 or more minutes. The reasons, while beyond the scope of this discussion, may lie in the neural mechanisms through which superficial heat modulates pain. It has been hypothesized that more prolonged (20-40 min) stimulation of neural pathways may be necessary to affect pain signaling in the dorsal horn.

Electrotherapy

Electrotherapy is complex and multifaceted and is the subject of entire books. In athletic training, electrotherapy can be divided into four categories: **transcutaneous electrical nerve stimulation (TENS)**, **iontophoresis**, stimulation of **denervated** muscle, and microcurrent. The most widespread use of electrotherapy involves TENS, which can be applied for pain relief or to stimulate contraction of normally innervated muscle. Iontophoresis is a technique in which a direct current is used to drive medication across the skin into deeper tissue. Although the patient perceives the electrical current since the objective is not to influence neural activity, iontophoresis is not TENS. Injury to peripheral motor nerves results in denervation of muscle. It is possible to stimulate contraction of muscle directly with electrical current, but the parameters of the stimulus differ from those needed to stimulate contraction through depolarization of the motor nerves. Since the motor nerve is damaged and cannot depolarize, stimulation of denervated muscle is not considered TENS, as there is not a target *nerve* to depolarize. Microcurrent refers to a stimulus in which the average current falls below 1 milliamp; thus the units of current delivery are in the microampere range.

References to the use of electrical currents for the treatment of various disorders date to ancient times, and electrotherapy in athletic training has a rich history. The past two decades have seen an increasing focus on the effectiveness of treatments; and some applications of electrotherapy, while theoretically of potential benefit, may have little effect on the outcome of care. This is particularly true of iontophoresis of a variety of medications, as well as the application of microcurrent in the treatment of musculoskeletal conditions. Furthermore, while it is possible to stimulate the contraction of denervated muscle, it is not known what, if any, treatment protocol will improve the outcome of care. Such treatment does not speed or facilitate the regeneration of the motor nerve. TENS is the most commonly used form of electrotherapy in athletic training; and evidence indicates that TENS can reduce pain following acute musculoskeletal injury, reduce pain associated with some chronic conditions such as osteoarthritis of the knee, and enhance recovery of neuromuscular function following anterior cruciate ligament reconstruction surgery. Thus this section introduces TENS and focuses on treatments with TENS.

TENS

While TENS is only one part of the electrotherapy picture, it is a complicated subject. Over the years, several different waveforms (packages of electrical energy) have been developed, and much has been learned about how the nervous system functions and is influenced by electrical stimulation. Despite all of the advances, the mechanisms through which the body modulates pain messages are not fully understood. Moreover, some of the theorized benefits of particular waveforms and stimulus parameters have not been substantiated. Despite these complexities, the foundational concepts of TENS are fairly simple.

Nerves rest in a polarized state. When a peripheral nerve depolarizes, it no longer maintains an electrical charge but sends an impulse along its length to communicate with other nerves or muscle. When a nerve is exposed to an externally applied electrical current of sufficient strength, it depolarizes, which results in the same events as if it were depolarized through endogenous (body generated) means. Some types of nerves (larger-diameter nerves with more myelin covering) are more easily depolarized than others (thin, unmyelinated nerves). These differences in nerves allow the clinician to adjust the parameters of the stimulus and select how many types of nerves will be targeted. The clinician can also select how often the targeted nerves will be stimulated by adjusting the treatment frequency.

The body modulates pain through multiple mechanisms, including the increase of input from large-diameter afferent nerves. When tingling, without muscle activity, is perceived with the application of a TENS unit, it results from the depolarization of the large-diameter nerves originating in cutaneuous and subcutaneous tissues. The increase in impulses along these nerves arriving at the dorsal horn of the spinal cord results in the release of enkephalins that inhibit the pathways transmitting pain. This is the most common strategy for relieving pain with TENS. It is also possible to affect pain by using a stimulus that results in repeated muscle twitches (motor TENS) or a **noxious** localized stimulus over trigger points or acupuncture sites. These techniques stimulate pathways in the brain that descend to the dorsal horn, releasing enkephalins to block pain transmission. These techniques are used less commonly because they are not appropriate for some patients and are less well tolerated.

The use of TENS to cause a muscle contraction requires that the stimulus be sufficient to depolarize pools of alpha motor neurons. Each motor neuron serves a few to several hundred muscle fibers depending on the size and function of a muscle. When a motor neuron depolarizes, all of the muscle fibers in the motor unit contract. This stimulus also causes the depolarization of large-diameter sensory fibers; thus the patient also perceives a strong tingling sensation during the muscle contractions.

Waveforms and Parameters

TENS devices deliver currents that are pulsed rather than continuous. Alternating and direct current are by definition continuous, while the currents delivered by TENS devices are interrupted and are classified as pulsitile. Many TENS devices have several different pulsitile currents from which to choose. Table 16.2 describes the characteristics of common pulsitile currents, each differing in waveform or the shape of the package of electrical energy delivered.

TENS devices were developed in the 1960s following advances in neuroscience and neuroanatomy. These devices delivered a biphasic waveform in an effort to neutralize the net electrical charge and thus prevent irritation or injury to the skin. Once it was realized that the short duration and relatively low frequency of the stimulus would not irritate the skin, monophasic (high volt) currents were introduced to provide deeper current penetration and permit clinicians to select the polarity of the stimulus, as it was hypothesized that positive and negative currents might differ in their effect on the tissues. The use of electrical currents to stimulate muscle development and restore neuromuscular control was also popularized in the late 1960s and 1970s with the introduction of "Russian" current. Interferential currents were later developed in an effort to target specific tissue and allow for deeper penetration of current.

The development of the various waveforms has likely led to more confusion than advances in patient care. Provided that the waveform does not deliver a gradual buildup in the electrical energy delivered within each pulse (no commercial TENS device has such a waveform), the shape of the waveform has not been shown to affect treatment responses. The response to treatments depends on the electrical energy delivered in the first phase (monophasic waveforms only have one), which is defined as the *phase charge*, and the frequency at which the pulses are delivered. Recall that nerves differ in how easily they can be depolarized with an electrical current. The more resistant a nerve is to depolarization, the greater the phase charge needed to cause depolarization. Table 16.3 summarizes the recommended stimulus parameters for the various applications of TENS. Also refer back to table 16.2 to review the limitations in adjustment of phase duration associated with the various commonly available waveforms.

Table 16.2 **Parameter Limitations Associated With Commonly Available Waveforms on TENS Devices**

Waveform	Description	Phase duration
High volt	Peak amplitude >150 V Low average current Monophasic, twin peak waveform	Fixed at 60-80 µs
Biphasic	May be symmetrical or asymmetrical square wave	In a wide range (e.g., 60-400 µs)
Interferential	Stimulating current (alternating pulses with varying amplitude) produced through interference of two alternating currents of different frequencies	Carrier Phase 2,000 Hz 250 µs 4,000 Hz 125 µs 5,000 Hz 100 µs
Premodulated	Same as interferential except that interference does not occur in tissue (stimulating current modulated in the unit)	Same as interferential
Russian	2,500-Hz alternating current modulated into packages of millisecond (e.g., 10 ms) duration	200 µs

Table 16.3 **Parameters Used in the Clinical Application of Electrical Stimulation**

Goal: TENS pain control	Phase duration	Amplitude	Pulse frequency	Target nerve fiber
Sensory	<150 µs	Submotor	60-120 pps	A-beta
Motor	200-300 µs	Strong motor	<10 pps	A-delta
Noxious	>300 ms	Painful	High (150) or low (1-4)	C fiber
Neuromuscular stimulation	250 µs	Motor	50 pps	A-alpha

In summary, the clinician has several decisions to make when using TENS devices. Understanding the principles of electricity, the structure and function of the peripheral nervous system, and the effects of electrical currents on the nervous system is essential for the most appropriate and effective use of TENS in clinical practice. This section and the guidelines provided form a foundation for such understanding. More advanced texts and course work will help you develop a more thorough understanding of TENS and the clinical research to guide clinical applications. Such resources will also further your understanding of the other forms of electrotherapy introduced earlier and address concerns about effectiveness that have emerged from clinical research.

Safety

TENS devices are very safe provided that a few precautions are observed and contraindications recognized. To prevent injury caused by electrical shock, all modalities, including whirlpools, ultrasound devices, and TENS units powered by electrical circuits, must be connected to ground-fault interrupted electrical circuits. Devices that are battery powered must be used in a manner consistent with manufacturers' recommendations. With use of TENS, electrodes must not be placed over the **baroreceptors** of the carotid sinuses at the anterior aspect of the neck, as this may cause changes in blood pressure. TENS is also contraindicated during pregnancy and for patients with cardiac pacemakers or cardiac arrhythmia. While the use of TENS in these patients is unlikely to cause harm, too little is known about the potential effects of exposure to TENS on fetal development; and without careful monitoring, it is not possible to be certain that TENS is not affecting pacemaker function.

Ultrasound

Ultrasound has multiple uses in health care, including imaging and physical rehabilitation. Different frequencies of ultrasound are used for each application. The ultrasound units used in athletic training and physical therapy emit sound energy at frequencies between 800 KHz (800,000 Hz) and 3.3 MHz (3,300,000 Hz). Most ultrasound units can transmit sound waves at frequencies of around 1 or 3 MHz. Some units are adjustable to 1, 2, and 3 MHz. The frequency affects how deeply the sound waves penetrate and warm tissues, with lower frequencies resulting in deeper penetration.

Ultrasound machines (figure 16.8) use electrical current to create a mechanical vibration in a crystalline material housed in the ultrasound head of the unit. Vibration of the crystalline material produces a wave of acoustic energy (ultrasound). The sound energy emitted from the ultrasound head travels through tissues and is absorbed.

As with electrotherapy, you can alter the treatment parameters of ultrasound depending on the desired effect. Fortunately, the number of adjustable parameters is smaller. You can control the amplitude of the sound waves and therefore the amount of sound energy being emitted from the sound head. The sound energy emitted by the crystal is measured in watts (W). The dose of sound energy delivered is based on the amount of energy that is being emitted divided by the radiating area of the crystal measured in square centimeters (cm^2). Thus, ultrasound dose is measured in W/cm^2. You can also adjust the duty cycle, the duration of treatment, and as noted previously, the frequency.

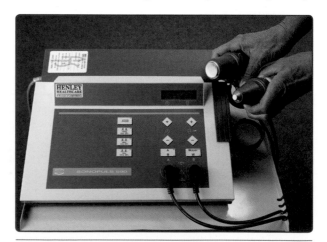

Figure 16.8   Ultrasound machine.

Duty cycle refers to the process of interrupting delivery of the sound wave so that periods of sound wave emission are interspersed with periods of interruption. Figure 16.9 depicts pulsed and continuous ultrasound. Often you can choose from among several duty cycles. To calculate the duty cycle, the time during which sound is delivered is divided by the total time the sound head is applied. For example, if ultrasound is transmitted for 150 ms out of every second of treatment, then the duty cycle is 150/1,000, or 15%. When the emission of sound energy is not interrupted, the duty cycle is 100%, and the ultrasound is referred to as continuous ultrasound.

Much has been learned regarding the treatment duration needed to elevate tissue temperatures to beneficial levels. An interaction among the frequency, dose, and treatment duration has also been found. The greatest

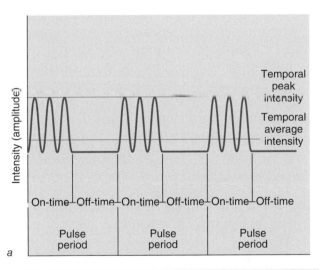

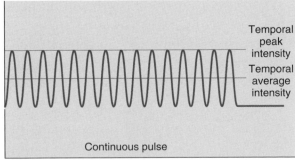

a

b

Figure 16.9 *(a)* In pulsed ultrasound, energy is generated only during the "on" time. Duty cycle is determined by the ratio of "on" time to pulse, in this case 50%. *(b)* Continuous ultrasound.

heating occurs with continuous ultrasound delivered at a frequency of 3 to 3.3 MHz at a high intensity (e.g., 2 W/cm^2). With these parameters, tissue temperature increases of greater than 4° C have been reported in less than 5 min. If the tissue to be heated is deeper (e.g., piriformis muscle), a lower frequency (1 MHz) is necessary, with 10 to 12 min of treatment required to approach a 4° C increase in tissue temperature (Draper, Castel, and Castel 1995).

The parameters just outlined are predicated on treatment over an area no greater than two or three times the effective radiating area (ERA) of the crystal and a slow, controlled movement of the ultrasound head (figure 16.10). The ERA is printed on each device. When larger areas are treated, the amount of acoustic energy reaching any single area is decreased. In addition, heat buildup is allowed to dissipate from the target tissue. Thus, there is less temperature increase during treatment and therefore less change in tissue elasticity and local blood flow during and after treatment.

Treating larger areas such as the lower back has little or no effect on the tissues, although there may be a placebo effect. Thus, ultrasound should not be applied over large areas. Currently, the best recommendation for treatment technique suggests covering a treatment area two or three times the ERA with the sound head covering less than 2 in./s.

Moving the sound head slowly prevents hot spots from developing in areas of peak amplitude and helps you maintain good contact with the skin or gel pad surface. With higher-quality crystals, the sound head can be moved more slowly, resulting in more uniform heating and greater patient comfort. Rapid, sloppy movement of the sound head with frequent breaks in contact between the skin or gel pad decreases the thermal response to treatment.

Unfortunately, it is now apparent that ultrasound devices differ in the energy field produced within and between manufacturers (Johns, Straub, and Howard 2007a, 2007b; Straub, Johns, and Howard 2008). Thus, while it is possible to provide guidelines for

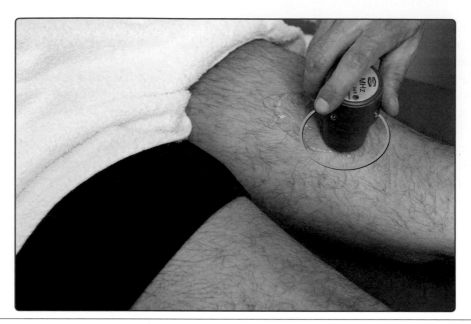

Figure 16.10   Treating an area two or three times the effective radiating area.

treatment parameters, the extent of heating and patient reports of discomfort can vary among devices even with selection of the same parameters. Thus, the intensity (W/cm^2) must be reduced if the treatment becomes uncomfortable, and well-tolerated treatments may not be heating tissue to the extent desired.

Thermal Effects of Ultrasound

Many of the benefits of ultrasound have been attributed to tissue heating. Warmed tissues are more easily stretched, and ultrasound is commonly used in conjunction with stretching and mobilization techniques to enhance tissue and joint mobility. An increase in temperature also increases metabolic activity, which in turn increases local blood flow. An increase in local blood flow may also occur independent of temperature increase during ultrasound. At this time, however, it is not clear whether the increase in blood flow is of clinical benefit.

Safety and Effectiveness

Ultrasound is a relatively safe, easy-to-use therapeutic modality with few contraindications. Of greatest concern is the use of ultrasound in individuals with cancer and the impact of ultrasound on fetal development. Ultrasound has been reported to promote growth (Sicard-Rosenbaum et al. 1995), and perhaps metastasis, of malignant cells in laboratory animals and should not be used near tumors. The impact of therapeutic ultrasound on fetal development in humans is not fully known. Thus, therapeutic ultrasound should not be applied near the abdomen during pregnancy or to women of childbearing age who could be pregnant. The energy delivered to the tissues with therapeutic ultrasound is much greater than with diagnostic ultrasound, a common practice during pregnancy. Ultrasound also should not be applied over an infection or to patients who may have a deep vein thrombus (DVT).

Despite considerable confusion in the literature over the years, the work of Gersten (1958) and Lehmann and colleagues (1966) provided evidence that ultrasound can be applied safely over metal implants such as plates and screws. However, because low-frequency ultrasound is used to loosen prostheses for removal and revision, and because the long-term impact of ultrasound on joint replacements is not fully known, it should not be used over joint replacements.

Ultrasound should not be applied over the heart or in the area of a cardiac pacemaker.

Ultrasound should also not be applied over the eyes or genitalia. The use of ultrasound directly over open epiphyses should be minimized, because the impact of such exposure is not fully known and may involve accelerated closure of epiphyses. However, adolescents and children rarely experience problems for which ultrasound is indicated. Exposure of the spinal cord to ultrasound should be minimized. In patients who have had a **laminectomy**, do not apply ultrasound directly over the area of the cord that is no longer protected by bone. Although these precautions and contraindications should be observed, they rarely affect the selection of ultrasound as a therapeutic modality.

The limited evidence of effectiveness of ultrasound in the treatment of musculoskeletal conditions is of considerable concern. The lack of effectiveness reported in the treatment of conditions such as tendinopathy, plantar fasciitis, and low back pain is likely multifactorial. As noted previously, devices differ in the energy produced by the sound head. In some studies the parameters or the administration technique was inconsistent with those typically recommended. In the case of tendinopathy, once labeled and treated as an inflammatory condition, new understanding of the pathology may explain a lack of response to treatments with ultrasound. Perhaps improved technology and new research will better define a role for ultrasound in the treatment of musculoskeletal conditions. At this time, however, it is important to appreciate that while ultrasound can increase tissue temperature, there is little evidence that treatments with therapeutic ultrasound used in athletic training and physical therapy improve the outcomes of care for the vast majority of patients with musculoskeletal conditions.

Laser

LASER is an acronym for **l**ight **a**mplification of **s**timulated **e**mission of **r**adiation. Four classifications of lasers are used in communication, manufacturing, and medicine as well as many other fields. Lasers range from class 1 lasers, which are incapable of producing damaging radiation and are thus safe for the eyes, to high-power class 4 lasers that pose significant hazards if used improperly. Lasers used to treat injuries to the musculoskeletal system and the skin are class 2 and 3 lasers, incapable of generating tissue heating above 36.5° C. These therapeutic lasers, which are used to stimulate tissue healing and manage pain, have been called cold lasers, low-power lasers, and low-intensity lasers. Currently, low-level laser therapy (LLLT) is the term most commonly used to refer to treatment with these devices. The clinical application of LLLT requires an understanding of the unique characteristics and generation of laser light.

Low-level lasers have been used extensively in physical medicine outside of the United States for many years. Since 2002, the Food and Drug Administration (FDA) has granted the premarket notification (510(k)) for the use of LLLT for specific clinical applications. The 510(k) allows a specific laser device to be marketed for use in the treatment of the specified conditions. Approval means that the approved laser can be sold, but that the only claim the manufacturer can make is for the indication described in the 510(k). For example, low-level laser has been approved for

- "adjunctive use in providing temporary relief of minor chronic neck and shoulder pain of musculoskeletal origin" (U.S. Department of Health and Human Services Food and Drug Administration website, www.accessdata.fda.gov/cdrh_docs/pdf3/k032816.pdf) and
- "adjunctive use in the temporary relief of hand and wrist pain associated with Carpal Tunnel Syndrome" (U.S. Department of Health and Human Services Food and Drug Administration website, www.accessdata.fda.gov/cdrh_docs/pdf2/k020657.pdf).

The parameters including the wavelength of light and power of the approved devices differ but are specific to the approvals cited. Several other companies have received premarket notification approvals for their devices for the same applications. Approval for additional applications will depend on clinical research submitted to the FDA. It is important to note that the clinical literature has described the use of LLLT for many conditions, including a number that are relevant to athletic health care—for example, wounds and abrasions, epicondylalgia, and tendinopathy. Moreover, the use of laser for conditions for which the FDA has not given approval does occur. The clinician should be aware of federal and local regulations regarding the use of LLLT as well as the liabilities of unapproved applications.

Light Energy

The acronym LASER provides insight into how laser light is produced. Central to understanding laser is the photon. A **photon** is a particle of radiant energy. Laser is a process of stimulating the release of photons by stimulating the atoms making up a liquid, solid, or gas (lasing medium) to produce photons, then amplifying the energy to high levels before permitting it to be released from the laser device.

Visible light occupies a small band of the electromagnetic spectrum. The electromagnetic spectrum is the total range of energy expressed in relation to the wavelength and frequency. Electromagnetic energy con-

sists of photons that travel at the speed of light: 300,000,000 m/s. The wavelength and therefore the frequency of photons differ. Long wavelengths such as radio waves are measured in meters, while gamma rays are measured in femtometers (10^{-15} m). Photons of different wavelengths have different energy levels (figure 16.11). Photon energy is proportional to its frequency—the higher the frequency, the higher the photon energy. Thus high-energy photons are in the gamma, X-ray, and ultraviolet end of the spectrum and are capable of causing atom or molecular ionization that damages tissue. Low-level laser therapy devices produce light that is visible (wavelength 400-760 nanometers [nm]) or in the infrared (>700 nm) range. Laser light is very wavelength specific and therefore energy specific.

LASER Light Production

An atom has a nucleus consisting of protons and neutrons, with electrons orbiting about in designated shells or valence levels. When energy is applied to an atom, it may be absorbed, causing one of the electrons to move and orbit in a higher shell. An atom in this state is labeled as "excited" and is unstable. The electron will return to a normal level of orbit (called ground state) as soon as possible. When this occurs, the energy that caused the excited state is released as a photon (packet of light). In a normal state, electrons are absorbing energy and releasing

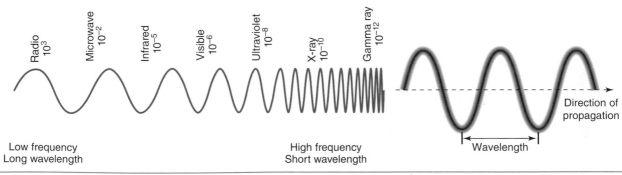

Figure 16.11 The electromagnetic spectrum is a continuum of energies that are categorized by their wavelength and frequencies, which are inversely proportional. As the frequency increases, the wavelength shortens; and when the frequency is low, the wavelength is long. The visible spectrum is within the electromagnetic spectrum and has wavelengths between 400 and 760 nm.

photons continuously as the atoms attempt to remain in their most stable form (**spontaneous emissions**; see figure 16.12).

How is the light amplified? When a quantity of atoms is retained in a chamber (lasing chamber) and excited by the application of energy, photons are released in this confined area. As a photon strikes another excited atom, it stimulates the release of an additional photon as the electron returns to its resting orbit. As this occurs, the original photon is unaffected and continues to influence other atoms. Thus, as more and more photons are generated, increasing amounts of light energy are produced (**amplification**). A lasing chamber is constructed with a semipermeable (also referred to as semireflective) mirror at one end. When the ability of the mirror to reflect light is exceeded, some laser light escapes from the chamber through the mirror (figure 16.13). The wavelength of the photon depends on the material being stimulated. If helium-neon gas is stimulated, the photons will have a wave length of 632 nm; if gallium-arsenide is stimulated, the wavelength of the photons is 904 nm. Two important points now emerge. First, all of the atoms being stimulated in laser device are the same; in other words, the material in a lasing chamber is pure. Thus, all of the photons in the chamber are of identical wavelength, which results in the special properties of laser light to be discussed shortly. Secondly, the great variety of applications of laser stems from the fact that different materials result in the release of photons of unique wavelength and frequency. Thus, if a high-frequency, short wave length photon is released, the photon contains more energy. This would characterize a thermal laser in comparison to a low-level laser used in rehabilitative medicine that does not cause heating of tissues.

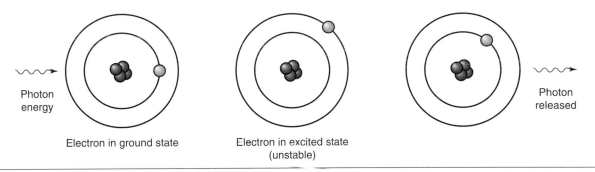

Figure 16.12 Energy (photon) causes an atom to become excited, and an electron moves to a higher valence level. All matter seeks its most stable form, and energy is required for an atom to be in an excited state. The matter releases an equal amount of energy (photon) as the atom goes back into its ground state. This process occurs naturally (spontaneous emission).

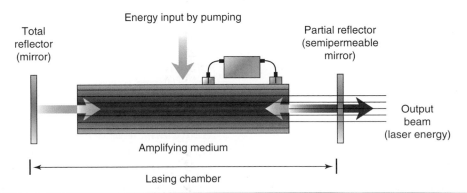

Figure 16.13 Basic production of a laser. Energy is applied to a closed chamber to allow amplification of photons. The energy is released at one end in the form of a laser.

Properties of LASER Light

What is unique about laser light? Laser light has three related properties: **monochromaticity**, **coherence**, and **collimation**. *Monochromic* means that the light is of one color or one wavelength that is specific to the energy level of the photon. The wavelengths of light energy range from 100 to 10,000 nm (billionths of meters). If the wavelength is less than 400 nm, the light falls into the ultraviolet spectrum. Visible light has wavelengths of 400 to 700 nm. The infrared spectrum lies between 700 and 10,000 nm. Two points can be drawn from this information. First, not all lasers emit light in the visible spectrum; secondly, when the light of a laser is visible, the light is of a single color since it is monochromic.

"Coherent" means that all of the waves of light energy are of the same length and are traveling in a similar phase relationship. This characteristic increases the wave amplitude characteristic (constructive interference). Furthermore, all of the energy is traveling in the same direction. This leads to the third characteristic of lasers, which is collimation.

"Collimation" refers to the degree to which the beam remains parallel with distance. A perfectly collimated beam would have parallel sides and would never expand at all. A laser beam does diverge somewhat and even obeys the inverse square law as the distance from the laser source is increased. The divergence of laser is minimal and varies with the type of laser (gas vs. diode), and it can be modified with the use of lenses. The collimation of the laser is a safety concern for both the patient and practitioner as the energy is concentrated to a thin beam. When the energy is focused on a small part of the retina, damage can result whether the laser is visible or not. Properties of laser and white light are compared in figure 16.14.

Dosage and Safety

Laser devices differ in wavelength and therefore the depth of presentation. The characteristics of helium-neon and gallium-arsenide

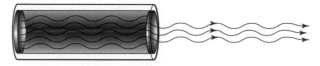

Coherent laser

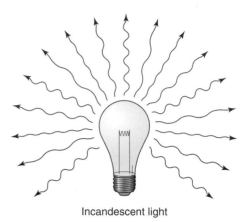

Incandescent light

Figure 16.14 Contrast the light emitted from a laser to that emitted from a light bulb. White light contains many different colors and therefore many wavelengths of light. Since the waves are of different lengths, they cannot remain in phase and they diverge. Thus, the light from a single bulb can illuminate a large area. The light emitted from a laser does not readily diverge, allowing travel over long distances and greater penetration.

lasers are reviewed here. Clinicians should review and understand the characteristics of each laser they use so as to maximize safety and the potential for effective treatment.

A helium-neon (HeNe) laser emits red visible light with a wavelength of 632 nm. The power output of modern helium-neon lasers is up to 25 mW. The depth of penetration with this wavelength is from 6 to 10 mm. A HeNe laser is commonly used in superficial wound care. The relationship between the wavelength (and thus color of light) and penetration is represented in figure 16.15.

A gallium-arsenide (GaAs) laser is a semiconductor laser that emits infrared energy at a wavelength of 904 nm, which is invisible to humans. The output of GaAs lasers is up to 100 mW, and the depth of penetration has been reported to be 30 to 50 mm. This type of laser is being applied to deeper tissues such as tendons and ligaments.

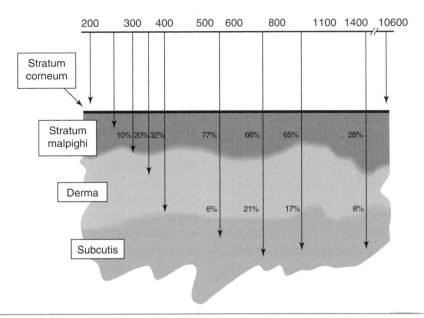

Figure 16.15 Depth of penetration. Wavelength of the laser is associated with the color (infrared, red, and so on) and the depth of penetration. Some laser energy is absorbed in the superficial, subcutaneous area, which decreases its ability to penetrate to deeper tissues.

Image from Lawrence Berkeley National Laboratory. Available: http://www.lbl.gov/ehs/pub3000/Skin_Effects.jpg.

The total amount of energy delivered to the tissue is measured in joules/cm². The energy delivered is dependent on the length of exposure of an area to laser as well as the characteristics of the laser. Thus the time over which laser is applied to the tissues is also critical. Fortunately, devices are programmed to automatically set the treatment time based on the desired quantity of energy delivery. Doses reported in the literature can provide some guidance for selecting a laser and appropriate parameters. For example, there are reports of benefit and lack of benefit when laser is used as an adjunctive treatment in patients with lateral elbow tendinopathy. In a systematic review of clinical trials, Bjordal and colleagues (2008) reported benefits from laser treatments at 904 nm at doses of 0.5 to 7.2 joules/cm². Detailed discussion and recommendations for the treatment of multiple conditions with the various laser devices available are well beyond the scope of this chapter. The doses reported in clinical trials fall well within the range of safety suggested by Tume and Tume (1994), who stated that adult doses should not exceed 50 J and that the maximum dosage for children

under 14 years of age is 25 J. It is important to note, however, that the benefits or lack benefit reported in clinical trials of LLLT cannot be generalized to all devices and applications. The foundation provided here should help prepare you to critically appraise the literature and ultimately elect to use laser when the clinical evidence suggests a high probability of benefit.

Although laser may conjure up visions of *Star Wars*, LLLT has been used for treatment of many neuromusculoskeletal conditions in many countries, and no adverse effects have been reported in over 1,700 publications (Denegar, Saliba, and Saliba 2010). As with any modality application, however, it is still important to ensure a proper diagnosis and have a thorough understanding of that diagnosis prior to treatment. There are also a few concerns specific to laser.

• *Eye safety.* Never look into the aperture of the laser. The cornea transmits light energy, and the eye focuses the light on the retina. Wavelengths over 700 nm are invisible; therefore, the light reflex response will be absent. This could result in retinal damage. Eye protection should be provided for both the clinician and the patient if the classification of the laser is 3b or higher. Laser warning signs should be present. It is also recommended that the laser probe be kept in contact with the skin whenever possible. Safety keys are provided with many laser units to help avoid indiscriminant activation of the laser.

- *Posttreatment reactions.* Fatigue has been reported after laser treatments (Tuner and Hode 2002). This was short-term and was more common in patients suffering from chronic pain. Pain may also be reported the day after treatment. This is believed to be due to an activation of tissue healing mechanisms that have become dormant (Tuner and Hode 2002) and should be a positive response sign, especially in a chronic injury condition.

Contraindications and Precautions

Because LLLT can inhibit cell function when applied in high doses, laser therapy should be applied at appropriate dosages. A number of contraindications warrant special consideration.

- *Pregnancy.* No published research addresses the effect of laser therapy on an unborn child. As a precautionary measure, laser therapy should be avoided in pregnant women.
- *Cancer.* No mutagenic effects have been reported with the use of LLLT. Cancerous cells in vitro have been stimulated to grow, but in vivo studies resulted in a reduction in tumor size that was attributed to an enhanced immunological system (Wohlgemuth et al. 2001). Only oncologists should treat cancer patients.
- *Thyroid gland.* Thyroid gland activity has been modified by laser energy; therefore treating over this area should be avoided (Hernandez, Santisteban, and del Valle-Soto 1989).
- *Children.* No studies have identified any impact on open growth plates. Since there

are limited studies on the use of LLLT in children, the treatment should not be performed unless the benefits clearly outweigh the potential for risk in the presence of open growth plates. Generally the maximum recommended dosage for children is less than 25 J (Tume and Tume 1994).

Clinical Applications of Laser

Although the means for generating laser light are well understood and the response of patients with specific conditions to treatments with laser devices is the subject of numerous studies, the mechanisms responsible for the effects of treatments are not fully understood. Laser can facilitate the healing of slow-healing or nonhealing wounds (Enwemeka et al. 2004; Woodruff et al. 2004) and even speed the healing of skin abrasions in healthy individuals (Hopkins et al. 2004). Laser has also been reported to relieve the symptoms of carpal tunnel syndrome (Shooshtari et al. 2008) and lateral epicondylalgia (Bjordal et al. 2008) and to facilitate the treatment of Achilles tendinopathy (Stergioulas et al. 2008) when used in conjunction with an eccentric exercise regimen. The mechanisms behind these responses have not been fully explained and require further investigation. It is again important to note that not all studies have concluded that LLLT is effective even in the conditions mentioned here. As more research is conducted, clearer guidelines regarding patient and parameter selection to assist in decision making will emerge.

Summary

It is likely that new applications and new laser devices will continue to be developed. Low-level laser therapy has been used for treatment of many neuromusculoskeletal conditions; however, the efficacy of all applications has not been carefully assessed. Research will continue to generate data concerning success rates in treating specific conditions, as well as optimal dose, length of exposure, and frequency of treatment. Clinicians seeking to use lasers must understand the physical principles, types, and classifications of lasers; strive to remain current with the research literature; and observe established safety procedures and contraindications.

Mechanical Energy and Manual Therapies

The therapeutic modalities discussed previously in this chapter involve heat, cold, electricity, ultrasound, and laser applied to either affect neural activity, heat deep tissue, or influence cell activity. Modalities, including the hands, can be used to affect mechanical forces in an effort to achieve treatment goals. This section provides an overview of traction, compression, and manual therapies. Indications, precautions, and contraindications for these treatments are summarized in table 16.4.

Traction

Mechanical traction involves using a machine or apparatus to apply a traction force to the body (figure 16.16), whereas with manual traction the force is applied by the hands. Most traction treatments are administered to distract or separate segments of the cervical or lumbar spine. However, gravity reduces the separation during sitting or standing. Despite the inability to generate more separation,

Table 16.4 Indications and Contraindications for Traction and Intermittent Compression

	Indications	Precautions and contraindications
Cervical traction	Pain Muscle spasm Hypomobile facet Disc herniation	Positive vertebral artery test Positive alar ligament test Acute neck injury (fractures, sprains with joint instability) Advanced rheumatoid arthritis Bone cancer Increased pain or radicular symptoms with treatment Advanced osteoporosis
Lumbar traction	Pain Muscle spasm Disc herniation Hypomobile facet Nerve root impingement	Pregnancy Claustrophobia Internal disc derangement Fractures, sprains with joint instability Bone cancer Increased pain or radicular symptoms with treatment Advanced osteoporosis Hiatal hernia
Intermittent compression	Swelling and edema	Thrombophlebitis Infection Acute fracture Pulmonary edema and congestive heart failure
Manual therapies	Pain Muscle spasm Edema Loss of motion	General: Symptoms of organic disease or cancer must be followed up before a modality, including a manual procedure, is administered. Addition precautions and contraindications for manual therapies include the following: Infection Skin lesions Joint instability Bone-on-bone end feel and advanced arthritis Recent fracture or surgery Advanced osteoporosis Mobilization of cervical spine in the presence of advanced rheumatoid arthritis Deep vein thrombosis

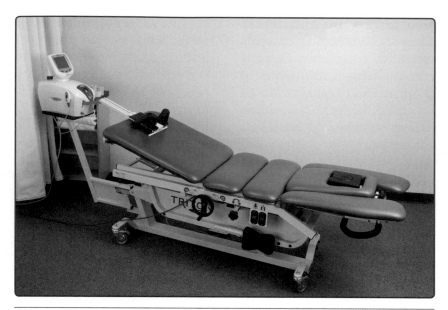

Figure 16.16   A splint traction table.

some patients experiencing symptoms of spinal nerve compression may get relief of symptoms with traction treatment.

Although the use of mechanical traction is limited, an understanding of the principles and applications of manual and mechanical traction is useful.

Cervical Traction

Distraction of the cervical spine can benefit some patients with cervical pain and dysfunction. This author prefers to perform manual traction (see figure 16.17) before mechanical traction is considered. Manual traction allows you to carefully control force application and head position to maximize the relief of symptoms. Manual traction also allows you to combine manual techniques. If manual traction relieves pain or **radicular** symptoms, you can move to mechanical traction for longer treatments that require less of your time. While you cannot precisely quantify the traction force that you apply through your hands, a force of 15 to 25 lb will result in a perceived elongation of the cervical spine. The best approach is to increase the mechanical force gradually until the individual reports relief similar to that experienced with manual traction.

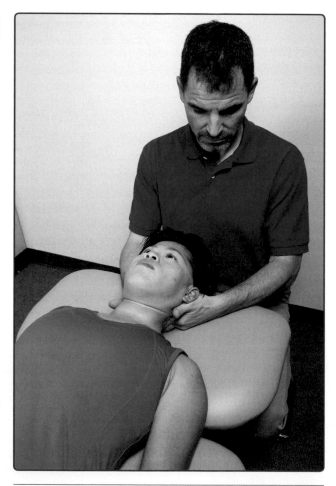

Figure 16.17   Manual cervical traction.

Mechanical Traction Technique

For people who respond well to manual traction, this is an option that requires less of your time. The patient should be positioned supine, with the neck flexed and side bent to a position of greatest comfort (figure 16.18). To apply the device, position the individual's head so that the pads of the head support align with the base of the occiput; then adjust the pads securely at the base of the occiput. If the pads are too tight, the person will complain of pain. If they are too loose, they will slide and pinch the ears, and little traction force will be transferred to the spine.

You can select continuous or intermittent traction. Intermittent traction, in which the maximum traction force is applied for a set time period (typically 30 s) and then the force is reduced, is more comfortable and better tolerated in most cases. The period of reduced force, or rest period, is usually about the same as that for the maximum force. The traction force during rest is usually 50% of the maximum traction force.

As noted previously, the amount of traction force should be gradually increased to provide a tolerable distraction. Begin with 15 lb on smaller individuals and people with more pain and 20 to 25 lb on larger individuals with more long-standing pain. Treatment time can be adjusted up to 20 to 30 min depending on the individual's response. Greater amounts of cervical flexion up to approximately 30° will direct the distraction force to lower cervical segments.

Precautions and Contraindications to Cervical Traction

Mechanical cervical traction is not appropriate for everyone and could result in catastrophic injury if applied inappropriately. Trauma to the head and neck may damage bone, ligament, and musculotendinous structures, resulting in laxity or instability. Fracture and injury to the stabilizing soft tissues must be ruled out or allowed to heal before you use traction. One additional consideration of extreme consequence is fracture of the dens or odontoid process of the second cervical vertebra (axis) (figure 16.19). Trauma, especially with a whiplash mechanism, can fracture the dens. Unfortunately, this fracture is not always recognized and may not be particularly painful. If traction

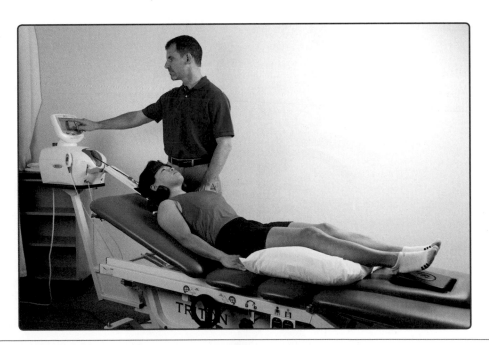

Figure 16.18 Cervical traction with a Chattanooga traction unit.

is applied in the presence of a dens fracture, dislocation of the first or second cervical vertebra, an often fatal injury, could result.

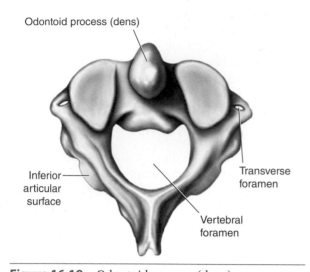

Figure 16.19   Odontoid process (dens).

Reprinted from R. Behnke, 2005, *Kinetic Anatomy*, 2nd ed. (Champaign, IL: Human Kinetics), 123.

It is important that patients be thoroughly evaluated following trauma that can result in damage to the structures of the cervical spine before any treatment decisions are made.

Another concern related to cervical traction involves the potential to place the head in a position that compromises the vertebral arteries. The vertebral arteries pass through the foramen in the transverse processes of the fifth through second cervical vertebrae. These vessels ascend to the circle of Willis, which distributes blood supply to a large area of the brain (figure 16.20). Prolonged positioning of the head can lead to an insufficient blood supply to the brain and pose the risk of stroke. The clinician must be certain that the patient does not have compromises to either vertebral artery before applying cervical traction. Traction is also contraindicated in some individuals with osteoporosis and rheumatoid arthritis, conditions that may

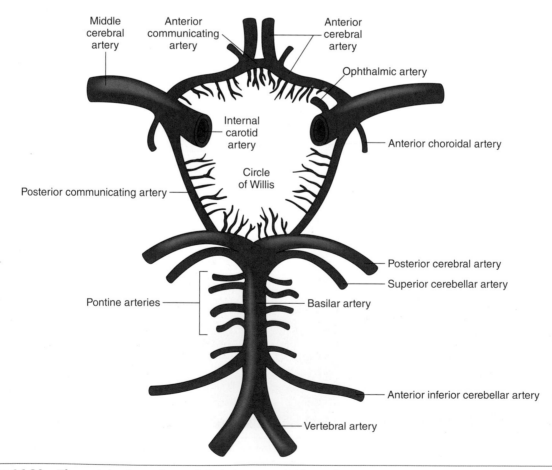

Figure 16.20   The vertebral arteries and their intracranial branches.

render the bone or connective soft tissues of the cervical spine unable to withstand traction forces. If you have any concerns when treating people with these conditions, consult with the referring physician. It is much better to err on the side of caution than risk injury to the cervical region.

Lumbar Traction

Distraction of the lumbar spine can also be accomplished with mechanical traction. The traction forces can separate or distract the facet joints and relieve pressure on spinal nerves. Most physically active individuals with disc pathology need help to find a resting position that alleviates symptoms. Most disc injuries involve the posterior lateral aspect of the disc. Lumbar extension is believed to encourage the nucleus to migrate anteriorly, away from the spinal nerves. Thus, lying prone with a tolerable extension of the lumbar spine often alleviates the radicular symptoms associated with disc injury. The advantage of finding positional relief is that the individual can control symptoms at home.

Because of the nature of managed care and its success in treating low back problems without mechanical lumbar traction, this technique is not used often. However, it may be very useful in a subgroup of patients, as described by Fritz and colleagues (2007), with signs of nerve root compression whose symptoms peripheralize with lumbar extension or a crossed straight-leg raise.

Setup

Setting up lumbar traction for a patient and positioning the patient appropriately are rather involved (figure 16.21). Careful instruction

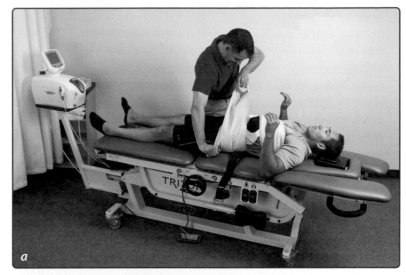

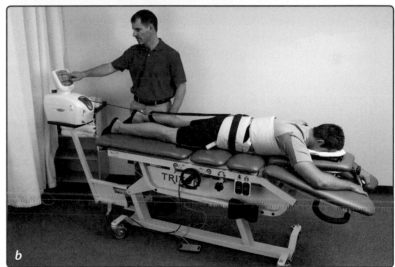

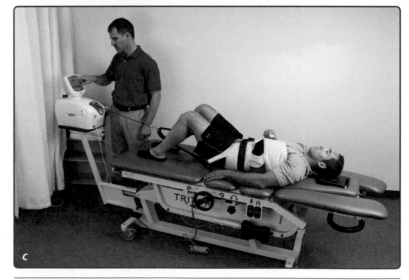

Figure 16.21 (a) Placing lumbar traction harnesses. (b) An individual in the prone position. (c) An individual in the supine position with hip flexed to approximately 90°.

and practice are needed to ensure patient comfort and safety. Once the belts are positioned, traction forces are administered in either a continuous or an intermittent mode. Intermittent traction (30-45 s on, 15-30 s rest) is better tolerated. Shorter "on" times (15 s) have been suggested for treating facet dysfunction and longer "on" times (60 s) for disc injury. Traction may be applied with the patient in prone or supine. Unfortunately, little research supports the efficacy of mechanical lumbar traction or provides well-substantiated treatment parameters.

An initial traction force of 25% of body weight is a reasonable starting force. If the initial force is tolerated, increase the traction force up to 50% of body weight. Treatment times usually range from 10 to 20 min, depending on the nature of the problem and the response to treatment.

Precautions and Contraindications

There are fewer contraindications for lumbar traction (summarized in table 16.4 on p. 403) than for cervical traction. Pregnancy, hiatal hernia, and advanced osteoporosis are absolute contraindications. Fractures and medical conditions, such as cancer, that affect the integrity of the connective tissues also contraindicate mechanical traction. Occasionally individuals experience a significant increase in pain during traction, in which case traction must be terminated. This is particularly common in persons suffering from internal disc derangement.

Intermittent Compression

Intermittent compression involves the use of a pneumatic device that intermittently inflates a sleeve around an injured joint or limb. Intermittent compression devices are used to reduce edema and posttraumatic swelling. Intermittent compression is easy to administer. A compression stocking is applied to the limb to be treated (figure 16.22). Once the stocking is in place, the intermittent compression unit is adjusted for duty cycle and maximum pressure. No duty cycle has been established as the most effective. Inflation times of 30 to 40 s are well tolerated when interspersed with 20- to 30-s "off" or deflation periods.

There is some disagreement regarding the optimal inflation pressure. Manufacturers have developed guidelines for various conditions (Fond and Hecox 1994). The maximum pressure recommended in treat-

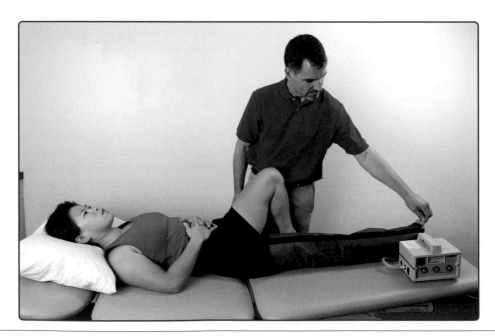

Figure 16.22   Intermittent compression pump with sequential air filling.

ing posttraumatic edema is 50 to 90 mmHg (Fond and Hecox 1994; Hooker 1998). A setting just below diastolic blood pressure is well tolerated by physically active individuals and appears to reduce edema. Once the duty cycle and pressure have been set, the injured individual remains with the affected limb elevated throughout a 20- to 30-min treatment.

There are few contraindications for intermittent compression. Certainly all situations in which tissue motion poses a risk, such as healing fractures and gross joint instability, would contraindicate intermittent compression. Infection, DVT, pulmonary edema, and congestive heart failure also contraindicate intermittent compression.

Intermittent compression is a relatively safe but passive approach to reducing posttraumatic edema. There is also concern that reductions in swelling observed immediately following treatment are not sustained when the affected limb is returned to a gravity-dependent position (sitting, standing, walking) (Tsang et al. 2001). Thus, the injured person will likely improve faster by performing pain-free active exercises to encourage lymphatic drainage during treatment in the clinic or athletic training room, and three to four times daily at home, as long as the swelling persists.

Manual Therapies

Manual therapies, including various forms of massage, mobilization, and provider-guided movements, are commonly used in the treatment of musculoskeletal conditions. The topic of manual therapy is often not considered in the context of therapeutic modalities. Furthermore, learning these techniques requires specific instruction and extensive practice beyond the brief introduction provided here. Such preparation will also include a review of contraindications for the various techniques that must be observed to ensure patient safety. The purpose of this presentation is to discuss the similarities in treatment goals between some of the modality applications discussed previously

and some manual therapy techniques. For example, massage may be performed in an effort to reduce pain and muscle spasm or tone. While mechanical energy is directed to the patient with the provider's hands, the modality involves energy transfer in the same vein as the machine modalities described throughout this chapter. Moreover, the relief of pain and muscle hypertonus occurs through a response of the nervous system to the stimulus. Manual therapies also have applications in restoring motion and neuromuscular control that further promote full recovery from injuries.

The skilled clinician selects the modalities and treatment techniques that—based on the best available evidence and their experience and expertise—offer the best opportunity to achieve the patient's goals. Recognizing manual therapies as modalities expands the choices available. In some cases manual techniques offer distinct advantages; in others, heat, cold, and electrotherapy, for example, may offer greater opportunities for self-directed treatments outside of the clinical environment. The choice between manual therapies and other modalities is not an either-or decision. Combining treatment strategies may result in the most effective and cost-efficient plan of care.

Biofeedback

Biofeedback involves the use of instrumentation to bring about conscious awareness of physiological events. Electromyographic (EMG) biofeedback is the form of biofeedback that is most commonly used in the treatment of musculoskeletal impairment. Electromyographic biofeedback differs from the modalities discussed in this chapter in that it is a device to record electrical activity of muscle rather than a modality that transfers energy to the body. Electromyographic biofeedback can help patients regain volitional control of muscle to increase force production or help them learn to decrease tension in muscle. Since no energy transfer occurs, the application of EMG biofeedback is safe as long as active muscle contraction is not contraindicated. Electromyographic biofeedback is also often better tolerated than neuromuscular electrical nerve stimulation because of the discomfort associated with electrically stimulated muscle contractions.

Some practice on the part of the clinician is needed in order to best utilize EMG biofeedback. However, for patients struggling with neuromuscular control, EMG biofeedback offers clinicians a well-tolerated and usually effective treatment option.

CASE STUDY

Janet, a collegiate ice hockey player involved in preseason conditioning, presents with low back pain. She complains of 4/10 pain with normal daily activity and reports that she has not trained in the past 2 days due to increasing pain with jogging and resistance training. She was evaluated by the team physician and athletic trainer, who together concluded that the pain was mechanical and that evidence based on her age, flexibility, positive prone instability test, and painful movements was sufficient to recommend a lumbar stabilization exercise program.

Think About It

1. Is the application of a therapeutic modality appropriate in caring for Janet? How might a modality help Janet now?

2. What factors would you consider in selecting a modality if it is deemed to be appropriate? Which modality would you select? Why?

3. Would the application of a therapeutic modality help Janet participate in a therapeutic exercise program? When should treatment with a therapeutic modality be discontinued?

Learning Aids

SUMMARY

This chapter provides an overview of the therapeutic modalities commonly applied by athletic trainers. It is essential that these modalities be applied safely and that patients with contraindications for a particular modality application be identified. Beyond the concerns of safety, the athletic trainer must know how to operate devices and perform techniques, must be able to articulate the physical and physiological principles forming the rationale for a treatment, and increasingly needs to make treatment decisions based on the evidence derived from clinical trials. It is no longer appropriate

to apply a treatment based on what theory suggests may be the result; instead one must apply treatments with an understanding of the likelihood and extent of benefit gleaned from the best available research. Practice patterns related to the use of therapeutic modalities by athletic trainers and other health care providers have changed over time, and the rate of change has increased in this age of evidence-based medicine. Thus, it is not sufficient to learn how to use the devices and perform the techniques described in this chapter. The athletic trainer must also be prepared to access and appraise the clinical literature so that the evaluations performed, recommendations made, and treatments rendered reflect best practices as defined by the ever-growing and changing scientific base from which we practice.

KEY CONCEPTS AND REVIEW

▶ **Identify the most common indications for therapeutic modality application.**

Pain relief, restoration of neuromuscular control, swelling management, treatment of adhesions in conjunction with manual therapy, acceleration of repair in selected circumstances (e.g., use of low-intensity pulsed ultrasound in fracture care)

▶ **Describe the common forms of heat and cold, the main treatment goal, and general precautions and contraindications for each.**

The common forms are ice pack, cold pack, cold water circulating unit, immersion and whirlpool, ice massage, moist heat pack, and warm water whirlpool. The goal of most applications of cold and superficial heat is to relieve pain. Cold application is contraindicated in individuals with cold urticaria, Raynaud's phenomenon, cold-induced hemoglobinuria, and cryoglobulinemia. Caution must be exercised to prevent thermal burns with superficial heating, as well as to prevent contamination of open wounds with any modality application.

▶ **Identify the parameters that need to be considered when TENS is applied to relieve pain or recruit muscle contraction.**

Phase duration, stimulus amplitude, and frequency

▶ **Describe the parameters, precautions, and contraindications for ultrasound.**

Parameters include frequency, with 1 or 3 MHz the most common options; amplitude of the sound waves, resulting in an increase in energy delivery measured in Watts per square centimeter; the duty cycle; and duration of treatment. Ultrasound is contraindicated for individuals who have cancer or are pregnant.

Ultrasound also should not be applied over an infection or to patients who may have a deep vein thrombus (DVT). It should not be used over joint replacements; over the heart or in the area of a cardiac pacemaker; or over the eyes or genitalia. In patients who have had a laminectomy, ultrasound should not be applied directly over the area of the cord that is no longer protected by bone.

▶ **Identify two FDA-approved uses of LASER.**

1. "adjunctive use in providing temporary relief of minor chronic neck and shoulder pain of musculoskeletal origin"
2. "adjunctive use in the temporary relief of hand and wrist pain associated with Carpal Tunnel Syndrome"

It is important to note that the clinical literature has described the use of LLLT for many conditions, including a number that are relevant to athletic health care, for example wounds and abrasions, epicondylalgia, and tendinopathy. The effectiveness of these and other applications of LLLT has not been well established.

▶ **Describe the advantages and disadvantages of manual versus mechanical cervical traction.**

Manual traction allows you to carefully control force application and head position to maximize the relief of symptoms. Manual traction also allows you to combine manual techniques. If manual traction relieves pain or radicular symptoms, you can move to mechanical traction for longer treatments that require less of your time.

▶ **Identify the uses, setup, precautions, and contraindications for lumbar traction.**

The traction forces can separate or distract the facet joints and relieve pressure on spinal nerves in patients with a disc injury. Once the belts are positioned, traction forces are administered in either a continuous or an intermittent mode. An initial traction force of 25% of body weight is a reasonable starting force. If the initial force is tolerated, increase the traction force up to 50% of body weight. Treatment times usually range from 10 to 20 min, depending on the nature of the problem and the response to treatment. Pregnancy, hiatal hernia, and advanced osteoporosis are absolute contraindications. Fractures and medical conditions, such as cancer, that affect the integrity of the connective tissues also contraindicate mechanical traction.

▸ **Identify two of the many forms of manual therapy.**

Manual therapies include various forms of massage as well as joint mobilization.

▸ **Describe how EMG biofeedback can be applied in rehabilitation.**

Electromyographic biofeedback is used to record electrical activity in a muscle. Audio and visual signals corresponding to the level of electrical activity provide the patient and clinician with immediate feedback on the success of efforts to improve recruitment. This feedback fosters effective motor unit recruitment and improved force development.

CRITICAL THINKING QUESTIONS

1. A volleyball player suffered an inversion mechanism ankle sprain when he landed on a teammate's foot in a blocking drill. A tournament is coming up in 10 days, and the player has expressed a strong desire to be ready for the next game. The team physician has evaluated the injury as a Grade I sprain involving the anterior talofibular ligament and has cleared the patient to participate with the ankle supported if he is able. Discuss the modalities you might use to reduce pain and promote therapeutic exercise.

2. A female basketball player is struggling with getting her quadriceps to function after an arthroscopic knee surgery. Discuss the role that therapeutic modalities might play in helping her regain strong volitional quadriceps contractions.

CHAPTER 17

Therapeutic Exercise Parameters and Techniques

Peggy A. Houglum, PhD, ATC, PT
Kirk Brumels, PhD, AT, ATC

OBJECTIVES

After reading this chapter, the student should be able to do the following:

- Describe the methods used to measure range of motion of a joint.
- List five stretching techniques that can be used to increase range of joint motion.
- List four common manual therapy techniques used to treat neuro-musculoskeletal conditions.
- Describe the two types of muscle activity.
- Understand the difference between open kinetic chain (OKC) and closed kinetic chain (CKC).
- List the three principles of strengthening.
- Identify the three main components of proprioception.
- Describe plyometrics and list the three phases involved.
- Understand the difference between functional activities and sport-specific activities.
- Identify the four goals for functional and sport-specific exercise.

This chapter delves into basic techniques for restoring or developing range of motion and flexibility, muscular strength and endurance, coordination and agility, soft tissue and joint mobility, and functional and activity-specific exercises. These techniques are used to restore the critical physical attributes needed for recovery and participation in physical activity. It is important to remember the principles of rehabilitation and tissue healing discussed in chapter 15 when you implement these techniques or exercises. Effective rehabilitation occurs when all areas of rehabilitation are addressed and tissue healing is not disrupted. The rehabilitation needs and desires will be specific to each case and patient that you encounter. Understanding the diagnosis, getting to know your patient, setting short-term and long-term goals, and implementing appropriate techniques and exercises to meet those goals are all important for complete rehabilitation and recovery.

Range of Motion and Flexibility

The terms *range of motion* and *flexibility* are often used interchangeably, but there is a difference between them. **Flexibility** is the ability to elongate or stretch and range of motion is the amount of mobility within a joint. Although flexibility and strength are related and when one is deficient the other may also become deficient, they are not the same. Clinically, **range of motion** measurements are used to quantify both range of motion and flexibility. Although there is a technical distinction between the two, clinical interpretations make differences less clear. For this reason, we use the terms *range of motion* and *flexibility* interchangeably in this text.

Measuring Range of Motion

Before you can determine whether a joint has deficient range of motion, you first know the normal range of motion. Only then can you decide whether stretching exercises should be included in the therapeutic exercise program. There is no consistent agreement on expected and normal ranges of motion within the scientific community. In addition, many controllable and uncontrollable factors affect range of motion. Normal range of motion is different for each joint, each patient, and each sport and position. Therefore, each patient's normal range of motion requirements of the injured segment should be determined by comparison with the contralateral body part and the demands of the patient's individual activities.

Range of motion is usually measured with an instrument known as a **goniometer**. The goniometer is essentially a protractor with a stationary arm and a movable arm, as shown in figure 17.1. It can measure up to either 180° or 360°. Many varieties of goniometers have been designed to measure different joints. Houglum (2010) provides a thorough discussion on how to conduct goniometer measurements.

To measure accurately with a goniometer, the most common tool for evaluating range of motion, placement of the protractor and arms is important. The arms of the goniometer are placed along the length of the two limbs forming the joint. If the protractor is placed correctly, the pivot point should be lined up over the axis of motion of the

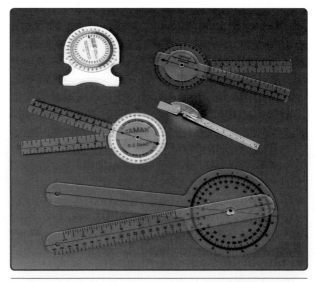

Figure 17.1 Goniometers come in different sizes to measure various body segments. They most often measure up 360° or 180°.

joint. For correct alignment, the limbs being measured should be exposed. With some exceptions, the goniometer is placed along the central lateral aspect of the limb. Figure 17.2 demonstrates measuring techniques for some joints.

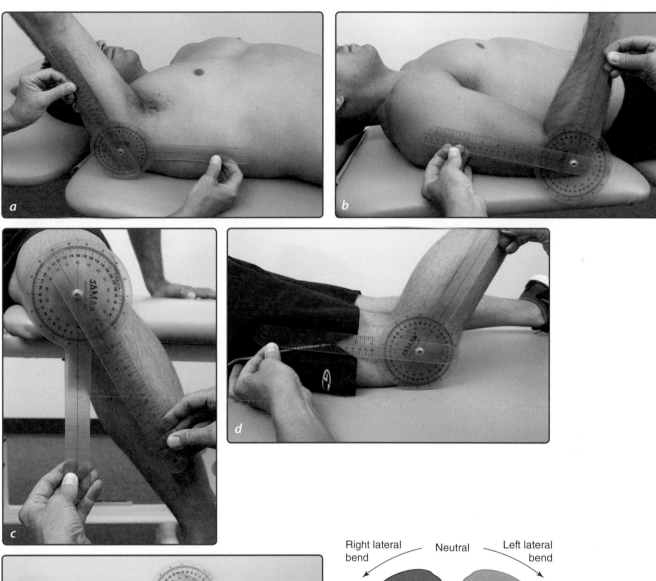

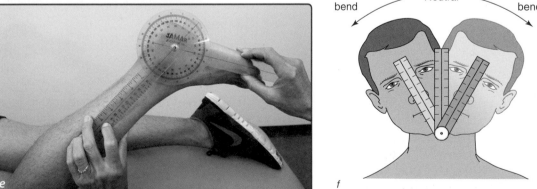

Figure 17.2 Goniometer placement for measuring *(a)* shoulder flexion, *(b)* elbow flexion, *(c)* hip medial rotation, *(d)* knee flexion, *(e)* ankle plantarflexion, and *(f)* cervical lateral flexion. The center of the goniometer is placed over the joint's center (axis of motion). For reliable measurements, alignment of the goniometer's stationary and movable arms and fulcrum must be accurate.

Range of motion is measured in either a 180° or 360° system using either a 180° or 360° goniometer. In the 360° system, 0° is overhead and 180° is at the feet. In the 180° system, 0° is at the start of the range in the anatomical position and 180° is at the end. Either system is valid and can be used to measure range of motion. The most common system used for musculoskeletal injuries is the 180° system.

A rehabilitation clinician's ability to accurately measure range of motion depends on her training, experience, and attention to detail. Even an experienced clinician with good equipment can expect accuracy only within 3° to 5° of true values. It is therefore vital to be as consistent as possible. Careful attention to the placement of the goniometer arms and making sure that the axis of the goniometer coincides with the joint's axis of rotation are very important to ensure accurate measurements. Check the goniometer placement, adjust the patient's position if necessary to achieve correct body segment alignment, and then check again before recording your final measurement to help ensure accuracy. Consistent measurements depend on your attention to these details. If your technique is good, your measurements should be reliable. If your technique varies, your results will be inconsistent and of no use to you, the patient, or anyone else.

Recording Range of Motion

Range of motion records are indicated first by the joint and motion measured and then by the type of motion measured: active range of motion (AROM) or passive range of motion (PROM). Degrees are most often recorded based on a 180° scale. If a patient is unable to achieve full extension (0°), the point at which the patient is able to move is recorded along with the end point of motion in the opposite direction. For example, if a patient is lacking 15° from full extension and is able to flex the knee to 100°, the record will show knee extension-flexion = 15° to 100°. Sometimes a clinician records the number of degrees lacking from extension

as a minus (–) number, such as –15°. This can be misleading, however, in that it may also be interpreted as 15° of hyperextension.

Goniometric Terminology

Goniometric measurements involve terms that allow practitioners to communicate with each other. Knowledge and use of these terms is important for reproducible measurements and accurate sharing of information among health care practitioners of different backgrounds and clinical expertise. The following are terms that are frequently used to refer to range of motion, flexibility, and goniometric measurements.

sagittal plane—The anterior–posterior vertical plane that the longitudinal axis passes through and that divides the body into right and left halves.

frontal (coronal) plane—Any vertical plane that divides the body into front and back parts.

transverse (horizontal) plane—A plane that divides a section of the body into upper and lower parts. It is parallel to the horizon.

flexion—Bending a joint so that the two body segments approach each other and decrease the joint angle.

extension—Straightening a joint so that the two body segments move apart and increase the joint angle.

abduction—Lateral movement of a limb or segment away from the midline of the body or part.

adduction—Lateral movement of a limb or segment toward the midline of the body or part.

medial rotation—Rotation of a joint around its axis in a transverse plane toward the middle of the body. Although not as correct, this motion is also called *internal rotation*.

lateral rotation—Rotation of a joint around its axis in a transverse plane away from the midline of the body.

Although not as correct, this motion is also called *external rotation*.

supination—Movement of the palm forward or upward into the anatomical position. Also, the multiplanar rotation of the subtalar and transverse talar joints that includes plantarflexion, adduction, and inversion.

pronation—Movement of the palm backward or downward so that the palm faces in a posterior direction, opposite the anatomical position. Also, a multiplanar rotation of the subtalar and transverse talar joints that is the combination of dorsiflexion, abduction, and eversion.

inversion—Inward-turning motion of the foot that causes the bottom of the foot to face medially.

eversion—Outward-turning motion of the foot that causes the bottom of the foot to face laterally.

dorsiflexion—A flexion of the ankle that causes the dorsum (top) of the foot to move toward the leg so that the angle of the ankle decreases.

plantarflexion—An extension of the ankle that causes the dorsum (top) of the foot to move away from the leg so that the angle of the ankle increases.

radial deviation—A movement of the wrist toward the thumb side of the forearm. Also called *radial abduction*.

ulnar deviation—A movement of the wrist toward the little-finger side of the forearm. Also called *ulnar abduction*.

opposition—A diagonal movement of the thumb across the palm of the hand to permit it to make contact with one of the other four fingers.

depression—A downward movement of the scapula.

elevation—An upward movement of the scapula.

protraction—A forward movement of the scapula. Also called *scapular abduction*.

retraction—A backward movement of the scapula. Also called *scapular adduction*.

upward rotation—A movement of the scapula that causes the glenoid to face forward and upward. The inferior angle of the scapula moves laterally away from the spine, and the scapula slides forward.

downward rotation—A movement of the scapula that causes the glenoid to face downward and backward. The inferior angle of the scapula moves medially, and the scapula slides backward.

horizontal flexion—A motion of the shoulder in a transverse plane toward the midline of the body. Also called *horizontal adduction*.

horizontal extension—A motion of the shoulder in a transverse plane away from the midline of the body. Also called *horizontal abduction*.

Stretching

When an individual has an injury that results in deficient range of motion, several techniques can be applied to restore range of motion, depending on your preference and skill, the type of tissue restriction involved, the extent of the injury, and the duration of the loss of motion.

Probably one of the most common methods of increasing range of motion is stretching exercises. Regardless of the type of stretch used, the application of heat beforehand produces a better stretch. Heat can be applied either passively or actively. An example of a passive heat application is the use of a hot pack. A better method is active heat application, in which the patient performs a warm-up activity, such as exercising on a stationary bike, stair climber, or upper body ergometer, before stretching. A hot pack provides superficial heat, but an active exercise increases the deeper tissues' temperature more effectively and more safely than a passive modality (Saal 1987).

Types of Stretching

Stretching exercises can be divided into active stretching, passive stretching, and a combination of the two. The choice of stretching technique depends on the tissues involved, the stage of healing, the patient's motivation, the time and facilities available, and other factors related to the injury.

Active stretching includes flexibility exercises that are performed by the patient without outside assistance from either another person or a machine (figure 17.3).

Passive stretching includes a variety of methods, including short-term and long-term stretches. Passive stretching involves the use of equipment or another person, and the patient does not assist in the stretch (figure 17.4). In a typical example of a short-term passive stretch, the clinician moves the injured part through its range of motion and applies a stretch at the end of the motion while the patient remains relaxed. The proximal segment of the joint being stretched should be stabilized to prevent its movement while a firm pressure is applied to the distal segment. A steady pressure is applied until the slack of soft tissue is taken up and the joint is tight. The joint is then moved slightly beyond this point. The patient should feel a stretch or tension, but not pain. The most effective stretches involve the steady application of force over a period of time. This is a long-term passive stretch and is applied at a lower level of force than a short-term stretch. It is also applied for several minutes before being released.

The combination of active and passive stretching is often referred to as neuromuscular facilitation or **proprioceptive neuromuscular facilitation (PNF)**. Although PNF can be used as a strengthening technique, it also is useful for gaining range of motion. Of the various PNF techniques used to increase motion, the most frequently used are the hold–relax, contract–relax, and slow reversal-hold-relax techniques.

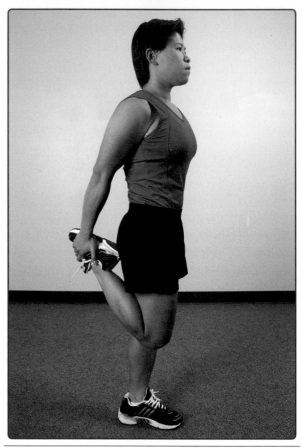

Figure 17.3   Active stretch.

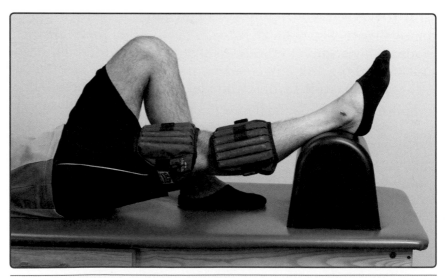

Figure 17.4   The patient does not assist in passive stretch. The stretch here is provided by gravity and is further assisted with weights on the leg.

Two technique patterns are used in PNF: agonistic and antagonistic. The **agonistic muscle pattern** occurs when the muscle is contracting toward its shortened state. The **antagonistic muscle pattern** is diagonally opposite to the agonistic pattern and occurs when the muscle is approaching its lengthened state. Each pattern of movement involves three planes of motion: flexion-extension, abduction-adduction, and medial rotation–lateral rotation. For example, if an agonistic pattern of motion included flexion, adduction, and lateral rotation, the antagonistic pattern would include extension, abduction, and medial rotation.

In each of the descriptions that follow, it may be easiest to visualize an example. Think of a hamstring muscle that is tight and suppose that you are trying to improve its flexibility. In this example, the hamstrings group is the antagonist and the quadriceps group is the agonist.

• The **hold–relax technique** uses a maximal isometric contraction of the antagonist (hamstrings) in all three planes of movement at the end of the agonist (quadriceps) range, followed by a relaxation of the hamstrings. The agonist is then used actively without resistance to increase motion of the antagonist (hamstrings). This technique is used to relax muscle spasm.

• The **contract–relax technique** is used with patients who have limited range of motion. With the patient's restricted joint placed at the end range in the agonistic (quadriceps) pattern, the clinician provides isotonic resistance against the antagonist muscles (hamstrings) to allow diagonal and rotational motion to the end range. When the patient relaxes the muscle, the clinician moves the part passively into the agonist muscle pattern to stretch the antagonist (hamstrings). The process is repeated several times.

• The **slow reversal-hold-relax technique** uses concentric contraction of the agonist (quadriceps) into the range-limited motion of the hamstrings followed by an isometric contraction of the antagonist (hamstrings). This is followed by relaxation of the antagonist (hamstrings), then concentric movement by the agonist (quadriceps). The clinician provides maximal isometric resistance against the rotational component of the movement.

Table 17.1 summarizes the three PNF techniques for improving flexibility.

Another type of stretching—ballistic stretching—is the use of quick, bouncing movements through alternating contraction and relaxation of a muscle to stretch its antagonist. This type of stretch is not used much in rehabilitation because of the damage it can cause to already injured tissue.

Assistive Devices in Stretching

In addition to equipment such as weights, pulleys, and straps for providing prolonged stretch to areas of limited motion, many devices are commonly used to help people regain range of motion.

• *Continuous passive motion machines.* A **continuous passive motion (CPM)** machine is sometimes used following surgery

Table 17.1 PNF Techniques to Improve Flexibility

Technique	Muscle activity
Hold-relax	Muscle is brought to end motion, isometric contraction of tight muscle, relax, stretch via contraction of opposing muscle.
Contract-relax	Muscle is brought to end motion, isotonic contraction of tight muscle, relax, passive movement to end range.
Slow reversal-hold-relax	Opposing muscle contracts to bring tight muscle to end range, isometric contraction of tight muscle, relax, stretch via contraction of opposing muscle.

to restore range of motion. Although now used less frequently, a CPM can help counteract the deleterious effects of immobilization and reduce pain and edema after surgery. Continuous passive motion machines are designed for a variety of joints, including the knee, ankle, elbow, wrist, and shoulder. An example of a knee CPM is seen in figure 17.5.

• **Splints.** Splints also assist in prolonged stretching of restricted joints. After injury, the collagen and connective tissue that produce scarring become progressively more difficult to stretch, and prolonged stretching for more than 20 min is often needed. In such instances, splints that apply a low-level, continual stretch force are often most beneficial. They commonly use a three-point lever

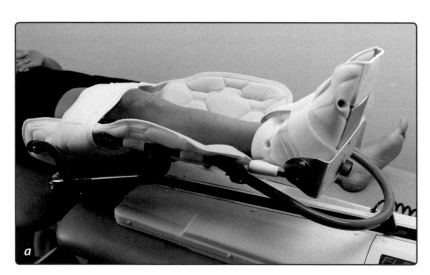

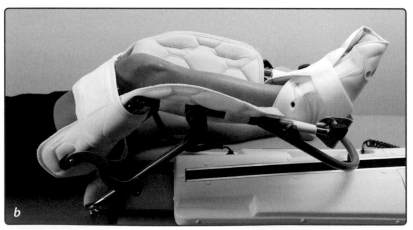

Figure 17.5 Continuous passive motion machine: Range of motion limits for *(a)* extension and *(b)* flexion can be set at desired levels as necessary.

and spring system to provide a low-level, continual load.

Indications, Contraindications, and Precautions for Stretching

Before applying a stretch to increase range of motion, you must know when stretching is indicated, when you should not use stretching, and what precautions apply. The choice of stretching technique depends on the tissues involved, the stage of healing, the patient's motivation, the time and facilities available, and other factors related to the injury.

• **Indications.** As part of the patient evaluation performed in rehabilitation, the clinician determines deficiencies in range of motion, the structures causing the loss of motion, and the status of the tissue. Is the loss a result of recent scar tissue formation, adherent and mature scar tissue, spasm, edema, postural deformities, or weakness of opposing muscles? If ligaments, capsules, muscles, fascia, skin, or other soft tissue is shortened because of scar tissue or adhesions, stretching exercises are indicated. Stretching is also indicated in the presence of contractures and structural deformities from injury or posture changes over time.

• **Contraindications.** Although stretching is usually safe, it is contraindicated when certain conditions are present. One of these is a recent fracture where immobilization is necessary for healing and movement is detrimental to healing. Others are a bony block that restricts motion, infection in a joint, acute inflammation in a joint, extreme and sharp pain with motion, and conditions in which tightness of soft tissue actually contributes to an area's stability.

• *Precautions.* Precautions should be taken to ensure the most effective application of the stretch and to prevent harm from the stretch. Before applying any treatment, you should always explain to the patient what you will do and the sensations and outcome to expect. A patient who is apprehensive and unable to relax will not receive an effective stretch treatment.

Manual Therapy Techniques

Manual therapy is the use of hands-on techniques to evaluate, treat, and improve the status of neuromusculoskeletal conditions. A variety of structures, including joints and soft tissue, are affected by procedures that fall into the category of manual therapy. The various procedures in this category are defined according to the tissues and structures they influence.

Many medical professionals consider manual therapy techniques subjective because little quantitative research has addressed the efficacy of such techniques. It is difficult to create an objective research design with these treatments because the specific application, direction, duration, and amplitude of a force can vary from one health care provider to another. With these variations come a variety of outcomes, so a truly objective assessment of treatment effectiveness is difficult, if not impossible. Most of the benefits recorded are considered anecdotal because of their subjective basis. Manual therapy techniques, however, deserve attention and application because clinical report outcomes are often overwhelmingly positive.

There is no cookbook method for applying manual therapy. You must be able to use your skills of observation, palpation, analysis, and technique application. As with other aspects of rehabilitation, analysis and deduc-

tive reasoning are skills vital to a successful outcome of manual techniques. Depending on the specific injury and resulting impairments, you may choose to use more than one manual therapy technique. Evaluation and deductive reasoning allow you to select treatment techniques that can best reduce the impairment and improve the functional ability of the injured patient.

Massage

Massage is the systematic and scientific manipulation of soft tissue for remedial or restorative purposes. Massage affects various systems of the body through its influence on reflex and mechanical processes to produce desired results. Many types of massage are used in a number of applications to achieve a variety of goals. Even though massage is used in nonmedical situations, it still produces a physiological effect. This section briefly describes the range of techniques most commonly used in the treatment of injuries.

Effects of Massage

Massage produces reflex physiological and mechanical effects in the area treated. Repetitive pressure stimulation without irritation to the skin causes transmission from peripheral receptors to the spinal cord and brain, which results in relaxation of muscles and dilation of blood vessels. Mechanical effects improve blood and lymph flow, promote mobilization of fluid, and stretch and break down adhesions to ultimately assist in reducing edema and improving tissue mobility. The overall end result is relaxation of muscles, dilation of local capillaries, increase in lymph flow to reduce edema, reduction of pain, and improvement in soft tissue movement. The specific effects vary depending on the type of massage.

Types of Massage

Although there are many different massage techniques, three primary techniques are used in treating injuries to achieve the effects mentioned earlier.

• *Effleurage.* **Effleurage**, or stroking, is a massage that is performed by running the hand lightly over the skin's surface. The stroke moves distally to proximally (figure 17.6). Effleurage is used to assist in venous and lymphatic flow to decrease edema and aid in muscle relaxation. If the technique is used primarily to treat edema, it should be performed with the part in a position such that gravity can assist the flow. The pressure should be applied firmly and deeply but not heavily. The direction should be toward the heart.

• *Petrissage.* Compression and kneading fall under the category of **petrissage**. In this technique, the tissue is grasped and released with varying degrees of pressure so that the mechanical effects of movement between the skin's underlying structures reduce edema (figure 17.7). This technique is often preceded and followed by a stroking technique for relaxation. Petrissage is used to promote circulation, relax muscle, mechanically assist fluid exchange, and improve mobility of muscle tissue.

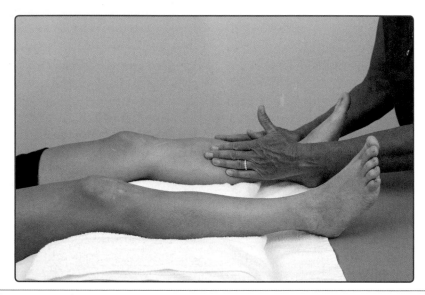

Figure 17.6   Effleurage: Stroking motion begins distally and moves proximally toward the heart. Elevating the segment during treatment further assists in edema reduction.

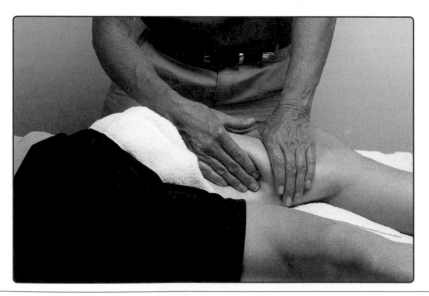

Figure 17.7   Petrissage: Skin and underlying tissue are kneaded and lifted to improve tissue mobility, relax muscle, and promote circulation.

• *Friction.* **Friction** massage is a deep-pressure movement of superficial soft tissue against underlying structures (figure 17.8). Sometimes the underlying structure is bone or another hard surface, and sometimes it is soft tissue, such as muscle or fascia. The intent is to loosen scar tissue and adhesions of deeper parts, such as tendons, ligaments, and joint capsules, to improve movement and gliding of these structures. Friction also helps to stimulate circulation of the local area. It usually is applied through firm pressure by either the thumb or finger pads in a crisscross or circular motion.

Indications, Contraindications, and Precautions for Massage

Before using massage, you should evaluate its appropriateness for your rehabilitation goals and make sure that it is appropriate for the current stage of tissue healing. In addition, you should critically evaluate the indications, contraindications, and precautions for the massage technique you will be using. To be effective, it must be beneficial and indicated.

• *Indications.* The indications for massage are related to its effects. Relief of pain, muscle relaxation, reduction of swelling, and mobilization of adherent scar tissue are all appropriate indications for the use of massage. The specific technique selection is based on the findings of the evaluation. Recent edema secondary to trauma is an indication for effleurage and petrissage massage techniques. Friction massage is indicated when scar tissue restriction of superficial tissue can be palpated.

• *Contraindications.* Massage is contraindicated when the technique may aggravate the condition or cause additional harm to the patient. Contraindications include the presence of infection, malignancies, skin diseases, blood clots, and any irritations or lesions that may spread with direct contact.

• *Precautions.* When you apply massage, both the patient's skin and your hands should be clean. Your hands should be warm, and your nails should be trimmed so as not to cause a laceration or abrasion. Rings, watches, and wrist jewelry should be removed for the same reason. A lubricant is used to reduce friction with the application of effleurage. Less lubricant is used with petrissage, and still less is used with friction massage.

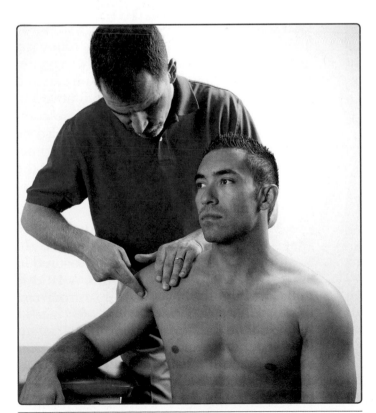

Figure 17.8 Friction massage across the biceps tendon loosens adhesions and stimulates circulation.

Myofascial Release

Myofascial release is a close relative of massage. They both involve manual contact with the patient, and they both use the sense of touch to evaluate the problem and the effectiveness of the treatment. They also both include the use of pressure and tissue stretch to produce results.

There are many different techniques of myofascial release, but they all are essentially variations of the same principle: The use of manual contact for evaluation and treatment of soft tissue restriction and pain has the eventual goal of relief of those symptoms to improve motion and function. There are different names for these techniques: myofascial release, myofascial stretching, strain-counterstrain, Rolfing, and soft tissue mobilization.

Muscle Energy

Like many manual therapy techniques, muscle energy techniques have their origin in osteopathic medicine. **Muscle energy** is the use of muscle contraction to correct a joint's malalignment. Muscle energy techniques are used to treat joint malalignments. These techniques involve the precise and controlled voluntary contraction of a muscle against a counterforce provided by the rehabilitation clinician, followed by a passive stretch. Muscle energy theory is based on the premise that joint malalignments occur when the body becomes unbalanced. Malalignment may be the result of a muscle spasm, a weakened muscle overpowered by a stronger muscle, or restricted mobility. The muscle contraction used to correct a malalignment may be **isometric**, **concentric**, or **eccentric**. The patient controls the magnitude of contraction, and the clinician positions the patient and provides the resistance to change the alignment of the treated joint.

Joint Mobilization

Joint mobilization is one of the most commonly used manual therapy techniques in the treatment of restricted joint motion. **Manipulation** and mobilization are not new concepts. Hippocrates (460-355 B.C.) used these techniques in his medical practice and recorded various methods of manipulating bones and joints. Through the years a variety of approaches to manipulation and mobilization have been developed. More recent schools of thought have been influenced by the teachings of manual clinicians such as Geoffrey Maitland (1991), Freddy Kaltenborn (2002), James Cyriax (1977), James Mennell (1964), and Stanley Paris (1988).

Joint mobilization is on a continuum with manipulation. They both involve passive movement of a joint, but mobilization is under the patient's control in that voluntary contraction of a muscle will stop the movement. Manipulation is at such a speed that the patient is unable to stop the motion. Mobilization is frequently performed by rehabilitation clinicians, but manipulation is not. Manipulation is most commonly performed in chiropractic applications and is beyond the scope of this book.

As with many manual therapy techniques, the exact effects of joint mobilization are unknown; however, a few investigators have recently provided evidence to demonstrate the efficacy of joint mobilization for specific conditions. Though most reported benefits remain anecdotal, many clinicians report consistent, positive results from their treatments; it is therefore assumed within the allied health and medical world that the techniques produce some biochemical, biophysiological, or biomechanical benefits.

Muscular Strength, Power, and Endurance

To effectively rehabilitate patients following an injury, it is important to help them regain or redevelop muscular strength, power, and endurance. Although many rehabilitative and functional exercises address all three components of muscle function, it may also be important to work on just one area at a time. Therefore it is imperative to understand the differences in function and ways of developing these areas.

- **Muscle strength** is the maximum force that a muscle or muscle group can exert. In healthy individuals it is usually measured in 1RM, the 1-repetition maximum. A 1RM is the weight that a muscle or muscle group can lift for only one repetition.

- **Muscle power** is strength that is applied over a distance for a specific amount of time. Power is involved in most athletic events and is strength incorporated with speed. Power is represented mathematically by the formula $P = F \times D/T$, where P = power, F = force, D = distance, and T = time.

• **Muscle endurance** is the ability of a muscle or a muscle group to perform repeated contractions against a less than maximal load. A muscle's endurance, or ability to prolong activity, depends on the status of the energy systems available and the forces resisted. With advanced conditioning levels, circulatory and local metabolic exchanges improve.

Muscle strength and muscle endurance can be placed on a continuum of exercise. High-intensity, low-repetition exercise, at one end of the continuum, emphasizes primarily strength gains. Low-intensity, high-repetition exercise, at the other end of the continuum, produces primarily muscle endurance gains.

Muscle Activity

Although some authors refer to the types of muscle activity as muscle contraction, this is not entirely accurate. Contraction implies a shortening of the muscle, but as you will see, a muscle does not always shorten when it acts. Therefore "muscle contraction" is referred to here as muscle *activity* or *movement*. There are two types of muscle activity, static and dynamic. Static activity is also called isometric. Dynamic activity is divided into isotonic and isokinetic. Isotonic activity can be further divided into concentric and eccentric movements involved in open or closed kinetic chain activities and movements.

Static Activity

Static, or **isometric**, **activity** is produced when muscle tension is created without a change in the muscle's length. Static activity is used not only in therapeutic exercise but also in daily activities and sport participation. The disadvantage of isometrics is that strength gains are isolated to only within 20° of the angle at which the isometric is performed. It is important to remember to caution the patient to avoid a **Valsalva maneuver** during isometric exercises. The Valsalva maneuver occurs when the patient holds his breath, causing an increase in intrathoracic pressure. This can in turn impede venous return to the right atrium, leading to an increase in peripheral venous pressure (increasing blood pressure) and reducing cardiac output because of lowered cardiac volume. If you see a patient holding his breath during exercise, remind him to breathe avoid the Valsalva maneuver risk.

Dynamic Activity

The term *dynamic* in relation to activity implies a change in the position of a muscle. **Dynamic activity** is further divided into specific types.

• Isotonic activity is dynamic in that it involves a change in the muscle's length. If the muscle shortens, the activity is called concentric. If the muscle lengthens, the activity is called eccentric. Although you can isolate muscle activity to produce either concentric or eccentric motion, most sport and daily activities involve the use of both concentric and eccentric actions.

• Isokinetic activity is a dynamic activity in that it involves motion. It differs from isotonic activity, however, in that the velocity is controlled and maintained at a specific speed of movement. *Isokinetic* means "having the same motion" and refers to the unchanging speed of movement that occurs during these activities. Whereas the speed of motion remains constant, the amount of resistance provided to the muscle varies as the muscle goes through its range. Isokinetics is sometimes called **accommodating resistance** exercise because of the change in resistance given throughout a range of motion.

Open and Closed Kinetic Chain Activity

A kinetic chain is a series of rigid arms linked by movable joints. This is a mechanical description of the body. **Open kinetic chain (OKC)** and **closed kinetic chain (CKC)** within the body are identified in terms of the distal segment of the extremity, the hand or foot. The kinetic chain is open when the distal segment moves freely in space. A kinetic chain is closed when the distal segment is weight bearing and the body moves over the hand or foot. Generally, OKC athletic activities produce high-velocity motions such as throwing a ball, swinging a racket, or the swing phase of the leg during running or kicking a ball; CKC activities are functional weight-bearing activities such as squatting, pushing with arms extended, or handstands that compress the joint and thus place lesser shear forces on the joints. This decreased shear force means that CKC exercises are generally safer to use earlier in a therapeutic exercise program.

Both the OKC and CKC systems involve a relationship between one joint and the others within the chain. This is important to remember in therapeutic exercise, because if you ignore the other joints within the chain when rehabilitating an injured joint, success of the program will be elusive. Function of one joint is not exclusive: The function of one joint determines the function of the other joints within the chain.

Strength Equipment

Many types of equipment are available to provide strength gains in both rehabilitation and conditioning programs. Most equipment can be used for both purposes. Cost varies greatly also—from very little to several thousand dollars. What you decide to use in your therapeutic exercise programs depends on your familiarity with the equipment, availability, budget, and the specific needs of the injured patients. Regardless of the amount or kind of equipment you have, you can design a very comprehensive, progressive, and appropriate therapeutic exercise program for every patient you treat. Your imagination and knowledge are ultimately the determining factors in the quality of the program you create.

The following sections deal with the most common items of equipment available on the market. Most are items you will become familiar with before you complete your curriculum.

Manual Resistance

Manual resistance equipment is the least expensive therapeutic exercise equipment. The only requirement is you. **Manual resistance exercise** is an exercise in which the rehabilitation clinician applies manual force to produce either static or dynamic resistance. Manual resistance can be applied isometrically if movement is not desirable, if pain occurs with motion, or if the patient's muscle has a specific area of weakness within a range of motion. Manual resistance can also be applied concentrically or eccentrically, through part of the motion or the full motion.

Body Weight

Exercise using body weight also requires no equipment. The patient's own body weight provides the resistance, as shown in the push-up example in figure 17.9. A variety of exercises for the upper and lower extremities and the trunk can be used, along with progressions, to offer an adequate system of therapeutic exercises.

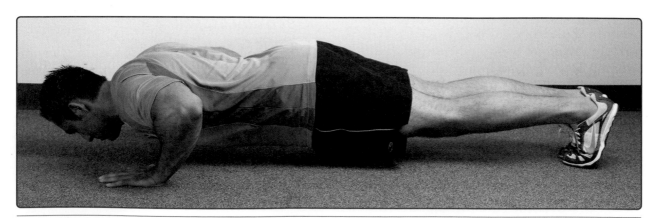

Figure 17.9   Push-ups are a classic body weight exercise.

Rubber Tubing and Bands

Rubber tubing and bands provide dynamic resistance exercises via the elastic elements of their makeup (figure 17.10). They are packaged in large and small rolls, so strips can be cut to varying lengths; they also come in a range of resistance levels, indicated by different colors. Although various companies market the bands with their own color indicators, the most familiar spectrum corresponding to resistance levels from lightest to heaviest is tan, yellow, red, green, blue, black, silver (gray), and gold (butterscotch). The color-coding scheme for tubing is similar.

Free Weights

When most people think of strengthening, they think of free weights. Free weights include cuff weights, barbells, and dumbbells. They come in a variety of sizes and styles. The weight is either attached to the body part or held by the patient during the exercises. Cuff weights typically cannot be changed in size. Some can be modified by the addition of preset weighted tubes or packets that are placed in a pocket on the cuff. The cuffs are attached to ankles or wrists.

Some dumbbells and barbells are adjustable: Various weights can be placed on the bar and are secured with collars (figure 17.11). Other dumbbells and barbells are fixed and their weight cannot be changed. *Dumbbells* refers to weights that are used in

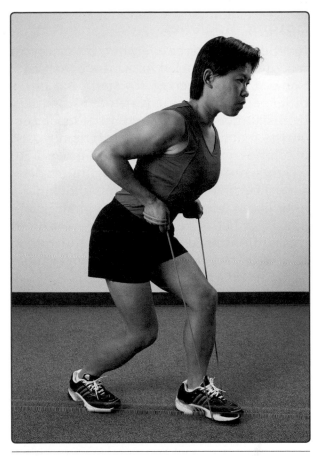

Figure 17.10   Rubber band bent-over row exercise.

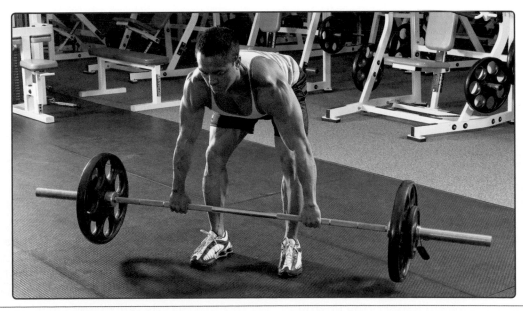

Figure 17.11   The barbell used in the bent-over row is an example of a free-weight or isotonic exercise.

one hand, are usually smaller, and are either fixed weights or adjustable. *Barbells* refers to a larger free-weight system that requires using both hands.

Isotonic Machines

In addition to free weights, a variety of machines can be used for isotonic exercises. Some have a fixed lever system that offers different amounts of resistance. Changes in resistance occur differently, depending on the machine. The most commonly used machines provide altered resistance with weights, resistance bands, or hydraulic pressure. This category of equipment includes a long list of machines made by many companies. A list of generic examples includes hydraulic devices, multiple-station units, individual freestanding stations, and rubber cord resistive machines.

Isokinetic Machines

Isokinetic machines (figure 17.12) offer resistance at a constant speed, so the amount of resistance varies through the range of motion. This is sometimes referred to as *accommodating resistance*. To produce a constant speed, the machine offers a matching resistance when the patient attempts to push the arm of the machine as hard as possible. For an isokinetic exercise to produce the desired results, the patient must resist the machine with maximal effort.

Isokinetic exercise machines have been available since the early 1970s. They were very popular during the 1970s and 1980s. Several manufacturers produced isokinetic equipment during the 1980s. Today, emphasis has moved away from using isokinetic equipment for exercise, but it is still used to objectively evaluate and compare muscular strength, power, and endurance of an injured body part to preinjury levels or to the nonaffected side.

Proprioceptive Neuromuscular Facilitation

Proprioceptive neuromuscular facilitation (PNF) has been helpful in restoring flexibility,

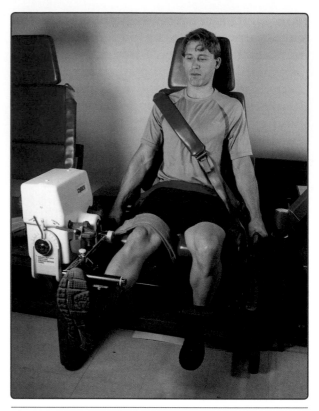

Figure 17.12 Strength evaluation and isokinetic testing using an isokinetic machine.

strength, and coordination of injured muscles and joints. We discussed PNF techniques for flexibility earlier; this section deals with the use of PNF for strength development. The underlying significance of this technique is in its use of combinations of primitive movement patterns performed with a maximum amount of resistance applied throughout the range of motion. Exercise techniques based on PNF use impulses from the afferent receptors in various parts of the body to stimulate the desired motion. The techniques were originally found to be useful in the treatment of neuromuscular disorders, but over time they have also proven beneficial for application to orthopedic disorders.

The premise underlying PNF is that central nervous system stimulation produces mass movement patterns, not straight-plane movements. Natural motion does not occur in straight planes but in mass movement patterns that incorporate a diagonal motion in combination with a spiral movement. In other words, all major parts of the body move in patterns that have three components (see figures 17.13 & 17.14). These diagonal patterns (identified as Diagonal 1 [D1] and Diagonal 2 [D2]) include the components of flexion-extension, adduction-abduction, and medial-lateral rotation. Houglum (2010) provides additional information on PNF patterns.

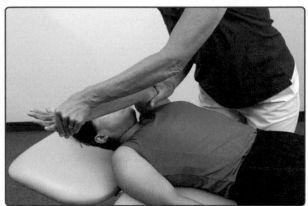

Joint	D1 flexion	D2 flexion
Shoulder:	Flexion	Flexion
	Lateral rotation	Lateral rotation
	Adduction	Abduction
Forearm:	Supination	Supination
Wrist:	Radial flexion	Radial extension
Fingers:	Flexion	Extension

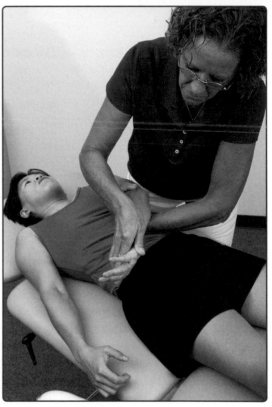

Joint	D2 extension	D1 extension
Shoulder:	Extension	Extension
	Medial rotation	Medial rotation
	Adduction	Abduction
Forearm:	Pronation	Pronation
Wrist:	Ulnar flexion	Ulnar extension
Fingers:	Flexion	Extension

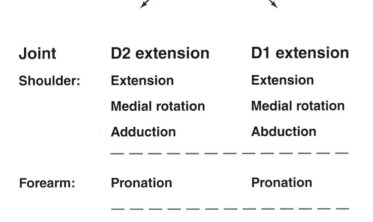

Figure 17.13 Upper extremity proprioceptive neuromuscular facilitation patterns.

Joint	D1 flexion	D2 flexion
Hip:	Flexion	Flexion
	Adduction	Abduction
	Lateral rotation	Medial rotation
Ankle:	Dorsiflexion	Dorsiflexion
	Inversion	Eversion
Toes:	Extension	Extension

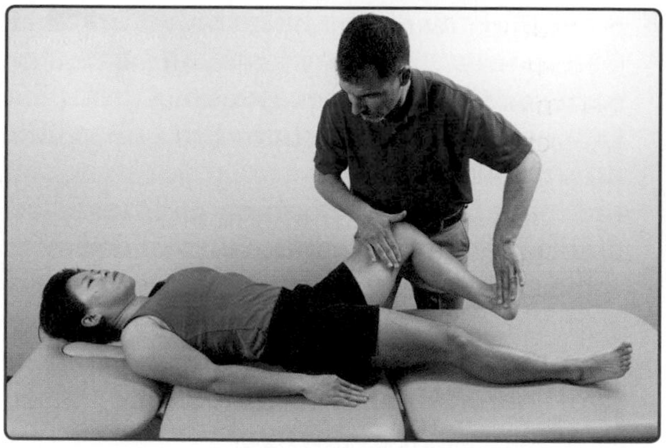

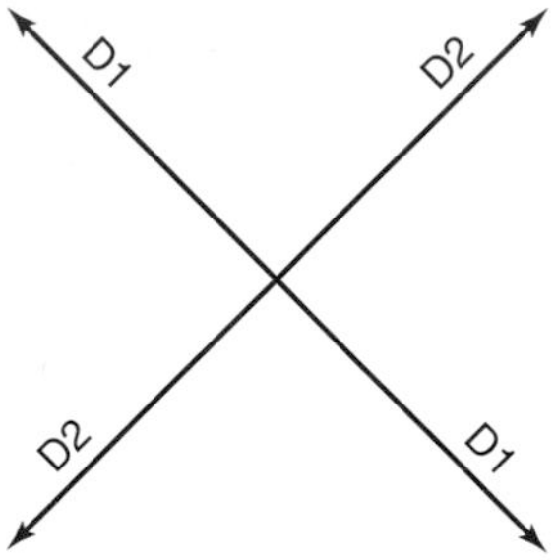

Joint	D2 extension	D1 extension
Hip:	Extension	Extension
	Adduction	Abduction
	Lateral rotation	Medial rotation
Ankle:	Plantar flexion	Plantar flexion
	Inversion	Eversion
Toes:	Flexion	Flexion

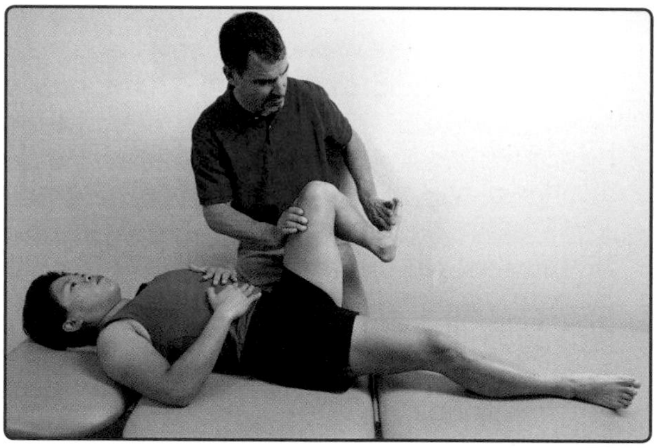

Figure 17.14 Lower extremity proprioceptive neuromuscular facilitation patterns.

Principles of Strengthening Exercises

Once a therapeutic exercise program starts, strengthening exercises at some level should begin. However, the exercises must be appropriate for the patient, the injury, and the time frame. You should adhere to several important principles when initiating strengthening exercises as part of the therapeutic exercise program.

No Pain

There should be no pain during strengthening exercises. Delayed pain or postexercise pain should be avoided. Postexercise pain accompanied by postexercise edema is an indication that the exercises have been too severe. It is advisable to reduce the severity of the exercise or even postpone the application of a strengthening exercise if you observe these symptoms. Pain produces a reflex withdrawal of muscle activity so that the muscle will not produce a maximal output. Progression of strengthening exercises should be gradual and within the patient's tolerance. If you increase resistance too much too quickly, the body may experience an inflammatory response. Increased edema and pain are key signs of inflammation.

Attainable Goals

Goals for the patient should be challenging but attainable. This means that it should be possible for the patient to move the selected weight for the required number of repetitions and sets and to perform the specific exercise. Most patients are goal oriented and are determined to achieve any goal set for them by themselves or by others. If goals are not achievable, the unrealistic expectations placed on the patient will serve only to frustrate both you and the patient. If you discover during the course of the exercise routine that you have set too high a goal, it is best to adjust the goal. Occasionally you may need to adjust goals according to the patient's response to the previous exercise session.

Progressive Overload

Providing a **progressive overload** of exercises is key to muscle strengthening. To continue to produce strength gains, the load must be progressively greater. This concept is sometimes referred to as the **overload principle**: As a muscle's strength increases, the muscle must be overloaded.

When it is not possible to actively exercise the injured area, **cross-training** can produce strength gains. Cross-training occurs when the contralateral part is exercised, resulting in strength gains on the opposite extremity. The results depend primarily on the amount of resistance provided to the exercising extremity: The greater the effort of the extremity, the greater the results. This is a useful technique that you can apply in therapeutic exercise programs when the patient's injured area is restricted, perhaps because it is in a cast or splint, and exercise of the part is limited.

Exercise Progression

A progressive overload can be applied with the use of various systems of progression. Several programs have been advocated by a number of professionals over the years and have been used rather widely in rehabilitation.

One progression system is the **DAPRE** (**D**aily **A**djusted **P**rogressive **R**esistive **E**xercise) technique (Knight 1985). This is a complex system of daily exercise (6 days a week) progression that meets the individual's ability to tolerate increased resistance. Table 17.2 illustrates the establishment of a repetition maximum and number of repetitions along with the determination of the next session's exercise weight.

The essential element of DAPRE is that on the third and fourth sets of exercise, the patient performs as many repetitions as possible. The number of repetitions the individual can perform on the third set determines the amount of weight to be added for the fourth set of the day as well as for the next treatment session.

The intent of the program is to have the patient perform as many repetitions during the set as possible. The goal is five to seven repetitions. If the patient does 8 to 12 repetitions, the weight change is minimal; but if the patient performs 15 to 20 repetitions, the weight change is significantly larger. This program continues until the strength of the injured part is within 10% of the strength of the noninjured counterpart. At that time the emphasis shifts to other deficiencies such as muscle endurance or coordination, and the DAPRE program is continued twice a week to maintain strength.

Proprioception

Agility, balance, and coordination unite to allow an individual to move accurately, quickly, and efficiently. These three parameters are a complex unit that depends on strength and flexibility as its foundation. If a muscle is too weak to move a body part, it

Table 17.2 DAPRE System of Strength Progression

Technique

Set	Repetitions	Weight
1	10	50% of working weight
2	6	75% of working weight
3	As many as possible	100% of working weight
4	As many as possible	Adjusted from third set*

Adjustment guidelines

Number of repetitions performed during prior set	Fourth-set weight adjustment based on third set	Next-day weight adjustment based on fourth set
0-2	wt; redo set	wt; redo set
3-4	by 0-5 lb	Keep the same
5-7	Keep the same	by 5-10 lb
8-12	by 5-10 lb	by 5-15 lb
13 or more	by 10-15 lb	by 10-20 lb

*See adjustment guidelines.

The number of repetitions performed on the third set determines the weight used on the fourth set. The next treatment day's starting weight is determined by the number of repetitions performed on the fourth set of the previous treatment session.

Based on Knight 1985.

cannot be expected to control the movement of that part. Likewise, an extremity must have the flexibility and muscle endurance necessary to allow it to function and meet the demands of athletic activity. If a muscle has limited flexibility so that it lacks the full motion required for an activity, or if a muscle is unable to work long enough to perform an activity correctly without premature fatigue, the muscle will be unable to coordinate the segment properly for that activity.

Agility, balance, and coordination are also controlled by what are collectively referred to as proprioceptors (figure 17.15). **Proprioception** is fundamental to correct performance, and correct performance requires good agility, balance, and coordination. In other words, proprioceptors play a vital neurosensory role in the patient's motor skills and are a key factor in the ability to perform tasks with dexterity, mastery, and proficiency. It is certainly necessary for individuals to have good flexibility as well as muscle endurance and strength in order

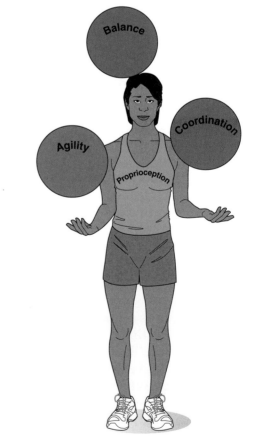

Figure 17.15 Components of proprioception.

to perform well, but proprioception is crucial if the individual is to execute any skill with accuracy, consistency, and precision. To know how to influence proprioception in any performance, we must first understand what proprioceptors are and how they affect execution skill.

Proprioception is the body's ability to transmit position sense, interpret the information, and respond (without conscious effort) to stimulation through appropriate execution of posture and movement. Neuromuscular control of proprioception is produced by the input received from receptors within skin, joints, muscles, and tendons. These proprioceptors play an important role in the maintenance of posture, the conscious and unconscious awareness of joint position, and the production of motion. Proprioception is what allows us to know the position our fingers are in without looking at them. It is what maintains our balance when we stand. It is what enables us to write smoothly. It is what enables us to jump, run, and throw. It is what permits us to change our delivery when we miss the goal on a jump, to move from an asphalt to a gravel surface, and to correct the overshoot of our target with our throw. Although we must first have the flexibility, muscle strength, and endurance to be able to perform these activities, it is proprioception that gives us the agility to change the direction of movement quickly and efficiently, the balance to maintain our stability, and the coordination to produce the activity correctly and consistently.

Proprioceptors are afferent nerves that receive and send impulses from stimuli within skin, muscles, joints, and tendons to the **central nervous system** (CNS). Some of these impulses transmit information regarding the tension of a muscle and the relative position of a body part to control muscular activity. Some of these proprioceptive elements, such as Golgi tendon organs and muscle spindles, have been discussed in previous chapters. Other afferent elements also provide input to the CNS and determine a patient's performance ability.

An individual's agility, balance, and coordination are determined by the reception and interpretation of information and the response initiated by proprioceptors. The proprioceptors are located in the skin, muscles, tendons, and joints.

Balance

Balance is fundamental to most activities. Balance is required to perform a simple activity such as standing. Correct performance requires the maintenance of balance. An individual who does not have good balance is in danger of injury. If balance is not restored following an injury, the risk of reinjury significantly increases.

Balance is the body's ability to maintain equilibrium by controlling the body's center of gravity over its base of support. Balance is important in both static and dynamic activities. Standing and sitting are static balance activities. Examples of dynamic balance activities include walking, running, and dancing.

Balance is influenced by strength and by input from the CNS. It is because strength influences balance that strength is emphasized before proprioception in a therapeutic exercise program.

Coordination

Coordination is another proprioceptive function fundamental to athletic activities. **Coordination** is the complex process by which a smooth pattern of activity is produced through a combination of muscles acting together with appropriate intensity and timing. Several muscles are involved in a coordinated activity. Some muscles are stimulated to produce an activity while others are simultaneously inhibited. At the same time, other muscles are stimulated to provide synergistic or stabilizing responses to permit the desired motion to occur. Each muscle must provide an accurate response both in timing and in intensity in order for the activity to be coordinated. If a muscle is too weak to provide the appropriate response, the activity will be uncoordinated and undesirable.

Agility

Agility is the ability to control the direction of the body or a segment during rapid movement. Athletic agility requires a number of qualities: flexibility, strength, power, speed, balance, and coordination. It involves rapid change of direction and sudden stopping and starting.

Agility is a highly advanced skill that requires a base of flexibility, strength, and power. Adequate flexibility provides a base for speed and power. Since power is needed for agility and power is force times distance divided by time (F × D/T), one can increase power by increasing the distance through which the body part moves. Greater flexibility produces greater power. Power is important because the greater the power, the more quickly a patient is able to move.

Strength is also a component of agility. A patient who has good strength can control the inertia that forceful movement creates. Strength is a controlling factor in a patient's maneuverability.

In order to be effective, speed must be accompanied by coordination. Coordination, as we have seen, is important for proper execution of an activity.

As with coordination activities, therapeutic exercise for agility should begin with simple exercises and progress to more complex activities as skill level improves. Ladder or dot drills are common examples of agility exercises (figure 17.16). The ultimate goal of agility exercises is for the patient to perform all agility activities involved in her sport. Execution of simple activities, including simple drills, is used in the early stages of agility exercises. These activities are usually components of an athletic skill and are performed at slower than normal speeds. As the patient improves, the activity becomes more complex and the speed more closely resembles that in normal sport participation.

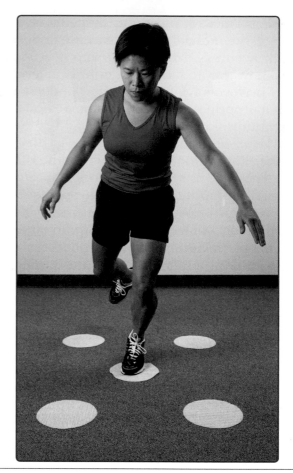

Figure 17.16   Dot drill exercise.

Plyometrics

When the patient has achieved goals in flexibility, strength, balance, coordination, and agility, the next step is to finely tune his abilities in preparation for specific sport skills and other activities. Most sport activities require explosiveness, rapid changes in direction and speed, and the ability to absorb and produce forces quickly—all performed automatically, economically, and efficiently. Goals established to demonstrate these parameters must be achieved before the patient moves on to sport-specific activities, as patients must have certain levels of strength, flexibility, and proprioception to participate safely in plyometric exercises.

Athletic skills are the combined result of natural talent and proper training. Injured patients possess the same inherent talent they have always had, but the effects of pre-injury training diminish following injury and inactivity. The capacity to perform athletic skills at preinjury levels must be restored through therapeutic exercise and retraining before the patient is able to return safely to sport competition.

A relearning by the neuromuscular system must occur for the patient to return to normal sport performance levels. The relearning process uses what is commonly referred to as **plyometrics**. Plyometrics not only is a precursor to functional activities but also can include specific functional sport activities. Plyometrics is the use of a quick movement of eccentric activity followed by a burst of concentric activity to produce a desired powerful output of the muscle. In other words, a plyometric exercise is one that facilitates a muscle to produce a maximum strength output as quickly as possible. It is a brief, explosive style of exercise that can be modified through intensity, volume, recovery, and frequency. Power production is the ultimate goal in plyometrics. Again, recall that power is force times distance divided by time ($F \times D/T$). The quicker the time, the greater the power.

Plyometric Exercise Phases

Plyometric exercises can be divided into three phases: the eccentric phase, the amortization phase, and the concentric phase. All three phases are important to plyometric performance. The eccentric phase prepares the muscle; the amortization phase transitions the muscle; and the concentric phase is the outcome.

Eccentric Phase

The eccentric phase occurs when the muscle is prestretched as it actively lengthens. The slack is taken out of the muscle, and its elastic components are put on stretch. This is the preparatory phase that "sets" the muscle as the individual gets ready to perform the activity. This phase uses muscle spindle facilitation so that the quality of the response is determined by the rate of the stretch. The muscle's activity directly correlates with the quantity of the stimulation: The greater the stimulation, the greater the muscle's response. The eccentric phase is the most important phase of plyometric activity because it increases the stimulation to provide for this increased muscle response.

Amortization Phase

The eccentric phase is followed immediately by the **amortization** phase, which is simply defined as the amount of time it takes to move from eccentric to concentric motion. This phase should be quick. If too much time is spent here, the elastic energy is dissipated as heat and is wasted. A prolonged amortization phase also inhibits the stretch reflex. The concentric motion that results when the amortization is slow is weaker than intended. The amortization phase is the transition phase. The quicker the transition from eccentric to concentric activity, the more forceful the movement will be. The force produced is a result of the combination of the stretch reflex and the elastic energy released. In essence, the force produced is also influenced by the amount of time it takes to make the transition from eccentric to concentric activity, so the transition time must be quick for the plyometrics to produce maximum force.

Concentric Phase

The final phase, the concentric phase, is the result of the combined eccentric and amortization phases. The concentric phase is the outcome phase. If the eccentric activity has been quick and the amortization has occurred rapidly, the concentric phase will produce an increased force production with a greater speed.

Plyometric Program Considerations

Because plyometric activities are generally more intense than other types of exercises, you must consider several special issues regarding their application in therapeutic exercise programs. If the patient has satisfied the preplyometric considerations and has the flexibility, strength, and proprioceptive elements required for plyometric activities, she must also meet criteria involving factors such as age, appropriate body weight, competitive level, surface, footwear, and proper technique in order to participate safely. In addition, plyometric exercises must be performed on an appropriate surface, and progression and goals must be determined appropriately.

Functional and Sport–Specific Exercise

Too frequently the injured patient's program focuses on restoring flexibility, strength, power, and endurance, and the sport-specific demands are forgotten. During the later stages of the therapeutic exercise program it becomes important to prepare injured patients to withstand the specific stresses of their sport and meet its skill demands; it is also essential for them to have confidence that they can return to full participation.

Functional and sport-specific activities, exercises provided in the final phase of rehabilitation, prepare the patient to return to normal, preinjury participation. The rehabilitation clinician must understand and appreciate not only the patient's sport or occupation but also his responsibilities and customary activities.

Once the basic parameters of flexibility, strength, endurance, and proprioception have been restored, specific exercises mimicking necessary skills are added to the program. This will restore the injured patient's confidence in his performance ability and also provide an avenue for renewing the skills lost following the injury.

Definitions and Goals

Before we can discuss specific functional programs and sport-specific activities, we must understand what they are and what their basis and goals are. Once you realize how a therapeutic exercise program progresses to its functional and sport-specific exercise portion, it will become clear when and how to apply functional exercises to this final phase.

Definitions

This phase of the therapeutic exercise program has two components: functional exercise and sport-specific exercise. **Functional activities** are exercises that precede sport-specific activities in a rehabilitation program. They commonly involve multiplanar activities and provide greater stresses and demands than strength exercises. They may include precursor activities to sport-specific exercises such as walking prior to running or underhand tossing prior to throwing. They prepare patients for the more advanced skill demands they will experience in sport-specific activities. **Sport-specific activities** are exercises that include drills involved in a specific sport. They differ from functional activities in that they are specific to sport performance.

An additionally important element that must be included in any phase, including this one, is functional evaluation. **Functional evaluation** is an assessment of the patient's ability to perform an exercise or skill drill safely and correctly before she is allowed to advance to the next level. In other words, each time the patient achieves the established short-term goal, an assessment of the patient's performance is made before the patient advances to the next progression. When the patient has fulfilled all requirements of the rehabilitation program goals, the final functional evaluation takes place before the patient resumes full participation. In order to safely advance to each therapeutic exercise level, the patient must pass the functional tests. The functional tests vary according to the patient's level within the therapeutic exercise program. Examples of these tests are discussed later.

Goals

Functional and sport-specific exercise has four goals. The first two have to do with functional performance and the last two with sport-specific performance. The first goal is to attain full functional levels of flexibility, strength, endurance, and coordination. The second is to achieve full functional ability so that normal speed, power, control, and agility are restored. The third goal is to restore the patient's self-confidence about performance as well as confidence in the injured body segment. The final goal is to return the patient to full participation safely and efficiently at a level at least equivalent to the preinjury level.

The first and second goals are achieved through the therapeutic exercise program for basic and advanced functional activities. These are discussed in the next section. The third goal is achieved through the advancement of exercises and the success that the injured patient experiences at each level. Success builds self-confidence, and failure makes self-confidence elusive; so it is important that the clinician provide exercise goals that are challenging yet achievable. Being both injured and unable to participate in normal activities often causes an injured patient to become unsure of his abilities. Not participating also leads to loss of some of the skills that were so natural before the injury. To reestablish in the patient a preinjury level of self-confidence in his athletic skills, it is necessary to incorporate into the therapeutic exercise program a progression of specific exercises that mimic the skills the patient will need to resume normal-level functions.

The final goal is achieved when all the other goals have been met. This goal is the end result and final goal of any therapeutic exercise program. To achieve it, the rehabilitation clinician must include both functional and sport-specific activities in the therapeutic exercise program. A final functional evaluation takes place before the patient returns to full participation, but it is the patient's ability to participate successfully in the normal activities that is the final test of a therapeutic exercise program.

Contribution to Therapeutic Exercise

Functional and sport-specific exercises are a part of the total rehabilitation process. In that sense, they make a vital and unique contribution to the patient's preparation and return to competition. They must place unique combinations of stresses on the patient to produce unique results. The following sections deal with eight of these demands and the corresponding results.

Normal Motion

Exercises are designed to reproduce the specific motions of the patient's normal activity. They are individually designed for the demands of each patient so that they mimic the normal activity that the patient will perform. Normal activity requires normal motion. If normal motion is lacking, the patient places undue stress on areas that must compensate, and these areas are at risk for additional injury. For example, if a tennis player does not have the normal shoulder flexion and lateral rotation needed to serve, she may develop a low back injury from hyperextending the lumbar spine to hit the ball overhead.

Multifaceted Muscle Activity

Several different types of strengthening activities are used in functional exercises. They commonly include a mixture of isometric, concentric, and eccentric activities because most functional activities include these types of movements. The muscle must have the strength, coordination, and control to quickly change from one type of movement to another and to effectively produce the summation of forces. Even in the simple activity of running, the lower extremity muscles undergo a rapid change of concentric and eccentric activity in their roles as accelerators, decelerators, and stabilizers during different parts of the running cycle.

Multiplanar Motion and Multiple Muscle Group Performance

Functional activities are not performed in straight-plane movements. They involve the simultaneous use of all three planes of motion. They also include the use of many muscle groups that are recruited at one time to produce the desired activity. Exercises must mimic these functional activities by incorporating many muscle groups working in multiple planes.

Multiplanar motion is performed in a coordinated manner through the simultaneous facilitation and inhibition of many muscles. Even an activity like throwing a ball not only involves the shoulder, elbow, wrist, and hand muscles but also requires coordinated multiplanar motions from trunk and lower extremity muscle groups.

Stabilization and Acceleration Changes

Functional motion requires that some muscles work to stabilize a part while other muscles work to either accelerate or decelerate or to change quickly from stabilization to acceleration or deceleration. If sport-specific exercises are to mimic specific sport activities, muscles must be trained to perform these fluid changes that are part of even basic activities. To use the example of a throw, the trunk must be stabilized if the shoulder is to have a platform from which to propel the ball. Even during an activity such as walking, the hip and leg muscles stabilize and limit lateral movement as the body is propelled forward.

Proprioceptive Stimulation

Proprioception is the awareness of body movement and position and is vital to performance. Proprioceptive skills, basic and advanced, must be finely tuned and must be prepared to meet the activity demands to which the patient will be returning. Exercise performance requires the use of proprioception, and improvement of the patient's functional performance directly correlates to his proprioceptive development.

Agility and Power Development

Agility and power are essential requirements for most sports. Agility is necessary in order for the basketball player to dribble the ball downcourt, for the volleyball player to dive and pass the ball to the setter, and for the hurdler to time each jump correctly. Power allows the sprinter to reach the finish line before the other competitors, the football defensive lineman to sack the quarterback, and the crew team to sprint to the end of the race. Agility and power are required in a gymnast's floor exercise routine, an ice skater's triple-Lutz jump, and a water polo player's scoring a goal. Agility and power must improve as the patient increases her ability to perform sport-specific activities. Progressive and functional sport-specific exercises steadily stress and therefore increase the patient's ability to perform at an agility and power level sufficient for appropriate skill execution and level of competition.

Sport-Specific Skill Development

Functional exercises—from the early basic exercises to the more advanced sport-specific exercises—have as their goal the injured patient's return to sport participation. The sport-specific exercises used in the later stages of rehabilitation are specifically designed with this goal in mind. These exercises mimic the sport activities and place the same demands on the injured patient that he will encounter when returning to participation. The specific skills needed to perform the rehabilitation exercises are the same skills that are needed to perform within the sport.

Confidence Development

As the patient succeeds in performing those sport-specific exercises that mimic the demands of the sport, confidence returns. By the time the patient is ready to resume sport participation, she has demonstrated an ability to perform the skills that participation requires. This gives her the self-confidence to perform without hesitation and also to meet the demands of the sport with confidence in the injured part.

Basic Functional Activities

In a good therapeutic exercise program, functional exercise and functional evaluation take place from the very beginning. The basic functional exercises that begin an injured patient's therapeutic exercise program follow a progression to build the foundation for improvement in more specific skill activities. The program starts with exercises for achieving basic parameter goals such as flexibility, strength, endurance, and proprioception. To some extent, these can be considered functional exercises because they are used to attain a goal that is necessary for specific performance. For example, in order to jump hurdles, a runner has to gain a functional degree of flexibility in the hamstrings. In order to compete, a wrestler must have full functional flexibility in the shoulders. A pitcher needs functional muscle endurance to pitch a game. A gymnast must be able to stork stand on the ground before he can stand on a balance beam.

Basic functional exercises have been discussed previously. At this point, the progression and sequence of the exercises should seem logical to you. Exercises for flexibility, strength, endurance, and proprioception follow a logical sequence. Each parameter requires a coherent progression of exercises that provides increasing stress as the area adjusts to and becomes able to tolerate greater stresses because of improvements already made.

Functional evaluation tools use objective criteria. For example, gains in range of motion are evaluated by goniometry, and strength gains are evaluated by manual muscle testing or the use of objective tools such as isokinetic equipment or grip dynamometers. Once you have determined that a patient has reached specific goals, you advance the individual to the next goal.

Sport-Specific Activities

Functional progression of advanced parameters involves advancement to specific skill activities. A patient must start with fundamental skill functions and progress to advanced skill functions after having mastered some of the basic skills. Advanced functional activities include plyometrics and specific skill-drill exercises. In addition to flexibility, strength, muscle endurance, and proprioception, they require the more advanced skills of agility, speed, power, and control. Depending on the requirements of the advanced skill, some advanced functional exercises can be started earlier in the program while the patient is still working to achieve proficiency in basic skill execution. For example, patients can start basic coordination exercises such as bouncing a basketball before they have achieved full range of motion or full strength.

As with the evaluation of functional performance of basic exercises, evaluation of advanced functional exercises involves periodic examination and assessment and a logical progression. Patients should have good static and dynamic balance before performing plyometric exercises. They should be able to perform plyometric exercises before specific skill activities are incorporated into the therapeutic exercise program. These are all logical, commonsense concepts. The skill of the rehabilitation clinician is a factor in determining exactly when the progressions should occur and what they should be. This skill is based on knowledge about tissue healing; knowledge of the influences of the stresses applied by various exercises and activities; observation of the patient's reaction to the stresses; knowledge of exercise sequences; and knowledge of the specific demands, skills, and requirements of the injured patient's sport or work tasks. The rehabilitation clinician's skill is also based on good judgment and common sense about how much stress to apply and when during the therapeutic exercise program to apply that stress.

The rehabilitation clinician determines on an individual basis how complex the initial functional exercise should be and how quickly the complexity should increase. You must consider the factors already outlined and make the best judgment. Remember, it is always better to err on the side of caution when advancing the patient so that progression continues consistently forward, without regression.

Advanced functional exercises and sport-specific exercises are more complex, more challenging, and more rigorous than the basic functional exercises. This is generally so because multiple planes of motion, more muscle groups, more complex and simultaneous movements, and more agility are required for correct execution. Because of the increased demands that such activities impose, there are also precautions that one must respect in assigning advanced therapeutic exercises to a patient.

Functional Evaluation

Evaluation of function is an ongoing process. Throughout the therapeutic exercise program, the rehabilitation clinician evaluates the patient's ability to perform both basic functional and sport-specific exercises. Advances in the program take place only after

the patient is able to successfully perform to expected levels at each evaluation step. The final functional evaluation occurs before the patient is allowed to return to full participation. At this time the functional evaluation is highly individualized and is based on the specific demands of the patient's activity. The patient's performance in the evaluation determines her readiness to return to sport participation. Final functional examination includes highly specific drills and tests the person's performance skill. These examinations should be as objective as possible and mimic the individual's sport as much as possible. For a gymnast, the functional examination may include dismounts, tumbling skills, or apparatus skills. For a basketball player, the functional examination includes dribbling, shooting, cutting, or passing drills. For a football defensive lineman, the functional examination includes assessment of skills such as blocking, lateral or forward movements, agility, or quick changes of direction. Because specific skill activities vary greatly from job to job or sport to sport, or among positions within a sport, you must

CASE STUDY

Sally is the athletic trainer for the Nottingham University Tigers, the defending national champion track and field team. Bruce, the star sprinter for the team, has been rehabilitating from a hamstring strain suffered 4 weeks ago. Bruce is doing well with his range of motion and strengthening exercises. He has also been doing some jogging and distance running, in addition to bicycling, to improve his muscular endurance and cardiovascular fitness. He has been cleared by the team physician to begin a functional and sport-specific rehabilitation program with the goal of full return to sprinting over the next 2 weeks.

Think About It

1. Describe a progressive and functional running program for the next 2 weeks.

2. Are plyometric exercises indicated? If so, how would you implement them? If not, why not?

3. Describe any sport-specific exercises you would prescribe for Bruce.

4. What other rehabilitation exercises would you implement or continue for Bruce over the next 2 weeks and for the remainder of the season?

be familiar with the specific requirements for the patient. You may need to obtain the supervisor's or coach's help in defining functional exercises and tests for some specific activities. It is the goal of the final functional examination, however, to demonstrate to the patient, the medical team, and the supervisor or coach that the individual is able and ready to withstand the stresses of full participation.

The functional tests for determining readiness to return to full participation must fulfill certain criteria, some of which have been previously mentioned. One criterion is that the examination tool should be as objective as possible. A test should be repeatable so that it can be used both in the initial examination and in the final examination to measure changes and assess whether or not the patient has achieved the appropriate goals. Functional tests should provide useful information to the patient and medical team about the progress and status of the patient's performance. They should also be able to show whether or not the functional exercise program is providing the advancement of parameters necessary for return to participation.

In the final functional examination, your observation and assessment of the patient's performance is critical. Any activity should be performed without hesitation, and the use of each extremity should be appropriate, with no favoring of the injured limb. The patient should move quickly, stabilize appropriately, and demonstrate self-confidence with all maneuvers. On the basis of the patient's performance, you should be unable to identify which extremity has been injured.

Learning Aids

SUMMARY

The goals of therapeutic exercise are to evaluate and improve range of motion, muscular strength, muscular power, muscular endurance, proprioception, agility, balance, coordination, and functional or sport-specific exercise ability. Multiple techniques can be used to reach these goals, and it is up to the athletic trainer to assess the current status of the patient and implement techniques and exercises to facilitate goal attainment. The basic exercises that begin an injured patient's therapeutic exercise program follow a progression to build the foundation for improvement in more specific skill activities. Step-by-step evaluation determines when the patient should advance to the next stage in the process leading up to functional and sport-specific exercises. These are used to attain full functional level of performance, restore the patient's confidence, and return the patient to sport participation.

KEY CONCEPTS AND REVIEW

▶ **Describe the methods used to measure range of motion of a joint.**

To measure accurately with a goniometer, the most common tool for evaluating range of motion, placement of the protractor and arms is important. The arms of the goniometer are placed along the length of the two limbs forming the joint. If the protractor is placed correctly, the pivot point should be lined up over the axis of motion of the joint. For correct alignment, the limbs being measured should be exposed.

▶ **List five stretching techniques that can be used to increase range of joint motion.**

Active stretching, passive stretching, assisted (using an appliance) stretching, ballistic stretching, proprioceptive neuromuscular facilitation

▸ **List four common manual therapy techniques used to treat neuromusculoskeletal conditions.**

Massage, myofascial release, muscle energy techniques, joint mobilization

▸ **Describe the two types of muscle activity.**

Static activity, or isometric activity, is produced when muscle tension is created without a change in the muscle's length. Dynamic activity is further divided into specific types. Isotonic activity is dynamic in that it involves a change in the muscle's length. If the muscle shortens, the activity is called *concentric*. If the muscle lengthens, the activity is called *eccentric*. Isokinetic activity is a dynamic activity in that it involves motion. It differs from isotonic activity, however, in that the velocity is controlled and maintained at a specific speed of movement.

▸ **Understand the difference between open kinetic chain (OKC) and closed kinetic chain (CKC).**

The kinetic chain is open when the distal segment moves freely in space. Kicking and throwing a ball are open kinetic chain activities. A kinetic chain is closed when the distal segment is weight bearing and the body moves over the hand or foot. The weight-bearing phase of running and a handstand are closed kinetic chain activities.

▸ **List the three principles of strengthening.**

No pain, attainable goals, progressive overload

▸ **Identify the three main components of proprioception.**

Balance is the body's ability to maintain equilibrium by controlling the center of gravity over its base of support. Coordination is the complex process by which a smooth pattern of activity is produced through a combination of muscles acting together with appropriate intensity and timing. Agility is the ability to control the direction of a body or segment during rapid movement.

▸ **Describe plyometrics and list the three phases involved.**

Plyometrics is the use of a quick movement of eccentric activity followed by a burst of concentric activity to produce a desired powerful output of the muscle. In other words, a plyometric exercise is one that facilitates the ability of a muscle to produce a maximum strength output as quickly as possible. It is a brief, explosive exercise. Power production is the ultimate goal in plyometrics. The three phases are the eccentric phase, the amortization phase, and the concentric phase.

▸ **Understand the difference between functional activities and sport-specific activities.**

Functional activities are exercises that precede sport-specific activities in a rehabilitation program. They commonly involve multiplanar activities and provide greater stresses and demands than strength exercises. They may include precursor activities to sport-specific exercises such as walking prior to running or underhand tossing prior to throwing. They prepare the patient for the more advanced skill demands they will experience in sport-specific activities. Sport-specific activities are exercises that include drills used within a specific sport. They differ from functional activities in that they are specific to sport performance.

▸ **Identify the four goals for functional and sport-specific exercise.**

The first goal is to attain full functional levels of flexibility, strength, endurance, and coordination. The second is to achieve full functional ability so that normal speed, power, control, and agility are restored. The third goal is to restore the patient's self-confidence regarding performance as well as confidence in the injured body segment. The final goal is to return the patient to full participation safely and efficiently at a level at least equivalent to the preinjury level.

PRACTICE!

For hands-on practice in this area, go to the web resource and complete the following:

Level 2.12, Module M1: Range of Motion and Flexibility Exercises

Level 2.12, Module M3: Isometric Resistance Exercises

Level 2.12, Module M5: Daily Adjustable Progressive Resistive Exercise

CRITICAL THINKING QUESTIONS

1. One of the star players on your college basketball team had ankle reconstruction in the off-season and is now returning to practice in his fourth and final year of participation. Everyone believes this player will get a chance to play in the WNBA if she has a great senior season. You have been watching her during practice and you are amazed at the number of times she has ended up on the floor. Over the next two practices, as you monitor for this, you find that some other players are on the floor two times per practice, none more than two times, and most not even once. Your star player was on the floor at four times in one of the two practices and seven times in the other. Discuss your thoughts about why she may be falling down so often. You are sure her strength is good since you have been testing her on the isokinetic dynamometer, and all indications are that she is back to 90% to 100%. Describe therapeutic interventions you would use to help her stay on her feet during practice.

2. One of the running backs on the football team ruptured his patellar tendon doing plyometric jumps from a 30-in. platform. Now that he is back to full participation and full weight room workouts he is faced with doing plyometrics again with the team. He has come to you to express his hesitation to return to plyometrics and asks your advice. Explain what you will tell him and give your rationale for your decision.

CHAPTER 18

Pharmacology in Athletic Training

Susan Kay Hillman, ATC, PT

OBJECTIVES

After reading this chapter, the student should be able to do the following:

- Define and list examples of generic versus trade name drugs.
- Discuss why drugs are classified as nonprescription, prescription, or controlled substances.
- Identify the methods of administering medicinal drugs to patients.
- Define *agonist* and *antagonist* as related to medicinal drugs.
- Identify the various sources one could use to find information on drugs.
- Explain how to find information on the USOC or the NCAA banned drug lists.
- Discuss the inflammatory process and describe how drugs may affect that process.
- Identify the more common side effects of anti-inflammatory drugs and the steps that may be taken to reduce these unwanted outcomes.
- Describe the effects of analgesics and discuss reasons to limit their use in sport participation.
- Identify ways in which a fungal infection may be controlled with medicinal drugs.
- Describe ways in which a laxative may be misused.

It is critical for athletic trainers to learn the basics of **pharmacology**, just as it is to understand the effects of any other treatment. With knowledge of which medicinals are used for specific problems, the way a drug works, and some of the mechanics of its action, the athletic trainer may better communicate with the individual taking the medicine, as well as with the prescribing physician, and thereby maximize the therapy for the individual.

In this chapter we focus on the application of pharmacology to specific problems frequently encountered in sports medicine settings. In no way should the reader construe this information as comprehensive or infer that this bit of knowledge sufficiently prepares anyone to prescribe or dispense medicinal drugs. This information will serve as a basis upon which to build an understanding of drug therapy and will give you some understanding of how and why drugs work. See Ray and Konin (2011) for more information on methods of organizing plans to legally and safely store medication within the sport treatment facility.

Drug Nomenclature and Classification

Pharmacology can be confusing to athletic trainers because of the variety of names given to drugs. Each drug can be identified according to its chemical, generic, or trade name. The chemical name, usually a long and difficult one, refers to the specific chemical structure of the compound. The generic name, also called the "official" or "**nonproprietary**" name, is usually shorter and is often derived from the chemical name. The trade name is the name the manufacturing company assigns to the compound. You might accurately surmise that several companies manufacture an identical generic product but assign different names to it. For instance, ibuprofen is the common name or generic name for the **analgesic** (painkiller) known by the trade names Advil, Nuprin, Motrin, and the less familiar trade name of Rufen.

One very important aspect of understanding drugs is understanding the drug classifications. There are two general classifications of medicinal drugs: nonprescription or over-the-counter (OTC) drugs and prescription drugs.

Nonprescription or Over-the-Counter Drugs

Nonprescription drugs can be purchased by consumers directly from store shelves. In general, OTC medications are used for minor problems. These medications are judged to be safe or free of major side effects when taken in the recommended dosage. One must be careful when suggesting that an individual use an OTC medication. Always advise the person to follow the dosage recommendations on the product and to check with a pharmacist or physician before combining any medications. Too often, individuals self-medicate using OTC products that if taken in combination with other compounds can exert unwanted or even hazardous side effects.

Prescription Drugs

Classification as a prescription drug indicates that the individual needs a prescription for the medicine. The physician determines that the drug is necessary to treat an illness or condition. The physician also interviews the patient regarding the use of other drugs and provides information about drug interactions. In addition to the prescribing physician, the issuing pharmacist often reviews the effects, side effects, and precautions with the consumer at the time the medicine is issued.

Prescription drugs are further classified according to their potential for abuse. The government holds tight controls on the use of prescription drugs—hence the term **controlled substances**. These drugs, with their potential for abuse, are further categorized into one of five schedules (schedules I-V).

Schedule I drugs are the drugs with the highest potential for abuse and are approved for use in only a very limited number of patients; the schedule II, III, and IV drugs are successively less likely to be abused; and schedule V drugs have the lowest relative abuse potential. Table 18.1 gives examples of drugs on each schedule.

There are rules for prescribing, dispensing, and renewing prescriptions for all five types of controlled substances. The patient must have a written prescription for the controlled drug and must obtain the drug in person. These steps are necessary to prevent false ordering of these dangerous drugs as well as for ensuring that the drug is given to the proper person. If the team physician has drugs in his office, these drugs are kept under tight security in an area that is double locked for added safety.

The Study of Drugs

Pharmacology is the science of drugs. Researchers focus on two distinct areas when studying drugs: **pharmacotherapeutics** and **toxicology**. If we look at the roots of these two words we see a continuum, from therapeutic to toxic. We may all know cases in which a prescribed drug was used in excess of the dosage specified and had a toxic effect. The toxic effect is usually not lethal (although sufficient dosages may cause a life-threatening condition), but the effect is

Table 18.1 | **Controlled Substances by Schedule Classification**

Schedule	Qualifications for designation	Drugs in schedule
Schedule I	(A) The drug or other substance has a high potential for abuse. (B) The drug or other substance has no currently accepted medical use in treatment in the United States. (C) There is a lack of accepted safety for use of the drug or other substance under medical supervision.	Opium Experimental opiate derivatives Hallucinogenic substances
Schedule II	(A) The drug or other substance has a high potential for abuse (B) The drug or other substance has a currently accepted medical use in treatment in the United States or a currently accepted medical use with severe restrictions. (C) Abuse of the drug or other substance may lead to severe psychological or physical dependence.	Opiates (i.e., methadone) Methamphetamine
Schedule III	(A) The drug or other substance has a potential for abuse less than that of the drugs or other substances in schedules I and II. (B) The drug or other substance has a currently accepted medical use in treatment in the United States. (C) Abuse of the drug or other substance may lead to moderate or low physical dependence or high psychological dependence.	Stimulants Depressants Nalorphine Narcotic drugs Anabolic steroids
Schedule IV	(A) The drug or other substance has a low potential for abuse relative to the drugs or other substances in schedule III. (B) The drug or other substance has a currently accepted medical use in treatment in the United States. (C) Abuse of the drug or other substance may lead to limited physical dependence or psychological dependence relative to the drugs or other substances in schedule III.	Barbital Meprobamate Methylphenobarbital Phenobarbital
Schedule V	(A) The drug or other substance has a low potential for abuse relative to the drugs or other substances in schedule IV. (B) The drug or other substance has a currently accepted medical use in treatment in the United States. (C) Abuse of the drug or other substance may lead to limited physical dependence or psychological dependence relative to the drugs or other substances in schedule IV.	Not more than 200 mg codeine per 100 ml or per 100 g Not more than 100 mg opium per 100 ml or per 100 g

not desirable and usually not therapeutic; it is thus called an unwanted effect. The subjects of toxicology and pharmacotherapeutics are extensive and are far beyond the scope of this chapter. Therefore the discussion here is limited to the major therapeutic effects, as well as some of the unwanted effects, of common drugs used in athletic health care.

Pharmacokinetics

As indicated by the word "kinetics" (kinetic = movement) in the term, **pharmacokinetics** is the study of how medicines move. Pharmacokinetics can be broken down into four subcategories: absorption, distribution, metabolism, and elimination. Looking briefly at the basics of each of these will help you better understand specific medicinals discussed later in this chapter.

Before absorption can occur, the drug must enter the body. There are two primary ways in which a drug is administered: **enteral** and nonenteral. The enteral route is termed **alimentary** or enteral because of its pathway into the body via the alimentary canal, or digestive system. Routes of enteral administration include oral, sublingual, and rectal. The nonenteral route is termed **parenteral** because entry into the body is through a pathway other than the alimentary canal. This method usually allows the drug to be delivered directly to the target site, making the quantity of drug actually reaching the target more predictable. Routes of parenteral administration include inhalation, injection, and topical and **transdermal** application.

Drug Absorption

Absorption is the movement of the drug across a cell's membrane. Movement across a membrane is usually accomplished by some method of diffusion or transport (see figure 18.1). Generally, the smaller the drug compound, the more easily it moves across a cell membrane, thus allowing greater distribution. Additionally, if the drug is lipid soluble, it breaks down or binds with fats and thus is able to gain access to more tissues, leading to greater distribution.

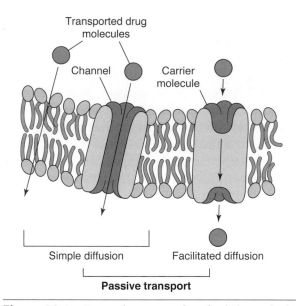

Figure 18.1   Some drugs are absorbed through the membrane by simple passive or facilitated passive diffusion.

If there is a difference in chemical concentration on two sides of a permeable membrane, the chemical will move from the area of high concentration to the area of lower concentration. This is termed passive diffusion, a method of transporting substances across the cell membrane. "Passive" emphasizes the fact that the movement occurs without any energy expenditure; the driving force is the pressure difference on the two sides of the membrane.

Diffusion at cell junctions must occur if a compound is to be administered through the alimentary canal but needs to be distributed to an area outside the canal (e.g., the nervous system or muscular system). The diffusion of the compound occurs in the space between cells; this space may either allow or prohibit the passage of drugs, as in the case of the blood–brain barrier. The capillary walls in the brain produce a barrier to many water-soluble compounds, yet the barrier is permeable to lipid-soluble substances. This is one of the reasons that some drugs can affect the central nervous system quite readily (such as anesthetics) while others are rather ineffective in that role.

In general, the more lipid soluble the drug is, the more tissues will be affected (wider distribution) and the more potential the drug will have to exert an effect on the central nervous system.

Drug Distribution

Once the drug is absorbed from its point of entry, the circulatory system distributes the drug throughout the body, thus the "distribution." The extent to which the drug reaches the systemic circulation is termed bioavailability, which is expressed as the percentage of the drug that reaches the bloodstream. Once the drug is in the systemic circulation, further distribution into body tissues may be necessary to allow it to reach the target area. Furthermore, many drugs have to cross cell membranes and tissue barriers to reach the desired target.

Drug Transformation and Elimination

Basically, the process of drug transformation involves making substances soluble for excretion from the liver or urinary tract. The process that determines whether a compound is excreted in the **bile** (liver) or the urine is complicated and depends on the patient's internal physiology. Drugs processed through the kidneys are excreted in the urine, while drugs processed through the digestive tract are eliminated from the body into the stool. Most drugs, especially water-soluble drugs, are excreted into the urine. The acidity of the urine can affect the rate of elimination of a drug. The acidity of the urine can be changed by diet, drugs, or kidney disorders. This is an important concept in the treatment of poisoning or drug overdose. In these cases, the acidity of the urine is changed if the patient is given other drugs (such as an antacid like sodium bicarbonate or an acid like ammonium chloride) to speed up the elimination of the toxic drug. The kidney, liver, lungs, and gastrointestinal tract all can help in the process of transformation, each with the task of making the substance soluble and ready for elimination.

The effectiveness of drugs that are fat soluble may be altered when they are converted to a water-soluble state in the liver. Some drugs may become more potent when they are converted in the liver. Other drugs may require transformation in the liver in order to become therapeutic. Some drugs are not metabolized at all and may be excreted totally intact. Still others are transformed into other compounds that have some other therapeutic or even a toxic effect.

Aspirin is among the drugs that must be transformed in order to produce any therapeutic value. Drugs like this are called **prodrugs**. Another particular drug (not to be named) is marketed in the United States as a muscle relaxant but undergoes a transformation in the liver into a potent and very addictive compound that is frequently abused. Many other drugs possess these metabolic characteristics, complicating the study of pharmacology even further.

The amount of time needed to reduce the drug concentration in the body to 50% is termed the drug **half-life**. Knowledge of the half-life of a drug is important for understanding how often the drug is administered. Usually, after administration of the drug for five half-lives, a steady state is achieved in which the amount administered is equal to the amount eliminated. The half-life and the steady state of a drug are the factors that lead a physician to prescribe a loading dose of a drug—a first dose that is twice the normal dose. The loading dose allows the concentration to reach effective levels more rapidly.

Pharmacodynamics: How the Drug Works

The word **pharmacodynamics** can be broken down into "pharmaco" and "dynamics." Dynamics relates to the Greek word *"dynamikos,"* meaning powerful. Thus, pharmacodynamics refers to the power the drug has on the body, or the way it exerts its effect. Drugs act by binding to specific target receptors on the cell's exterior. When a drug binds to a receptor, it triggers a cellular process and thereby activates the therapeutic response (see figure 18.2).

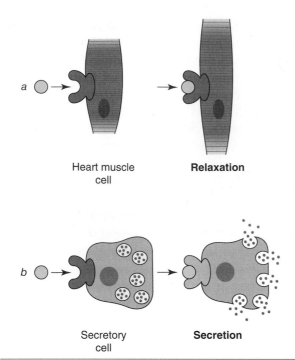

Heart muscle
cell   **Relaxation**

Secretory
cell   **Secretion**

Figure 18.2 Some drugs act by binding to specific target receptors in the cell's membrane.

Molecular biology of the cell by ALBERTS ET. AL. Copyright 2008 Reproduced with permission of GARLAND SCIENCE - BOOKS in the format Textbook via Copyright Clearance Center.

Similarly to muscles, drugs have **agonists**[2] and **antagonists**[2]. Just as an agonistic muscle produces a change, an agonist drug acts with the receptor site to produce a change. There are also drugs that work in the opposite fashion. These, called antagonists, exert an inhibitory action on the receptor cell. This action suppresses the activity of the cell that is the cause of the patient's discomfort or disorder. For example, if you stepped into a patch of poison ivy, you might break out in an allergic response like itching and hives. You could use a topical antihistamine like Benadryl cream that would block the histamine (allergic) reaction, and your itching and hives would go away quite quickly. The reason is that Benadryl (diphenhydramine) binds with the body tissues that cause the allergic reaction, inhibiting the cell function.

Efficacy refers to how effectively a drug works. Certainly we would all prefer to take a drug if we could be assured of its efficacy in treating the condition. The ability of the drug to produce an effect is not always related to

the drug's **potency**. The potency of a drug is a measure of the dose of the medicinal needed to produce a specific effect. A more potent drug is not a more effective drug; it would have the same effect as another drug, but with the more potent drug the effect can be achieved with a lower dose. Tolerance to a drug simply indicates that the body cells have built up a kind of resistance to the drug so that increased amounts are needed to achieve the same effect. This tolerance makes the drug appear less potent, but actually the drug has become less efficient because of changes in the cell.

III Effects of Medications

To understand how and why particular drugs work, one must also consider the nondesired effects of a drug. Nondesired effects include adverse or side effects (see the sidebar Therapeutic Side Effects), allergic (and anaphylactic) reactions, and drug interactions.

Drug Adverse Effects

Often drugs produce undesired effects or effects unrelated to the reason for taking the medication; these are called adverse effects. The adverse effects of a drug are often highly predictable, and most patients tolerate them quite easily. While a drug is being tested for Food and Drug Administra-

THERAPEUTIC SIDE EFFECTS

It may be interesting to note that an **antihypertensive** drug (drug used to reduce high blood pressure), minoxodil, has a side effect of causing **hypertrichosis** (the growth of body hair). Although it may seem odd to mention this, there's a reason. Minoxodil, marketed under the trade name Rogaine, is used topically to actually stimulate hair growth—an example of a drug that is used therapeutically for its side effects.

tion (FDA) approval, researchers record and track common adverse effects. If the drug is considered safe and is approved, then the drug manufacturer is required by law to list the adverse effects on the packaging material or on product inserts. Occasionally, however, adverse effects may not be anticipated or in individual cases may be different from the ones listed. Remind those you are working with to check the product inserts, call their physician, or talk to a pharmacist if they have any questions or concerns regarding adverse effects. Also, educate yourself about the unwanted side effects of medications your clients are taking.

Drug Allergies

Adverse drug reactions have become an increasingly common medical problem with the use of increasing numbers of therapeutic and diagnostic agents. In the United States, these reactions affect an estimated 1 to 2 million people a year. Adverse drug reactions are believed to be the most common cause of iatrogenic (caused by the treatment itself) illnesses, and up to 30% of hospitalized patients may experience such a reaction (see figure 18.3). These reactions can be divided into two broad categories: toxic and allergic. Most adverse reactions, including unwanted side effects, overdoses, and drug interactions, are toxic. Only 6% to 10% are allergic reactions, but these are the most serious. Death is reported in 1 of every 10,000 cases.

A patient is said to have a drug allergy when the medicine produces a response different from what is expected. For example, a product called Zomax was taken off the market a short time after it was introduced because many people who took this aspirin-like product developed severe itching and hives, signs of allergic response. Severe allergenic reactions may involve anaphylactic responses that include bronchospasm, hypotension, shock, and death if not treated quickly. It is always important to know of any allergies in those you work with, and keeping that record on the individual's chart as well as on the preparticipation physical is recommended. The allergic response is much different from an unwanted side effect: An adverse effect is something that a majority of the people who take the medication will report, but an allergy is a definite contraindication to use of the medicine.

Drug Interactions

Drug interactions are also factors that play a big role in our understanding of drug effects. A drug interaction is just what the name implies: an interaction between two drugs. This happens when drugs that are metabolized stimulate or depress the **metabolism** of other drugs. These interactions may be agonistic (compounding the effect of the medication, also termed synergistic) or antagonistic (canceling the effect of the medication). For example, alcohol is a drug and should not be consumed while the individual is taking a prescribed drug, because alcohol is agonistic with many drugs and increases the potential for side effects of the medication. As an example of the opposite, or antagonistic, effect, there have been reports—although

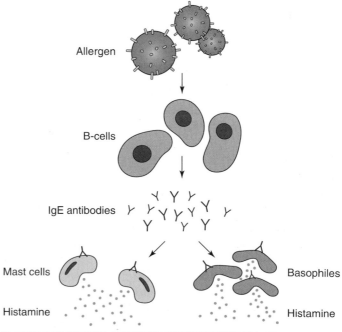

Allergen

B-cells

IgE antibodies

Mast cells

Histamine

Basophiles

Histamine

Figure 18.3   An allergic reaction mechanism in the body.

the research has not been conclusive—that some antibiotics decrease the effectiveness of oral contraceptives in certain women. Thus the synergistic (agonistic) effect compounds the effect or side effects of a drug, while the antagonistic effect could reduce or even cancel the effect of the drug.

Sources of Drug Information

The idea of drug receptors and agonistic or antagonistic effects of drugs is much more complex than this very simplified discussion indicates. The student of pharmacology investigates the exact cells with which the drug interacts and the extent to which the action occurs. For our purposes, knowledge that the system exists helps us understand why a particular drug works the way it does; yet for additional information, there are places to turn.

- *Physician's Desk Reference.* *Physician's Desk Reference (PDR)* is a text commonly available in sports medicine departments. The *PDR* is an exhaustive reference for prescription drugs, classifying each drug by trade name and generic name as well as providing a pictorial guide to aid in the identification of medicinals. The information on each drug includes dosage parameters, effects, and side effects: all the information included in the product information provided by the manufacturer. One of the difficulties with this reference is that it does not list all generic drugs—and generic drugs are often the ones that the consumer chooses.

- *Facts and Comparisons.* *Facts and Comparisons* is a reference similar to the *PDR*, but it includes many of the generic drugs. One tremendous benefit of *Facts and Comparisons* is that it is published in a binder into which one can easily insert the updates provided monthly.

- *Product information.* The pharmacist preparing the prescription often supplies product information. Cooperation with a local pharmacist may allow the athletic trainer nearly immediate information on any drug of interest.

- *Web information.* Information is abundant at Gold Standard Multimedia (www.goldstandard.com/) and is available to aid the practitioner in understanding various drugs. Just as with the printed drug references, this website includes product information, drug references, and more advanced material for members. Coaches and administrators interested in learning more about banned substances can join Drug Free Sport (www.drugfreesport.com) and access the Resource Exchange Center (REC). One can submit the name of a drug and receive confidential information on the banned status of substances including dietary supplements. Many organizations subscribe to this service and attest to its value.

- *United States Anti-Doping Agency (USADA).* A wide variety of drugs have been found to be potentially dangerous to the patient or to offer an unfair advantage in sport. Sport organizations have stepped forward to control the use of these drugs. Both the National Collegiate Athletic Association (NCAA) and the United States Olympic Committee (USOC) publish their own banned drug lists. (For the NCAA list, go to www.ncaa.org/, click in the search box, and type "banned substances." For the USADA list, go to http://usada.org/drugline/.) In addition, both organizations make their drug-testing policy clear to competing athletes, including such aspects as the frequency of testing and the ramifications of positive tests; for example, look at http://usada.org/files/active/athletes/athlete-handbook.pdf or the USADA main website at http://usada.org/.

Although the prescription and dispensation of medicinal drugs are out of the scope of practice of the athletic trainer, every health care practitioner should be aware of actions and side effects of the majority of drugs in categories commonly used in athletic medicine. In your investigation of medicinal drugs, you may see discussions of dosage. In medicine, abbreviations are used to denote the number of doses per day. Table 18.2 identifies the common abbreviations used to indicate dosage schedules.

Table 18.2 Abbreviations for Dosage as Used in Pharmacology

Abbreviation	Latin term	Meaning
bid	bis in die	Twice daily
tid	ter in die	Three times daily
qid	quater in die	Four times daily

Drug-Testing Policies and Procedures

As mentioned previously, each organization (USOC, NCAA, National Football League, and so on) establishes its own drug-testing policy governing all participants on those teams. Many individual schools and teams establish their own drug-testing programs.

In general, drug testing is done with a urine test. The urine is collected under same-sex observation of the void (emptying of the bladder). Student-athletes are typically informed of the test and escorted immediately to the testing site. After the void, the urine is packaged, identified, and sent to an analysis laboratory for testing. When individuals are unable to void, they are required to stay in the testing area and it is suggested that they drink the beverages provided until they feel the urge to urinate. All beverages provided in the testing center must be in individual, closed containers and should be free of caffeine.

Positive test findings are reported to the designated team authorities, and the appropriate sanctions are levied. These sanctions vary according to the particular drug-testing policy of the group, school, team, or league.

The NCAA tests athletes at random times during the school year as well as at championship events. Event testing is usually done at the conclusion of the contest, whether it is the first or the final round of the tournament. The athlete(s) are met at the conclusion of the contest by a courier. This courier is responsible for staying with the athlete from the time the individual is informed that she must report to the drug-testing area until she is signed in by the NCAA-appointed drug-testing staff. Once the drug test is complete, the urine is analyzed and any positive findings are reported to the conference, to the person's coach, and often to the school athletic director. Positive drug-testing results obtained in championship events are often devastating to the individual as well as the team and school because the student-athlete has disobeyed conference rules, the team will forfeit if it won the event, and the student-athlete will be stripped of eligibility to compete for the next 365 days.

Drugs Specific to Athletic-Related Conditions

As an athletic trainer, it may not be as important to understand pharmacology as deeply as you understand anatomy, yet some knowledge of each of the types of drugs you may encounter can prove beneficial in caring for patients. The following sections present drugs according to a general classification of their action. Each subsection provides general information about the drug, followed by details on how the drug is administered, its adverse effects, and the implications for the athletic trainer. The other aspects of pharmacokinetics (absorption, distribution, transformation, and elimination), pharmacodynamics, and drug interactions are typically areas the athletic trainer depends on the physician to understand. These areas are not within the scope of this chapter.

Inflammation and Drug Treatment

As an athletic trainer, you will encounter individuals with inflammation, the most common effect of injury or overuse. This is a vascular response to physiological tissue damage. This vascular response prevents, or at least limits, the spread of injury-causing agents to the adjacent tissues. In addition, the process of inflammation serves to dispose of cellular debris and sets the stage for the repair process to begin (see figure 18.4). When trauma occurs, the offended tissue becomes an active inflammatory site. Initially, a short period of vasoconstriction occurs to prevent further bleeding. Shortly after this period is a release of chemical mediators (histamine, bradykinin, thromboxanes, leukotrienes, and prostaglandins) that cause a vasodilation of the vessels in the area. With vasodilation comes an increase in the permeability of the vessel walls, allowing white blood cells to enter the injury site. Increased membrane permeability leads to an increased flow of cellular fluid into the area, causing localized edema (swelling).

Drugs that are able to block or inhibit this series of events are classified as anti-inflammatory agents. Anti-inflammatory drugs can be classified as **nonsteroidal** or steroidal. Within the nonsteroidals is the category of salicylates.

Nonsteroidal Anti-Inflammatory Agents: Salicylates

Aspirin and other salicylates are, worldwide, the most frequently used drug in the treatment of pain, fever, and inflammation. Aspirin is the main member of the family of salicylates and the first nonsteroidal anti-inflammatory drug (NSAID) that was introduced. Aspirin remains the standard by which the other NSAIDs are compared. Aspirin is a prodrug, which means that it is inactive until it is metabolized or broken down into its constituent parts. In the case of aspirin, this chemical breakdown process occurs in the liver.

One of the most distinct characteristics of aspirin is that it permanently binds to platelets (a type of small cell within the blood that helps it to clot), effectively terminating the platelet's synthesis of thromboxane. Since a platelet's life span is at least 7 days (8-10 days), the anticoagulant effects of aspirin continue for approximately 1 week to 10 days after the dosage is discontinued.

Aspirin is often combined with other ingredients to modify its effect. If aspirin is too harsh for the patient's intestinal mucosa, the salicylate may be buffered. The agent used to buffer the aspirin is usually an antacid product that neutralizes the stomach's acidity and thus decreases the potential for gastric irritation. Another additive takes the form of an external coating of the tablet that will slow down the rate at which the medicine dissolves, leading to a slower release of the aspirin's effect (delayed release). Caffeine added to aspirin products has become a staple on the market (Excedrin Migraine) for headache sufferers. The addition of caffeine acts to elevate mood as well as to constrict blood vessels that may be distended, causing the increased headache pain.

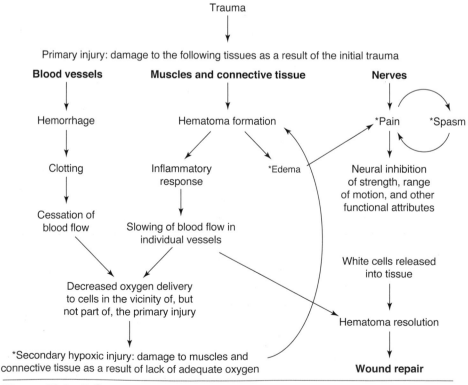

Figure 18.4 Inflammatory response to trauma.

Many varied types of aspirin products are marketed, all with specific claims regarding their effectiveness against pain or their ability to reduce pain without stomach upset. People should fully evaluate each product for its actual effectiveness before subscribing to its claims.

Routes of Administration

Enteric aspirin products are administered by mouth and may include tablets, capsules, chewable tablets, chewing gum, and liquids. Think about a patient who has incurred a broken jaw. Some forms of salicylates may be less desirable for this individual (especially if the jaw was wired shut); thus the liquid administration would be the best choice.

Another enteric aspirin product is a suppository. A salicylate suppository may be chosen for a patient who is vomiting and thus unable to ingest the aspirin.

Adverse Effects of Salicylates

As mentioned earlier, aspirin binds with blood platelets; this can be considered an adverse effect of the drug. In people who are elderly, aspirin is often used to thin the blood in an attempt to reduce the chance of blood clots in the brain or heart. In this case, the binding with platelets may be a desired effect and not an adverse effect; but in the young, athletic population, thinned blood could be problematic. Since trauma is associated with bleeding and aspirin can decrease the availability of platelets, bleeding can be prolonged. Bruising and bleeding in the joints can be increased; thus it is not advisable to administer aspirin in the active population.

Gastrointestinal (GI) irritation as well as GI damage has long been recognized as the primary problem with aspirin. This GI effect may be attributable to irritation of the gastric mucosa caused by the drug, or to the inhibition of prostaglandins that protect the stomach from acidic conditions. Some patients have more difficulty than others with GI irritation when taking aspirin; people who have a history of ulcers are the most affected. Coating is sometimes employed in an attempt to delay dissolution of the drug until it reaches the small intestine. This coating, called enteric coating, not only delays dissolution and release but also delays the therapeutic effects of the drug—and still does not preclude irritation of the duodenum (first part of the small intestine). Buffering of the tablet has also been used to blunt the drug's acidic effects on the gastric mucosa. Taking the aspirin with a meal also buffers the acidic effect, but this too delays the onset of desired effects. A last resort, or a choice for patients with known stomach ulcers, is to combine the aspirin therapy with a second drug designed to prevent or treat, or both prevent and treat, GI irritation. This dual therapy is certainly not required in all patients but may be the only alternative in some gastric-sensitive patients.

Hepatic (liver) and renal (kidney) disorders, although rare, can be produced in patients with preexisting diseases or in those using NSAIDs for prolonged periods or in high doses.

Aspirin overdose, known as aspirin intoxication or poisoning, may occur with doses of 10 to 30 g, but this figure is highly patient specific and quite variable. The overdose is usually accompanied by headache, tinnitus (ringing in the ears), hearing difficulties, confusion, and GI irritation. Children are much more vulnerable than adults to aspirin overdose, especially if treated with adult doses of the drug.

Aspirin has also been associated with a rare condition known as Reye's syndrome. Reye's occurs in children and young teens, often after they have had chicken pox or influenza. Symptoms associated with Reye's syndrome include high fever, vomiting, liver dysfunction, and a decreasing level of alertness that progresses rapidly and often leads to delirium, convulsions, and coma and has the potential to cause death. There is no definite link between aspirin and Reye's, but it is recommended that aspirin and other NSAIDs not be used to treat fever in children and teenagers.

A small percentage of the general population exhibits an aspirin intolerance or hypersensitivity. These individuals have allergic reactions of bronchospasm, urticaria (hives), and severe rhinitis (inflammation of the nasal mucosa) within a few hours of ingesting aspirin. A potential exists for cardiovascular shock in these people, so in this group the use of any NSAID is contraindicated.

Some studies have shown that aspirin and some common NSAIDs inhibit the synthesis of certain components of connective tissue, with implications for the healing of cartilage, tendons, ligaments, and bone. These studies have not fully established this negative connection; therefore continued research is necessary.

Implications for the Athletic Trainer

The main concern about the use of aspirin and other salicylates in the physically active population is the effect on the blood's clotting mechanisms. Since activity is often associated with trauma (micro- and macro-), bleeding is not uncommon. If salicylate drugs are being used and trauma occurs, the chance of excessive bleeding is increased.

Another concern one would have about the use of salicylates is irritation of the stomach. If a person takes a salicylate immediately after a workout or competition, the natural buffers from a meal may not be present, thus increasing the likelihood of gastric upset.

It is always wise to fully evaluate the severity of the pain and the other treatment options available before recommending any anti-inflammatory drugs for the physically active individual.

Nonsalicylate, Nonsteroidal Anti-Inflammatory Drugs

All NSAIDs have the properties of analgesia, antipyresis, and **anticoagulation** as well as an ability to control inflammation. The level at which the NSAID exerts these effects is drug and dose dependent. A plethora of NSAIDs exists, with more being introduced on a frequent basis. Most commonly, NSAIDs are grouped according to their chemical similarities.

A relatively recent development in the treatment of inflammation occurred in the late 1990s. This development focused on the cyclooxygenase-2 (COX-2) inhibitors, medications that target prostaglandins, one of the main chemical mediators that cause inflammation. It has been established that the body produces two main types of prostaglandins: the COX-1 and -2 prostaglandins. The COX-1 prostaglandins are produced by the stomach and other body tissues. These prostaglandins are credited with protecting the gastric mucosa, thus preventing or limiting stomach upset. The COX-2 prostaglandins are effective in the inflammatory process. The traditional NSAIDs have some effect on both the COX-1 and the COX-2 pathways, while the newer NSAIDs, called the COX-2 inhibitors, primarily inhibit the inflammatory pathway without disturbing the protection of the gastric lining through the COX-1 pathway.

The number of NSAIDs on the market makes the doctor's decision on which drug to use a bit challenging. Few clinical differences are found among the various groups or families of NSAIDs, although some reports indicate that the side effects and adverse reactions are greatest with a family of NSAIDs called fenamic acid compounds. The therapeutic effect of any NSAID is patient specific and is based on the clinical response rather than some predetermined indication. Generally, if an individual is being treated with a compound from one group without improvement, the prescribing physician changes the medication to a compound in another family of NSAIDs. It is not unusual, in patients not responding to one compound, to try two or more drugs before finding an effective choice. Each NSAID family targets its effect on a specific part of the inflammatory process. Specific drugs within that family act in the same way. The sports medicine professional should have easy reference to information on each NSAID family. See the sidebar Groups of Nonsteroidal Anti-Inflammatory Drugs for a listing of generic names for each NSAID classification.

More differences have been reported in evaluation of the cyclooxygenase inhibition characteristics of the drug. The COX-2 inhibitors are much less apt to cause stomach upset and thus can exert their anti-inflammatory

GROUPS OF NONSTEROIDAL ANTI-INFLAMMATORY DRUGS

Acetic Acids

Diclofenac
Etodolac
Indomethacin
Ketoralac
Sulindac
Tolmetin
Enolic acids
Oxyphenbutazone
Phenylbutazone
Piroxicam

Fenamic Acids

Meclofenamic acid
Mefenamic acid

Propanoic-phenolic Acids

Fenoprofen
Flurbiprofen
Ibuprofen
Ketoprofen
Naproxen
Suprofen

Carboxylic Acids

Aspirin
Choline magnesium salicylate
Salicylate
Diflunisal
Magnesium salicylate
Salicylamide
Salsalate
Sodium salicylate

COX-2 Inhibitors

Celecoxib
Rofecoxib
Meloxicam
Valdecoxib

Each classification of NSAID consists of a variety of products. This listing represents some of the many products available. Products are listed (by generic name) under the family or group name.

influence without the unwanted gastric effects. In future years, the COX-2 inhibitors will certainly come to be the NSAID of choice for most sport-related trauma.

Yet another way to classify the NSAID family of drugs is by their availability without a prescription. The NSAID groups available over the counter include ibuprofens (Advil, Motrin, and Nuprin), the ketoprofen group (Orudis and Actron), and the naproxen group (Aleve and Naprosyn).

Administration

Nonsteroidal anti-inflammatory drugs are generally administered by mouth, in the form of a tablet, capsule, or liquid. Anti-inflammatory drugs are available for use in the eye; these are called ophthalmic preparations. Some NSAID drugs, such as Toradol, are administered intramuscularly initially and then with oral doses.

Adverse Effects of Nonsteroidal Anti-Inflammatory Drugs

Similar to the salicylates, the NSAIDs in the COX-1 inhibitor group are often associated with gastric irritation, nausea, and vomiting. This unwanted effect of the drug can be virtually eliminated with use of the COX-2 inhibitor NSAIDs. If GI disturbances are a problem, the patient may be able to reduce the symptoms by ingesting the drug only with a full meal and by ingesting large quantities of fluids.

Some drugs in the NSAID category are associated with central nervous system (CNS) effects such as frontal headache, dizziness, vertigo, and mental confusion.

The NSAID phenylbutazone (Butazolidin) has been reported to be poorly tolerated by many, with adverse effects occurring in approximately one-half of all patients treated (Mycek, Harvey, and Champe 2000, p. 411). **Aplastic anemia** is the most significant and serious of the unwanted effects. Other adverse effects are similar to those with other NSAIDs.

Implications for the Athletic Trainer

Since inflammation is probably the most common complaint of the patient, anti-inflammatory drugs use is quite frequent. With that in mind, it is important for the athletic trainer to understand the adverse effects common to NSAID use and report those conditions to the prescribing physician. When a patient is undergoing any treatment for a sport injury, it is wise to frequently reevaluate the signs and symptoms so that a change can be made (whether in medication or in the physical therapy plan) to attempt to produce some improvement.

Patients should be reminded of the importance of taking the NSAID with a meal and of following the directions on the prescription. Failure to follow the directions often leads to adverse effects from the drug.

Anti-Inflammatory Drugs: Corticosteroids

Interest in developing adrenal steroids (corticosteroids) originated in the 1930s when scientists were investigating the function of the adrenal glands in an effort to develop synthetic compounds with the same effects as the normal adrenal function. Some but not all effects were reproduced, and research continued until investigators in 1949 observed a dramatic decrease in the symptoms of arthritic patients with administration of the steroid cortisone (a glucocorticoid). Cortisone and corticotrophin were successful as anti-inflammatory agents, but interest in discovering other functions and products of

the adrenal gland continued. In 1953, further research uncovered a drug named aldosterone, a **mineralocorticoid** produced by the adrenal gland, which was found to be a major factor in the maintenance of the body's fluid and electrolyte balance.

Adrenal steroids have proven quite successful (although the effect is temporary) in the management of rheumatoid arthritis, but the drugs are not without side effects. The number and severity of the side effects are the primary reason behind the limited use of the drug. In most medical communities, oral steroid anti-inflammatory agents are used only when the NSAIDs fail or in occasional cases in which immediate results are required, but then only for the short term and usually in the form of a dose pack. The dose pack allows an immediate loading of the drug into the person's system; a gradual decrease in the amount of steroid taken then follows until the dose pack is finished (about 5 days to 1 week).

There are two adrenal steroid compounds: **glucocorticoids** and mineralocorticoids. The mineralocorticoids are most commonly used to supplement a patient's deficient adrenal production. The glucocorticoids are the compounds most frequently used in athletics, mainly because of their excellent anti-inflammatory action. The effect on the patient's inflammatory symptoms includes reduction of tissue heat, reduction of **erythema**, control of swelling, and decrease in local tenderness. The glucocorticoids are also effective in suppressing immune responses in some diseases like asthma.

The glucocorticoids affect the inflammatory process through inhibition of prostaglandin and leukotriene production as well as by impairing the function of macrophages and leukocytes. Both functions, and others like them, effectively suppress the body's inflammatory response.

The glucocorticoids used most commonly in athletics are cortisone, hydrocortisone (Cortaid), prednisone, methylprednisolone (Medrol), and dexamethasone (Decadron) (table 18.3). Usually the particular drug is chosen due to its duration of action.

Table 18.3 Common Injectable Glucocorticoids Used in Athletics

Generic name	Trade name (if any)
Cortisone	
Dexamethasone	Decadron
Hydrocortisone	Cortaid
Methylprednisolone	Medrol
Prednisone	

Adverse Effects of Glucocorticoids

Among the adverse effects of glucocorticoids is the common ill effect associated with glucocorticoid injection in and around a joint. The strong catabolic effect of a glucocorticoid is not limited to the target structure and has been implicated as the cause of actual tendon rupture.

Implications for the Athletic Trainer

Although the athletic trainer does not prescribe corticosteroids, it is essential that you understand what they are and their intended effects. It should not be a surprise if an individual reports to you that the doctor gave him "steroids" if the physician has failed to fully explain the drug therapy. It would be wise to educate the patient regarding the difference between anabolic (muscle building) steroids and corticosteroids (anti-inflammatory drugs).

In all cases of adrenal steroid use in and around joints, the sport therapist should keep a record of the area of injection, the strength of the steroid, and the patient's response. Always consult the physician when someone reports having received a "cortisone" injection so that you can establish all the facts of the treatment provided.

It is also important to keep excellent records in the patient chart when you know that a corticosteroid has been prescribed and what strength and type of corticosteroid was administered. This information will become critical if more conclusive evidence is found to relate corticosteroids with soft tissue (especially muscle) injury.

Pain and Analgesics

Pain is one of the more common complaints heard in athletic medicine. The pain may be the result of acute trauma or chronic irritation or may be **iatrogenic** (caused by the treatment) following surgery. Regardless of the cause, the first concern should always be to alleviate the effect of the offending factor.

If the causal factor of pain is inflammation, an anti-inflammatory agent may affect the pain at the same time that it decreases the inflammation. In some cases, however, the pain must be controlled in order to allow the individual to function more freely or allow the healing process to continue, or both. Understanding pain and the physiological processing of **noxious** (painful) stimuli, as seen in figure 18.5, is an asset when the time comes to study the therapeutic treatment of pain, a topic of prime concern in Houglum (2010) and Denegar and colleagues (2010). For now, we concentrate only on the control of pain using pharmaceutical medications; the other texts discuss the complex nature of the physiology of pain.

It is important to understand the difference between medicating people to allow them to function normally in life, and perhaps even in rehabilitation, and medicating individuals to allow them to continue to participate in the activity that caused the injury. Remember that pain is a signal. Pain usually prevents an individual from continuing in a harmful activity. Masking this signal through the use of analgesics is not only risky; it may be strictly contraindicated in some conditions. Additionally, every participant, coach, and sports medicine professional should be aware of the potential dangers associated with the misuse of analgesics. No game or contest should be more important than the individual's health and well-being.

Pain medications run the gamut from the OTC products available in the local drugstore and supermarket to the strictly controlled narcotic drugs that are highly regulated and quite potent. Certainly we all recognize the difference between the analgesic needed for a mild headache and the medication that may

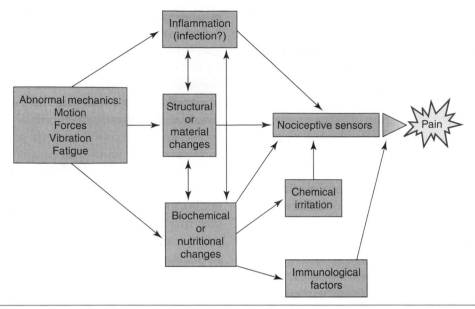

Figure 18.5   A possible pain control mechanism.

Reproduced with permission from White AA III: The 1980 Symposium and Beyond, in Frymoyer JW, Gordon SL, eds.: *New Perspectives on Low Back Pain*. Rosemont, IL, American Academy of Orthopaedic Surgeons, 1989.

be required after reconstructive surgery. This wide range of products provides the physician with many choices in the pharmaceutical management of pain. Most physicians would agree that pain should be managed with the least harmful, least addictive drug possible. Here we consider two main types of analgesics: narcotics and nonnarcotics.

Narcotic Analgesics

The two main types of analgesics are both used for pain, yet the stronger, more addictive narcotic pain relievers are reserved for severe pain such as postoperative pain or pain from serious tissue damage.

Narcotic pain relievers have a limited use for most sport injuries. Moderate to severe pain, such as acute pain following a significant injury or surgery, is often treated with prescription drugs rather than the OTC agents. Narcotic analgesics of the opioid family provide excellent relief from this more severe pain because of their ability to bind within the central nervous system and interrupt nociceptive (pain) transmission. Opioid analgesics, however, have a negative side: They can cause physical as well as psychological addiction. This fear of addiction is typically not a concern in the treatment

of acute traumatic injury because the duration of use of the narcotic drug is very short. Long-term use of narcotic painkillers, on the other hand, should be avoided because of the increased risk of drug dependence. In the mid-1990s a very prominent NFL star openly admitted to having become addicted to pain medications taken during the football season. Following this public announcement, most individuals and sports medicine specialists began looking more critically at their use of pain medications. Masking pain to allow someone to participate is certainly not condoned by the medical community and should never be done without careful protection of the injured area to avoid exacerbation of the problem.

Among the opiates, three specific drugs are familiar to the general public: morphine, codeine, and heroin. Heroin is not used for sports medicine needs and is not discussed here. Morphine is used to relieve moderate to severe pain and is often used as the standard with which other prescription analgesics are compared. Codeine is frequently the analgesic of choice for oral preparations of medicinals to control postsurgical or severe pain.

Endogenous opioids are a group of opioids that are produced in the human body and are often referred to generically as **endorphins**, yet there are actually three groups of endogenous opioids: endorphins, dynorphins, and enkephalins. Endogenous opioids are manufactured in the brain and released as the body attempts to control pain. They have specific receptors in the central and peripheral nervous systems, giving them a very direct avenue of action; yet endogenous opioids are not as potent as the exogenous opioids. Exogenous opioids such as morphine, codeine, and heroin are either natural (from a plant), semisynthetic (from a plant and also manufactured), or synthetic (manufactured).

Opioid receptors have been the subject of much detailed research since their discovery. That there is more than one type of opioid receptor has been well documented. It has also been documented that the different receptors allow different effects to occur. Not only are the effects of the opioids controlled by the receptors, but the side effects also vary according to the particular receptor.

Nonnarcotic Analgesics

Generally, the nonnarcotic analgesics are the same drugs as the NSAIDs (including aspirin and salicylates), since the NSAIDs are able to work in both capacities (analgesic and anti-inflammatory). Salicylates, ibuprofen, and acetaminophen are the most common names associated with OTC analgesics. Salicylates and ibuprofen products are NSAIDs; acetaminophen is the only nonnarcotic that is not also an NSAID.

Both the analgesic and the anti-inflammatory actions of salicylates are believed to be caused by peripheral inhibition of prostaglandin synthesis as with the other NSAIDs. However, in contrast to other NSAIDs, aspirin may also inhibit the action and synthesis of other mediators of inflammation.

Antipyretic effects of salicylates are a result of inhibition of prostaglandin synthesis in the hypothalamus rather than at the local site as in their other actions. Aspirin also may increase the blood flow to the skin and cause sweating, thus dissipating heat associated with a fever.

Another analgesic that is not an anti-inflammatory is acetaminophen (Tylenol, Datril, Pamprin, and Panadol). Acetaminophen is a weak prostaglandin inhibitor in the peripheral tissues. Its effect is similar to that of aspirin in diminishing pain or fever, but it is not at all helpful in the reduction of inflammation. Acetaminophen is the analgesic of choice when the patient is allergic to aspirin or has intolerance to salicylates. Children with viral infections may be treated with acetaminophen without the risk of Reye's syndrome associated with use of aspirin products.

Acetaminophen is very useful in the treatment of mild to moderate pain and is provided in OTC strengths of 325 and 500 mg in tablet, capsule, and liquid-preparation forms. In Europe, paracetamol is the equivalent to acetaminophen and is quite readily available. Liquid acetaminophen preparations are also available, which is helpful when acetaminophen is needed for intraoral injury or for surgery involving the jaw or mouth.

A narcotic agent to increase the drug's potency may supplement acetaminophen. This combination, such as Tylenol III or Tylenol IV, is often used for the treatment of severe pain associated with fractures, dislocations, or other trauma, including surgery. The narcotic (usually codeine) adds the analgesic effect of the narcotic pain reliever to that of the acetaminophen; the narcotic-supplemented acetaminophen is therefore a high-level analgesic limited in its use to patients with severe pain. Acetaminophen with codeine (Tylenol III, Tylenol IV) is a controlled prescription drug because of the narcotic; thus its use is strictly monitored.

Administration of Analgesics

Analgesics have a wide variety of routes of administration, probably because of the wide variety of situations in which pain is the dominant complaint.

Analgesics are most commonly taken by mouth in either a pill, capsule, or liquid form but may also be given transdermally by iontophoresis or a specialized patch, by injection into a muscle, or intravenously. You may hear of a patient having an analgesic "pump" following surgery. This most often involves one of the narcotic pain relievers, and the pump allows the patient to administer small doses of the drug as the pain dictates, always with the machine preventing an overdose of the medicine.

Adverse Effects of Analgesic Therapy

The most common unwanted effects of opioids include drowsiness, dizziness, blurred vision, nausea, vomiting, and constipation. Addiction to opioid drugs, as previously stated, is also a risk from both a physical and a psychological point of view. There is clear, documented evidence that morphine causes a physical addiction—as evident in the severe withdrawal symptoms experienced by addicts when the drug is no longer available. At first the patient feels uneasy or nervous and may experience depression. Physical signs of addiction occur during withdrawal and include sweating, nausea, and vomiting. Muscle tremors and twitching are also associated with narcotic withdrawal. Withdrawal symptoms can last anywhere from 36 h to 5 days. After this withdrawal period, the person may still have a strong psychological addiction to the drug, such as a strong desire or craving for a "fix." Psychological addiction can last for years and is often thought to be the most difficult part of the addiction and withdrawal process.

As we discussed earlier, aspirin inhibits platelet function, but the body's blood-clotting mechanisms usually begin to return to normal within 36 h after the last dose of the drug. Other salicylates have minimal effect on platelets, and acetaminophen has no effect on the platelets.

Gastrointestinal irritation is fairly common with the use of many of the NSAIDs and salicylates but less common with the COX-2 inhibitor classes. Aspirin and buffered aspirin products have approximately the same absorption rate; however, the incidence of bleeding is reported to be higher with plain aspirin tablets than with the buffered products. Gastrointestinal mucosa injury is seen less often with coated aspirin than with plain aspirin or buffered aspirin. Patients with erosive gastritis or peptic ulcer should avoid salicylates because of the possibility of exacerbating the condition.

Tinnitus and hearing loss associated with salicylate therapy are dose related and usually completely reversible, typically subsiding within 24 to 48 h after the dose is reduced or discontinued.

Implications for the Athletic Trainer

It is important to understand the types of analgesics available for the treatment of pain. Although you will not prescribe drugs, you should be able to inform the patient regarding the type of analgesic prescribed or what might be expected following a surgical procedure. Additionally, understanding of the various alternatives for pain medication may prove beneficial in helping patients decide wisely when selecting an OTC analgesic for minor pain.

Anesthetics: General and Local

It is probably obvious that a surgical patient will most likely need both sensory sedation and full muscle relaxation in order for the surgeon to perform the needed procedure. This is accomplished by the use of general **anesthesia**. The vast area of general anesthetics is complex and beyond the scope of this book; a simple explanation is that a combination of drugs is needed to prepare for, achieve, and bring the patient back from anesthesia. General anesthetics are drugs that are very general in their action; they cause the patient to become unconscious, amnesic, and totally relaxed muscularly. Because of the multiple systems involved in sedating a patient for surgery, several drugs are combined to achieve and maintain the specific anesthetic goal.

From time to time the surgeon elects to use a local anesthetic rather than a general anesthetic. Local anesthetics are capable of blocking all nerves, thus acting on both sensory and motor functions. Although motor paralysis may at times be desirable, it may limit the ability of the patient to cooperate, as in obstetric delivery and in some surgeries of the nervous system (when the motor function of the nerve must remain intact but the sensory fibers are being cut). In most cases of local anesthesia used in athletic medicine, both the sensory and motor functions are affected. Minor surgery or suturing of open wounds is usually accomplished under local anesthesia. Only the area of concern needs to be affected, and the local anesthetic provides just sufficient results. An individual in need of dental work typically receives a local anesthetic to decrease the associated pain. This anesthesia is not limited to the sensory nerve, and the person often returns from the appointment showing signs of facial muscle paralysis.

The choice of a local anesthetic for a specific procedure is typically based on the duration of the action needed. Procaine (Novocain) and chloroprocaine are short acting; lidocaine (Xylocaine), mepivacaine (Carbocaine, Isocaine), and prilocaine (Citanest) have an intermediate duration of

action; and tetracaine (Pontocaine), bupivacaine (Marcaine), and etidocaine (Duranest) are long-acting drugs (see table 18.4).

In the treatment of superficial abrasions, several preparations are available to reduce the sensitivity of the exposed nerve endings. Some of the topical preparations on the market are Benzocaine, Nupercainal, and Xylocaine (available in ointment, cream, jelly, and solution forms).

Administration of Anesthetics

General anesthetics are administered either by inhalation or as an intravenous preparation; local anesthetics can be administered via injection or applied topically (iontophoresis or cutaneous application without a driving current).

Adverse Effects of Anesthetics

Knowledge of the adverse effects (see table 18.5) associated with anesthesia can help us understand the reason behind many of the operative precautions that are exercised. The

Table 18.4 Pharmacokinetic Properties of Local Anesthetics

Anesthetic agent	Rate of onset of anesthesia	Duration of action
Novocain	Rapid	Short
Xylocaine	Slow	Moderate
Carbocaine, Isocaine	Slow	Moderate
Citanest	Slow	Moderate
Marcaine	Rapid	Long
Pontocaine	Rapid	Long
Duranest	Rapid	Long

Table 18.5 Skeletal Muscle Relaxants Used in Surgery

Drug	Main effects	Side effects
Depolarizing drugs (succinylcholine)	Skeletal muscle paralysis following muscle fasciculations. All skeletal muscles are involved, including respiratory muscles.	Cardiac arrhythmia Hyperkalemia with a possibility of cardiac arrest Increased intraocular pressure Increased intragastric pressure and potential of vomiting Postoperative muscle pain
Nondepolarizing drugs (tubocurarine)	Skeletal muscle paralysis with small muscle paralysis first and respiratory paralysis last.	Hypotension (low blood pressure)

anesthesiologist has several duties in keeping the individual sedated during a surgical procedure; this function, although often noticed but given relatively little attention by the untrained observer, is actually extremely critical to a safe and comfortable sedation during surgery. The adverse effects are numerous but are clearly understood, allowing steps to be taken to avoid problems during surgery. Specific adverse effects include cardiovascular effects (hypotension and arrhythmia), increased intragastric pressure, intraorbital pressure, postoperative muscle pain, and histamine responses (itching and hives).

Implications for the Athletic Trainer

Rest assured that without specialized training, you will not find yourself administering general anesthetics; yet it is good to understand both the things you may observe when attending surgery and the things the patient is undergoing during the operative procedure.

In many college and professional athletic facilities, the team physicians keep at least two injectable local anesthetics on hand, typically one shorter-acting (Xylocaine) and one longer-acting (Marcaine) anesthetic. In these settings you may be asked to set up the physician's area with the injectables; thus an understanding of the various types of anesthetics may be critical if the physician asks you to set out short- or long-acting supplies only. The addition of a vasoconstrictor (epinephrine) to the local anesthetic decreases the rate of absorption of the anesthetic and thus the duration of action.

Central-Acting Muscle Relaxants

A variety of compounds are available to reduce muscle spasm associated with local injury. Some of the numerous generic names (and trade names) are carisoprodol (Soma), chlorzoxazone (Parafon Forte; chlorzoxazone and acetaminophen), cyclobenzaprine hydrochloride (Flexeril), diazepam (Valium), methocarbamol (Robaxin), and orphenad-

rine (Norgesic; orphenadrine with aspirin and caffeine).

Often the drug treatment of muscle spasm involves a muscle relaxant with an analgesic that is added in an effort to provide pain relief. Regardless of the type of skeletal muscle relaxant used, the mechanism of action is not well understood; yet the overall effect is sedation. All the drugs have some general depressant activity on the central nervous system, and the ability of the compound to selectively relax skeletal muscle has not been proven.

Administration of Muscle Relaxants

Most muscle relaxants are administered orally or by injection.

Adverse Effects of Muscle Relaxants

Because of the sedative action of these drugs, the primary side effect is drowsiness with the addition of some dizziness. Nausea, lightheadedness, vertigo, ataxia, and headache may occur depending on the patient and the specific muscle relaxant used. Some physicians feel that the side effects and central action of the skeletal muscle relaxant are sufficient reason not to prescribe them for the student-athlete. In cases in which the muscle spasm is severe and must be blocked to allow the patient to sleep comfortably, the physician may prescribe a relaxant to be taken at bedtime.

Implications for the Athletic Trainer

It is wise to understand the effect of skeletal muscle relaxants and to advise the individual accordingly. The sedative effect—although not the specific effect one might want—often reduces local muscle spasm associated with athletic injury. It is important to remind someone taking a muscle relaxant that the drug has a strong sedative effect and that use during the day might interfere with normal daily activities. Because of the specific nature of physical therapy and the general effects of the drug therapy treatment, it is also important to emphasize the need for compliance with any physical therapy prescribed.

Nonorthopedic Medicinals

The general group of nonorthopedic medicinals is truly open-ended. The number of drugs available equals the variety of medical problems that one might encounter. Some categorization is obviously necessary. We will examine some of the drugs used for common, nonorthopedic problems that affect all individuals, namely, drugs for upper respiratory system problems, drugs to combat infections, and drugs for digestive tract disturbances.

Medications for Upper Respiratory Tract Conditions

Unfortunately, the common cold is very tenacious, lasting about a week regardless of the therapeutic measures taken. Among the few things one can do is to reduce or control the symptoms: runny nose, congestion, sore throat, and the like. Two types of drugs are available to help with the congestion or runny nose effects: decongestants and **antihistamines**. A persistent cough can present an irritating problem both in daily life generally and in sport activity. Suppression of the cough reflex has long been a recognized action of opioids, particularly codeine; but this is not a favored drug to use because of its addictive potential and also because it often leaves the patient with a feeling of euphoria or drowsiness. Four main nonnarcotic preparations are prescribed for management of the congestion or cough (or both) associated with an upper respiratory illness or allergies: decongestants, antihistamines, **antitussives**, and **expectorants**.

Decongestants

Decongestants are used for sinus congestion with or without nasal discharge. Allergies and the common cold are often seasonal; they also vary with area of the country. Decongestants used to treat these symptoms are members of the alpha-1-adrenergic agonist family of medicines. Some of the more common decongestants are pseudoephedrine, ephedrine, epinephrine, and oxymetazoline. Various companies manufacture decongestants under different trade names (see table 18.6).

Administration of Decongestants

The alpha-1-agonists may be taken systematically (oral forms) or applied locally to the nasal mucosa via aerosols.

Adverse Effects of Decongestants

The primary adverse effects of decongestants include headache, dizziness, nervousness, nausea, and cardiovascular irregularities, all of which become more apparent with continued use. The decongestant usually does not cause tiredness or lethargy; on the contrary, some individuals feel that the alpha-1-agonist actually produces a feeling of heightened arousal or a "buzz."

Implications for the Athletic Trainer

Since it is within the law to provide a single dose of an OTC medication, you may find that this is within the scope of your job. If it is, and patients see you for a decongestant, it is very important that you record the drug and dosage provided. Situations have happened in which the patient finds that the decongestant gives her a "buzz," and soon the

Table 18.6 Grouping of Decongestants Used in Athletics

Generic grouping	Common trade names	Dosage form
Pseudoephedrine	Actifed, Sudafed, and others	Oral: tablets and liquid
Ephedrine	Primatene tablets	Oral: tablets and liquid
Epinephrine	Primatene Mist	Nasal spray
Oxymetazoline (or phenylephrine)	Neo-Synephrine, Afrin	Nasal spray and tablets

patient is depending on the sports medicine staff to provide the dose. Without a good record system, the patient may see several different people on the health care staff and obtain a single dose from each. This multiple dosing is certainly dangerous and a bad situation to allow to develop.

Antihistamines

Antihistamines are used for a number of problems in athletics. Not only are they helpful in the management of allergic responses to hay fever; they are often used for their strong secondary effect, sedation. The antihistamines can be used to produce a mild sedation that is helpful in management of the restless individual who is unable to fall asleep.

The numerous antihistamines vary in the degree of sedation they cause, which is often the adverse effect that limits the use of this type of drug. Newer antihistamines do not cross the blood–brain barrier and thus exert less of the sedative effect but are quite effective in producing the desired effects of drying up the mucosal vasculature and decreasing congestion. Table 18.7 shows some of the more commonly used antihistamines; as you may notice, some of the trade names are those associated with preparations that help with sleeping. As noted earlier, this is a side effect of the antihistamine; but because the effect is so strong, the drugs are marketed for their secondary effect. One might regard an antihistamine as actually two drugs in

one, although caution is warranted if sleep or drowsiness is not a wanted effect.

Administration of Antihistamines

Antihistamines are usually taken orally, as either a pill or a liquid.

Adverse Effects of Antihistamines

Although antihistamines often produce drowsiness, this may not be classified as an unwanted or adverse effect. Nonetheless, one must include drowsiness in the classification of adverse effects when discussing medications for the upper respiratory tract.

Dry mouth, decreased coordination, tightness in the chest, dizziness, and blood pressure changes are reported as additional adverse effects of antihistamines.

Implications for the Athletic Trainer

When suggesting an OTC product for the patient to purchase, it is prudent to inform the person of potential drowsiness. If the patient needs to study, drive, or be alert for some other reason, the choice of antihistamine becomes more important.

Antitussives

Antitussives are used to suppress coughing, but usually only for the short term. Opioids are analgesics, but can cause cough suppression. Due to the addictive nature of opioids, they are usually not prescribed as a main antitussive. The antitussives chosen varies according to the physician's, phar-

Table 18.7 Common Antihistamines

Generic name	Trade name(s)	Sedative effect
Brompheniramine	Dimetane	Low
Chlorpheniramine	Chlor-Trimeton	Low
Clemastine	Tavist	Low
Loratadine	Claritin	Low
Terfenadine	Seldane	Low
Diphenhydramine	Benadryl, others	High
Dimenhydrinate	Dramamine	High
Doxylamine	Unisom	High

macist's, and patient's personal preferences. Frequently the patient or parent searching for something to control a cough is met with such an array of choices that the decision becomes quite difficult. Some of the more common of these drugs are listed in table 18.8. In a 2008 Cochrane review it was reported "There is no good evidence for or against the effectiveness of OTC medicines in acute cough" (Smith, Schroeder, Fahey, 2008)

Administration of Antitussives

The oral route of administration of antitussives is well known to most people. Cough syrups, lozenges, and pills are all commonly used in an attempt to reduce a cough.

Adverse Effects of Antitussives

Antitussives may cause drowsiness or a feeling of dizziness in some people, while in others they may cause restlessness and nervousness. Additionally, they may result in constipation, especially if taken for several weeks.

Implications for the Athletic Trainer

Many patients do not realize the differences between cough and cold medications such as expectorants, cough suppressants, or decongestants. Educating patients about the antitussives will help them make the best purchase for their symptoms. When a patient has a cough for weeks on end, it may be important to help the person find a health care provider who will be able to prescribe stronger medication than what is available for general, OTC purchase.

Expectorants and Mucolytics

The substances called expectorants and **mucolytics** are grouped together pharmacologically but are quite different in effect. The mucolytic drugs help to decrease the viscosity of respiratory excretions, while expectorants serve to facilitate the production and ejection of the mucus. Typically these types of agents are used to decrease the accumulation of thick, viscous secretions that clog respiratory passages. Often the expectorants and mucolytics are used in conjunction with antitussives and decongestants. Some physicians feel that the effects of the drugs are no better than that provided by a household humidifier. The only mucolytic drug currently in use is acetylcysteine, yet the number of products known as expectorants is great. The most common expectorant, guaifenesin, is used in many OTC preparations. The way guaifenesin works is unclear, yet the FDA recognizes its positive effects.

Administration of Expectorants and Mucolytics

Most expectorants and mucolytics are provided in the oral forms. Cough syrups are well labeled with the word "expectorant."

Adverse Effects of Expectorants and Mucolytics

The primary adverse effect is GI upset, and this is exacerbated if the syrup is taken on an empty stomach. Other unwanted effects include insomnia, headache, vertigo, skin rash, and breathing problems.

Table 18.8	Common Antitussives (Cough Suppressants)	
Generic name	Trade name(s)	Action
Codeine	Many	Direct inhibitory effect on brain stem cough center
Hydrocodone	Triaminic Expectorant DH	Similar to action of codeine
Dextromethorphan	Many	Similar to action of codeine
Caramiphen	Tuss-Ornade	Antihistamine
Benzonatate	Tessalon Perle	Anesthetic to respiratory mucosa

Implications for the Athletic Trainer

Expectorants and mucolytics have a special role in the management of the common cold. When evaluating the types of medicinals to help abate the symptoms of cough and congestion, one must pay attention to the type of cough. Coughs that sound as if they are producing movement of phlegm from the lungs are called productive coughs. These types of coughs may benefit from the use of mucolytic and expectorants, while the harsh, raspy cough that sounds dry usually does not benefit from this type of therapy.

Bronchodilators (Beta-Adrenergic Agonists)

There are a number of **bronchodilators** on the market; most, if used by persons with asthma, are in the form of an inhaler. Bronchodilators, which are often beta-adrenergic agonists, cause smooth muscle relaxation, effectively opening the constricted airways. Albuterol is the product most commonly used in athletic health care; two trade names of albuterol are Proventil and Ventolin (inhalers). Following inhalation, the effects are seen within 5 to 15 min and last from 3 to 6 h.

The use of inhalants is intended for those who have asthma, yet some physicians prescribe an inhaler when mucus is plugging the respiratory airways. The active agent in the inhaler is actually the critical factor, yet the method of administration (inhalation) allows the drug to be delivered directly to the respiratory tissues with minimal side effects. A person who has asthma may be prescribed anti-inflammatory agents as well as bronchodilators to reverse the bronchial constriction associated with the condition.

The classification "asthmatic" encompasses a wide range of involvement. Some people experience bronchoconstriction only when exercising (exercise-induced **bronchospasm**), while others experience constriction of the air passageway day in and day out. Changes in environmental conditions and minor colds affect the person with asthma much more than people without this condition. Patients experiencing more severe forms of asthma, or those in an acute episode, may be given the anti-inflammatory drugs (cortisone preparations) in an effort to control the swelling in the bronchioles once the bronchodilator opens the passages sufficiently. Products such as Azmacort and Flovent are steroid preparations that either prevent the narrowing or relax the smooth muscle of the air passages. These preparations may be on the banned drug list for college and Olympic sports, and it is prudent to investigate the legality of such a drug prior to use in a competitive individual.

Administration of Bronchodilators

Most often the drug is provided in a metered-dose inhaler: Each time the canister is activated it emits a metered dose. For severe breathing problems, a "breathing treatment" is employed in which a nebulizer mixes the drug into a fine mist; the drug is then dispensed over a period of about 10 min, providing improved distribution of the drug into the bronchioles.

Adverse Effects of Bronchodilators

One of the most disconcerting side effects with use of inhalers is its effects on the heart. After a breathing treatment, people often experience a "racing heart" or other cardiac irregularities. Inhaler treatment may also be followed by a central nervous system effect that gives the individual a sense of nervousness. Long-term use of bronchodilators may cause inflammatory conditions of the pharynx due to the medicine's coming into contact with the back of the throat.

Implications for the Athletic Trainer

The major problem with the use of bronchodilators is the patient's hand–breath coordination. The individual must maximally exhale and then time the depression of the canister with an inhalation. Too often, the timing is good but the inhaler is aimed so that the drug is placed at the back of the throat. Occasionally a breathing treatment is needed and is administered in the team physician's office by the physician or paramedics.

Infections and Antibiotics

When we talk about infection, we should stop for a moment and ask ourselves why an infection has occurred. A small amount of prevention may be all that is needed to avoid the use of medicinal drugs. A good rule is that all open wounds must be well cleansed with soap and warm water. Some irritants or bacteria enter the skin or other tissues, and no outward sign of injury is noticed until infection is present. When infection develops, medicinal drugs may be needed.

There is some confusion surrounding the terminology used to refer to drugs for treating infections. It helps to think of the infection in terms of the cause and to know that the name of a drug for treating infection has the prefix "anti-" followed by the term for the offending element—that is, antibacterials, antifungals, and so on. The term antibiotic denotes an agent used to kill an organism. Here we discuss the antibiotics in terms of their specific function—either antibacterial or antifungal.

Antibacterial Agents

Topical antibacterial agents are often used in athletics after cleansing of an open wound. Although use of the antibacterial in this situation is mostly prophylactic, the agent can be effective for treating some superficial wound infections. The most proper way to deal with an infection is to take a culture and employ sensitivity studies to determine what type of bacterium is causing the infection. Since some bacteria are resistant to specific agents, treatment with these agents will be ineffective. Unless the infection is full-blown, the athletic trainer may adequately treat superficial wounds with one or more of the products commonly available over the counter.

Antibacterial agents used topically usually contain a mixture of antibacterial agents and include a variety of trade name products; the more common are Neosporin, Polysporin, and Bacitracin, among many others with similar names.

An interesting side note concerns a "trainer's trick" to care for the superficial wounds caused by artificial turf. Obviously, with all turf burns, the most critical factor in preventing infection is thorough cleaning of the wound. This very often is extremely difficult because of the irritation of many nerve endings on the abraded skin. Reducing the sensitivity of the skin prior to cleaning the wound often allows one to fully cleanse the skin surface. This is easy to do during the competition at the same time that one covers the open wound. Simple application of a topical anesthetic in lieu of an antibiotic allows the anesthetic to desensitize the area while the patient completes the contest; afterward, the person can shower and clean the wound with less discomfort. The products used to aid in the anesthetic action include the true anesthetics available in cream or ointment form and the anesthetic creams designed for hemorrhoid treatment, which provide both the antibacterial and the anesthetic effect.

Antibacterial agents, regardless of the tissue infected, are classified according to their effect, whether it be via inhibition of the bacterial cell's wall and its function (penicillins and cephalosporins), via inhibition of bacterial protein synthesis (aminoglycosides, erythromycin, and tetracycline), or, finally, via inhibition of the bacterial DNA/RNA function (sulfanilamides). Some of the trade names associated with the antibacterials are listed in table 18.9.

Administration of Antibacterials

Topical applications are the most familiar form of application of antibacterials used in athletics. Systemic infections may be treated with oral antibacterials, and severe infections may be treated with injectable forms of the medicines.

Adverse Effects of Antibacterials

Medical professionals have warned against the overprescribing of antibacterials in young patients due to the potential of an increased resistance to the drug. Other unwanted effects include diarrhea, nausea and vomiting, rash, injection site inflammation, and seizures.

Table 18.9 Common Antibacterial Agents

Action	Generic name	Trade name(s)
Cell membrane synthesis inhibition	Penicillin	V-Cillin K, Amoxil, many others
	Cephalosporin	Keflex, Keflin, Ultrase, Suprax, many others
	Bacitracin	Bacitracin ointment
Protein synthesis inhibition	Erythromycin	E-Mycin, EES, Erythrocin, others
	Tetracycline	Achromycin V, Vibramycin, others
DNA/RNA inhibition	Fluoroquinolone	Cipro
	Sulfanilamide	Gantrisin, Silvadene

Implications for the Athletic Trainer

The antibacterial agents often used by the athletic trainer are those administered topically. Rarely do drugs administered topically cause systemic intolerance; thus there are no precautions to their use, short of an allergic response. In the case of treatment of superficial abrasions such as turf burns, thorough cleansing of the wound and application of a topical antibacterial agent are strongly recommended.

Antifungals

Fungal infections are much like bacterial infections; however, the agents used to treat bacteria will not affect fungi, and agents effective against fungi are not effective against bacteria. Primarily, the antifungal agents work by disrupting fungal membrane functions. Most healthy individuals do not develop the fungal infections associated with people whose immune system has been suppressed.

When oral antifungal medications are used for tenacious infections such as those under the nail bed (toenails are especially prone to fungal infections), the physician may advise the person to take the medication just prior to exercise. The reason is that the antifungal medication is distributed to the nail bed through perspiration; so the more the person perspires, the more effective the treatment can be. Unfortunately, these nail bed infections are usually quite tough, and eradication using oral antifungals can take months.

Not infrequently, people are bothered by fungal infections in areas of high moisture such as the groin, feet, and hands. The individual should be educated regarding good hygiene to control or prevent fungal infections. Control entails keeping the area as dry as possible, taking care to wear only clean garments over the affected tissues, and, if necessary, beginning the application of an antifungal agent.

The person with a fungal infection needs to apply the antifungal medication to the affected area two or three times daily. With regular application of an antifungal cream or ointment, the fungus can be brought under control within 2 or 3 weeks, after which time the person may be able to switch to a powder form. Too often people notice the problem and self-treat it with the powder antifungal, only to minimally control the spread rather than effectively treat the fungus. Some products are prescription drugs and others are over the counter; some products are combined with a topical corticosteroid that may provide more rapid improvement than is possible with the antifungal alone. Some of the topical antifungals are listed in table 18.10.

Administration of Antifungals

Antifungal agents are of two varieties: oral medication (pills) and topical medication (cream, ointment, and powder). The oral medications are used for subcutaneous (below the skin) and systemic mycoses (diseases caused by fungi), whereas superficial mycoses are easily treated using topical agents.

Table 18.10 Common Topical Antifungal Preparations

Generic name	Trade name(s)
Clortrimazole	Clotrimazole Cream 1% (prescription), Lotrimin
Miconazole	Micatin, Monistat
Naftifine	Naftin (not good against yeasts)
Tolnaftate	Tinactin

Adverse Effects of Antifungals

The topical antifungals are fairly free of adverse effects; the oral form of the drug has a variety of unwanted effects such as headache, neurological changes, liver disorders, and some degree of photosensitivity.

Implications for the Athletic Trainer

Careful observation of the skin and nail beds of the patient may be the first step in caring for fungal infections. Refer the patient to a physician for diagnosis and proper medical care, especially when topical antifungal OTC medications do not seem to manage the problem. Subungual (under the nail) infections and infections that appear to be spreading must be treated by a physician. Educating patients about the treatment measures may help them to make the proper decision about consulting a physician.

Drugs for Treatment of Gastrointestinal Problems

Physically active patients have problems similar to those of the population in general; GI disturbances are not uncommon. The patient may be under great stress, resulting in diarrhea or upset stomach. Travel and changes in eating habits may cause constipation, or, conversely, loose stools or actual diarrhea. All digestive system problems are manageable if they are recognized; it is just a matter of having the patient report the problem.

Antidiarrheals

Two classes of drugs are used to treat diarrhea: opioids (Lomotil, Imodium) and nono-pioids (Donnagel). Both effectively slow the movement of food through the GI tract. One aspect to note, however, is that antidiarrheals produce bowel "paralysis"; and if the diarrhea is associated with an infection, the infection may continue to proliferate, creating a potential for bowel rupture secondary to the expanding infection. Caution is always in order when one is treating diarrhea with no known etiology.

Some of the products used to treat diarrhea are also adsorbents (not "absorbents"). Adsorbents attach other substances like bacteria to their surface without any chemical action, but there is question about how effective they are in decreasing stool production and water. Kaopectate and Pepto-Bismol are among these products (bismuth salicylate), which also decrease gastric acid secretion and may aid in quieting an upset stomach.

Administration of Antidiarrheals

Antidiarrheals are available for oral consumption in liquid form as well as tablets or capsules.

Adverse Effects

In addition to the effect of bowel paralysis, the antidiarrheals often cause constipation if taken for a prolonged period. The opioid antidiarrheals, like other opioids, may cause drowsiness and dizziness as an unwanted side effect.

Implications for the Athletic Trainer

Often patients are quite shy about reporting bouts of diarrhea, so it becomes important to understand the seriousness of the condition if and when a patient confides in you. Not only should you understand the treatment and precautions regarding diarrhea; you also need to understand the sequelae of the condition. Whenever excess water is lost through the bowel, the body quickly enters a state of fluid depletion. Care must be taken to replenish fluids and electrolytes in the patient who is experiencing diarrhea.

Laxatives

Although constipation is a less frequent problem in the young, healthy population, it may be a problem in the athletic arena (more among the coaches and administrators than the participants!). The two main types of products used to reduce constipation are bulk-forming laxatives and bowel stimulants.

Bulk-forming laxatives (Metamucil and the hyperosmotic agents) absorb water in the lower GI tract and stretch the bowel, stimulating peristalsis. Most of these products contain dietary fiber to aid in more regular action of the bowel. Bowel stimulants act to irritate the intestinal mucosa or the **splanchnic nerves** serving the bowel. This type of laxative includes Dulcolax, Ex-Lax, and other commonly available products.

Administration of Laxatives

The bulk-forming laxatives are for oral consumption, coming in convenient wafer form or a powder that one mixes with water or another beverage. The bowel stimulants are usually administered rectally via suppository or enema application methods.

Adverse Effects of Laxatives

The unwelcome effects of oral laxatives include feelings of bloating or cramping of the bowel. Some reversal of the constipation can occur, resulting in diarrhea. Nausea, flatulence (intestinal gas), and increased thirst have been reported. The rectally administered laxatives have been known to cause rectal area discomfort including bleeding, blistering, burning, itching, or pain.

Implications for the Athletic Trainer

Unfortunately, the laxatives are a group of drugs that may be misused by some. College athletic trainers have found gymnasts and wrestlers using laxatives to clear the bowel in an attempt to decrease body weight. This practice is dangerous because the medication interrupts the body's normal physiology. The large intestine is responsible for removing fluids from the waste material; and with a bowel stimulant or laxative, the large intestine is so irritated that fluid absorption is aborted and the waste expelled. Dehydration can result from the misuse of a laxative, predisposing the individual to additional

harm especially during exercise in a warm environment such as a wrestling room. Those responsible need to use care in both drug inventory and dispensation procedures so that it is easier to recognize any misuse of these medications.

Antiemetics

Emesis, or vomiting, is sometimes troublesome for individuals with pregame anxiety or motion sickness. The antiemetics most often used for this type of problem include dimenhydrinate (Dramamine) and meclizine (Antivert, Bonine). Some antacids and adsorbents also help in soothing the gastric mucosa and decreasing the irritation that is causing the vomiting.

Administration of Antiemetics

Except in the case of a medical condition causing frequent vomiting (such as with chemotherapy), emesis can be controlled with oral medications.

Adverse Effects of Antiemetics

The typical products used for emesis, unfortunately, are apt to cause drowsiness or a headache, neither of which would be welcome during an athletic competition.

Implications for the Athletic Trainer

Medical conditions unrelated to simple anxiety can also cause vomiting. Early stages of pregnancy, for example, may cause vomiting as well as medical problems such as heat exhaustion, appendicitis, food poisoning, head injury, and various diseases. The underlying cause of vomiting must be understood and evaluated, and caution must be exercised in treating patients who have recurrent bouts of vomiting.

Antacids

Some people experience occasional minor gastric upset due to their eating habits. The drugs used to decrease the stomach irritation actually neutralize stomach acids. Antacids contain a combination of a carbonate or hydroxide and an aluminum, magnesium, or calcium that work together to control the gastric pH.

Others have gastric ulcers or irritable bowel syndrome (IBS) that may require medications designed to block the release of gastric acid. Such preparations include Tagamet, Pepcid, and Zantac.

Administration of Antacids

The most common form of antacid is the chewable tablet, and many of these tablets are readily available without a prescription. Other oral forms include powders or tablets that are to be dissolved in water or other fluid, liquid forms, and chewing gum. Medications for IBS are most often in tablet or liquid form but can be administered by injection or intravenously for severe medical conditions.

Adverse Effects of Antacids

When antacids are taken as directed, very few adverse effects are noted. If the medicine is taken in large doses or over a long time, minor unwanted effects can occur, including a chalky taste, mild constipation or diarrhea, thirst, stomach cramps, and whitish or speckled stools. Unwanted effects such as those that may accompany Tagamet, Pepcid, and Zantac administration include headache, dizziness and diarrhea, or nausea and vomiting.

Implications for the Athletic Trainer

Products to settle the stomach are sometimes used in an attempt to counteract poor eating habits, and the health care specialist should educate patients so they can attack the problem at the cause—that is, nutritional habits—and not depend on the quick-fix antacid. Chronic use of antacids has a potential to contribute to kidney stones. Evidence is insufficient to establish a causal relationship, but this is still reason enough to convince a person to stop using these products if at all possible.

Learning Aids

SUMMARY

The study of pharmacology can be overwhelming, but with diligence, the health care practitioner will become familiar with actions and interactions of various medications. Some pharmaceuticals are more commonly used in some settings than in others, but those commonly used in the particular setting you work in should be the ones with which you are most familiar. It is never a problem to refer to *PDR* or other drug references to learn more about a medication. It would serve our patients better if we all did that.

KEY CONCEPTS AND REVIEW

▸ **Define and list examples of generic versus trade name drugs.**

By generic drug, we mean a drug that is referred to by its "official" or nonproprietary name. This name is often derived from the chemical name but is much shorter and simpler. An example of a generic drug is acetaminophen; a trade name of acetaminophen is Tylenol. There can be as many trade names (proprietary names) as there are companies that make the product.

▸ **Discuss why drugs are classified as nonprescription, prescription, or controlled substances.**

Nonprescription (OTC) drugs can be obtained from the store shelf. Taking the OTC drug as indicated on the label should pose no difficulties for most patients (unless the patient has an allergy to that medication). Over-the-counter drugs are usually sufficient for minor problems. Prescription drugs are more powerful drugs that must be selected by the physician (or other certified professional such as a physician's assistant). To avoid adverse drug interactions, the prescribing health care practitioner interviews the patient about allergies and other medications being taken. Prescription medications can be refilled with the permission of the physician. Controlled substances are those drugs that have a high potential for abuse. There are rules for prescribing, dispensing, and renewing prescriptions for the five types of controlled substances. These drugs must be kept in a secure area of the facility, and those responsible must keep thorough records of any controlled drugs dispensed.

▶ **Identify the methods of administering medicinal drugs to the patient.**

Drugs can be administered via the digestive system (enteral), meaning that the drug is taken in (by mouth, under the tongue [sublingually], or rectally) and then enters the appropriate organ or system from that point of origin. Nonenteral methods of administration include delivery by injection (including IV, intra-articular, intramuscular), application to the skin (topical), inhalation, and transport through the skin (transdermal).

▶ **Define *agonist* and *antagonist* as related to medicinal drugs.**

An agonist to a drug assists with the same function as the drug does. The effect of taking two agonistic drugs is an enhancement of the primary effect. The antagonist is opposite in its effect or counterproductive to the effect of the primary medication. Taking both the drug and an antagonist to it cancels or decreases the effectiveness of the primary drug.

▶ **Identify the various sources one could use to find information on drugs.**

One can obtain information about a particular drug by asking a pharmacist for patient information on the drug. Other sources include books containing drug information such as the *PDR* and *Facts and Comparisons*.

▶ **Explain how to find information on the USOC or the NCAA banned drug lists.**

Information on policies on the use of various drugs can usually be obtained from the governing body for the athletic group. For instance, to find out what drugs are banned for Olympic athletes, you can contact the USOC and request its banned drug list; for information regarding banned drugs in college athletics you can contact the NCAA. The Internet is an excellent way to obtain contact information for these organizations.

▶ **Discuss the inflammatory process and describe how drugs may affect that process.**

Prostaglandins and thromboxanes are implicated in the production of pain, inflammation, fever, and excessive blood clotting. Prostaglandins are produced by the synthesis of arachidonic acid that is ingested in our normal diet. The pathway by which the prostaglandins are produced is called the cyclooxygenase pathway. Nonsteroidal anti-inflammatory drugs act by blocking the cyclooxygenase pathway, which affects the production of prostaglandins and thus decreases inflammation, pain, fever, and excessive blood clotting.

▶ **Identify the more common side effects of anti-inflammatory drugs and the steps that may be taken to reduce these unwanted outcomes.**

In general, the major side effect of NSAIDs is stomach upset. Some agents are less irritating to the stomach mucosa or do not cause as much bleeding from the irritation. The best method of prohibiting or limiting this side effect is to always take the NSAID with food or milk. Some people insist that an antacid taken in conjunction with the NSAID reduces gastric upset, but this has not be proven scientifically. The patient should always be cautioned not to take the anti-inflammatory drug on an empty stomach.

▶ **Describe the effects of analgesics and discuss reasons to limit their use in sport participation.**

Analgesics work on the same basis as the anti-inflammatory drugs, by blocking the cyclooxygenase pathway—effectively blocking the production of prostaglandins. The main reason for not using analgesics during sport participation is that pain often signals structural damage. Without the nociceptive input (pain), the participant may continue to stress the injured tissues, exacerbating the condition.

▸ **Identify ways in which a fungal infection may be controlled with medicinal drugs.**

Fungal infections may present a superficial problem (skin fungus) or a subcutaneous problem (under skin layers). Fungal infections that are not superficial are difficult to treat with the standard OTC antifungals that are effective for the superficial problems. Systemic fungal infections are treated with an oral antifungal. In addition, superficial fungal infections are resistant to the powder form of many OTC antifungals. It is important to educate infected participants about use of the antifungal creams and ointments in order to eradicate the fungus, and then to suggest use of the powder to keep the environment unfavorable for the fungus to return.

▸ **Describe ways in which a laxative may be misused.**

Loss of body weight is very important to some participants. Unfortunately, laxatives can help people artificially reduce their weight. This misuse of laxatives can lead to serious health concerns and should be avoided.

PRACTICE!

For hands-on practice in this area, go to the web resource and complete the following:

Level 2.7, Module H1: Medication Resources

Level 2.7, Module H2: Medication Physiology

CRITICAL THINKING QUESTIONS

1. One of your swimmers has been having shoulder impingement symptoms. You evaluated him and offered some exercises to help balance the shoulder muscles. He was also referred to the physician for evaluation. In that evaluation, the doctor mentioned that the exercises were very important and that the patient should begin a course of anti-inflammatory medication. You know that the patient has had an irritable stomach in the past. Explain what adjustments may be made in the prescribing of an anti-inflammatory drug for this individual.

2. A freshman soccer player has been doing strengthening exercises for her previously sprained ankle. One day you notice that she tossed her backpack in a corner of the exercise area and some bottles fell out. Concerned about her knowledge of drugs, you ask what the bottles contain. She answers by showing you three bottles: Bayer aspirin, Tylenol, and Orudis. You ask her if she is taking all three of the pills and how much of each, and she says only that it depends on the day. Explain the appropriate use of each of these in an active individual and give recommendations for which one(s) this player might want to use to help in controlling the ankle inflammation and pain.

3. Several members of your college track team come to you asking how they can find information on "banned drugs." They explain that they are asking you because they didn't want the head athletic trainer to think they were "doing drugs." They say they just want to be sure they are not doing anything that might disqualify them from the upcoming track meet sponsored by TAC (The Athletic Conference). Explain how you could help these individuals.

Health Care Administration

The health care administration (HA) portion of the NATA BOC (2011) competencies is covered in this part of the *Core Concepts in Athletic Training and Therapy* text. The two chapters in part V discuss concepts related to health care administration; other areas of this text that pertain to topics in the health care administration competencies are found in the introduction and chapters 13 and 14.

Chapter 19 introduces the reader to management functions such as establishing vision and mission statements, understanding strategic planning, and budgeting. It also covers information management and documentation.

Chapter 20 provides information on insurance; third-party reimbursement; and primary, secondary, and self-insurance coverage. Other topics include credentialing laws, elements of negligence, and various legal concerns for the athletic trainer.

COMPETENCIES

Health Care Administration (HA):
HA-3, 4, 6-10, 12, 17-20, and 25-27

CHAPTER 19

Management Strategies in Athletic Training

Richard Ray, EdD, ATC
Eric J. Fuchs, DA, ATC, EMT-B

OBJECTIVES

After reading this chapter, the student should be able to do the following:

- Understand and develop vision and mission statements for a sports medicine program.
- Understand the principles underlying sports medicine strategic planning.
- Understand the components of the staff selection process, including federal laws and regulations.
- Understand the different kinds of budgeting processes and apply them to an athletic training setting.
- Understand the importance of documentation as part of a complete information management system in sports medicine.
- Understand and describe the different types of information to be managed in a typical sports medicine program.

Effective managerial practices are essential to providing quality, integrated, and comprehensive health care to our patients. Athletic trainers' management responsibilities often include developing a comprehensive management plan for overseeing clinical outreach services and implementing a quality collegiate sports medicine program. They frequently extend to supervising assistant athletic trainers or graduate assistants or working as part of a planning team to build a new stadium or facility that will include space for an athletic training room. Athletic trainers must learn how to recognize and develop managerial skills and strengths in themselves and their staff to successfully complete the various management tasks they will face during their career.

Vision and Mission Statements

The first step an athletic trainer must take when planning for a new sports medicine program or the improvement of an existing program is to develop a succinct description of what the program should eventually become—a **vision statement**. The vision statement should be both ambitious and compelling (Block 1987). It should spell out the athletic trainer's hopes and aspirations for the program. The vision statement contains four distinct elements. First, the statement identifies the provider of the service. Second, it identifies the specific service to be provided. Third, it identifies the target clients. Finally, the statement includes a quality declaration that identifies aspirations for how internal and external audiences will receive the program. The vision statement should become the ultimate standard by which the program is judged. Although these elements might seem self-evident, they are important because of the way they function in the next step—the mission statement.

A **mission statement** serves as a blueprint for every program activity and service. The statement should be comprehensive enough to describe the program but simple enough that everyone knows it well. Pearce (1982) has defined the mission statement as "a broadly defined but enduring statement of purpose that distinguishes a business from other firms of its type and identifies the scope of its operations in product and market terms." Spallina (2004) has characterized the mission statement as "a brief statement describing what the leadership wants the program to become in order to remain viable and competitive." Gibson, Newton, and Cochran (1990) have suggested the following components of a mission statement. Adapted for a sports medicine program, they include

- the particular services to be offered, the primary market for those services, and the technology to be used in delivery of the services;
- the goals of the program;
- the philosophy of the program and the code of behavior that applies to its operation;
- the "self-concept" of the program based on evaluation of strengths and weaknesses; and
- the desired program image based on feedback from internal and external stakeholders.

Planning

The athletic trainer has long been thought of as a jack-of-all-trades. Although athletic trainers' roles have become more specialized since sports medicine clinics began in the late 1970s, most athletic trainers still handle a variety of job-related activities (see figure 19.1). Because the job has so many aspects, the athletic trainer must develop planning skills.

Planning is an athletic trainer's best hope for accomplishing sports medicine program goals. Without planning, he leaves the ultimate success or failure of the sports medicine program to chance (Castetter 1992; Young 2007). The importance of functioning **operational plans** for the sports medicine

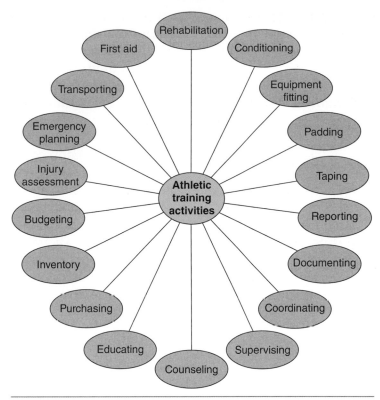

Figure 19.1 Job-related activities of the athletic trainer.

program should not be underestimated. One of the most common pitfalls in every type of organization is the failure to effectively translate the strategic vision for the program into workable, useful operational plans (Garofalo 1989). Three often misunderstood types of operational plans are policies, processes, and procedures.

Policies

Castetter (1992) has defined **policy**[1] as a plan for expressing the organization's intended behavior relative to a specific program subfunction. By definition, policies are broad statements of intended action promulgated by boards empowered with the authority to govern the operation of the organization. Policies are not intended to answer detailed questions about how the sports medicine program operates. They are intended as road maps to guide an athletic trainer in developing and operating a sports medicine program in accordance with the desires of the policy board. Athletic trainers should be

consulted in the development or modification of institutional policies that affect the sports medicine program. A well-managed organization with a sports medicine program should have policies in place that express the intended behaviors of the program.

Processes

Processes are the next step down from policies on the hierarchy of operational plans. **Processes** are the incremental and mutually dependent steps that direct the most important tasks of the sports medicine program. Each process should relate to at least one, and possibly many, of the policies that govern the program. Each policy will undoubtedly have several supporting processes.

Procedures

Procedures provide specific interpretations of processes for athletic trainers and other members of the sports medicine team. They are not abstract. They should be written in clear and simple language so that different people will interpret them in the same way. Procedures are the lowest level of the planning hierarchy.

An example of how policies, processes, and procedures are linked might look like this:

Policy 1.0

The policy of Memorial Hospital is to provide sports medicine services at the site of athletic practice and competition for the three Ashton County high schools.

Process for the Injury Rehabilitation Subfunction

The sports medicine team, including the physician, athletic trainer, and physical therapist, shall work together to provide patients or clients with a rehabilitation program appropriate for their injuries. Consideration will be given to the location of the rehabilitation program (home, school, or hospital), the equipment required to attain the desired rehabilitative effect, the insurance coverage provided by the student's family, and the insurance coverage provided by the school.

Procedure for Discharge From Rehabilitation

Physical therapists or athletic trainers shall discharge patients and clients from rehabilitation only after consulting with the attending physician. Discharge shall occur when the critical long-term goals, established when the patient was admitted, have been met. All discharged clients shall be given oral and written instructions in the long-term care of their injuries.

Practices

Even the most well-considered procedure often leaves room for an athletic trainer to make professional judgments about how to handle particular administrative tasks. The ways in which administrative tasks are actually accomplished are known as **practices**. Practices should never contradict the directions provided for in the procedure they are intended to support. For example, a sports medicine clinic might have a written procedure requiring that all therapeutic modalities be calibrated and safety inspected once per year. This sound procedure is consistent with professional standards. The athletic trainer-administrator still has several decisions to make. Which vendor will she contact to service the equipment? What time of the year will she choose to have the equipment serviced? Should she send all the equipment out at once, send half of the inventory at one time, or stagger the schedule for the various pieces of equipment? The decisions she makes are examples of practices. Practices are important because they allow the athletic trainer to make decisions based on changing conditions, without violating the letter or spirit of the policies and procedures manual. The sports medicine program should assess its practices from time to time for congruence and conformity to the procedure they support. In addition, the practices in the sports medicine program must be consistent with professional standards and state and federal laws. For example the National Collegiate Athletic Association (NCAA) publishes sports medicine guidelines for its member colleges and universities to consider and review (see sidebar Topics on Which the NCAA Has Issued Sports Medicine Guidelines); the National Athletic Trainers' Association (NATA) publishes and regularly updates position statements on how athletic trainers should manage various medical conditions or on prudent standard of care guidelines an athletic trainer should follow. The NATA has published position statements on topics ranging from emergency action planning to lightning safety guidelines.

Policies, processes, and procedures are usually communicated to employees in the form of a policies and procedures handbook. This document is important. Not only does it educate employees regarding the procedures they are to follow; it also serves as a legal foundation for action if they do not. Poorly written or incomplete procedure handbooks are frequently the basis for employee action against employers because they are often viewed as a kind of contract.

TOPICS ON WHICH THE NCAA HAS ISSUED SPORTS MEDICINE GUIDELINES

For the most recent versions of these guidelines, see the *NCAA Sports Medicine Handbook* at http://ncaa.org/health-safety.

Sports Medicine Administration

Medical Evaluations, Immunizations, and Records

Dispensing Prescription Medication

Lightning Safety

Institutional Alcohol, Tobacco, and Other Drug Education Programs

Emergency Care and Coverage

Medical Disqualification of the Student-Athlete

Skin Infections in Wrestling

Prevention of Heat Illness

Assessment of Body Composition

Nutrition and Athletic Performance

Nontherapeutic Drugs

Nutritional Ergogenic Aids

Menstrual Cycle Dysfunction

Weight Loss—Dehydration

Blood-Borne Pathogens and Intercollegiate Athletics

The Use of Local Anesthetics in College Athletics

The Use of Injectable Corticosteriods in Sports Injuries

Cold Stress

Brachial Plexus Injuries

Concussion and Second-Impact Syndrome

Participation by the Impaired Student-Athlete

Participation by the Pregnant Student-Athlete

The Student-Athlete With Sickle Cell Trait

Protective Equipment

Eye Safety in Sports

Use of Trampoline and Minitramp

Mouth Guards

Use of the Head as a Weapon in Football and Other Contact Sports

Guidelines for Helmet Fitting and Removal in Athletics

Large organizations, such as hospitals and universities, commonly have more than one handbook. One contains all of the organization's policies (remember that policies are statements passed by the board in control of the organization). Another contains procedures intended to apply to all employees of the organization, regardless of which department they work in. Human resources procedures are typically codified in procedure manuals.

It is important that your mission and vision statement be projected and associated with a professional image. One way to do this is with dress code procedures. Athletic trainers need to be acutely aware of their personal appearance, from dress to grooming. Remember the saying "You never get a second chance to make a first impression." As athletic trainers, we never know when someone will become injured; but once an injury occurs, our interaction with the patient, coach, parents, and others can be dramatically affected by our appearance and dress. (See the sidebar Dress Code Procedure.)

Human Resource Management

Athletic trainers are professionals who are oriented in general toward providing clinical services. Most have never had any training in how to manage human resources. Some athletic trainers excel at this aspect of administration without any formal understanding of human resource systems, but they are the exceptions. The most complicated tools the athletic trainer will ever work with are

DRESS CODE PROCEDURE

All members of the university sports medicine staff shall be professionally attired at all times during their work shift. Staff members and students shall wear a university-approved name badge at all times when on duty. The first badge shall be provided at university expense. The cost of replacement badges is the responsibility of the staff member. Athletic trainers (staff and students) on duty shall wear a uniform shirt approved by the head athletic trainer. Each staff member will receive two uniform shirts per year. Additional uniform shirts are the responsibility of the staff member. All staff members shall wear a uniform jacket when covering outdoor events during cool weather. The jackets are the property of the university and may be checked out from the clothing locker in the main athletic training room storage room. The following clothing is prohibited at all times, regardless of setting:

- Blue jeans
- Sweatshirts
- Unkempt clothing
- Clothing with holes

Questions regarding this procedure should be directed to the head athletic trainer.

people. Without a system for managing those assets, a sports medicine program is unlikely to accomplish its mission. This section focuses on the human resource function of a sports medicine program and the skills that athletic trainers need to be successful in this area. Athletic trainers often find themselves involved in the hiring process as either a candidate, a search committee member, or the hiring official. Regardless of your position in the process, knowing and understanding the human resource hiring process is essential.

Staff Selection

The basis for human resource management in sports medicine is **staff selection**. Although the term *staff selection* might imply only identifying and hiring new athletic trainers, it has a much broader meaning in law. The Equal Employment Opportunity Commission's *Uniform Guidelines on Employee Selection Procedures* (1978) defines *staff selection* as any procedure used as a basis for any employment decision. Athletic trainer hiring, promotion, demotion, retention, and performance evaluation are all considered selection activities by law (see figure 19.2). To comply with the *Uniform Guidelines*, athletic

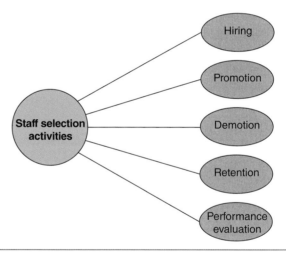

Figure 19.2 Staff selection activities in sports medicine.

trainers must be sure that their employment practices do not adversely affect any group protected under the law. The only exception to these rules occurs when an organization can prove that it discriminates because of "business necessity." The following sections provide practical suggestions for athletic trainers with staff selection responsibilities.

Position Description

A formal document that contains information about the required qualifications for a job, as well as the work content, accountability, and scope of the job, is known as a **position description**. The position description is an important communication link between the athletic trainer and the supervisor that creates a common understanding of the role the athletic trainer should play in the program. The athletic trainer's position description should be divided into two sections: the job specification and the job description (see figure 19.3). The **job specification** describes the qualifications an athletic trainer should have to fill the role (Haddad 1985). The **job description** lists the responsibilities for which the athletic trainer will be held accountable (U.S. Small Business Administration 1980). Each responsibility should be assigned a weight so that the athletic trainer understands which duties are considered the most important (Fowler and Bushardt 1986). Figure 19.4 provides an example of a sample position description.

Athletic trainers who write position descriptions struggle with several important questions. Should the items be specific or general? Should the document describe what ought to be or what is? Although no definitive answers to these questions would meet the needs of every situation, general guidelines do exist. When delineating the duties and responsibilities of the athletic trainer, being as specific as possible is generally useful. Explicit descriptions are important because they provide clear direction for the athletic trainer.

The program head should perform a final check on all position descriptions. The combination of input from the supervisor and the subordinate into the position description is more likely to result in a balance between the needs of the employee and those of the sports medicine program. In any case, the position description should reflect only the characteristics of the job, not ambiguous personal characteristics like loyalty, initiative, and trust. The position description should be reviewed and modified as needed, at least once a year, to reflect changes in the athletic trainer's qualifications or the work environment (Bruce 1986).

Recruitment and Hiring

Attracting and retaining qualified, competent staff members is crucial to the overall success of a sports medicine program. Recruitment of athletic trainers and other allied health care professionals should be viewed from two perspectives: the long-range need for human resources within the sports medicine program and the immediate staffing needs.

The long-term staffing plan depends, to a significant degree, on the strategic plan of the sports medicine program. How is our client base likely to change? How will the accomplishment of our goals and objectives affect our need for staffing? The long-range recruiting plan should consider a number of factors, including the likelihood of promotion or transfer of present staff members, upcoming retirement plans, and the projected availability of athletic trainers and other allied health care workers in the labor pool. All these factors are important.

The other perspective in the recruitment process is the immediate need for staffing the sports medicine program. Immediate staffing needs typically arise because of four types of changes in the makeup of the present staff: radical program changes, termination (for either personal or professional reasons), retirement, and death. Each of these can result in the immediate need to fill a vacant position. Neither long-term nor immediate staffing needs of the sports medicine unit can be fulfilled unless those needs are successfully integrated into the overall institutional or departmental staffing plan.

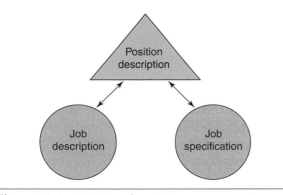

Figure 19.3 Position description components.

Position Description

Job title: Assistant Athletic Trainer

Date: July 1, 2012

Department: Intercollegiate Athletics

Status: Salaried nonfaculty

Incumbent: Judy Armstrong

Supervisor: Linda Black, Head Women's Athletic Trainer

Written by: David Lewis, Coordinator of Sports Medicine, and Judy Armstrong

Approved by: James Wilson, Director of Intercollegiate Athletics

Job Specification

Factor	Job Specification	Person Specification
Education	Requires minimum of bachelor's degree	Must have a bachelor's degree
Certification	Requires credentials consistent with Ohio law and recognized national standards	Must be BOC certified, hold a valid Ohio license, and be certified in CPR
Working conditions	Requires travel over weekends and holidays and exposure to all kinds of weather	Must have flexible schedule and be in good physical condition
Physical demands	Requires lifting of injured patients, manual dexterity, and administration of CPR	Must be able to lift heavy weights and have functional use of all four extremities

Job Description

Job Responsibilities	Relative Importance (1 = low 5 = high)
Coordinates and delivers athletic training services to members of the field hockey and gymnastics teams including, but not limited to, coordination of physical exams, evaluation and treatment of injuries at practices and games, design and supervision of rehabilitation programs, counseling within the limits of expertise, and prepractice and game taping	5
Refers injured patients to appropriate physicians according to guidelines in the *Standard Operating Procedures*	5
Submits injured patient status reports to coaches by 11:00 a.m. of the day following the injury	4
Maintains computerized injury and treatment database according to guidelines in the *Standard Operating Procedures*	3
Coordinates NCAA Injury Surveillance program by conducting in-service training for student athletic trainers, collecting and checking the accuracy of individual and weekly injury report forms, and mailing completed forms to the NCAA by Monday of each week	3
Prepares annual injury and treatment report for all sports by June 1	3
Exhibits behaviors in strict compliance with the NATA *Code of Professional Practice*	5
Performs other duties not specifically stated herein but deemed essential to the operation of the sports medicine program as assigned by the Coordinator of Sports Medicine or the Head Women's Athletic Trainer	Varies

Figure 19.4 Sample position description.

Hiring practices vary greatly from organization to organization, but there are common steps for recruiting and hiring sports medicine personnel. Most organizations use a system that resembles the following 10-step process.

1. ***Request for position.*** Such requests should be detailed enough to document need, based on both present and forecasted program conditions.

2. ***Position request approval.*** Athletic trainers should try to anticipate the data that administrators will need to make a decision.

3. ***Position vacancy notice.*** The athletic trainer might be required to advertise the position vacancy to satisfy collective bargaining agreements and state and federal guidelines; positions should be posted internally and externally according to established protocols.

4. ***Application collection.*** A common practice is to appoint a committee of interested persons with a legitimate stake in hiring the athletic trainer to screen applications, which should be sorted into three groups: unqualified applicants, qualified applicants with complete application files, and apparently qualified applicants with incomplete application files.

5. ***Telephone interviews.*** Telephone interviews before on-site interviews are useful for weeding out unsuitable applicants and providing additional information not readily communicated in application letters or resumes. Remember that some questions asked during an interview are legal and others are illegal (see the sidebar Examples of Legal and Illegal Interview Questions).

6. ***Reference checks.*** This aspect of the recruitment and hiring process is important because it allows the athletic trainer to validate the information supplied by the candidate. Notes from all conversations should be kept in the applicant's file for future reference by other members of the search committee.

7. ***On-site interview.*** Only those applicants who are obviously well qualified for the job should be interviewed on-site. Most visits should include a number of interviews with institutional stakeholders. The visit should typically be 1 or 2 days in length, depending on the level of responsibility of the position.

8. ***Recommendation and approval for hiring.*** Supporting documentation, including the candidate's resume, transcripts, letters of recommendation, and interview notes, should accompany the recommendation for hiring; and search committee members should be sure they make a final recommendation for hiring based solely on the qualifications of the candidate and not on personal characteristics unrelated to the job.

9. ***Offer of contract.*** Only the person who is authorized to negotiate a contract with the candidate should call and orally extend an offer of employment. If the parties can agree on terms of employment over the telephone, the authorized institutional representative should prepare a formal employment contract consistent with institutional rules, collective bargaining agreements, and state and federal laws.

10. ***Hiring.*** After a candidate has signed a written employment contract, the institution should send a letter to the other applicants thanking them for their interest in the position and informing them that the position has been filled.

Finding Your Job

Everything presented up to this point in this section was written from the perspective of the athletic trainer-administrator who is looking for just the right person to join his staff. Because many readers of this text are entry-level athletic training students who aren't yet in a position to be doing the hiring, it seems fitting to include a few tips for helping you find your first job. Although the preceding material will help you understand the recruiting and hiring process from an employer's point of view, you should consider a few additional things when looking for a job.

Identifying Job Openings

If you are a student just getting ready to graduate and enter the workforce, one of

EXAMPLES OF LEGAL AND ILLEGAL INTERVIEW QUESTIONS

Illegal Question	Legal Question
Are you a U.S. citizen?	Could you, after employment, submit verification of your legal right to work in the United States?
Do your religious beliefs allow you to work on Sundays?	Weekend and holiday work is a condition of this position. Is that acceptable to you?
Are you married? Do you have children?	Weekend and overtime work is a condition of this position. Is that acceptable to you?
Do you have any illnesses or disabilities?	Can you perform the essential job functions of this position with or without accommodation?
Did you serve in the military? What kind of discharge did you receive?	Did you serve in the military? Were any of the jobs you performed similar to those in this position?
Where did you learn to speak Spanish?	Do you speak any languages other than English that would be useful in this position?

the questions you have undoubtedly asked is, "Where can I find a job as an athletic trainer?" Athletic training positions are advertised in many places. The career center at your university may have a database of recently posted positions. Similarly, your professors probably receive many letters every month advertising athletic training positions in all kinds of settings. The classified "Help Wanted" section of your local newspaper is usually not a rich source of athletic training positions, but you may find local schools, hospitals, or companies advertising there from time to time. Other ways to identify potential athletic training jobs include the following:

- Networking
- Cold calling
- Web-based databases
- Conventions and job fairs

Making Contact

After you have identified a list of potential employers, the next step is to make sure that they become aware of your interest, background, credentials, and skills. A well-prepared resume and cover letter are the most common ways to accomplish this, but you can and should use other methods to help you stand out from the crowd. Depending on how your cover letter and resume were delivered, it is usually a good idea to follow up with either an e-mail message or a phone call to make sure that the potential employer received them. Yate (2002) suggested that this contact experience should have four goals:

- Get the employer's attention
- Generate interest in your application
- Create a desire in the employer to know more about you
- Encourage the employer to take action on your application

Here are a few steps that will help you accomplish those goals:

- Express your enthusiasm for the opportunity to work in the organization.

- Fill the employer in on any additional experiences that you may have had since sending in your materials.
- Remind the employer of the special skills or experiences you have that help you stand out from the crowd.
- Ask the employer if she has any preliminary questions she would like to ask you.
- Thank her for her time.
- Stay in touch with all potential employers in this way until the position is filled or you have accepted another job.

Interviewing

Interviewing for a job can take several forms. Employers sometimes conduct preliminary interviews by telephone before arranging face-to-face interviews with the most promising candidates. As suggested earlier, some employers conduct interviews at conventions and job fairs, whereas others prefer to bring the applicant to the employment site. Whatever the interview technique or location, your first task as the interviewee is to prepare. Although you'll certainly need to be able to answer the employer's questions during the interview, you should also be able to summarize your experiences, qualifications, and skills in approximately 30 s. You should be able to articulate your professional philosophy. Be prepared to explain how you deal with difficult problems, using examples from your past. Find out as much as you can about the organization before the interview—the organization's website is a great place to start this part of your preparation. All this takes planning and practice. You should arrange for a videotaped mock interview so that you can practice and receive feedback. Many career counseling centers on college campuses offer this service.

First impressions are critical. Although the employer has seen your cover letter and resume, the interview is probably the first time he will meet you in person. Employers should certainly be concerned about your knowledge, skills, and experience as important predictors of future job performance;

but they will also be developing an impression of how well you are likely to fit into the culture of the organization. They will determine in a relatively short time whether they like you—and whether the other employees with whom they work will like you as well. The following tips will help you develop a good first impression with prospective employers:

- Dress professionally for the interview.
- Learn as much about the organization as you can before the interview.
- Be enthusiastic.
- Be courteous.

Closing the Deal

An interview creates a first impression in the mind of the employer. You should take steps to build on that first impression after the interview ends. After the interview, you should repeat in modified form the steps you took to contact the employer before the interview. Here are a few things you can do to help the employer remember you after you drive away from the interview:

- Send thank-you notes.
- Send postinterview references.
- Keep in touch.
- Don't burn bridges.

Personnel Deployment

The cost of employing people makes up the largest portion of the budget for most service-oriented enterprises, including those in which athletic trainers typically work. If an educational institution, health care facility, or business that employs athletic trainers is to operate effectively and efficiently, it must deploy the right number of staff at the right times and in the right places. Too often, employers hire athletic trainers and, without doing adequate planning for reasonable workloads that yield effective patient outcomes, expect them to manage every aspect of the patient or employee health care needs.

Nelson, Altman, and Mayo (2000) recommend that institutions consider the following five elements when planning staff deployment:

- *Activities to be performed.* What jobs are critical to the successful operation of the sports medicine operation? When and where do these tasks take place? The answers to these questions should flow from the goals and objectives of the sports medicine program.

- *Required abilities.* What level of professional competence is required for each of the identified tasks? Which professional credentials, licenses, or certifications are required by law or commonly accepted standard?

- *Number of required staff.* How will the number, timing, and location of tasks, along with rules governing reasonable workloads, affect the number of personnel required to accomplish the mission?

- *The way in which the staff currently uses its time.* Are the athletic trainers currently in place using their time efficiently? Effectively? Are they working on the right kinds of tasks given their level of training and expertise?

- *Finding staff to accomplish the goals of the program.* Are resources available to hire additional athletic trainers if they are needed? Can athletic trainers be reassigned to achieve greater efficiency? Can other personnel assume some of the duties now assigned to athletic trainers? Too often the first impulse—especially in athletic training, in which understaffing has been a chronic problem for many years—is simply to hire more staff to accomplish the mission of the sports medicine program. The athletic trainer-administrator has the responsibility, however, to accomplish the mission at the least possible cost.

Performance Evaluation

Performance evaluation is the process of placing a value on the quality of an athletic trainer's work. Performance evaluation is important for at least two reasons. First, it can help a supervising athletic trainer make valid and reliable distinctions between athletic trainers who are performing at or above program expectations and those whose work is unsatisfactory. Second, a properly implemented system of performance evaluation helps the athletic trainers being evaluated identify areas of weakness and eliminate or reduce them. Remember, however, that any performance evaluation instrument not based on a specific athletic trainer's weighted job description and not designed for a particular purpose is useless. Performance evaluation is *not* the annual completion of a form. Performance evaluation is a process carried out throughout the entire year that involves mutually establishing goals, creating performance standards for accomplishing those goals, measuring the level of accomplishment, mutually understanding how well the athletic trainer met her goals, and mutually developing plans to remediate performance deficiencies and continue professional development. Measuring performance often requires the input of the athletic trainer being evaluated, the athletic trainer's peers, the supervisor, the clients, and the consulting physicians. Any performance evaluation instrument not built on these principles would be so riddled with caveats as to render it meaningless.

Financial Resource Management

Athletic trainers are often very good about stewardship of the financial resources they are allotted to provide high-quality medical care. It's important to realize that while being a good steward is often expected, athletic trainers sometimes need to advocate for increased funding and know how to demonstrate the necessity using data from previous budgets. Therefore an understanding of budgets and the budgeting process is paramount.

Budgeting

Budgeting financial resources is a process that organizational leaders ask program heads to accomplish. Athletic trainers and others responsible for planning and delivering sports medicine services must develop skills in planning and implementing budgets so that needed services are delivered in an effective, timely manner and allocation of financial resources is consistent with the strategic plans of both the institution and the sports medicine program.

A **budget** is a plan for the coordination of resources and expenditures (Horine 1991). A budget also serves as a tool for estimating receipts and disbursements over a period of time (Mayo 1978). Beyond its practical uses as a restraint on resource waste and as a predictive tool for the financial health of a sports medicine program, a budget is a quantitative expression of the athletic trainer's management plan. As such, it is both a strategic plan for how the sports medicine unit will function over a given period and an operational plan for how it will accomplish its goals.

Although many practitioners think of budgeting as a task that begins and ends in a narrow time frame during a particular part of the year, the wise athletic trainer views budgeting as a continuous process of prioritizing, planning, documenting, and evaluating the goals of the sports medicine unit and translating those goals into concrete plans for how to expend available resources. Because athletic seasons stretch over all 12 months and new programs of all types are added to the athletic trainer's responsibilities, the budgeting process requires constant attention to the status of funds and ongoing evaluation for the next budget cycle.

Jones and Trentin (1971) have suggested that budgets be used as the primary tools for planning and controlling a program. This approach helps athletic trainers differentiate between the concepts of budgeting and forecasting. Forecasting is the process of predicting future conditions based on various statistics and indicators that describe the past and present situations. Typically, only a few people near the top of the organizational chart perform forecasting. Because budgeting is a type of planning, however, it requires input from the grass roots of the sports medicine program. An effective budget considers the input of all employees about using the financial resources to meet documented program needs as opposed to simply allocating funds according to past traditions.

Types of Budgets

Most sports medicine budget planning is based on one of six budgeting models (Ray 1990). The six most common budgeting methods are zero-based, fixed, variable, lump-sum, line-item, and performance budgeting. Each of these methods can be an effective way to help athletic trainers plan the financial activity of their programs, depending on the particular circumstances and nature of the programs they direct. The **spending-ceiling model**, also known as the *incremental model* (Wildavsky 1975), is the budgeting circumstance most often desired by sports medicine program directors. This method requires justification only for expenditures that exceed those of the previous budget cycle. Sports medicine programs in financial crisis are often forced to combine their primary budgeting method with the spending-reduction model. Under the **spending-reduction model**, department heads, including directors of sports medicine programs, must reduce their budgets to preserve institutional funds. This budget method requires the most imagination and creativity of all the budget models. Because financial resources tend to be reduced periodically in most sports medicine settings, the wise athletic trainer identifies those goods and services that could be cut without seriously affecting the program and patient services. If a financial crisis does arise, the athletic trainer will be prepared and know where to make cuts.

Each of the following budgeting methods can be used in either a spending-ceiling or spending-reduction mode:

• ***Zero-based budgeting.*** Zero-based budgeting is an administrative method that requires unit directors to justify every expense without reference to previous spending patterns. This method requires close attention to documentation of actual program needs.

• *Fixed budgeting.* Fixed budgeting is an appropriate process for sports medicine programs in financially stable environments. This method requires an athletic trainer to project both expenditures and program income, if any, on a month-by-month basis to determine total program costs and revenues for the fiscal year.

• *Variable budgeting.* Variable budgeting requires that expenditures for any given time period be adjusted according to revenues for that period. Unfortunately, the athletic trainer who coordinates the activities of a sports medicine clinic is rarely able to predict the monthly balance of expenditures to revenues with perfect accuracy.

• *Lump-sum budgeting.* In lump-sum budgeting, a parent organization provides an athletic trainer with a fixed sum of money and the authority to spend that money any way he sees fit.

• *Line-item budgeting.* Line-item budgeting requires that athletic trainers list anticipated expenditures for specific categories of program subfunctions. Typical line items for a sports medicine program include expendable supplies, equipment repair, team physician services, and insurance (see figure 19.5).

• *Performance budgeting.* Performance budgeting breaks the functions of a sports medicine program into discrete activities and appropriates the funds necessary to accomplish these activities. This method is typically used by large organizations to manage divisional budgets and is less likely to be used at a departmental level.

Athletic trainers have a financial responsibility to maintain control over the inventory of sports medicine equipment and supplies. They can usually accomplish this by inventorying regularly, centralizing storage of supplies, automating the inventory process, restricting access to storage areas, and implementing reminder systems.

Information Management

In today's climate in which health care providers are being pushed to move all medical

Acct. No.: 213702		Dept.: Sports Medicine		Responsible person: Stan Curtis	
Object code	Account description	09-10 Expense	10-11 Budget	11-12 Request	Percent change
3110	Travel	229.25	300.00	300.00	0
3205	Supplies	7,632.32	9,000.00	9,475.75	5.3
3305	Printing	89.29	100.00	100.00	0
3315	Speakers	0	1,500.00	1,500.00	0
3320	Stipends	5,997.96	6,300.00	6,300.00	0
3360	Postage	257.65	300.00	300.00	0
3530	Repairs	313.15	500.00	500.00	0
3650	Phone	428.89	475.00	500.00	5.3
3720	Uniforms	430.00	500.00	500.00	0
3850	Periodicals	150.00	150.00	150.00	0
4035	Insurance	200.00	250.00	300.00	20.0
4100	Dues	90.00	100.00	100.00	0
Department total		$15,818.51	$19,475.00	$20,025.75	2.8

Figure 19.5 Sample line-item budget for a school-based sports medicine program.

records to electronic record systems, medical record management and documentation play a critical role in any athletic trainer's employment setting. Insurance reimbursement requirements for records, along with the need for athletic trainers to demonstrate that their clinical practices are evidence based and that quality patient outcomes support their clinical practices, necessitate that athletic trainers strive for excellence in their patient charting, whether it takes the form of electronic or written medical records.

Why Document?

Although documentation is only one of the information management tasks that athletic trainers must accomplish, it is common to all employment settings. Why is this skill so important? Why should busy athletic trainers concern themselves as much as they do with this task? There are many reasons. Medical documentation helps protect the legal rights of both the physically active patient and the athletic trainer by providing a written record of the care that the athletic trainer has provided. The adage "If it isn't written down, it didn't happen" is an increasingly appropriate guiding principle for all athletic trainers (Hawkins 1989). Medical documentation serves as a memory aid for athletic trainers and other professionals involved in the care of patients. In many cases, the law requires medical documentation for compliance with state licensure or certification. Additionally, in school-based programs, the medical records may be considered educational records and must be maintained according to **FERPA** (Federal Education Rights Privacy Act). Medical documentation is required to meet professional **standards of practice**. The Board of Certification Standards of Professional Practice require documentation of physician referral, initial evaluation and assessment, treatments, and dates of follow-up care for all clients or patients cared for in a *service program* typical of most educational settings. Medical documentation improves the quality of communication among the various professionals involved in the patient's care. Reimbursement decisions by third-party payers, such as insurance companies and health

maintenance organizations, are based on medical documentation. Medical documentation should be part of the basis for deciding when to discharge a patient from an athletic trainer's care (Kettenbach 2009, 1995). Well-written and well-organized medical documentation should serve as a tool for problem solving in difficult cases. This documentation should be written with the following list in mind to aid in legal protection in the event a patient or client decides to take legal action:

- Legal protection
- Memory aid
- Legal requirements
- Professional standards
- Improved communication
- Insurance requirements
- Discharge decisions
- Improved care

Physical Examination Forms

The physical examination results should come first in the medical record. The physical exam normally occurs first chronologically, and the results can be a quick reference for athletic trainers or physicians. Some states mandate the use of specific physical examination forms for high school student-athletes. In other states and settings, athletic trainers can choose from a wide variety of forms. The form chosen should call for the following information (see figure 19.6):

- Personal data (name, address, date of birth, and so forth)
- Health history
- Vital signs
- Physician's review of systems
- Special procedures (blood and urine analyses, X rays, echocardiograms, and so forth)
- Functional tests (joint strength, aerobic capacity, and so forth)

Injury Evaluation and Treatment Forms

Injury evaluation and treatment records should provide a concise account of the

ATHLETIC PHYSICAL EXAMINATION SUMMARY

1. Name: _____   M or F: _____ Age: _____ Date: _____
2. S.S. #: _____   Year in school: FR   SO   Jr   Sr
   Sport: _____   E-mail: _____ Cell phone: _____

Medical History Survey

3. Do you have now, or have had in the past, problems with:	Yes	No
a. Headaches, needing treatment		
b. Heart problems of any kind		
c. Breathing (e.g., asthma)		
d. Abdominal pain		
e. Dizzy spells		
f. Family members with heart disease		
g. Eyes (except glasses)		
h. Hearing or ears		
i. Racing heart or skipped heart beats		
j. Joint pain, swelling		
k. Knees—injury, giving out, swelling		
l. Spine—back or neck		
m. Broken bones		
n. Kidneys or bladder		
o. Chest pain		
p. Diabetes		
q. High blood pressure		
r. Cancer		
s. Operations or surgery		
t. Severe viral infection such as mono or myocarditis		
u. Skin disorders		
v. Other major injuries		
w. Drug allergies		
x. Eating disorder		

4. If you answered yes to any of #3, give details below by letter.

5. Have you ever been knocked unconscious? If yes, explain: Yes ___ No ___

6. Have you ever had a cervical spine injury? If yes, explain.   Yes ___ No ___

7. Do you have any permanent handicap or disability? If yes, explain: Yes ___ No ___

8. Are you under a physician's care at the present time? If yes, explain: Yes ___ No ___

9. Are you taking any medication or drug at this time? If yes, explain: Yes ___ No ___

10. Year of last tetanus. _____

11. Women—Do you have a monthly menstrual period?   Yes ___ No ___
    Date of last period: ____
    If no, explain:

12. Do you have any intense fear of gaining weight?   Yes ___ No ___

(For Examining Physician Only)

13. Eyes:
    Rt. Eye _____   Lt. Eye _____

14. General information:
    HT ___ WT ___ B/P ___ Pulse ___

Examination	Normal	Abnormal
15. Head		
16. Eyes		
17. Nose and throat		
18. Ears		
19. Neck		
20. Lungs		
21. Heart		
22. Abdomen		
23. Hernia		
24. G-U		
25. Extremity		
26. Shoulders		
27. Knees		
28. Other:		
29. Nervous		
30. Knee laxity		

31. Rt. ___ MCL ___ LCL ___ ACL ___ PCL ___
    Lt. ___ MCL ___ LCL ___ ACL ___ PCL ___

PHYSICIAN'S STATEMENT

32. Approved for sports   Yes ___ No ___

33. Approved pending further study.
    Explain:

34. Approved with limitations.
    Explain:

35. Disapproved.
    Explain:

36. Date _____
    Signature _____

Figure 19.6 Sample of a physical examination form.

Reprinted by permission of the Hope College Health Clinic, Holland, MI.

patient's progress from the time of injury until the time of discharge. These forms often constitute the bulk of the medical record. Although many athletic trainers maintain separate records of injury evaluations and treatments, each treatment should be easily linked to a documented injury. Athletic trainers can choose from five methods for documenting injury evaluation and treatment data: problem-oriented medical records (figure 19.7), **focus charting** (figure 19.8), **charting by exception**, computerized

PROBLEM-ORIENTED MEDICAL RECORD COVER SHEET DATABASE

Past Medical Hx.   Family Hx.

Social Hx.   **Habits**

Tobacco:

Alcohol:

Drugs:

Seat belts:

Exercise:

Nutrition:

Problems   Dates

1																
2																
3																
4																

Plans   Dates

1																
2																
3																
4																

Follow-up: See SOAP notes in record.

Figure 19.7 Cover page for problem-oriented medical record.

SPORTS MEDICINE FOCUS CHART

Name: Jones, Mike   Sport: Basketball

Date	Data	Action	Response
2/6/12	Probable 3° R ATF sprain	RICE x 20 min. Compression sleeve, ankle brace, crutches issued.	Pain decreased to 2/10. Patient understood home care instructions.
2/7/12	3° R ATF sprain	Cold whirlpool with AROM x 20 min. Form walking x 10 min. JOBST compression pump x 30 min.	Decreased limp with walking. Increased DF ROM to 5°.
2/8/12	3° R ATF sprain	Cold whirlpool with AROM x 20 min. BAPS in PE in seated position. JOBST compression pump x 30 min.	Discarded crutches. Swelling reduced to minimal level. PF/DF ROM equal to L. ankle.

Figure 19.8   Sample focus chart for use in recording injuries (data), treatments (action), and progress (response).

documentation, and **narrative charting**. A common method that athletic trainers use to document injury evaluation and treatment is the SOAP (Subjective, Objective, Assessment, and Plan) form (figure 19.9) and pneumonic.

Reports of Special Procedures

Reports of all special procedures should be included in the medical record. Although special-procedure reports should be entered into the medical record chronologically, each should be annotated to refer the reader back to an initial injury or illness assessment report. Special procedures include but are not limited to the following:

- Isokinetic strength tests
- Blood tests
- Urinalysis
- X rays or other imaging procedures
- Surgical reports
- Cardiac assessments (echocardiogram, graded exercise tests, thallium uptake scans, and so forth)

Communication From Other Professionals

An athletic trainer commonly receives written documentation of a patient's medical

INDIVIDUAL INJURY EVALUATION AND TREATMENT RECORD

Name: Jones, Mike   Sport: Basketball   Body part: R-Ankle

Date injury occurred: 2/5/12   Date injury reported: 2/6/12

Primary complaint: R-ankle pain   Secondary complaint: None

Subjective data: Pt. inverted R-ankle while playing basketball. Reports "a loud snap." No previous hx. of ankle injury. Otherwise normal medical hx. Pain w/ walking is 5/10. Pain at rest is 3/10. Pain to palpation over the ant. talofibular ligament. No other bony or soft tissue tenderness noted.

Objective data: Moderate swelling over lateral malleolus. No discoloration or deformity. Ankle is warm to touch. Lacks 5 deg dorsiflexion and 10 deg planter flexion in both AROM and PROM compared to L-ankle. Strength is 4+/5 for DF, PF, Inv. & Er. compared to 5/5 for L-ankle. Anterior drawer test is remarkably positive w/ mushy end point. Talar tilt test equivocal due to swelling. Neg. Klieger's test. Pt. walks w/ a noticeable limp and cannot bear wt. on the R-foot w/out assistance. Applied RICE for 20 minutes. Issued compression sleeve and ankle brace. Fitted crutches and provided instruction in crutch walking. Educated pt. on RICE techniques for home program. Provided pt. w/ ankle home care brochure. Pt. indicated he understood instructions.

Assessment: Probable 3° ATF sprain.

Plan: Will refer to Dr. Smith. Appt. arranged for 3:00 pm today. Applied RICE for 20 minutes. Issued compression sleeve and ankle brace. Fitted crutches and provided instruction in crutch walking. Educated pt. on RICE techniques for home program. Provided pt. w/ ankle home care brochure. Pt. indicated he understood instructions.

Evaluator's signature: David Black

Date	Treatments and progress
2/6/12	RICE x 20 min. Instructions for home care program. Crutches w/ instructions. Compression sleeve and ankle brace. Pt. tolerated tx. well. Pain at rest 2/10. Swelling reduced. DB

Figure 19.9   Sample evaluation and treatment form using SOAP note format.

status from physicians, physical therapists, and other health care professionals involved with the case. One type of documentation is the referral form (Gabriel 1981), sent with a patient when she is referred to the physician's office or the emergency room (see figure 19.10). The injured athlete referral form provides legally defensible proof that the

---

HOPE COLLEGE SPORTS MEDICINE MEDICAL REFERRAL

Name: _____   Sport: _____

Date: _____   Time: _____   Physician: _____

Athletic Trainer's Impression: _____
_____
_____
_____

Physician's Diagnosis and Recommendation: _____
_____
_____
_____

Recommended Activity Level (check all that apply):

    Bed rest _____   Attend classes only _____   Practice as able _____

    No practice or competition _____   No restriction _____

    Limited physical activity as noted above _____

Follow-Up Appointment   _____   _____
                       Date   Time

_____
Physician's Signature

Please instruct the student to return this form to the athletic training room.

_____

I hereby authorize _____ to release all records related to the injury/illness specified above to Richard Ray, Meg Abfall, Dr. Patrick Hulst, Dr. John Schloff, the Hope College Health Clinic, or any other representative of the Hope College medical staff. I further authorize the above-named health care provider to discuss my case with any representative of the Hope College medical staff. I waive any and all claims against the above-named health care provider, Hope College, and any of its employees or contractors in connection with the communication and disclosure of such information.

_____
Student's Signature

_____   _____
Date   Witness

Figure 19.10   Sample medical referral form.

Reprinted by permission of the Hope College Health Clinic, Holland, MI.

athletic trainer consulted with a physician as required by the Standards of Professional Practice and, in many states, by law. In addition, it improves communication between the athletic trainer and the physician by taking the burden of having to relay information off the injured individual.

The referral form should include the patient's name, sport, injury date, and appointment date and time. It should allow space for the athletic trainer to document the initial evaluation findings. The form should provide space for the physician to write a diagnosis and orders for treatment or rehabilitation. The athletic trainer and physician should date and sign their notes. Finally, the form should include a section that complies with the Health Insurance Portability and Accountability Act (**HIPAA**) (see the later section, "Release of Medical Information"). The patient signs the form, authorizing the physician to share the patient's medical information with the athletic trainer or other members of the sports medicine team. Ath-

letic trainers can ensure that referral forms are returned.

Emergency Information

Athletic trainers in high schools and colleges must frequently contact an injured student-athlete's parents or guardians, an urgent responsibility if the patient has a serious accident or illness. To do so, the athletic trainer usually uses the emergency information form in the medical record (see figure 19.11). This form should include patient information, such as name, address, phone number or numbers, date of birth, and Social Security or student identification numbers. The form should also include parents' names, addresses, and telephone numbers (home and business). Some athletic trainers have suggested that the form contain the patient's insurance information as well (Miles 1987). This form should be readily accessible in the medical record, perhaps affixed to the inside cover of the patient's folder.

EMERGENCY INFORMATION

Name: _____ Sport: _____

Date of birth: _____ Address: _____

Social Security or ID number: _____

Phone (Home): _____ (Work): _____ (Cell): _____

Parents' names: _____

       Address: _____

       Phone (Home): _____ (Work): _____ (Cell): _____

Person to contact in an emergency:

       Relationship: _____ Phone: _____

Name of insurance company: _____

Policy numbers: _____

Is this insurance company a health maintenance organization (HMO)? Yes ___ No ___

If so, list the HMO telephone number: _____

Figure 19.11 Sample emergency information form.

Adapted, by permission, from B.J. Miles, 1987, "Injuries on the road: Good information reduces problems," *Journal of Athletic Training* 22(2).

Release of Medical Information

Another commonly understood legal principle is that health care providers may not release a person's medical records without consent. This principle has been written into the federal legal code in the form of two laws: the Family Educational Rights and Privacy Act (FERPA) of 1974 (sometimes referred to as the *Buckley Amendment*) and the Health Insurance Portability and Accountability Act of 1996 (HIPAA). FERPA requires educational institutions to receive formal written consent from students (or, in the case of minors, their parent or guardian) before they can disclose educational records to a third party. The law also requires educational institutions to make available to students all records relating to their enrollment unless they specifically waive the right on a case-by-case basis.

HIPAA was enacted to help employees transfer their health insurance when they switched employers, to ensure that their health information would remain private, and to give people more access to their own health care information. HIPAA applies only to "covered entities." The law may cover athletic trainers in some settings but not in other settings. In general, athletic trainers are working in environments subject to HIPAA rules when each of the following three conditions applies:

- The person, business, or agency furnishes, bills, or receives payment for health care in the normal course of business.
- The person, business, or agency conducts covered transactions. Covered transactions are those activities normally associated with billing.
- The covered transactions are transmitted in electronic form.

Athletic trainers working in covered entities should be most attentive to seven areas with regard to HIPAA rules:

1. *Obtain consent for treatment.* Athletic trainers must provide patients with a written "Notice of Privacy Practices" that delineates the manner in which the health care agency intends to use and disclose a patient's health information. Patients must acknowledge in writing that they received this information except in emergencies that render the patient unable to provide written acknowledgment.

2. *Obtain authorization to release health information.* Athletic trainers working in covered entities must receive written authorization to share a patient's health information with persons who are not part of the chain of health care providers, including coaches, athletic administrators, scouts, and the media. The athletic trainer must obtain authorizations for each instance of information release; a blanket release signed at the beginning of the year or even at the initiation of the treatment will not suffice *(for athletic trainers not covered by the law, a blanket authorization is permissible)*. A valid authorization must include

- a description of the information to be disclosed,
- the persons authorized to disclose information,
- the persons to whom the information may be disclosed,
- the purpose of the disclosure,
- the expiration date of the authorization,
- the patient signature and date, and
- if signed by a representative, a description of that person's authority to act for the patient.

Authorizations are *not* valid under the HIPAA rules unless they include each of the following:

- A statement that the individual may revoke the authorization in writing, instructions on how to revoke the authorization, and a reference to the Notice of Privacy Practices mentioned earlier
- A statement that treatment, payment, enrollment, or eligibility for benefits may not be conditioned on obtaining

the authorization or, if such services are conditioned on the authorization, a statement that details the consequences of refusing to sign the authorization

- A statement informing the patient that the persons to whom the information is being provided could disclose his health information

3. *Release only the minimum necessary information.* HIPAA requires that athletic trainers and other covered entities limit the amount and frequency of information release to the minimum required to accomplish the purposes for which the information is being released.

4. *Safeguard patient information.* Although HIPAA allows for certain incidental disclosures of patient information (for example, someone in the clinic overhearing a conversation between two athletic trainers regarding a patient case), the rules require that reasonable efforts be made to safeguard such information. Good practices require maintaining charts and other patient documents in a secure manner.

5. *Observe state laws governing the treatment of a minor's health information.* Because HIPAA defers authority over access to the health records of minors to the individual states, athletic trainers must be familiar with their state's laws governing minors and their health records.

6. *Do not combine authorizations, except for research purposes.* The HIPAA rules generally require that the patient sign a separate authorization for each purpose for which patient information will be used or released. This rule does not apply when the information will be used for research purposes.

7. *Business associates must safeguard patient information.* Athletic trainers who refer patients to other entities must ensure that the entity to whom the referral is being made has policies in place to safeguard the patient's health information. The athletic trainer must have contracts with these entities that specify the nature of the safeguards.

Learning Aids

SUMMARY

Athletic trainers need to learn to become better managers of resources, which include personnel, budget, and time. Quality athletic training services are provided by a team of athletic trainers working efficiently together and with other health care providers and their patients to ensure a quality outcome for injuries and the rehabilitation or prevention programs provided. This cannot occur without good managerial leadership, which starts with the development of a mission and vision statement and proceeds to the recruitment of quality and well-qualified staff members. A quality athletic trainer manager understands how and when to provide needed support, resources, and an environment that allows staff members and others to successfully complete their jobs and roles. Athletic trainers must also be aware of HIPAA and FERPA with regard to medical records, and the impact these federal laws have on personnel and human resource management. Record keeping is vital to successful athletic training services; records include not only medical records, but also inventory, budgetary, and continuing education records of personnel, to mention a few.

KEY CONCEPTS AND REVIEW

▸ **Understand and develop vision and mission statements for a sports medicine program.**

Vision statements should be ambitious and compelling and should include hopes and aspirations of the program. They contain four distinct elements: identification of the provider of the service, the service to be provided, the target clients, and a quality declaration that identifies aspirations for how internal and external audiences will receive the program.

The mission statement is "a broadly defined but enduring statement of purpose that distinguishes a business from other firms of its type and identifies the scope of its operations in product and market terms." It is a written expression of an organization's philosophy, purposes, and characteristics.

▶ **Understand the principles underlying sports medicine strategic planning.**

The principles underlying sports medicine strategic planning are policies, processes, and procedures. Policies serve as road maps to guide the athletic trainer in developing and operating a sports medicine program in accordance with the desires of the policy board. Processes are the incremental and mutually dependent steps that direct the most important tasks of the sports medicine program. Procedures provide specific interpretations of processes for athletic trainers and other members of the sports medicine team.

▶ **Understand the components of the staff selection process, including federal laws and regulations.**

Staff selection is defined as the procedure for making employment decisions such as hiring, promotion, demotion, retention, and performance evaluation. Employment practices must not adversely affect any group protected under the law unless the organization can prove that they do so out of "business necessity." Ten steps commonly involved in the recruiting and hiring process are request for position, position request approval, position vacancy notice, application collection, telephone interviews, reference checks, on-site interviews, recommendation and approval, offer of contract, and hiring. Ath-

letic trainers must be able to differentiate between legal and illegal interview questions.

▶ **Understand the different kinds of budgeting processes and apply them to an athletic training setting.**

The six most common methods of budgeting are zero-based, fixed, variable, lump-sum, line-item, and performance budgeting.

- Zero-based budgeting is an administrative method that requires unit directors to justify every expense without reference to previous spending patterns. Athletic trainers will be required to create narrative explanations for each area of their programs, along with the financial basis for each of those functions.

- Fixed budgeting requires an athletic trainer to project both expenditures and program income, if any, on a month-by-month basis to determine total program costs and revenues for the fiscal year.

- Variable budgeting requires that expenditures for any given time period be adjusted according to revenues for the same period. Decreased revenues in any given month would result in decreased expenditures in order to achieve a balanced budget.

- Lump-sum budgeting is a model whereby a parent organization provides an athletic trainer with a fixed sum of money and the authority to spend that money any way he or she sees fit.

- Line-item budgeting requires that athletic trainers list anticipated expenditures for specific categories of program subfunctions. Supplies, services, continuing education, and insurance are common line items.

- Performance budgeting breaks the functions of a sports medicine program into discrete activities and appropriates the funds necessary to accomplish these activities. This method is typically used by large organizations to manage divisional budgets and is less likely to be used at a departmental level.

▶ **Understand the importance of documentation as part of a complete information management system in sports medicine.**

Medical documentation is important for several reasons. It helps protect the legal rights of both the physically active patient and the athletic trainer; it can serve as a memory aid; it may be required by law to conform to professional standards. Medical documentation also provides for improved communication, meets insurance requirements, aids in discharge decisions, and allows for improved care.

▶ **Understand and describe the different types of information to be managed in a typical sports medicine program.**

Information managed through a sports medicine program includes data obtained from the physical examination, injury evaluation, and treatment forms; reports of special procedures; communication for other professionals; and emergency contact information.

 PRACTICE!

For hands-on practice in this area, go to the web resource and complete the following:

Level 1.2, Module A3: Foundational Behaviors of Professional Practice 1

Level 1.3, Module B1: Administrative Policies and Procedures

CRITICAL THINKING QUESTIONS

1. You have just been assigned the position of head athletic trainer of your high school. One of your responsibilities is to develop the vision statement for your sports medicine program. Working with two classmates as your "team," write the vision statement.

2. The chapter refers to the adage "If it isn't written down, it didn't happen." It is important in any medical profession to keep accurate and complete records of the care provided. In the case of a patient lawsuit against an athletic trainer, give examples of how the quality and completeness of the documentation of care might affect the case. How would things differ if the documentation were incomplete and poor in quality?

3. One of your assistant athletic trainers recently accepted the position of head athletic trainer for a college near her hometown. You have started the process of finding a replacement. Explain what you would say if your assistant football coach came to you to tell you about his nephew who is just finishing his undergraduate degree in athletic training.

Reimbursement and Legal Considerations

Richard Ray, EdD, ATC
Eric J. Fuchs, DA, ATC, EMT-B

OBJECTIVES

After reading this chapter, the student should be able to do the following:

- Explain the difference between medical, health, and accident insurance.

- List the advantages and disadvantages of self-insurance, primary coverage, and secondary coverage.

- Define the basic legal responsibilities associated with third-party reimbursement.

- Define and discuss the legal principles most applicable to athletic training settings.

- Discuss the different types of credentialing laws that affect the practice of athletic training.

- Discuss the elements required to prove negligence on the part of an athletic trainer.

Throughout their careers, athletic trainers have opportunities to give their employers input on health, accidental, and medical insurance policies, whether primary or secondary, or to recommend selection of such policies. Athletic trainers in some states can bill for athletic training services, and many other states are working toward this goal along with the National Athletic Trainers' Association (NATA). Understanding third-party billing is important to the development of the athletic training profession and future athletic trainers. Athletic trainers need to be aware of the legal parameters for their clinical practice, which include state regulations, Board of Certification standards of practice, and the NATA code of ethics and standards of care, as part of their professional responsibility. Understanding the legal process and how to limit our exposure to legal action starts with learning and understanding the legal issues faced by practicing athletic trainers.

Understanding insurance and the associated forms can be challenging for today's athletic trainers; it is no simple matter to determine the right type and amount of insurance to have for their own family, let alone determine or recommend the types, coverage amounts, or plans needed for a school, an athletic program, or an event or for any other employer. This section provides an overview of this integral part of the athletic health care program.

Insurance Systems

Medical insurance is a contract between the holder of a **policy**[2] and an insurance company to reimburse a percentage of the cost of the policyholder's medical bills, usually after the policyholder has paid a deductible (Rowell 1989). **Health insurance**, on the other hand, is generally more comprehensive, in that it often includes provisions for maintaining good health rather than simply paying for illnesses and injuries.

Both of these insurance classifications should be distinguished from the type of policy most educational institutions buy for their student-athletes, athletic accident insurance, which is usually intended to supplement a student's family insurance plan and reimburses the cost of athletic accidents only (Chambers, Ross, and Kozubowski 1986). The insurance industry's definition of accident is different from the concept of injury as understood by most athletic trainers, coaches, parents, athletes, and other physically active patients. To an insurance company, accidents usually include acute, traumatic injuries, independent of any other cause or preexisting condition, that occur during practices and games. Specific exclusions in most accident insurance plans include injuries caused by overuse (tendinitis, bursitis, stress fractures, and so on), illnesses, and degenerative conditions. Some athletic accident insurance companies offer riders to cover the costs of chronic conditions, but riders generally increase the premium significantly.

A fourth type of coverage is catastrophic insurance, which usually takes effect after the first $50,000 in medical bills has been reached and provides lifetime medical, rehabilitation, and disability coverage for patients who have suffered long-term or permanent handicaps as a result of athletic injuries. Member institutions of the National Collegiate Athletic Association (NCAA) have received catastrophic insurance at no cost since 1991. Catastrophic insurance is also available to non-NCAA institutions and high schools through their national governing organizations.

Disability insurance is also available through many companies. This type of insurance is designed to protect patients against future loss of earnings because of a disabling injury or sickness that occurred while they were engaged in sport activities. The NCAA sponsors a disability insurance program for exceptional student-athletes in football, men's basketball, baseball, and ice hockey. The NCAA also sponsors a special assistance fund program that may be used to pay for some medical and dental expenses for Division I student-athletes.

Finally, some insurance companies provide coverage for specific kinds of health-related problems. Dental insurance and vision insurance are two examples. These policies can be bought separately or added to broader health care plans as riders.

Educational institutions designing a medical insurance system for their student-athletes can choose from three options: self-insurance, primary coverage, and secondary coverage (Hart and Cole 1992). As with any management option, each system has advantages and disadvantages, including cost.

Self-Insurance

Institutions that choose to self-insure are speculating that the amount they will pay out for medical expenses will be less than the amount they would pay for insurance premiums. The institution typically purchases no medical or accident insurance except for catastrophic coverage and pays medical bills incurred by student-athletes. National governing organizations such as the NCAA have rules that prevent educational institutions from paying for medical expenses not directly related to participation in intercollegiate or interscholastic athletics. Institutions that self-insure must be particularly careful to create and monitor procedures used to ensure compliance with these rules.

Self-insuring offers several advantages. Saving money is possible because the institution retains the potential profit that an insurance company normally earns. Processing claims is also simplified because there are no insurance claim forms to complete. Institutions have the flexibility to pay for procedures that a normal insurance policy might exclude.

Although cost can be an advantage with self-insurance, it can be a significant disadvantage as well. A large claim can deplete an institution's insurance fund, making it difficult or impossible to pay other, less costly claims. For that reason, it is large, financially healthy university athletic programs that typically choose self-insurance. The disadvantage of this method is that it ties up a substantial amount of money that the institution could use for more productive purposes. Institutions that self-insure can decrease their annual expenses by using a student-athlete's personal insurance as the primary source of coverage wherever possible. In this case, the institution becomes a secondary payer. The following sections discuss primary and secondary coverage.

Primary Coverage

Primary coverage is coverage under a medical or accident insurance policy that begins to pay for covered medical expenses as soon as the institution pays the deductible. The patient's (or the patient's parents') personal medical insurance is not a source for payment of medical bills arising out of athletic participation. Primary coverage simplifies and accelerates claims processing because the family does not need to be involved.

The disadvantage of primary coverage is the expense. Because the insurance company takes on all the risk for an institution's student-athletes, as opposed to sharing the risk with personal medical insurance payers, it must charge a substantially higher premium for the coverage.

Secondary Coverage

Secondary coverage, also known as excess insurance, is coverage under a policy that pays for covered medical expenses only after all other insurance policies, including the patient's personal medical insurance, have reached their limit. Most institutions select this type of insurance plan (Lehr 1992). The most obvious benefit of this approach is that institutions can lower their costs by spreading the risk associated with athletic injuries to other potential payers. Because personal insurance companies share the risk, the cost of secondary coverage can be as much as 60% lower than the cost of primary coverage.

The disadvantages of secondary coverage relate to claims processing. Because personal insurance serves as a primary layer of coverage, an institution must spend substantial time and energy communicating with parents and their insurance carriers to move claims along. This process can delay settling insurance claims, which can frustrate medical vendors that the institution wants to keep happy.

Third-Party Reimbursement

Athletic trainers are working hard to become recognized nationally and in many states to receive third-party reimbursement from insurance companies for the care they provide to patients. In several states, athletic trainers are able to receive third-party reimbursement for their services. As third-party reimbursement becomes the standard, athletic trainers need to know how it functions and know the regulations and legal issues involved. This section provides an introduction to third-party reimbursement, not a comprehensive review.

Third-party reimbursement is the process by which health care practitioners receive reimbursement from a policyholder's insurance company for services they perform. A **third party** is defined as a person, in this case a medical vendor, who has no binding interest in a particular contract (the insurance policy). Third-party reimbursement is the primary mechanism of paying for medical services in the United States. Hospitals and private-practice health professionals rely heavily on third-party reimbursement to generate the income that keeps their practices in business.

Third-party reimbursement is a growing but still relatively new practice for athletic trainers. Insurance companies, concerned about financial issues, have been slow to cover athletic trainers' services, even though the percentage of the population demanding those services is increasing. Access to payment for athletic training services through insurance companies is becoming more available now that more states credential athletic trainers. In addition, outcome studies conducted by NATA have demonstrated that athletic training services are

cost-efficient in the treatment of injuries in physically active populations (Albohm and Wilkerson 1999). As more state athletic trainers' organizations lobby their insurance commissioners and legislators for access to third-party billing (with the help of NATA), the number of athletic trainers who receive payment for their services in this way is likely to increase.

Although athletic trainers have historically lacked direct access to third-party reimbursement, they are often responsible for generating significant numbers of reimbursable dollars for the clinics and hospitals that employ them; therefore, they must understand this aspect of insurance. Many athletic trainers employed in sports medicine clinics perform tasks nearly identical to those performed by the physical therapists with whom they often work side by side. Athletic trainers working in high school outreach programs are often responsible for bringing in referrals to the clinics that employ them. Many of these patients pay for the services they receive by submitting claims to their medical insurance carriers.

Some athletic trainers in university sports medicine programs seek third-party reimbursement from their student-athletes' personal insurance companies. This practice is controversial, however, and has been criticized by some leaders in the profession, who say it creates the feeling that athletic trainers might prioritize their treatment of student-athletes based on insurance coverage (Godek 1992).

There are several models of third-party payment. Many health plans offer several models to their enrollees. Some companies even develop hybrid plans that mix the characteristics of the following models:

• Private medical insurance companies provide group and individual coverage for employees and their dependents. The medical insurance that these companies provide is typically the traditional type. This insurance model is also known as an indemnity plan (DeCarlo 1997). Patients in a **fee-for-service plan** are free to go to the medical provider of their choice. The plan reimburses a portion of the cost of covered services, and the patient is responsible for the copayment or deductible. The managed care models described next are rapidly replacing fee-for-service plans.

• **Health maintenance organizations (HMOs)** provide participating health care practitioners with a fixed fee for services rendered to members. A **capitation** (per person) system usually, but not always, determines fees. Health maintenance organizations that do not use a capitation system usually reimburse providers based on a fixed-fee schedule. Physically active patients insured by an HMO must use a primary care provider that participates in the HMO. A modest copayment is usually charged. Some HMOs provide services at medical facilities, whereas others provide care through a network of individual medical practitioners (**individual practice associations**, or **IPAs**).

• **Preferred provider organizations (PPOs)** operate similarly to HMOs but usually allow greater choice of health care providers and pay medical vendors on a fee-for-service, rather than a capitated, basis. Preferred provider organizations allow policyholders to choose any health care provider they wish but provide financial incentives for policyholders to use providers identified by the PPO. When physically active patients choose to see a medical provider who does not belong to the PPO, they can expect to pay for a greater percentage of the cost of the services. One variant of the PPO is the **exclusive provider organization (EPO)**, in which enrolled participants can receive benefits only from contracting medical providers (May, Schraeder, and Britt 1996; O'Leary 1994).

• A **point-of-service (POS) plan** is similar to a PPO. The primary difference between the two is that POS plans assign primary care physicians who act as gatekeepers by coordinating patient care. Most PPO plans do not.

• Government-sponsored programs provide coverage for the elderly (Medicare), the needy (Medicaid), and members of the armed forces and their dependents (TRICARE).

Legal Considerations in Sports Medicine

Athletic trainers have been aware for some time that they need a general understanding of certain legal principles to protect themselves and the institutions that employ them from the risk of lawsuit (Gieck, Lowe, and Kenna 1984). Wise athletic trainers, however, also realize that basic knowledge of legal principles, when applied thoughtfully and consistently, helps inform and improve their professional practice. These legal standards often provide extra incentive for athletic trainers to do what they ought to be doing routinely in their professional practice, regardless of the potential or likelihood of a lawsuit (Danzon 1985).

Of course, this chapter cannot provide definitive, comprehensive coverage of all the law related to the practice of athletic training. The aim is instead to introduce athletic training students to the legal issues they are likely to encounter in their professional practice. If an athletic trainer confronts a specific legal issue or problem, the best source of information is an attorney who is experienced in handling similar cases (Horsley and Carlova 1983). Effective policies and procedures, formed by consultation with both attorneys and insurance companies, also help guide athletic trainers through the minefield of legal perils they face daily.

Legal Principles

The common threat that confronts all athletic trainers who provide sports medicine services to patients is **malpractice**. According to Scott (1990, p. 6), health care malpractice is "liability-generating conduct associated with the adverse outcome of patient treatment. Liability may be based on

- negligent patient care,
- failure to obtain informed consent,
- intentional conduct,
- breach of a contract,
- use/transfer of a defective product, or
- abnormally dangerous treatment."

Torts

Although athletic trainers may enter patient–practitioner relationships that are implied contracts, unhappy patients are less likely to bring a legal action based on **breach of contract** than on an accusation that the athletic trainer committed a tort (Wadlington, Waltz, and Dworkin 1980). A **tort** is a legal wrong other than breach of contract for which a remedy will be provided, usually in the form of monetary damages. Actions based on tort law are pressed by plaintiffs in civil legal proceedings, whereas criminal cases are initiated by the government. All the legal grounds for malpractice, other than breach of contract, are based on tort law. Of the three types of tort (intentional tort, negligent tort, and strict liability tort), negligence, which focuses on the conduct of the practitioner, is the most common basis for malpractice actions.

Negligence

Athletic trainers are usually sued under a negligent tort theory (Leverenz and Helms 1990a). **Negligence** is a type of tort in which an athletic trainer fails to act as a reasonably prudent athletic trainer would act under the circumstances (Drowatzky 1985). Athletic trainers can demonstrate that their actions have been both reasonable and prudent by adhering to certain standards in the performance of their duties. Standards emerge from several sources, including individual, societal, institutional, and professional values (Leiske 1985). Standards derived from individual and societal values are often implicit (for example, patients should be treated with respect). Standards derived from institutional and professional values are typically more explicit and are usually codified by policies and procedures.

Standards are also derived from the position statements of professional associations. For example, the "National Athletic Trainers' Association Position Statement: Fluid Replacement for Athletes" (2002) and the "Inter-Association Task Force on Exertional Heat Illnesses Consensus Statement" (2003)

create a professional standard that athletic trainers and others involved in the health care of physically active patients should adhere to during hot, humid weather. Similarly, the American Heart Association's statement on cardiovascular preparticipation screening of competitive athletes creates a standard to which team physicians and athletic trainers should adhere when organizing and conducting preseason physical exams. The NCAA has established a comprehensive set of standards to which athletic trainers in college athletics should adhere (see *2010-2011 NCAA Sports Medicine Handbook*). For example, according to recent updates, all schools must have a concussion management plan on file requiring that any participant exhibiting signs or symptoms of a concussion be removed from competition, not be allowed to return to play that day, and be evaluated by a physician or his or her designee prior to return to play. The NCAA guideline on concussion notes that neuropsychological testing has proven an effective tool in assessing neurocognitive changes following concussion and can serve as an important component of an institution's concussion management policies (*2009-2010 NCAA Sports Medicine Handbook*). The NCAA Guidelines incorporates some of the guidelines and recommendations from the "Consensus Statement on Concussion in Sport" (2008). As another example, the NCAA now requires that all NCAA Division I athletes provide proof of testing for sickle cell trait, undergo testing, or sign a waiver regarding testing (*2010-2011 NCAA Sports Medicine Handbook*).

Athletic trainers need to read and review the various organizations' handbooks, guidelines, and position statements, as these documents are used in courts of law to establish standards of care and the athletic trainer's scope of practice. The number of recent deaths of professional, college, and high school athletes due to concussions and heat, as well as sudden cardiac deaths, has given rise to rapid development of new policies and standards. Athletic trainers and all sports medicine professionals must keep up with these changes, as they directly affect the scope of practice of many health care professionals.

Athletic trainers can be negligent through either omission or commission. **Omission** is the failure to do something that one should have done under the circumstances. **Commission** occurs when an athletic trainer performs an act that she should not have performed. To prove that an athletic trainer was negligent, the aggrieved patient must be able to substantiate the following five components (Ciccolella 1991):

- Conduct by the athletic trainer
- Existence of duty
- Breach of duty
- Causation
- Damage

Conduct

To substantiate a charge of negligence, the plaintiff must be able to prove that the athletic trainer, by either commission or omission, did something that links him to the case. Nonactions, such as thoughts, attitudes, or intentions, cannot render the athletic trainer negligent. Only when athletic trainers take an action (or fail to take an action) can the plaintiff successfully accuse them of negligence.

Duty

When does an athletic trainer owe a duty to a patient? Generally, athletic trainers employed by educational institutions have a duty to provide athletic training services to student-athletes actively engaged in those institutions' athletic programs. Athletic trainers employed by professional sport teams have the same duty toward team members. This duty has its legal origin in the athletic trainer's contract, in which she agrees to provide these services in return for payment. Whether a high school or university athletic trainer owes a duty to the student who is injured in an intramural basketball game or a physical education class is less clear and depends on the responsibilities defined by the employment contract. For this reason, athletic trainers should have an employment contract with a clearly written position description delineating their specific responsibilities.

Athletic trainers employed by sports medicine clinics have greater leeway in deciding whom they will accept as patients. Consequently, patients they owe a duty to should, in theory, be only those patients they choose to treat in their clinics. Enough exceptions to this general rule exist, however, that sports medicine clinic owners should consult with their attorneys to find out whom they might owe a duty to and under what circumstances. For example, sports medicine clinics that have a contract to provide services to an HMO might have a duty to provide services to the HMO's subscribers.

Abandonment is another issue related to duty that affects athletic trainers. Once an athletic trainer chooses to provide services to an injured patient, whether a duty originally existed or not, the athletic trainer does not have the legal freedom simply to walk away from the case except under certain circumstances. An athletic trainer cannot forsake even patients who do not cooperate or who fail to pay their bills unless he provides adequate warning and enough time for the patient to find alternative care.

In general, the duties owed by an athletic trainer to clients and patients are those described in the Board of Certification (2010) (BOC) *Role Delineation Study 6th Edition*. The courts have identified several specific duties, which include having an effective emergency action plan, complete with necessary first aid supplies and communication capabilities needed to communicate with on-site medical staff and emergency services. Additional specific duties an athletic trainer has as defined by the courts include the following:

- Maintain the confidentiality of the patient's medical records
- Provide adequate and proper supervision and instruction
- Provide safe facilities and equipment
- Fully disclose information about the patient's medical condition to the patient in question

Breach of Duty

The next step in proving negligence against an athletic trainer requires the aggrieved patient to establish by a preponderance of the evidence that the athletic trainer actually breached a duty owed the patient. The issue here is whether the athletic trainer exercised the **standard of care** that other reasonably prudent athletic trainers would have exercised under the circumstances. The athletic trainer can consult the standards of practice of various medical and athletic professional organizations to determine a standard of care if questions arise. Note that the standard of care does not require an athletic trainer to be the most knowledgeable or competent athletic trainer in the profession. If this were the case, nobody could meet the standard. Instead, the standard requires athletic trainers to perform their duties as other competent athletic trainers would under similar circumstances. In determining whether athletic trainers have met the standard of care, the laws of various states require that their actions be compared with those of other athletic trainers in one of the following three settings (Scott 1990):

- The same locality
- Similar communities
- The same or similar circumstances

The standard of care expected of athletic trainers in fulfilling their duties to their patients can depend on whether the state has credentialed the profession. Herbert (1990) posits that in those states without statutory credentialing, the athletic trainer might be held to the standard of care of other regulated health professionals, including physicians. Indeed, in *Gillespie v. Southern Utah State College* (669 P.2d. 861 [Ut. 1983]), an athletic training student was held to the standard of care of a physician in the treatment of a sprained ankle that later developed serious complications (Leverenz and Helms 1990b).

Causation

After an aggrieved patient has demonstrated that an athletic trainer breached a duty to exercise reasonable care, the patient must prove that the breach was in fact the legal cause of the injury (or made the original injury worse). The courts use two tests to determine causation. First, the plaintiff must prove **actual cause**. Actual cause is established if the patient can demonstrate that the athletic trainer's actions were a considerable determining factor in the damage claimed. The athletic trainer might be found only partially responsible for causing or aggravating the injury. If more than one defendant was responsible for causing or aggravating the injury, each defendant might end up paying a portion of the damages, consistent with that defendant's percentage of fault as determined by the court.

The second causation test is the requirement to demonstrate the existence of **proximate (legal) cause**. Proximate cause exists when an athletic trainer acts in a way that leads to harm or injury to another or to an event that injures another. Inherent in the notion of proximate cause is the **foreseeability** of the harm allegedly perpetrated by the athletic trainer. The requirement that harm must be foreseeable is positive for athletic trainers—they are not penalized for results that were improbable or unlikely.

Damage

The final step in establishing negligence is to determine whether the aggrieved patient actually suffered damages. If an athletic trainer breached a duty without causing any harm, no negligence occurred. An athletic trainer who oversteps her level of training by suturing a wound, for example, cannot be found negligent unless the plaintiff can prove that he suffered harm as a result (but a charge of practicing medicine without a license would probably have merit). Although physical damage is the most common and easily proven, the law recognizes other forms of damage as well. Emotional distress and loss of consortium (injury to the marital relationship) are just two examples (Herbert 1990).

Athletic trainers need to be constantly aware of potential liability associated with the practice of the profession. Athletic trainers must practice within their scope, maintain appropriate medical records, and comply with the BOC and state regulatory authorities. The better an athletic trainer understands the legal processes, the better prepared she will be to provide a defense if needed.

Reducing the Risk of Legal Liability

In addition to the certification requirements of the BOC, most states regulate the practice of athletic trainers. These state regulatory or practice acts represent an important step in assuring the protection of the public and for the advancement of the profession.

Credentialing

Athletic trainers must become familiar with the practice acts that regulate the profession. Both practicing athletic trainers and athletic training students should have such understanding because the law is likely to define different roles and responsibilities for these two groups. Athletic training practice acts vary a great deal among states and define "athlete" and "athletic trainer" differently. Some limit the scope and setting in which an athletic trainer may practice. Some allow athletic trainers to charge a fee for service, whereas others prohibit fee-for-service billing. Some limit the types of therapeutic modalities that athletic trainers can use. Most have specific educational requirements that may or may not correspond to those required for certification by the BOC. Most state laws require physician supervision. Some states also allow other health professionals, such as physical therapists, chiropractors, and dentists, to supervise an athletic trainer under certain circumstances. In states without specific credentialing for athletic training, an athletic trainer should obtain a copy of the state's **medical practice act** to determine the scope and setting of practice that the law permits athletic trainers and other health care providers.

Four types of credentialing laws regulate the practice of athletic training: licensure, certification, registration, and exemption. Athletic trainers practicing in states with athletic training practice acts should review the state law to determine what type of credentialing they require, as each type has different implications. In addition, the definitions and level of restrictiveness of each type of credentialing vary from state to state.

• *Licensure.* **Licensure** is the most restrictive form of governmental credentialing. The intent of licensure is to protect the public by limiting the practice of athletic training to those who have met the requirements of a licensing board established under the law. Licensure laws generally prohibit unlicensed individuals from calling themselves athletic trainers. More importantly, they prohibit unlicensed persons from performing the tasks reserved for athletic trainers under the law. Some states that license athletic trainers accept the equivalent of the BOC standards, but many have different requirements as well. Licensing boards are powerful legal entities because they are usually authorized to set the rules, in accordance with the law, that govern who may practice and who may not. They also set the fee required for license applications and renewals. Licensure is the most desirable of the four regulatory options for athletic trainers.

• *Certification.* **Certification**[2] is a less stringent form of professional regulation than licensure. A person who is certified is generally recognized to have the basic knowledge and skills required of practitioners in the profession. Both states and professional associations can certify health care practitioners. The BOC, for example, is the recognized certifying agency for ensuring that athletic trainers have the basic knowledge and skills to carry out their duties as defined by the *Role Delineation Study.* Athletic trainers who meet the requirements for BOC certification and maintain their certification are entitled to use the board's credential. Some states also certify athletic trainers. States get the authority to certify athletic trainers from a credentialing law passed by the state legislature and signed by the governor, the same process that gives them the authority for licensure. Unlike licensure, however, state certification usually protects only an athletic trainer's title, not the specific tasks that he performs. Noncertified persons could not call themselves athletic trainers, but they could perform the duties of an athletic trainer.

• *Registration.* **Registration** is another form of professional regulation that is less restrictive than licensure. In states that have registration laws, athletic trainers are required to register with the state before practicing. Some states allow a grace period during which athletic trainers may practice without being registered, as long as they begin their application for registration within the period established by the state's board. Because the registration law prohibits unregistered persons from practicing, it becomes a form of title protection for an athletic trainer. States that require registration may or may not require screening devices such as examinations, although most prescribe the educational requirements necessary to register as an athletic trainer.

• *Exemption.* Some states have provided the legal basis for athletic trainers to practice by exempting them from complying with the practice acts of other professions (e.g., physical therapist, physician assistant). Although **exemption** is often viewed as the least restrictive form of professional regulation, athletic trainers might still be required to meet a variety of standards, usually related to educational background or certification by the BOC, to qualify. In addition, athletic trainers are required to act according to the standards of the profession and the boundaries of their training.

Risk Management

Athletic trainers have been concerned with issues of legal liability for many years. As larger numbers of athletic trainers moved into management positions or took on management responsibilities along with their clinical duties, the broader construct of risk management became more important. Although athletic trainers are still concerned with the basics of avoiding legal liability in their clinical practices, they are increasingly called upon to help their schools, professional teams, clinics, and companies manage the risks that form the foundation for this liability.

What Is Risk Management?

At its most fundamental level, **risk management** is a process intended to prevent financial loss for an organization. In a broader sense, however, the goal of risk management is to prevent losses of all kinds (financial, physical, property, activity, time) for everyone associated with an organization, including its directors, administrators, employees, and clients (Culp, Goemaere, and Miller 1985). This broader application is warranted, because losses experienced at one level of an organization are usually felt at other levels. For example, if an individual successfully wins a large monetary award as a result of a lawsuit, the institution or business will have less money available to distribute until it meets the court-required obligation. This affects budgets across an institution or business in many cases.

As van der Smissen (2001) points out, risk management is more than the act of developing safety checklists. A comprehensive risk management program involves careful analysis of the risks facing the program or organization and the development of a plan for addressing those risks. She recommends using four general strategies for managing risk:

• *Avoidance.* When an activity, procedure, or event is so risky that dire consequences are likely, the organization may simply choose to avoid the activity. Avoidance is an especially appropriate risk management approach when the negative consequences of a particular activity have high costs.

• *Transference.* When activities are associated with high financial risk but low frequency (for example, catastrophic sport injury) or lower financial risk but high frequency (for example, fractures, joint injuries requiring surgery), a common method to reduce the risk of these activities is to transfer all or part of the risk to another entity. The organization usually accomplishes this by purchasing insurance designed to cover the financial loss associated with certain well-defined risks. Exculpatory clauses in waivers signed by patients, clients, or their parents are another example of a method to transfer the risk associated with sport participation to the participants and away from the organization, although this method has many flaws.

• **Retention.** Every organization—including organizations in which athletic trainers work—has activities or sponsors programs that have a level of risk deemed acceptable in light of the organization's mission. These risks are viewed as part of the cost of doing business. To eliminate the activities associated with these risks would fundamentally change the nature of the organization. The organization accepts and retains risks like these. These risks are still associated with a predictable level of financial cost, however, and the organization must account for it in the organization or program budget. Ideally, the organization should establish a reserve fund to cover costs that rise above predicted levels.

• **Reduction.** Careful development, implementation, monitoring, and evaluation of policies and procedures can reduce risks. Ideally, every risk that an organization knowingly retains should be accompanied by one or more policies and procedures designed to reduce the frequency and financial effect of that risk. For guidance on reducing risk in athletic programs, see the later section "Specific Risk Reduction Strategies."

Planning for Risk

Even the most prepared and conscientious organizations, despite their best efforts, experience unwanted events from time to time—including life-threatening emergencies. One of the most important roles that athletic trainers can play in helping the organization prepare for these events is to take the lead in developing emergency action plans. An **emergency action plan (EAP)** is a blueprint for handling emergencies that helps establish accountability for their management (Andersen et al. 2002; Gorse et al. 2010). Every organization that sponsors an athletic or physical activity program should have a written EAP (Gorse et al. 2010; Rehberg 2007). Indeed, the failure to have such a plan could constitute a breach of the institution's legal responsibility to conduct safe programs (Gorse et al. 2010).

The plan should cover every aspect of the program—including practices, games, and conditioning sessions. A variety of people, including every person or classification of person who will have a role in implementing the plan, should contribute to the EAP. Such persons typically include athletic trainers, athletic training students, team physicians, coaches, athletic administrators, campus safety officers, campus health center personnel, local law enforcement personnel, firefighters, emergency medical services personnel, athletic venue managers, and hospital personnel (Gorse et al. 2010; "Sideline Preparedness for the Team Physician" 2000; Rehberg 2007). The plan should be reviewed annually. In addition, it is helpful to test the plan from time to time by conducting a dry run involving the people who will be responsible for implementing the plan in an actual emergency. Each EAP should contain the following elements:

- A list of personnel involved in implementing the plan, including their roles, responsibilities, and a chain of command for decision making. Each person involved in implementing the EAP should have current training and certification in cardiopulmonary resuscitation (including use of an automatic external defibrillator), first aid, and bloodborne pathogen transmission prevention.

- The procedures to be followed in the event of an emergency, including communication and transportation procedures.

- Specific, venue-related directions that instruct personnel in the specific steps to be taken for each activity area. A map of each activity area indicating driveways, doors, gates, and telephone locations is critical. The plan should also include a list of the emergency equipment on hand at each venue.

- The hospital or clinic to which the injured patient will be transported, based on the extent of her injuries or medical condition. Hospital staff should be notified in advance of all contests and events that could result in emergencies requiring their services.

- A system for documenting the actions taken during an emergency and evaluating those actions to improve the emergency plan.

- A plan for directing athletic personnel during inclement weather, including a lightning safety plan (Gorse et al. 2010; Rehberg 2007; Walsh et al. 2000).

Specific Risk Reduction Strategies

Besides considering van der Smissen's (2001) general risk reduction strategies as outlined earlier, athletic trainers should think about implementing Rankin and Ingersoll's (2000) four-part strategy to help control risk in athletic programs:

1. Preparation for the activity
   - Administer preparticipation physical exams.
   - Monitor fitness levels.
   - Assess activity areas.
   - Monitor environmental conditions.
2. Conduct of the activity
   - Maintain equipment.
   - Use proper instructional techniques.
   - Provide adequate work–rest intervals.
3. Injury management
   - Have a physician supervise all medical aspects of the program.

- Evaluate and treat injuries correctly and promptly.
- Supervise student athletic trainers.

4. Records management
   - Document physician orders.
   - Document the treatment plan.
   - Document the treatment record.
   - Document the patient's progress.

Additional Strategies to Reduce Liability Risks

At the beginning of this section, we suggested that knowledge of legal liability would help improve the quality of care offered by an athletic trainer. To place that sweeping statement into context, consider the following suggestions as part of a strategy to avoid the threat of legal liability (Graham 1985).

- ***Build relationships.*** Develop and maintain good relations with patients, parents, coworkers, subordinates, and other health care professionals.

- ***Insist on a written contract.*** Have a written contract supported by a detailed position description that clearly delineates the athletic trainer's job functions.

- ***Obtain informed consent.*** Obtain informed consent for the services you perform. In the case of minors, obtain informed consent from their parents.

- ***Provide physical examinations.*** Be certain that every participant undergoes a physical examination by a state-licensed medical practitioner.

- ***Know the profession and its standards.*** Practice your profession unafraid, but keep in mind the standards of practice embraced by the profession.

- ***Document hazards.*** Make a documented attempt to reduce injuries by recommending or personally taking action to remove or modify potential hazards.

- ***Establish policies.*** Adopt and scrupulously adhere to policies and procedures designed to reduce the incidence of injury and to guide the actions of sports medicine personnel when injuries do occur. Keep all emergency first aid equipment in working order and available to those who might need to use it.

• *Document activities.* Document the details of all injuries, treatments, and reha-bilitative procedures so that a chronology of events can easily be determined after the fact. Maintain medical records until well after the statute of limitations for malprac-tice liability has expired (this varies from state to state).

• *Maintain confidentiality.* Maintain the confidentiality of the patient's medical record. When you wish to share the informa-tion with others, obtain written permission of the patient first.

• *Provide proper instruction.* When interacting with clients or patients, be certain that the instruction you provide allows for safe participation.

• *Supervise your staff.* Insist that every staff member adhere to prescribed program-matic procedures.

• *Participate in continuing education.* Take part in continuing athletic training edu-cation by attending seminars and symposia and reading sports medicine literature.

• *Recognize your qualifications.* Practice only within the limitations of the laws of your state and the boundaries of your training. In your actions, be consistent with the standard of care expected of other reasonably prudent athletic trainers.

• *Maintain insurance coverage.* All ath-letic trainers, certified and student alike, should have malpractice and liability insur-ance to safeguard their personal assets in the event of a legal action. Even if a malpractice suit is frivolous and eventually dismissed, the costs associated with defense are usually beyond the means of most athletic trainers.

Learning Aids

SUMMARY

As a health care provider, the athletic trainer needs to develop a working knowledge of the difference between medical, health, and accident insurance. Understanding the advantages and disadvantages of these vari-ous insurance options will allow an athletic trainer to develop, review, or recommend the best health insurance coverage options to employers. Athletic trainers today need to be aware of the situations that commonly present the most liability concerns for the profession. This includes understanding the types of state laws that affect the practice of athletic training, BOC's standards of practice, and standards of care associated with the athletic training profession through educa-tional standards and case law. This chapter provides an overview of medical, health, and accident insurance as it relates to a practicing athletic trainer. It also overviews legal issues related to the practice of athletic training that a clinically practicing athletic trainer must be aware of and work to mitigate whenever potential exposure exists or has been identi-fied.

KEY CONCEPTS AND REVIEW

▶ **Explain the difference between medical, health, and accident insurance.**

Medical insurance is a contract between the holder of a policy and an insurance company to reimburse a percentage of the cost of the policyholder's medical bills, usually after the policyholder has paid a deductible. Health insurance is generally more comprehensive; it often includes provisions for maintaining good health rather than simply paying for illnesses and injuries. Athletic accident insurance is usually intended to supplement a student's family insurance plan and reimburses the cost of athletic accidents only.

> ▸ **List the advantages and disadvantages of self-insurance, primary coverage, and secondary coverage.**

Self-Insurance

- Advantages: May help to save money, simplifies claims processing, has more flexibility (fewer restrictions)
- Disadvantages: Large claims may deplete budget, a substantial amount of money is set apart for insurance and cannot be used for more productive purposes

Primary

- Advantages: Simplifies and accelerates claims processing, does not involve patient's family
- Disadvantages: Cost is greater, premium for coverage is higher

Secondary

- Advantages: Costs less (up to 60% less), shares risk with other payers
- Disadvantages: Expense of time and energy to settle claims is greater, communication with family and their insurance company is necessary, processing of claims is often delayed

> ▸ **Define the basic legal responsibilities associated with third-party reimbursement.**

Athletic trainers must be aware of how third-party reimbursement functions, as well as the regulations and legal issues involved in the reimbursement process. Third-party reimbursement is the primary mechanism of paying for medical services in the United States. Access to payment for the athletic trainer's services through third-party payers is growing, and more states are credentialing athletic trainers. Athletic trainers need to be aware of the laws and regulations regarding reimbursement in the state that they are practicing in, as the legislation may be different from state to state.

> ▸ **Define and discuss the legal principles most applicable to athletic training settings.**

- Malpractice: Liability-generating conduct associated with the adverse outcome of patient treatment
- Breach of contract: An unexcused failure to perform the services specified in a contract, either formal or informal
- Tort: A legal wrong, other than breach of contract, for which a remedy will be provided, usually in the form of monetary damages
- Negligence: A type of tort in which an athletic trainer fails to act as a reasonably prudent athletic trainer would act under the circumstances

> ▸ **Discuss the different types of credentialing laws that affect the practice of athletic training.**

- Licensure: A form of state credentialing, established by statute and intended to protect the public, that regulates the practice of a trade or profession by specifying who may practice and what duties they may perform
- Certification: A form of title protection, established by state law or sponsored by professional associations, designed to ensure that practitioners have essential knowledge and skills sufficient to protect the public
- Registration: A type of state credentialing that requires qualified members of a profession to register with the state in order to practice
- Exemption: A legislative mechanism used to release members of one profession from the liability of violating another profession's practice act

> ▸ **Discuss the elements required to prove negligence on the part of an athletic trainer.**

Negligence can be through either the failure to do something when action should have occurred (omission) or the performance of an act or service that should not have been performed (commission). The elements necessary to prove negligence are conduct by the athletic trainer, existence of duty, breach of duty, causation, and damage.

PRACTICE!

For hands-on practice in this area, go to the web resource and complete the following:

Level 3.6, Module Q1: Regulation of Athletic Training Practice

Level 3.4, Module O4: Fiscal Management

CRITICAL THINKING QUESTIONS

1. The small community college you work for has an insurance policy that provides secondary coverage, using the patient's and family's insurance first; but patients often tell you that they don't have insurance, and the college has had to pay the medical bills in full. Design an agenda for a meeting you will chair to investigate options for how to manage this situation. Include on the agenda the people that should attend the meeting to participate in the decision-making for this issue. Include several options the group could consider for providing high quality athletic health care services at a reasonable cost to the college.

2. The equipment manager calls you saying a football lineman has tied a homemade neck roll to his football pads. The equipment manager asks you to take a look and give him your opinion—can the neck roll be left on, or should it be removed? What legal concerns do you have about a patient's use of a nonmanufactured piece of equipment for protection?

3. Your college athletic department has had severe budget cuts due to a depressed economy. The athletic director has informed you that the department is dropping the primary coverage insurance policy and picking up a secondary insurance policy. The transition will become effective in 30 days. What will you want to do to ensure that your patients' medical treatments will not be interrupted?

Advanced Athletic Training Concepts

This section of the *Core Concepts in Athletic Training and Therapy* text takes the reader to a higher level of understanding. Study of these three advanced chapters can easlly carry through to graduate courses. The competencies covered in these chapters are somewhat eclectic in that the readings will cover three different content areas: clinical examination and diagnosis (CE), therapeutic interventions (TI), and psychosocial strategies and referral (PS) (NATA BOC, 2011).

Chapter 21 presents the pathophysiology of tissue injury. The chapter reviews dense connective tissue and discusses the viscoelastic properties of tissue. Tendinopathies are presented and their pathology and histology discussed. The chapter also addresses the healing of articular cartilage and presents concepts of neuropraxia and neurotmesis.

Chapter 22 covers the psychology of sport injury. This chapter focuses on the injured individual and the psychological healing and rehabilitation that must occur. Other topics are psychological interventions, risk profiles, and the sport socioculture.

Chapter 23 focuses on evidence-based practice in athletic training. This chapter will give you an understanding of how to search the medical literature, how to develop an answerable clinical question, and how to appraise published research. You will learn how to integrate the evidence into clinical practice and how to measure your clinical outcomes.

COMPETENCIES

Clinical Examination and Diagnosis (CE): CE-8, 9, 11, 12

Therapeutic Interventions (TI): TI-1, 4

Psychosocial Strategies and Referral (PS): PS-1-3, 7-16

Pathophysiology of Athletic Injuries

Susan Saliba, PhD, ATC, PT, FNATA

OBJECTIVES

After reading this chapter, the student should be able to do the following:

- Identify tissues considered "dense connective tissue" and explain the components of such tissue.

- Explain why it is important to understand biomechanical models of the viscoelastic properties of tissue.

- Explain the pathology and histology of various tendinopathies common in athletics.

- Explain the potential for healing articular cartilage.

- Compare and contrast neuropraxia and neurotmesis.

When a patient sustains an injury, damage occurs in the musculoskeletal system. The pathophysiology of the injury, which encompasses the types of structures injured, the severity of the injury, and the mechanisms for healing, is important as the athletic trainer plans for the immediate disposition and care of the patient. Each tissue type has a unique ability to repair itself through the inflammatory reaction. Expectations of surgical management and the length of the immobilization and rehabilitative process arise from the study of how specific tissues deal with the application of stress (therapeutic exercise or activity). The degree of damage to the tissues also influences the outcome. Understanding the mechanisms of tissue healing and how the body adapts to outside forces is essential for athletic trainers designing and implementing rehabilitative programs.

The understanding of pathophysiology with respect to tissue injury, inflammation, and repair is essential to the athletic trainer's ability to plan and implement a comprehensive sport injury rehabilitation program. This chapter reviews the events of musculoskeletal tissue healing; more detail on the inflammatory process is presented both in *Therapeutic Exercise for Musculoskeletal Injuries* (Houglum 2010) and in *Therapeutic Modalities for Musculoskeletal Injuries* (Denegar, Saliba, Saliba, 2010). The chapter also presents a conceptual model for sport injury rehabilitation that incorporates rehabilitation phases, intervention goals, and progression criteria with respect to specific tissue types. While therapeutic exercise and rehabilitation theory are addressed in more depth throughout the Athletic Training Education Series, this chapter focuses on how specific tissue types respond to the application of forces (exercise) at various stages of the healing and repair process.

Pathophysiology

Pathophysiology is the study of an alteration in normal mechanical, physical, or biochemical functions that may result from disease or damage to normal tissues. In athletic training, most dysfunction arises from trauma or microtrauma to connective tissues that results in the pathological condition. In the disablement scheme, pathologies do not always cause impairments or loss of function, but the level of involvement often leads to some degree of disability with respect to physical activity. Furthermore, some disease processes may affect normal healing; the athletic trainer should be aware that cardiovascular disease, diabetes, and many types of polyarthritis can affect the normal process of injury repair. Additionally, pharmaceutical interventions such as oral steroids may affect the body's ability to return to function. All of these factors influence the overall health-related quality of life.

Pathology in the musculoskeletal system can arise from a traumatic event or from continuous overload to a structure. It is often relatively easy to follow a specific template for rehabilitation of a traumatic injury or a postoperative case since the exercises have been prescribed based on examination of the acute inflammatory process and the manner in which the tissues respond to forces. In an overuse injury, in contrast, the inflammatory process may start over continuously or be in varying stages of resolution, making it more difficult to determine the best course of action. In some overuse injuries, such as tendinosis, the inflammatory process has actually ceased (Rees, Maffulli, and Cook 2009; Sharma and Maffulli 2005). Rehabilitation incorporates the initial treatments applied to an injury, such as modalities or manual therapy techniques, as well as the prescription of therapeutic exercise. Individual texts in this series review specific rehabilitative techniques.

Connective Tissue Structure

Dense connective tissue comprises bone, muscles, tendons, ligaments, and fascia; one of its major functions is to hold the body together. Connective tissue has fibrous components and a ground substance. The fibrinous components, collagen and elastin, provide strength, extensibility, and resistance to tensile and torsional forces; the ground substance acts to hydrate the connective tissue matrix, stabilize the collagen, and resist compressive weight. Collagen has many forms, several of which have been recently discovered by researchers who study tissue engineering and the human genome. However, collagen types I, II, and III are the most relevant to athletic training since these types are involved in musculoskeletal injury and healing under normal circumstances.

Collagen is a highly organized chain of proteins whose structure was discovered in 1954. The collagen molecule, called **tropocollagen**, is made up of three intertwining polypeptide strands held together by hydrogen bonds. Tropocollagen is the term used for the triple helix. Collagen resists deformation; the fibers absorb forces by straightening, which results in maintenance of the tissue's shape (Egan 1987). **Type I collagen** is the strongest, most abundant collagen in the human body. Type I collagen is also the end result of the inflammatory process and is the constituent of mature scar tissue. **Type II collagen** is in hyaline cartilage, among other types of tissues, and has specialized functions. **Type III collagen** is the major component of granulation tissue and is produced by fibroblasts. This type of collagen is generated during the healing phase and is a precursor to type I collagen as the involved tissues strengthen and remodel. Type III collagen is less able to resist stress, and damage results if forces exceed its tensile strength.

The **elastin** component of connective tissue is a protein that helps the tissues regain their shape after being stretched or contracted. Ligaments, tendons, and fascia are all made of collagen and elastin (as well as skin), but each has a different proportion of collagen and elastin; thus, those tissues can be differentiated by their proportion. Structures that have a higher content of elastin are generally more elastic and thus have more ability to absorb shock. The

intervetebral discs, the arterial walls, and the skin are examples of tissues with high elastin contents. Stiffer tissues such as fascia have less elastin proportionally.

Finally, connective tissue contains an amorphous, viscous ground substance that acts as a supporter of cells, collagen, and elastin. The ground substance is made of water and a number of proteins, the organization and amount depending on the type of tissue. **Proteoglycans** have a protein core with a glycosaminoglycan (GAG) chain covalently attached to form a gel-like substance. Although there are several types of GAGs, chondroitin sulfate is an example of a proteoglycan associated with articular cartilage to help the structure withstand compressive forces. When combined with glycosamine, chondroitin sulfate is a common nutritional supplement used to promote articular cartilage health. Another proteoglycan is hyaluronan, which is a major constituent of synovial fluid. These proteoglycans provide lubrication to the joints, provide structure to the cells, and contribute to the overall difference of various connective tissues.

Biomechanical Responses of Connective Tissue

Although it is difficult to associate our tissues into the cellular components, it is important to understand the structural differences of specific tissues and understand how imposing forces (through activity or rehabilitation) affect those tissues. Understanding the cellular components and their responses to stress will give a therapist a much better understanding of why certain exercises or activities are permitted while others are prohibited. One can analyze a stress–strain curve to determine how different structures respond to an injurious force or how a tissue responds to imposed demands such as passive stretching. An engineer can induce a stress (force) to a dissected sample of tissue and measure the strain (change in length) that occurs. The force is plotted with the corresponding change in length to produce the curve known as **Young's modulus of elasticity** (figure 21.1). In connective tissue such as ligament or tendon, these graphs show how much force is needed to "take up the slack" or initiate a change in length (toe region), how much force is needed to elongate the tissue (linear region), and how much force will cause a mechanical failure (yield and failure region). The toe region for a ligament that is relatively stiff is small or nonexistent.

A stress–strain curve could be plotted for hamstring tightness, for example. As you perform the straight-leg raise, little force is needed to make the muscles taut. This low force represents the toe region. Then, as the force is increased, further range is gained in proportion to the force applied. This area is represented by the linear region. If you continue to apply the force, you may make permanent changes in the muscle length, meaning that gains in range of motion are attributable to the force applied (yield and failure region). However, if force application continues, the collagen fibers could rupture, resulting in injury. This area where there is a loss of mechanical integrity is represented by the yield point or failure. The graph can further describe tissues' stiffness by the slope of the linear portion (Magnusson et al. 2000).

We can see from this example that tissues respond to stress in much the way any solid structure does. Connective tissue has unique viscoelastic properties because of the combination of collagen, elastin, and the ground substance. Changes in tendon and ligament length also depend on the timing of the load. When we put a quick stretch on the hamstrings, tissue length changes relatively little (this phenomenon is also caused by reflexive muscle contraction). A long-duration, low-load stretch results in greater changes of tissue length. With a longer application of force, the viscosity of the ground substance permits more adaptation to the load. Furthermore, when the load is removed, the tissue takes a longer time to return to its resting length. Creep and stress-relaxation refer to the behavior of connective tissue under stress. **Creep** (figure 21.2) explains the benefit of the long-duration, low-load stretch for improving range of motion. The tissues change their length by continuing to elongate over time. This response is the basis for dynamic splinting and many of our stretching programs. Factors such as increasing tissue temperature, either via modalities such as ultrasound or with exercise, decrease viscosity of the ground substance, enhancing creep.

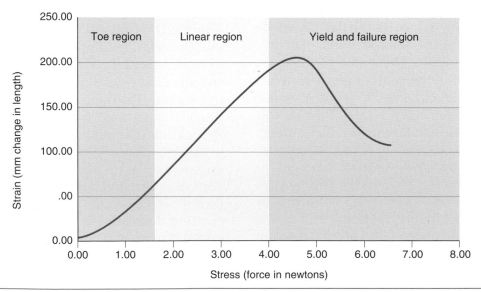

Figure 21.1 Young's modulus of elasticity. This graph represents general connective tissue properties; subtle changes in the graph will be seen depending on the type of tissue that is being tested. For example, the toe region for a ligament is very small or nonexistent, and ligaments are generally stiffer (have a more level slope) than tendons. Tendons are more elastic than ligaments and are able to change their length (strain) to a greater extent.

Stress-relaxation is a tissue's ability to relax or reduce tension in response to a constant deformation. As a constant stress is applied and the viscoelastic structure responds, the tension or stress within a muscle decreases over time (figure 21.3). The force does not have to increase within a treatment since the tissues are responding in a desirable manner (Magnusson et al. 2000). A comfortable, low-tension, long-duration stretch is the safest method to induce changes in length of connective tissue (Egan 1987).

A final biomechanical property of viscoelastic tissues is **hysteresis**. When a tissue is cyclically loaded, as in plyometrics or ballistic stretching, there is a gradual shift in the stress–strain graph that represents greater tissue length. Therefore, the loading and unloading of the tissues do not follow the same path (figure 21.4). Generally, after about 10 cycles there probably won't be any

more shift (figure 21.5). Although range of motion gains are more dramatic with cyclical stretching, injury can result if the force applied exceeds the mechanical limit of the collagen structure. This type of exercise should be reserved for previously strengthened tissues that have had time to adapt to the imposed demands.

Using these biomechanical models to examine how connective tissue responds to forces is exceedingly important for understanding injury mechanisms as well as for designing rehabilitation programs (Chandrashekar et al. 2008). As athletic trainers, we want to remove or apply forces to hasten the development of good, strong scar tissue so that an earlier return to safe function is possible. Knowledge of how certain tissue responds to stress helps guide the development of rehabilitation programs. When this is combined with understanding of the inflammatory process, athletic trainers can

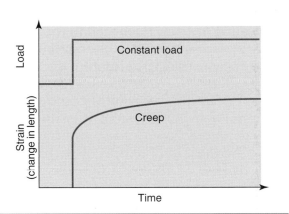

Figure 21.2 Creep in connective tissue.

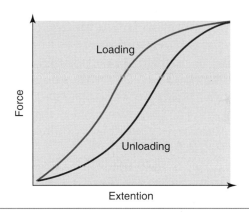

Figure 21.4 Hysteresis of connective tissue.

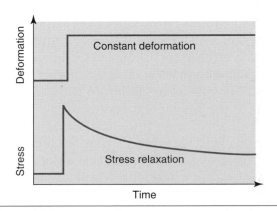

Figure 21.3 Stress-relaxation in connective tissue.

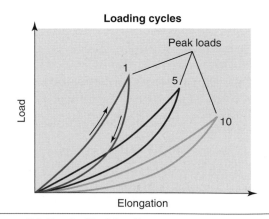

Figure 21.5 Cyclical loading.

predict when it is safest to eliminate activity and when to provide a controlled application of stress to help strengthen tissue.

When connective tissues are injured, the collagen can tear, resulting in a first-, second-, or third-degree injury. A sprain is an injury to a ligament or joint capsule, while a strain is an injury to a musculotendinous complex. In first-degree injuries, the fibers are stretched and localized inflammation is present, but the integrity of the tissue is maintained. A second-degree injury implies stretching and a partial tearing of the structure, also resulting in localized inflammation, but there may be some loss of tissue integrity. A third-degree injury is a complete rupture of the ligament or tendon causing a loss of integrity and function. Any external force that exceeds the tensile strength of the connective tissue, whether it is skin, bone, tendon, ligament, muscle, or nerve, results in an inflammatory process that ultimately ends with the development of a scar. The scar is produced by the body as a replacement for the lost tissue; however, its ability to perform the role of the original tissue is limited. For example, in healing, a laceration of the skin becomes a scar that has visibly changed from a wound; then to a scab as new cells are formed and the body eliminates the necrotic debris; then to a vulnerable vascular scar; and finally to a mature scar.

This process may take up to 1 year as the newly formed tissue adapts. In the skin, the scar prevents fluid loss and protects the body, but it may not have the mobility or the tensile strength of the original tissue. Likewise, an injured ligament may heal with scar or fibroblastic tissue that over time may adapt to provide some joint stability. However, once the structural integrity of the ligament has been lost, the ability of the scar to provide stability to the joint depends on the degree of injury, the change in length of the tissue (plastic change), and the stresses that are applied following the injury. High stress early may exacerbate instability, which is why surgical repair or reconstruction, immobilization, or both may be necessary. A lack of progressive stress later after injury may prohibit the scar from adapting in size and alignment to provide a functional replacement tissue. Health care professionals need to recognize when and how much stress should be applied to an injury to optimize return to function goals. Early in rehabilitation, stresses, including those applied through activity, are reduced to permit healing; later, graded stresses through therapeutic exercise are encouraged.

Inflammation

The inflammatory process is covered extensively by Houglum (2010) and Denegar and colleagues (2010). Each of these texts should be reviewed as a basis for the development of rehabilitation programs. Houglum (2010) emphasizes the mechanisms of connective tissue healing and repair, while Denegar and colleagues (2010) emphasize the cellular and vascular sequence of events during the inflammatory process and the ways in which physical agents can modify the development of swelling or pain. Each step in the inflammatory process is predictable, but the degree of the response varies. Although the process varies slightly in each tissue type, athletic trainers should thoroughly understand inflammation. Additionally, it is important to understand how overuse injuries occur and how the modification of activity and prescription of therapeutic exercise can encourage the resolution of a chronic injury.

In an acute injury, the phases of healing can be categorized into three periods with vastly different characteristics and therapeutic goals. An athletic trainer should be cautious about using only time as a way to determine the treatment. Injured active individuals often stress themselves during their functional activities, so the athletic trainer should pay more attention to the characteristics of the various healing phases than to a chronological time line. For example, some patients will be able to play basketball 3 days after sustaining a Grade II ankle sprain; however, this is likely to result in increased edema and pain. If the patient returns to play too soon, the athletic trainer should not assume that collagen healing occurs at day 21 because the new tissue is being constantly disrupted while painful play is permitted. Table 21.1 summarizes the phases of healing.

Immediately following an injury, the endothelial cells that line the blood vessels release several factors that initiate the inflammatory events. These cells cause an increase in blood flow to the area, potentiate pain, and draw leukocytes or white blood cells to the area. Ultimately these chemical events help to stop bleeding and isolate the injured area. This initial process, often called the inflammatory phase, is characterized by increases in pain, swelling, and protective spasm and lasts up to 4 days. The clinical goal during this time is to protect the injury from further harm and to lessen pain and swelling. Physical agents are often used in combination with gentle active range of motion and muscle contractions focused on regaining neuromuscular control. Many injuries require immobilization during this time for protection from further harm. Immobilization can restrict all motion, as when a hard cast is required for fracture healing; or a health care professional can choose a brace that permits motion during rehabilitation sessions. The latter is often the choice when safety permits, since complete immobilization can result in poorly organized scar tissue and a longer neuromuscular rehabilitation time. Examples of braces are the hinged knee brace, the walking boot, and the wrist cock-up splint. These devices should be worn during daily activities to protect the injury from stresses encountered throughout

Table 21.1 Chronology of Wound Healing

Phase	Time	Activity	Purpose or result
Inflammation	1 day	Neutrophil migration	Fight contamination Release growth factors and biologically reactive substances
Inflammation	1 day	Fibrin bridge creation	Redness, warmth, swelling, tenderness to touch
Inflammation	1-2 days	→ Monocyte migration	Phagocytose bacteria
Inflammation	2 days	Angiogenesis	Ingrowing fibroblasts
Inflammation	2-3 days	Production of type III collagen by fibroblasts	
Proliferation	4 days	→ Rapid increase in fibroblasts Increased epithelial cell mitosis Increased synthesis of extracellular collagen Increased proteoglycans	
Proliferation	5 days	→ Myofibroblast production	Wound contraction
Proliferation	5-7 days	Collagen synthesis, very active	
Remodeling	5-9 days	Reduction in fibroblasts Reduction in macrophages Reduction in wound vascularity → Reduction in fibronectin in proportion to the amount of type I collagen formed	Less redness
Remodeling	10 days	Wound contraction	
Remodeling	12 days	→ Conversion of type III collagen to type I	
Remodeling	6-18 weeks	→ Reduction in capillaries	Reduced fluid content, increased scar density
Remodeling	6-18 months	Completion of all healing	

→ = Key activities of each phase.

the day but can be removed for rehabilitation. It is important to explain to the patient when the brace should be removed, since compliance with the prescribed treatment is imperative for successful management of the condition.

The second phase of inflammation is often termed the proliferative phase since this is when fibroblastic cells are multiplying to produce scar tissue. Again, immobilization may be required depending on the degree of injury, especially when a muscle contraction or stretch could exceed the tensile strength of the newly forming tissue. For example, a tendon repair should be protected since the tension applied with certain movements may rupture the repair. This phase generally lasts from 4 to 21 days, although the duration may be much longer if sport or general activity is not controlled. Many individuals are able to play during this phase, but doing so may compromise or delay healing. The justification for participation depends on many factors and is generally guided by the judgment of the medical professional directing the care. Protective devices should be used, and therapeutic treatments and therapeutic exercise should be used in combination to continue to promote healing and strengthening of the injured tissues. A full examination is often required to address any compensatory adaptations that may result in another injury if early return is deemed safe. The rehabilitation program should take these biomechanical factors and deficiencies into consideration.

The final phase of inflammation, the remodeling phase, can last up to 1 year. The example of a skin wound can serve to emphasize the importance of ongoing rehabilitation. A laceration or surgical scar will close rather quickly (although sutures are often necessary) but remain red or pink for several months after the incision. If the wound is not protected with sunscreen, the scar may become hypertrophic or hyperemic. Generally, after a year, the scar blanches (appears white) as it devascularizes. The development of this mature scar is similar to the process that ligaments and other soft tissues go through in the remodeling phase.

The connective tissue formed from the fibroblasts continues to evolve from type III to type I collagen and aligns along patterns of stress; in this way the scar tissue increases its tensile strength. Thus, strengthening of the limb should continue long after one has assumed that the healing is complete.

Arthrogenic muscle inhibition (AMI) is a neuromuscular effect of injury that minimizes the ability to generate full strength and power of the muscles surrounding a joint (Pietrosimone et al. 2009). Arthrogenic muscle inhibition has been associated with injuries such as anterior cruciate ligament reconstruction and meniscus injuries and can be linked to osteoarthritis. This inhibition of the musculature is initially a protective mechanism but may limit full recovery if it is prolonged. Rehabilitation techniques that are incorporated during the remodeling phase may address AMI. Patients generally undergo supervised rehabilitation for a short time following the injury or surgery to meet functional goals such as walking or running. However, long-term strengthening is often necessary to address the physical needs of active individuals. A full musculoskeletal examination should identify weak or tight tissues that may lead to excessive stress on a joint. Rehabilitation or the strength and conditioning program should be individualized to address these factors for at least a year following injury. This procedure of evaluating the musculoskeletal system to determine deficiencies and applying appropriate intervention should follow the inflammatory phase guidelines.

With respect to rehabilitation, the clinician must examine each tissue type and understand the mechanisms of healing for each. Although injuries such as strains, sprains, fractures, and tendinopathies are discussed in greater detail in other texts (e.g., Shultz, Houglum, and Perrin 2010; Houglum 2010), this section discusses general factors related to the structure and function of various tissue types. Keep in mind the inflammatory process, as well as the structure and function of each tissue type, when determining how tissues will respond to the stresses placed upon them with therapeutic exercise and the return to activity.

Ligament

Ligament injuries are perhaps the most common of all athletic injuries, since a sprain, or injury to the joint capsule, is categorized as a ligamentous injury. The ligaments, combined with the bony architecture, provide static stability to the joint. When a ligament is torn, or even stretched, the stability of the joint may be compromised. Often an individual can strengthen the muscles surrounding a joint to help compensate for the lost stability. However, the specific ligament that is injured, the degree of injury, and the stresses placed on the joint may necessitate reconstructive surgery to enable the patient to regain the stability needed to permit function. Knowledge and experience help the athletic trainer to recognize the types of injury that require referral.

Injured ligaments undergo the same inflammatory response that all connective tissue does, resulting in edema formation with the eventual production of a scar. In a second- or third-degree injury, the athletic trainer should make an effort to eliminate stress on the ligament during daily activities and in the rehabilitation process. Bracing is often used during the early phase to help control aberrant joint movement. Within 1 week of the injury, fibrocytes and macrophages initiate the formation of collagen that is randomly aligned. The matrix continues to contain these cells until approximately 6 weeks (Viidik 1973). These cells diminish over 6 weeks to 12 months; and during a long maturation phase, the connective tissue scar forms around a joint. Often the matrix does not reach full tensile strength until 1 year.

Tendon

Tendons connect muscles to bone and transmit forces through the kinetic chain. The organizational structure of tendon is characterized by parallel bundles of type I and type III collagen. Tendon pathologies relate to the frequency, intensity, and direction of the load placed on the tendon, with eccentric stresses accounting for the majority of the offending forces. Most tendon injuries are characterized as overuse injuries and are termed tendinopathies. However, a tendon may rupture with an excessive concentric force that exceeds its tensile strength. Ruptured tendons require surgical repair in most cases, while tendinopathies, caused by repetitive stress, are treated with activity modification and therapeutic rehabilitation.

The categories of tendinopathies are presented in table 21.2. Discrimination or diagnosis of a particular type of tendinopathy often requires a histopathological analysis (Rees, Maffulli, and Cook 2009). Treating an overuse injury that is managed early in the inflammatory phase is much easier than treating an injury that has gone through inflammation and continues to degenerate. It may be necessary to reinstate the

Table 21.2	Categorization of Tendinopathies	
Diagnosis	**Pathology (microscopic)**	**Histopathology**
Tendinosis	Intratendinous degeneration (typically due to microtrauma)	Collagen disorientation with fiber separation and an increase in mucoid ground substance. May involve neovascularization and focal necrosis or calcification, and inflammatory cells are absent.
Tendinitis	Degeneration of the tendon with vascular disruption and inflammation	Same as for tendinosis but with indication of tears. Active inflammatory process with fibroblastic cell proliferation, bleeding, and granulation tissue.
Paratenonitis	Inflammation of the outermost layer of the tendon (paratenon) only	Mucoid degeneration of the outer layer with some inflammatory cells and fibrinous exudates.
Paratenonitis with tendinosis	Paratenonitis with degeneration	Degenerative changes as in tendinosis with mucoid degeneration, fibrin, and inflammatory cells in the paratenon.

inflammatory phase with an intervention such as stripping, thermal modalities, or other mechanisms so that eventual healing may occur. Most management strategies offer symptomatic relief but do not result in a resolution of the pathology. Despite remodeling, the biomechanical properties of the healed tendon may never match those of intact tendons (Sharma and Maffulli 2006).

In acute ruptures or lacerations with surgical repair, the inflammatory process is characterized by a proliferation of vascular and cellular events in the first 5 days. Collagen synthesis is maximal at 10 days, and fibroblastic production from the endotenon continues until the third to fourth week. Collagen synthesis ends at approximately 35 days, but the maturation and orientation require additional time. Protection from vigorous exercise is necessary for 2 months. Resistive exercises are generally permitted after 8 weeks, and the tissue continues to remodel for up to 6 months.

Bone

Injuries to the bone are referred to as fractures or stress fractures. Any disruption in the continuity of the bone or periosteum is a fracture. Fractures are further classified based on whether the skin covering the fracture is intact or not (closed vs. open) and the displacement and orientation of the fragments. Unlike other connective tissues, bone has the ability to regenerate, and injured bone is replaced with new bone cells. Also unlike other connective tissues, bone requires immobilization or fixation to heal since the newly produced matrix is easily disrupted during the healing phase.

Fractures result in an inflammatory phase lasting up to 4 days in which fibroblasts are produced; macrophages infiltrate; and, with the entrance of osteoclasts, the area is cleared of debris, fatty infiltrate, and other by-products of the injury. Osteoblasts, or the precursors to bone cells (osteocytes), are then stimulated to produce a callous. The fibrous callous forms within 3 to 4 weeks, and a shadow can be seen on radiographs. The ability of the callous to maintain alignment and function depends on the external stresses and the stability of the fracture. For example, in rotational fractures, a longer portion of the bone is fractured, so a longer healing time is required. Displaced fractures require reduction, that is, positioning in alignment during the immobilization. The greater space between the bone ends also results in the need for more healing time. Frequently a surgical intervention, or open reduction with internal fixation, places compression between the fractured ends of the bone, reducing the need for external immobilization. Between 4 and 6 weeks, the osteocytes fill in the matrix, and typically the tensile strength of the bone returns by 12 weeks.

Articular Cartilage

Articular cartilage injuries, which often accompany joint damage, may not be addressed during the acute resolution of the sprain. The articular cartilage is made of highly specialized cells that permit gliding of joint surfaces and a transfer of energy with both high and low loads and at various speeds (Moger et al. 2009). Synthetic articular cartilage cannot reproduce, and tissue engineers have not been able to regenerate natural articular cartilage. Most cartilage is composed of type II collagen; however, after an injury, type II collagen is often replaced with type I collagen, which is more typical of fibrocartilage. Osteoarthritis, or the breakdown of articular cartilage, often occurs as the result of joint trauma.

Injury to the articular cartilage may occur from progressive wear, especially wear attributable to a biomechanical compensation. Injury also may occur from trauma, and the depth and location of the defect will dictate the potential for healing. Some osteochondritis injuries require a removal of the osteochondrit since they are likely to result in a loose body within a joint, and some defects can be pinned in place or drilled to promote the formation of fibrocartilage. More recent procedures involve an arthroscopic transfer of healthy articular cartilage taken from a nonstressed area of the joint and implanted into the defect, similar to a skin graft. This procedure is most effective when the defect is small.

Articular cartilage injuries heal with the inflammatory reaction, initiating the proliferation of fibroblasts and collagen formation between days 5 and 14. Decisions regarding weight bearing are made during this time if joint protection is needed. Chondrocytes are apparent in 2 weeks, and type I collagen is formed within 8 weeks. Generally, the maturation process is complete between 4 and 6 months. Immobilization is strongly discouraged for articular cartilage injuries since the fluid transfer between normal cells requires movement.

Peripheral Nerve

Nerve injuries can occur as a result of stretching or traction, compression including contusion, or laceration. Injuries to the central nervous system, including concussions and spinal cord injuries, cannot be repaired because of the nature of the specialized cells in this system. Peripheral nerve injuries, however, may regain their function through the inflammatory process and a specialized process termed Wallerian degeneration. The Seddon classification system divides peripheral nerve injuries, in order of increasing severity, into neuropraxia, axonotmesis, and neurotmesis. A neuropraxia is a transient compression with very little damage to the actual nerve. This type of injury is often implicated in a "stinger" or brachial plexus injury, in the ulnar nerve at the elbow, or in the carpal tunnel. A localized inflammatory reaction occurs, but the continuity of the fibers is not disrupted. A neuropraxia can be compounded if the nerve is continually reinjured. The patient should be positioned in such a way as to reduce all nerve symptoms. For example, a patient with a lumbar disc injury should be told to avoid any position that reproduces peripheral symptoms to prevent permanent injury to the nerve. Furthermore, participation should be restricted when peripheral symptoms are present. In an

axonotmesis, a disruption in the nerve, the outermost fibers are still intact. Wallerian degeneration occurs with the inflammatory phases, causing a loss of sensory and motor function distal to the lesion. The degenerative phase lasts approximately 3 weeks, while the new nerve growth takes place at approximately 1 to 3 mm per day or an inch each month. The key to regeneration is that the neural tubes remain intact so that the new nerve growth is directed to the target organ (sensory or motor). Sunderland further classifies axonotmesis according to the damage to the connective tissues. Typically, these injuries have a good prognosis if permitted to heal.

The most severe peripheral nerve injury is the neurotmesis. This type of injury results in a complete disruption of the continuity of the nerve, including the supporting connective tissue. Surgical repair is required for healing, and the prognosis depends on the nature of the injury and the vascularity of the area. Scar tissue may also preclude a good result. Wallerian degeneration occurs both proximally and distally, and the rate of new nerve regrowth is similar to that for axonotmesis.

Patients with sensory dysfunction such as numbness, tingling, burning, or itching should be evaluated to determine (1) the location of the injury and (2) the specific nerve injured. For example, for a patient with numbness in the hand, the athletic trainer should identify the exact location of the numbness since the hand is supplied by three sensory nerves. Global numbness would have to come from a vascular injury unless multiple nerves are involved. The athletic trainer then determines the site of compression or injury—does it arise from a cervical disc, from pressure in the thoracic outlet, from the axilla, or from other sites as the nerve descends from the upper extremity into the hand? It is also important to discern whether the nerve is injured or whether the problem is a nerve root irritation.

Direct current stimulation has been suggested to improve function following a nerve injury. Long phase durations (of at least 1 s) are required to depolarize the muscle membrane when the nerve is no longer intact. Evidence supporting the use of direct current stimulation for denervated muscles is inconclusive. The treatment does not promote or

enhance nerve regrowth. However, some clinicians feel that the intermittent contractions help to preserve the protein component, particularly of the sliding filaments of the muscle, while active motion is not possible.

Learning Aids

SUMMARY

Connective tissue undergoes the inflammatory process when it is injured. The athletic trainer should understand the pathophysiology of the injury and be able to apply this understanding to a regimen that takes into consideration the activity restrictions for injuries and the additional stress of therapeutic exercise. Different tissue types respond to the inflammatory process and regain their tensile strength at different rates. The athletic trainer should be able to use the guidelines for each specific tissue type to implement the rehabilitation program and make a realistic suggestion for return to play based on the severity of the injury.

KEY CONCEPTS AND REVIEW

▶ **Identify tissues considered "dense connective tissue" and explain the components of such tissue.**

Dense connective tissue comprises the bone, muscles, tendons, ligaments, and fascia; one of its major functions is to hold the body together. Connective tissue has fibrous components and a ground substance. The fibrinous components, collagen and elastin, provide strength, extensibility, and resistance to tensile and torsional forces; the ground substance acts to hydrate the connective tissue matrix, stabilize the collagen, and resist compressive weight.

▶ **Explain why it is important to understand biomechanical models of viscoelastic properties of tissue.**

The viscoelastic models help explain how tissues respond to specific forces, particularly during return to activity and with rehabilitation. The goal for athletic trainers is to choose an exercise that will continually stress the structure in a method that will allow those tissues to become stronger, rather than to exceed the strength of the tissues as they heal. Ultimately the goal of the inflammatory process is to develop scar tissue that can withstand the forces of physical activity.

▶ **Explain the pathology and histology of various tendinopathies common in athletics.**

See table 21.2 for this information.

▶ **Explain the potential for healing articular cartilage.**

Articular cartilage does not heal. These highly specialized cells are able to distribute forces across the joint and lubricate the joint surface, however, damage to the cells results in degeneration of those joint surfaces. Osteoarthritis is the loss of articular cartilage. Any defect heals with fibrocartilage, however efforts to induce the formation of articular cartilage are continually being explored.

▶ **Compare and contrast neuropraxia and neurotmesis.**

- A neuropraxia is a transient compression with very little damage to the actual nerve. This type of injury is often implicated in a "stinger" or brachial plexus injury, in the ulnar nerve at the elbow, or in the carpal tunnel. A localized inflammatory reaction occurs, but the continuity of the fibers is not disrupted. A neuropraxia can be compounded if the nerve is continually reinjured.

- A neurotmesis results in a complete disruption of the continuity of the nerve, including the supporting connective tissue. Surgical repair is required for healing, and the prognosis depends on the nature of the injury and the vascularity of the area. Scar tissue may preclude a good result. Wallerian degeneration occurs both proximally and distally, and the rate of new nerve regrowth is similar to that for axonotmesis.

PRACTICE!

For hands-on practice in this area, go to the web resource and complete the following:

Level 2.4, Module E4: Body's Response to Injury

CRITICAL THINKING QUESTIONS

1. One of your sophomore basketball players tore her medial meniscus and cannot continue to participate. Her family flew her home to see their orthopedic surgeon, who wants to remove the torn piece of meniscus. The team's orthopedic surgeon feels it is important to attempt to save the entire meniscus, stating that removing the meniscus will put undue stress on the articular (hyaline) cartilage. Discuss the two options as you would present them to the patient and render your opinion.

2. The star center on the football team suffered a medial collateral ligament injury in the second game of the season, just 13 days ago. The patient is anxious to get back to playing, and the coach wants him to return as soon as possible. Explain the stage of the inflammatory process the player is in at this time and indicate the significance of this period. What are your thoughts on allowing the individual to return to play? Would you have any requirements for his participation? Explain your thinking.

Psychological Aspects of Sport Injury and Rehabilitation

Diane M. Wiese-Bjornstal, PhD, CC-AASP
Laura J. Kenow, MS, ATC
Frances A. Flint, PhD, CAT(C), ATC

OBJECTIVES

After reading this chapter, the student should be able to do the following:

- Outline the elements of the Sport Injury Risk Profile (SIRP).

- Explain the relationship between stress and athletic injury.

- Identify the psychological responses of patients to injury, including cognitions, affects, behaviors, and outcomes (CABO), using the model described in the chapter.

- Describe how characteristics of the sport injury socioculture affect participant health.

- Explain the Integrated Rehabilitation Model (IRM) as presented in the text.

- List and explain the psychological skills interventions that patients can use in sport injury situations.

- Outline the things that would help athletic trainers recognize psychosocial distress in a patient.

- List the steps an athletic trainer should take to establish a psychosocial referral network before it is needed.

- List the steps the athletic trainer could take to increase the likelihood that a patient will be receptive to psychosocial referral.

P hysical health is inseparable from the psychological and sociocultural aspects of patients' lives. Nowhere is this more evident, perhaps, than with sport injury. Some sport participants train in a culture that expects them to be tough and play through pain; once they are injured, the culture requires them to rehabilitate quickly and return to play without lingering fear or anxiety. Essential to the work of athletic trainers are effective understanding and recognition of these psychological, social, and cultural factors and how they affect sport injury prevention, rehabilitation, and recovery.

This chapter offers an overview of some of these many aspects of sport injury and rehabilitation. The first section offers insight into basic models of psychological influence on sport injury to build a base of understanding for the work of athletic trainers. The second section discusses interventions that athletic trainers might use and the effects of these interventions on physical and psychological recovery in the context of a comprehensive delivery model. The third section presents suggestions for the implementation of athletic training plans that provide for the effective management of psychological concerns, as athletic training rooms must be prepared to manage the psychological and sociocultural health of patients along with their physical health care needs.

Sport Injury Psychology and Socioculture

Before thinking about how the day-to-day work of athletic trainers might intersect with psychological and sociocultural factors, it is important to have a basic understanding of what those factors are and how they relate to sport injury. This section offers insight into the role of psychological and sociocultural factors in injury to set the scene for the specific psychological intervention and athletic training room management recommendations presented later in the chapter.

Sport Injury Psychology

The term **sport injury psychology** refers to psychological thoughts (cognitions), feelings (affect), actions (behaviors), and interventions that affect the risk of sport injury as well as the response, recovery, and return of participants (Wiese-Bjornstal 2010). In this section we explore these aspects of sport injury.

Sport Injury Risk

Why does sport injury happen, and what places one person more at risk for sport injury than another? The Sport Injury Risk Profile (SIRP; Wiese-Bjornstal 2009) view of the many factors affecting sport injury risk gives athletic trainers a means of understanding how psychological and sociocultural factors operate interactively with physical and environmental factors within the larger context of sport injury risk (see figure 22.1). Interventions directed at better managing these aspects have the potential to reduce risk of sport injury in the same way in which other more common athletic training interventions, such as changes in training and conditioning protocols or the use of protective equipment, reduce risks. In order to design and implement effective psychological and sociocultural interventions, athletic trainers must first understand the complex combination of influences on sport injury risk for individual participants on their teams and must recognize the ways in which psychological and sociocultural factors contribute to the risk.

The SIRP identifies specific examples of elements within each major contributor to the profiles that have been linked to sport injury risk. Participants all have their own unique profiles—combinations or constellations of risk factors that influence their personal risks for sport injury. There are likely both cumulative and interactive effects of these risk factors; in other words, the factors work together and in combination. Two broad categories of risk in figure 22.1 are personal and environmental. Personal

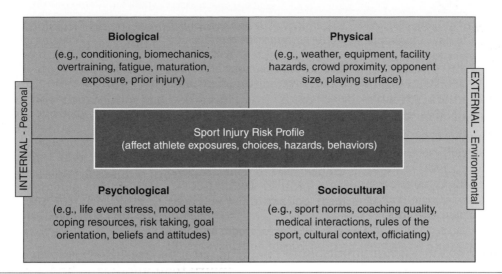

Figure 22.1   Sport Injury Risk Profile (SIRP).

From Wiese-Bjornstal 2008. Reprinted with permission of the author.

influences represent individual internal biological and psychological characteristics unique to each participant, while environmental influences encompass those arising from the physical and sociocultural external contexts in which that participant trains and competes.

Within each of these two broad categories of risk are two subcategories. Biological factors are internal; they represent the physical and physiological characteristics of individual participants and include such elements as physical condition, age, and existing muscular imbalances. Psychological factors represent internal mental characteristics of individual participants, including mood state, life stress, and risk taking. Physical factors encompass the external physical environments surrounding participation; environments precipitating injury occurrence might include things such as uneven surfaces, slippery conditions, and unsafe equipment. Sociocultural factors represent external sociocultural influences such as the quality and rigor of officiating, the quality and style of coaching, and the social pressure to play when one is hurt or fatigued. These risk factors influence sport injuries through their effects on participant exposures to potentially injurious situations, behavioral choices made, and hazards encountered.

Among all four subcategories, the role of participant developmental or life span level is apparent. Biological factors, for example, encompass developmental factors such as the physical vulnerabilities associated with growth (e.g., incomplete epiphyseal closure and risk of growth plate injuries in young active people; deterioration of joints in older individuals). Examples of psychological factors related to growth and development across the life span are the less diverse coping skills and capabilities of children, or the increased mental distress associated with chronic health conditions in the elderly. Examples of developmental level–related physical factors are the improperly sized or fitted equipment often used by young participants, or the reduced balance abilities of older patients leading to increased risk of a fall on slippery surfaces. Examples of sociocultural and age-related factors are the untrained volunteer coaches often working with young people, or the reduction in social interaction and support experienced by many older persons.

Another way of looking at psychological and sociocultural risk factors is through the conceptual model of stress and athletic injury (Andersen and Williams 1988). This model has guided much of the research on psychological and social influences on vulnerability to sport injury. The central psychological influence on the occurrence of sport injury, according to this model, is the **stress response**. Essentially, the more "stress" participants perceive, the more vulnerable they are to injury, particularly if they do not have sufficient **coping resources** for managing the stress. Stress-related changes that occur in patient attention and cognition (e.g., tunnel vision, attention turning inward toward personal thoughts rather than focusing outward on the risks in the sporting environment) and physiology (such as increased muscle tension and increased heart rate) can negatively affect individual behaviors and performance, which in turn increase the risk of injury.

Of all of the factors outlined in the model of stress and athletic injury, the most consistently supported finding is that individuals who report feeling significant stress from **major life events** (both sport and nonsport events, such as moving, death of a family member, divorce of parents, or starting a new school) are more likely to sustain a sport injury than those who report feeling less major life event stress. This seems to be particularly true if participants with high life event stress also report that they have limited coping resources to help them manage the stress. One can imagine a football quarterback, for example, so distracted by thoughts of his parents' impending divorce that he fails to see and prepare for the tackler about to hit him, leading to a **macrotrauma** injury that might have been prevented had he been "paying attention." Or, picture the swimmer with no one to talk to, training excessively to distract herself, whose neck and shoulder muscles are overly tense because she is worried about the health of her ill grandmother, thus altering her normal stroke mechanics and leading to **microtrauma** injury. These examples provide brief snapshots of how psychological and social factors contribute to sport injury risk.

It is clear that understanding why sport injuries happen requires an understanding of the complexity of the risk factors involved, including psychological and sociocultural factors. From the standpoint of the injury prevention role so important to the work of athletic trainers, it is imperative to understand the many risk factors so that the athletic trainer might design important risk reduction interventions, again including those that address potentially harmful sociocultural and psychological influences.

Sport Injury Response

Once sport injury happens, what then? Responses to sport injury are influenced by a wide variety of preexisting personal and social conditions such as personality, physical health status, nature of and prior experience with injury, sport type, time in season, and interpersonal relationships. Envision, for example, how a starting varsity basketball player might respond if she sustained a season-ending injury in the sectional championship game during her senior year of high school; then envision how a freshman substitute on the junior varsity team in a nonconference game near the end of the season might respond. Intuitively one would expect the starting senior in a playoff game to have more difficulty with her thoughts and emotions about the injury than the freshman, although of course there are many other possible variables affecting each individual. The point is that in order to better understand psychological responses to sport injuries, athletic trainers should consider important aspects of the personal and social atmospheres of participants.

What do patients think, feel, and do once sport injury happens, and how do these thoughts, feelings, actions, and outcomes cycle and change over the time course of rehabilitation, recovery, and return to play? Sport injury for most patients is a stressful life event (although, sadly, some patients express that they are almost relieved to be injured as it provides them with what they see as the only face-saving way to escape unrelenting pressures of sport imposed upon them by parents or others). Patients cycle through cognitions, affects, behaviors, and outcomes over the duration of the recovery, rehabilitation, and return process following

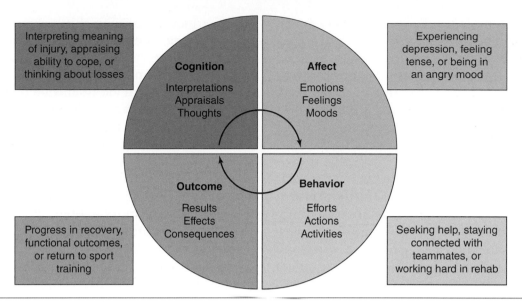

Cognition

Interpretations
Appraisals
Thoughts

Interpreting meaning of injury, appraising ability to cope, or thinking about losses

Affect

Emotions
Feelings
Moods

Experiencing depression, feeling tense, or being in an angry mood

Outcome

Results
Effects
Consequences

Progress in recovery, functional outcomes, or return to sport training

Behavior

Efforts
Actions
Activities

Seeking help, staying connected with teammates, or working hard in rehab

Figure 22.2 Dynamic cycles of psychological response to sport injury and rehabilitation: Cognition, Affect, Behavior, Outcome (CABO) model.

From Wiese-Bjornstal 2010. Reprinted with permission of the author.

sport injury. Figure 22.2 provides an illustration of the Cognition, Affect, Behavior, Outcome (CABO) model and these dynamic cycles of response to sport injury and rehabilitation.

The cognitions, or thoughts, of patients after injury and throughout the rehabilitation and recovery cycles involve evaluating a variety of aspects of the injury; this process is called **cognitive appraisal**. Patients might think about the sport injury cause (e.g., thoughts such as "Was it an accident?"), their personal abilities to cope with it (e.g., "Can I manage the rehab sessions along with my schoolwork?"), or the reactions of others such as coaches and parents (e.g., "Will my coach think I'm faking it?"). They also appraise their perceived recovery status (e.g., "I'm getting stronger every day") or the availability of social support (e.g., "I have some good friends who will listen to my fears when I get worried about the injury"). Both the negatives and the positives of the situation are appraised; perhaps patients think they have "lost" something due to the injury (e.g., starting position, scholarship, or status) or that they have gained something (e.g., a chance to review priorities, opportunity to develop skills and strengths in other

areas). Key aspects of cognitive appraisals reflect one's ability to cope with the injury and include assessments of the demands of the injury situation, the resources available to meet the demands, and the importance of meeting the demands. These many cognitive appraisals or thoughts influence affect, behavior, and outcomes after an injury.

Affective responses—the emotions, feelings, or moods of patients about sport injury—often arise from their cognitive appraisals, change throughout the injury and recovery process, and affect patient behaviors and recovery. Some of the most common negative mood states following a sport injury are anxiety or tension and depression; others include boredom, frustration, anger, and fatigue. Thoughts and feelings of stress and anxiety have been found to negatively affect mental health status and physiological recovery. Many patients, however, also respond to injury with more positive thoughts and feelings reflecting optimism, energy, and a sense of challenge. Emotions associated with loss, such as grief and sadness, are also possible particularly when patients appraise that they have indeed lost something that can never be regained. How patients feel about their injury affects what they do; for example, reflect on a male track athlete who is down, depressed, and discouraged about sustaining a season-ending injury. Would an athletic trainer expect that individual to show up for rehab each and every day and to complete all of the activities unsupervised giving his best effort? Most likely not, yet actions make or break the recovery.

What patients do, their observable behaviors or actions, have great bearing on their recoveries. Examples of overt **behavioral responses** following injury include such things as adherence to or compliance with treatment regimens, use of mental skills and strategies, use of social networks, risk-taking behaviors, and the effort and intensity with which the patient pursues rehabilitation. Cognitive appraisals (thoughts) and emotional responses (feelings) of the patients influence behaviors. Research shows us that patients who adhere to rehabilitation, use psychological skills to manage pain and direct energies, effectively use available social support, reduce risk-taking behaviors that inhibit rehabilitation, and pursue rehabilitation goals with optimum effort and intensity are more likely to recover from injury and return to previous athletic performance levels than are those who do not do so.

Anything athletic trainers can do to advantage these desired behaviors will also advantage patient recovery outcomes. A variety of **outcomes**—consequences, effects, and results—occur during response to sport injury cycles and natural healing processes. Outcomes include setbacks, plateaus, and other challenges as well as improvements and breakthroughs. Healing, health, functional, and performance outcomes coincide during the rehabilitation process. An evaluation of these outcomes by patients feeds back into further cognitive appraisals, thus continuing the cycles of response and recovery after a sport injury.

For example, think of the cycles that would be expected for an individual who thinks a sport injury is the worst thing that has ever happened to him and that his season is over. One might expect, based on his negative interpretations of the injury, that he would be feeling anxious, sad, and hopeless. Because of these feelings, most would not expect him to adhere to his rehabilitation protocol, which in turn would lead to less than optimal functional and healing outcomes. On the other hand, a patient who interprets an injury as something that will be challenging but possible to overcome would likely feel more vigorous and motivated. We would likely expect behaviors such as adherence and effort directed toward the rehabilitation and in turn better functional and sport performance outcomes.

These cycles of psychological response to sport injury are dynamic; that is, they change over time. Figure 22.3 provides an illustration of the psychological aspects of reaction, response, adjustment, and return (to play or life) phases over the life span of an injury. Temporal psychological response progression is not always linear; picture the cycles of response (figure 22.2) spiraling throughout the sport injury life span depicted in figure 22.3. The spiral progressions are like a Slinky toy, oscillating forward with progress toward psychological adjustment, but then regressing backward with a setback or reinjury. The goal for athletic trainers is to ensure that the Slinky bounces back and continues to make forward progress once again as the patient accommodates and strives for recovery.

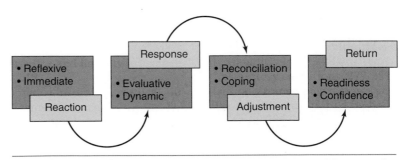

Figure 22.3 Psychological changes over a sport injury life span: the Reaction, Response, Adjustment, Return (RRAR) model.

From Wiese-Bjornstal 2009. Reprinted with permission of the author.

Sport Injury Socioculture

The term **sport injury socioculture** refers to social and cultural structures, climates, processes, and interventions that influence the sport injury risk, response, recovery, and return of participants (Wiese-Bjornstal 2010). To fully understand the psychological aspects of sport injury, it is necessary to consider the socioculture in which participants train and perform. Figure 22.4 provides an overview of some of the beliefs and actions characterizing the sport injury socioculture.

Some sport participants learn through socialization experiences that the expectation is for them to take risks, be "tough," and play through pain and injury. Athletic trainers might wonder whether, in fact, adherence to these expectations is voluntary or coerced, and may be concerned about times of incompatibility between health and sport performance. The willingness to sacrifice ethics, health, or common sense in pursuit of achievement in sport is highly visible through many actions of participants, such as the use of drugs to mask pain or training and competing with an injury despite medical recommendations to the contrary. The sport injury socioculture is also apparent in the norms of behavior when an injury occurs, such as the common practice of using participants or other coverage to shield the injured player from spectator view, kicking the ball out of bounds in soccer so as to allow an injured player to receive medical attention, or carrying an injured opponent around the softball bases. The counterpart socioculture and acceptability of aggressive or illegal behavior also relates to sport injury risk and response, with a significant number of injuries associated with illegal behavior (Wiese-Bjornstal, 2010).

The values of the sport world are such that coaches, teammates, fans, and the media often negatively judge athletes who refuse to play hurt. Sadly, some individuals responsible for protecting athletes play the role of motivator when sport injuries threaten competitive success. When administrators, athletic directors, coaches, and parents accept—and in some instances, advocate—continued sport involvement despite injury and contraindication to participate, the injured individual believes that playing with injury is honorable and praiseworthy. Continuing competition may be seen as worth the pain, hampered techniques, and potential for permanent injury.

So in order to fully understand the psychological consequences of sport injury, it is essential to consider the **normative culture** of sport that encourages ignoring or minimizing injury in pursuit of victory. Athletic trainers considering the many interventions they could use must take into account the ways in which the sport culture compounds the psychological complexity of sport injury.

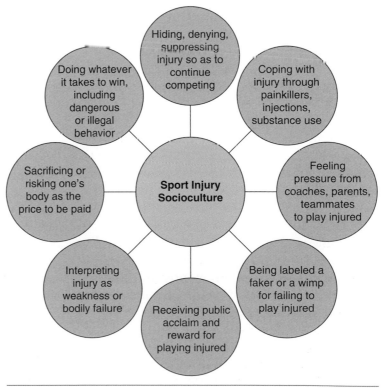

Figure 22.4 Beliefs and actions characterizing the sport injury socioculture.

Developed from Wiese-Bjornstal 2010. Reprinted with permission of the author.

Interventions for Psychological Recovery

Athletic trainers recognize that the body's healing process goes through specific phases entailing an **acute (inflammatory) phase** following the trauma, a **fibroblastic (proliferative) phase** of building, and a **maturation (remodeling) phase** (sometimes called sport specific or functional). By recognizing that the body responds to trauma in physiologically based stages, one can proactively apply various modalities and therapies. Athletic trainers know that with the fibroblastic (proliferative) phase comes the potential for setbacks in rehabilitation or for plateaus in the recovery. Thus athletic trainers can prepare patients for these possibilities, proactively. Athletic trainers also know that patients will want to push the limit in the maturation phase as they approach complete healing. They know that this is the time to balance challenging patients to move through functional progressions and holding them back so that they are not too aggressive in pushing their exercises. Because the athletic trainer is working proactively, he can anticipate the pitfalls of rehabilitation and avoid activities that may cause flare-up of an injury. This proactive approach enables him to augment and support the healing process.

Similarly, sport psychologists and athletic trainers can anticipate the psychological and sport-related challenges that their patients face (Flint 1998b). Rather than reacting to psychological issues, athletic trainers can anticipate and proactively aid the patient. For example, in the acute phase and depending on the injury, the patient is most likely going to be very negative about the situation that caused the injury and about what the future might hold with respect to a return to play. At this time there does not appear to be any light at the end of the tunnel. This is when psychological interventions geared toward negative thought stoppage and immediate goal setting might be most effective; this is the **proactive approach**.

Until recently, it has been primarily intuition that has guided what psychological interventions might be appropriate at specific times within the rehabilitation. Now, with the Integrated Rehabilitation Model (IRM, figure 22.5; Flint 1998a), it is possible to apply an anticipatory or proactive approach to the psychological and sport-related issues that patients face during their rehabilitation. This model provides a framework within which psychological interventions can be anchored so that they are relevant to the tissue healing process, psychological factors, and sport skills or return-to-play factors. Just as an athletic trainer knows that during the fibroblastic (proliferative) phase setbacks are common, we now know that physical events, like setbacks, will directly affect the patient's mood and motivation to continue with rehabilitation. In anticipation of the situation, the athletic trainer can educate the patient to be prepared for the challenge of overcoming the setback. Proactively, the athletic trainer prepares the patient and provides skills to deal with the specific physical and psychological challenge that is coming.

Another problem that we see in the rehabilitation process, particularly after a major injury and lengthy recovery, is a lack of congruence among all the factors involved in a successful return to play. Too often, patients are declared physically ready to return to play but are not prepared for competing either psychologically or in terms of sport factors such as new team offenses or strategies (Flint 2007b). A complete recovery from a sport injury involves much more than just physical rehabilitation. Sport psychological factors and sport-related influences must also be addressed so that the whole body is prepared for the return to sport. Using the physical healing framework upon which to base psychological and sport-related interventions allows for a proactive and logical protocol for a complete rehabilitation. The IRM provides such a framework, incorporating physical or physiological healing factors with psychological reactions to injury and

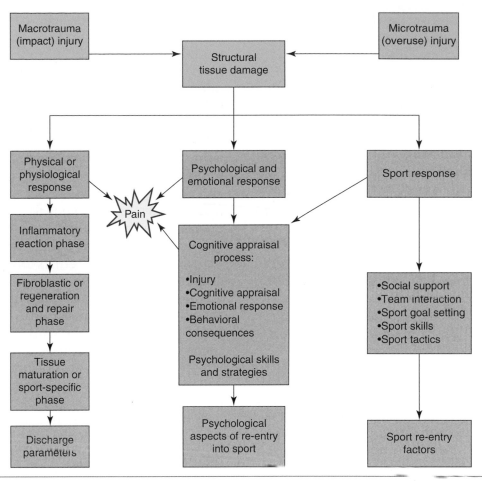

Figure 22.5 Integrated Rehabilitation Model (IRM).

Adapted from F.A. Flint 1998, *Sport psychology and rehabilitation*. Reprinted with permission of the author.

possible interventions along with sport-related features.

How can athletic trainers use the IRM to guide rehabilitation programs to work proactively with patients and ensure a complete recovery? More importantly, how do athletic trainers effectively integrate psychological interventions into their practice? Both of these are legitimate questions particularly in light of the fact that athletic trainers do not typically receive extensive education in sport psychology and are traditionally working overtime in crowded clinical practices. A look at the IRM will show how it might be used to provide a framework for timely psychological and sport-related interventions.

Integrating Physical, Psychological, and Sport Rehabilitation

In figure 22.5, depicting the IRM, the physical aspects of rehabilitation are listed in the first column: the acute (inflammatory) phase, the breakdown and building phase (fibroblastic or proliferative), and the maturation (sport specific or functional) phase. After the phases of healing are complete, the athletic trainer ensures that the discharge parameters are met before clearing the patient for a return to play.

The second column lists aspects of the psychological process, and the third column lists sport-related factors in rehabilitation. Associated with the acute onset of the injury (with macrotrauma or ongoing injury with microtrauma) is the cognitive appraisal of the injury by the patient. Myriad factors (e.g., winning vs. losing a game; first-time injury; season-ending injury) influence the patient in her reaction to the injury. So, along with potential swelling, pain, and loss of function in the physical response comes the cognitive appraisal—how the patient thinks and feels about the injury. At the same time, the patient may be hearing about the extent of the injury and perhaps about subsequent surgery. Concurrently, the team may be dealing with the loss of a key member of the team, replacing the injured athlete with another player, or adjusting team strategies due to the loss. Coaches and team personnel are typically occupied with adjustments that must be made to counteract the effect of the loss of an athlete. So, an acute physical reaction, a psychological reaction, and a sport reaction occur concurrently. The three aspects of the injury are linked; thus in all three, goal setting and other psychological interventions can also be linked.

In the next phase of healing, the proliferative phase, the patient is dealing with potential psychological negativity or depression, as well as a recognition that the team or sport associates are moving on. Here more than ever, one must draw or rely on the mental skills and personal qualities the patient possesses. Here also is the perfect opportunity to make the patient a participant in the healing process rather than a passive recipient of therapy. How can an athletic trainer make use of the skills and qualities of the patient within the physical aspects of the rehabilitation? Patients are used to goal setting and planning for success in sport. Thus, using goal setting in the physical rehabilitation planning, and including patients in the establishment of these goals, creates a sense of collaborative healing. Here, education on how the body heals, recognition of potential setbacks, and charting goals are ideal psychological interventions. As to sport-related actions, this is a favorable time to have coaches provide

input on what the patient can work on while away from the sport, explain if and how the patient can make a meaningful contribution to the team while injured, or update on new offenses and defenses.

The final phase of the physical rehabilitation (maturation or sport specific) marks the convergence of all three aspects of the recovery. Not only does the patient need to be physically ready to return to play; psychological readiness must be also considered. In addition, is the team ready for the teammate to be fully reintegrated? If the athletic trainer has not recognized that a patient is psychologically ready for a return to play, then no amount of physical training or encouragement will ensure a successful reentry. Doubts about reinjury or about where the patient now fits into the sport or team can make him tentative and potentially susceptible to reinjury. What kind of intervention at this point will help him overcome fear and a lack of confidence about being ready to return? One tool that athletic trainers use is functional progressions. Using sport-specific functional progressions is an ideal way to "ramp up" the patient to full participation, but also serves to build his confidence in the previously injured body part. Here again, athletic trainers may not recognize that they are using an intervention that has both physical and psychological ramifications. If the patient's coaches have been surveyed to see what specific skills can be included in the functional progressions, sport-related aspects of the final phase are also being integrated. Thus an integrated rehabilitation process has considered physical, psychological, and sport-related factors. In addition, the rehabilitation has been proactive rather than reactive in its design.

Psychological Skills Interventions

Psychological skills interventions are intentional actions used to improve the sport injury situation. These strategies are employed to achieve better cycles of psychological and physical responses and outcomes. Athletic trainers have a variety of intervention strategies at their disposal that can modify the patient's psychological response to sport injury for the better.

Mental Preparation

The same mental preparation that patients use to excel in sport can be used to overcome injury (Flint 2007a). Individuals routinely use visualizations, goal setting, and relaxation in their sport training, so the use of these psychological interventions, adapted for injury recovery, is logical. There is very clear consensus that the mental preparation of a patient is just as critical as the physical aspects of rehabilitation. If a patient has an optimistic and open approach to rehabilitation, it is more likely that she will comply with the rehabilitation and put forth an appropriate effort to aid in healing.

One of the most important aspects of an appropriate mental approach with the patient is the need to educate about the healing process. For patients who are new to rehabilitation and who have not experienced major injury previously, seeing atrophy, feeling trauma-related pain, and not having full body function are frightening experiences. By educating these patients in the intricacies of sport injury rehabilitation, athletic trainers can provide encouragement that a full recovery is possible. Patients who have been successful in sport will work hard in rehabilitation if they understand the process of healing and what needs to be done to safely return to sport.

Relaxation

Relaxation skills are often taught to patients to help them deal with the stresses related to injury and rehabilitation. Again, this is a reactive rather than a proactive approach since patients are already dealing with the stress of injury. Like sport skills, relaxation skills are best taught when stress levels are at their lowest. This allows for an integration of the new skills into the sport motor patterns without overlying stress. As the patient becomes more adept at using relaxation training, stress levels can be increased. Relaxation, like all other motor skills, requires

practice. A proactive approach to teaching relaxation is to add this skill to preseason training so that if an individual becomes injured, the skill is already integrated into his daily life. Trying to learn a new skill such as relaxation is much more difficult if that patient is already under stress. The challenges that he must face during recovery have been added to the stress of the injury itself, but at least he has a tool with which to deal with the additional stress.

As mentioned previously, relaxation is a motor skill that takes time to teach and requires practice. It appears that progressive relaxation (or Jacobsonian relaxation as named after its developer) is the most effective with athletes because of their inherent connection with their bodies. Athletes are "tuned in" to their bodies, and since progressive relaxation focuses on sensing the body's state of activation, this approach seems most applicable. This form of relaxation does not create a hypnotic state but rather leads to a releasing of tension in muscles. Patients are educated on how to sense the tenseness of muscles and then progressively release that tension. After a few sessions that provide education and practice, most athletes are ready to practice the skill on their own. A secondary benefit of teaching relaxation as a skill before the season starts is that being in a relaxed state is fundamental to the use of other psychological interventions, particularly imagery.

Imagery

Many people use visualizations as a means of either practicing physical skills or rehearsing plays before a competition. Athletic trainers can use this useful skill that participants already possess by educating patients about the healing process. Encouraging them to use their visualization skills to "see" the body healing itself (e.g., seeing new blood vessels, seeing debris being removed from the body) promotes the use of a powerful tool.

In the same way, patients can be taught the basics of how modalities work (e.g., ultrasound) so that they can use visualizations concurrently with modality use. Instead of sitting passively while receiving a modality treatment, the patient can visualize how the modality is affecting tissue. The efficacy of visualizations has been controversial; however, if patients believe that they are enhancing their recovery, visualization is a useful intervention.

Physical Recovery Confidence

While patients may overcome the physical aspects of the injury, if they have not fully dealt with the potential psychological side effects, the recovery will be incomplete and the return to play compromised. Patients who were injured may either fear reinjury while performing the actions that caused the injury or lack confidence in the previously injured body part. One of the tools that athletic trainers may use to help patients overcome these sensitivities is functional progressions. Functional progressions are small, incremental steps that are taken to build toward a complete skill or movement. Since confidence and the dispelling of a fear are difficult to achieve when a return to play is imminent, it is important that athletic trainers provide logical, stepwise progressions of skills or movements. In this way, patients can take the steps in their own time and gain confidence with the successful achievement of each step. These functional progressions typically take place during the maturation phase of the healing process, close to the timing of the reentry into sport (see figure 22.5).

Rational Emotive Therapy

This approach to managing anxiety, developed by psychologist Albert Ellis, can be very effective also in overcoming negative thought patterns regarding sport-related healing and recovery. This intervention helps patients examine beliefs they may have about the injury that are irrational or are not based on clear thinking. The approach has the patient recognize thoughts that may be inappropriately negative and then replace or refute these negative statements with more accurate and positive statements. For example, rational emotive therapy with a female basketball player who has torn her anterior cruciate ligament would have her refute negative statements like "I blew out my knee, and I'll never play again." The basic approach is to recognize what kinds of thought patterns are causing negative affect and then refuting or replacing the negative thoughts with more positive ones.

Goal Setting

Goal setting has been used by athletes and coaches for every aspect of sport development, from learning skills to preparing for important games. Athletic trainers may not recognize that they are using a sport psychological intervention when they do goal setting in their rehabilitation, but in fact they use goal setting every day in clinical practice. For example, in the acute phase when swelling appears, the athletic trainer applies compression and cold. This is a goal-setting approach, although it is rarely recognized as such. So, how can athletic trainers use a goal-setting intervention effectively with patients?

Since athletes are accustomed to goal setting and often use this approach to cardiovascular conditioning or strength gain, it should be a relatively simple task to educate them on an aspect of the healing process and then show them how the corresponding goal can be accomplished. For example, if decreasing swelling is one of the goals in the acute phase, educating the patient about how compression and cold help reduce swelling and giving him a home program may motivate him to comply with the instructions he is given. Explaining how a goal can be achieved and why the process works may encourage patients to follow home program instructions.

As can be seen from the rehabilitation goal-setting chart (Flint 2007b), goals can be established for every aspect of the healing process, including the physical, psychological, and sport-related aspects (table 22.1). While goals can be readily established for these various aspects of recovery, following guidelines on appropriate goal setting is important. For example, goals need to be measurable, performance oriented, and realistic. Setting goals with patients can help ensure a collaborative effort, which may encourage them to take ownership of achieving the goals. In addition, the goals need to be monitored and adjusted as the rehabilitation progresses. Athletic trainers do this every day as they establish baselines and adjust sets and reps in exercise programs. This intervention tool is easy to use and easily adapted to rehabilitation planning.

Patient Education

For patients who have never experienced a severe injury, gaining knowledge of what rehabilitation involves and what the future holds is critical. Patients who have not

Table 22.1 Rehabilitation Goal-Setting Chart

Physical or physiological goals	Psychological goals	Sport goals
Acute (inflammatory) phase (clinical goals) • Reduce swelling • Reduce pain • Protect from further injury • Maintain existing range of motion (ROM) • Educate on healing, nutrition, rehabilitation, psychological factors	**Cognitive appraisal process** • Increase knowledge of injury • Increase knowledge of available coping resources (particularly pain management) • Increase knowledge of support systems • Positive self-talk	**Initial injury phase** • Demonstrate support from coaching staff • Demonstrate support from other people
Fibroblastic (proliferative) phase (clinical goals) • Increase ROM • Maintain cardiovascular fitness • Increase proprioception • Regain muscle endurance • Promote specific tissue healing • Increase flexibility • Address scar tissue • Address other physical issues	**Psychological rehabilitation skills and strategies** • Relaxation, goal setting, rational emotive therapy • Knowledge of setbacks and plateaus • Healing visualizations	**Sport rehabilitation strategies** • Sport skills goal setting • Rehabilitation social support • Sport skill visualizations • Sport tactics and strategies visualizations • Potential team involvement
Maturation (remodeling) phase (functional goals) • Increase sport-specific strength • Increase power • Increase sport-specific functional activity • Increase sport-specific cardiovascular fitness • Increase proprioception • Increase agility • Address psychological issues	**Psychological preparation for reentry into competition** • Increase confidence in body parts via functional progressions • Increase confidence in performance skills • Increase knowledge about "flashbacks" • Performance visualizations • Reentry goals	**Preparation for sport reentry** • Ensure knowledge of team tactics and strategies • Ensure "game fitness" • Ensure understanding of team dynamics
Discharge parameters (from athletic trainer) • Minimum 90% strength (endurance and power) compared to opposite side • Full pain-free ROM • Full flexibility • Pain free • Full proprioception • Sport-specific cardiovascular fitness • Psychological issues addressed (or referred)		

Adapted from Flint, 2007. *Matching psychological strategies with physical rehabilitation.* Reprinted with permission of the author.

previously been involved in rehabilitation do not know what "rehabilitation" means. It is highly unlikely that they will buy into something that takes hard work without any rationale or explanation. In general, the more information a patient has about surgery and rehabilitation, the better the chances of a successful approach to recovery.

Typically, patients want to know about both procedural and outcome factors, especially if the injury recovery involves surgery. Procedural information includes information about what may happen during surgery, whether there will be pain, and what a scar might look like, as well as information about how to deal with the body's reactions to injury such as swelling and loss of range of motion. Outcome factors include long-term details such as success rates with recovery from this kind of injury and the length of time it may take to return to play. Patients who have just successfully recovered from a similar injury are often good sources of information.

Social Support Interventions

Social support refers to receiving help, comfort, and assistance from other people in challenging life situations such as sport injury. Social support interventions can take many forms, including injury recovery clubs, surgical clubs, and potentially modeling interactions. **Modeling** is a process of gaining knowledge and support from observing others and learning actions and attitudes through observation. Patients experiencing a major trauma, and perhaps surgery for the first time, will rely heavily on observations of others who have experience with these situations. Acquiring information and appropriate behaviors by watching others cope successfully with a medical situation is an ideal way to share knowledge about injury recovery.

Often patients feel isolated from their teammates and coaching staff. Prior to injury, these are the very individuals who typically provide social support in difficult times. Forming injury social support clubs (e.g., Anterior Cruciate Ligament [ACL] Club)

establishes a new support system with like individuals. The club could be a surgical recovery club or one that deals with specific injuries such as concussions. In many cases, these support clubs take the place of the patient's team and the participants form a bond based on shared experiences.

Modeling is a psychosocial intervention that is often used within medical settings without necessarily being recognized. For example, an athletic trainer points out someone who has already recovered from a specific injury to a patient who has just experienced the same injury. The patient who has just been injured sees someone who has recovered from the injury and has successfully returned to sport. This can be a very strong motivating factor in relation to the newly injured patient's commitment to the rehabilitation program. Research conducted using modeling in medical settings has shown remarkable results with the provision of behavioral cues to patients undergoing stressful medical procedures (Flint 1991; Kulik and Mahler 1987). Showing a patient someone who is similar in terms of position played, injury, surgical procedure, or size helps the viewer gain an understanding of how to act based on what the "similar other" does.

It could be said that two approaches to modeling can help patients overcome severe sport injury or surgery (Flint 2007a). Informal modeling happens every time an athletic trainer points out someone who has successfully returned to sport after a specific injury. Again, the viewer gains a sense that recovery from the injury is possible because the other patient has been able to recover. In a formal modeling situation, a patient might be intentionally paired with another patient who is one or two steps ahead in the recovery process. If the two patients do their rehabilitation at the same time, the one who is at an earlier step can see what to expect next and how the model copes with and overcomes rehabilitation challenges and setbacks. As one caveat to this approach, the athletic trainer may have to anticipate that setbacks in the model's rehabilitation could be discouraging to the viewer. There is always the chance that the model's rehabilitation will hit a snag and be delayed. Once the problem is overcome, however, this kind of example is very powerful because it shows the viewer how to cope with adversity in rehabilitation. Whether modeling is informal or formal, it is a very strong and motivating intervention in sport injury rehabilitation.

Psychological and sport-related interventions that help make patients active participants in the rehabilitation process rather than passive bystanders can only enhance the healing process. Motivating patients to "buy into" active participation in their own recovery creates a positive and collaborative rehabilitation.

Implementation of a Psychosocial Care Plan

How do athletic trainers implement a comprehensive system of care that accommodates the psychological needs of patients? Effective management involves attention to a holistic approach to such factors as sport injury care, an understanding of the appropriate roles of athletic trainers in mental health care, and the establishment of effective proactive plans to meet psychological needs.

Holistic Approach to Injury Care

As we have seen, sport injury creates not only physical changes for the patient but emotional and psychological changes as well. When working with the patient, it is important to bear in mind that a heart and a head are attached to the physically injured body. Therefore, holistic care for the patient, addressing needs of the body, mind and spirit, is essential. The athletic trainer's role in providing this care is outlined in the *Role Delineation Study* (Board of Certification [BOC] 2010) and *Athletic Training Educa-*

tional Competencies (National Athletic Trainers' Association [NATA] 2011).

Role of the Athletic Trainer

The BOC (2010) and NATA (2011) requirements lead to several specific recommendations for the role of athletic trainers in managing the psychological aspects of sport injury and rehabilitation. These include understanding their scope of expertise and counseling roles, recognizing psychological distress, working as part of a team, and making referrals to mental health professionals.

Expected Scope of Expertise

The BOC's *Role Delineation Study* (2010) defines the role of the athletic trainer by identifying the task knowledge and skill set needed to be a competent entry-level athletic trainer. Knowledge and skills relative to psychosocial aspects of the injury process are scattered across the five performance domains (injury/illness prevention and wellness protection; clinical evaluation and diagnosis; immediate and emergency care; treatment and rehabilitation; organizational and professional health and well-being) identified in the study. Since the *Role Delineation Study* functions as a blueprint for the development of the BOC national certification exam, psychosocial aspects of injury and referral must also be addressed within accredited athletic training education programs.

Athletic Training Educational Competencies (NATA 2011) guide the curricular development of athletic training education programs by outlining the minimal knowledge and skills to be mastered by students in their entry-level education. Psychosocial strategies and referral is identified as one of the eight content areas to be included in athletic training education. Combined with the knowledge and skills identified in the *Role Delineation Study* (BOC 2010), these competencies reflect the current practice expectations of athletic trainers relative to psychosocial issues and referral (see the sidebar).

SUMMARY OF PSYCHOSOCIAL INTERVENTION AND REFERRAL KNOWLEDGE AND SKILLS FOR ENTRY-LEVEL CERTIFIED ATHLETIC TRAINERS

Knowledge of

- Professional network for mental health referral
- Athletic trainer's scope of practice relative to psychosocial dysfunction
- Psychosocial aspects of pain perception and control
- Stress response model and its application to injury risk and occurrence
- Sign and symptoms of psychosocial disorders, including eating disorders, substance abuse, psychological adjustment to injury
- Psychological reaction to injury and illness
- Psychosocial aspects related to treatment, rehabilitation, reconditioning, and return to participation
- Basic principles of mental preparation, relaxation, visualization, and desensitization techniques

- Motivation and relaxation techniques for rehabilitation
- Response to catastrophic events and psychosocial referral needs for all involved parties
- Effective communication techniques

Skill in

- Making appropriate referrals for psychosocial issues
- Identifying signs and symptoms of psychosocial dysfunction
- Incorporating psychosocial techniques (motivation, visualization, imagery, goal setting, desensitization, stress management) into rehabilitation
- Communicating with mental health care professionals while preserving confidentiality of the patient
- Using appropriate counseling techniques

Developed by Kenow 2010. Reprinted with permission of the author.

Athletic Trainer as Front-Line Counselor

In managing psychosocial issues in the injury setting, athletic trainers often serve as frontline counselors. The daily contact athletic trainers have with sport participants helps foster a trusting relationship. With use of the communication and counseling skills described earlier in this chapter, athletic trainers' daily interactions with patients will nurture good rapport with them and create an athletic training room environment that is safe, supportive, and welcoming. Listening to patients in an open and nonjudgmental manner and showing empathy with their situation and challenges further helps to develop trust and rapport. Thus when injuries occur, patients are more likely to discuss their feelings and concerns.

The daily contact athletic trainers have with sport participants also places them in an ideal position to recognize small behavioral and emotional changes that may signal struggles to cope with certain aspects of injuries or sport participation. Competent athletic trainers are expected to recognize the presence of psychosocial difficulties and intervene to determine the extent and nature of the problems.

Recognizing Psychosocial Distress

Fortunately, psychosocial issues often manifest themselves in recognizable signs and symptoms, just as do physical problems. These signs and symptoms may include the following:

- Atypical behavior for the individual—the outgoing, energetic, boisterous person becomes withdrawn and lethargic
- Changes in appearance—the individual appears tired or fatigued or shows decreased regard for physical appearance or hygiene
- Rehabilitation difficulties—the patient shows a lack of compliance with the rehabilitation program or lack of effort during rehabilitation exercises
- Complaints of pain that seem incongruous with the amount of tissue damage the patient has suffered
- Psychophysiological complaints such as not sleeping or eating, tension headaches, or upset stomach

The observational skills that athletic trainers use to recognize signs and symptoms of physical dysfunction can also enable them to recognize these indications of psychological or emotional distress. Witnessing any of these signs or symptoms in individuals necessitates at least conversations with them to determine the underlying cause for these new behaviors.

Following such conversations, athletic trainers may feel comfortable using some of the intervention techniques previously described in this chapter to assist patients; but in other instances, they may recognize that the situation is beyond their scope of expertise or training, at which point referral may be required. Both the *Role Delineation Study* (BOC 2010) and *Athletic Training Educational Competencies* (NATA 2011) stress the importance of athletic trainers' recognizing the scope of their education and training and understanding the limits they face in independently handling some of the psychosocial issues in the injury process. Furthermore, the NATA code of ethics (2005) states that it is critical for athletic trainers to "provide only those services for which they are qualified

through education or experience and which are allowed by their practice acts and other pertinent regulation" (p. 2). Thus, when an athletic trainer's level of education or experience is exceeded, it is her ethical duty to make appropriate referrals.

Sports Medicine Team Approach to Injury Care

The previous discussion emphasizes the importance of a team approach to sport injury care. The sports medicine team is a collaboration of various health care professionals, each with their own areas of expertise and training, who function collectively to provide the best possible care for injured patients. Athletic trainers frequently establish a comprehensive referral network to address patients' physical needs. Unfortunately, the referral network of mental health care providers is often less comprehensive and in some cases absent. Ask an athletic trainer to list a good orthopedist for a knee injury and he will readily provide a name; ask him to list a good psychologist for a depressed injured patient and he may struggle to provide the same information.

Psychosocial Referral Sources

Mental health care providers should be an integral part of sports medicine teams and referral networks. A wide variety of mental health care professionals can provide beneficial assistance in the comprehensive care of patients recovering from sport injury. Table 22.2 provides a list of mental health professionals who could potentially be included in referral networks. Many of these professionals may be available to athletic trainers through on-campus or community resources.

Proactive Approach to Establishing a Referral Network

Athletic trainers are encouraged to take a proactive approach in developing relationships with mental health professionals rather than reactively seeking them out after a

Table 22.2 **Mental Health Professionals as Potential Referral Sources**

Title	Degree	Good source for:
Psychiatrist	MD	Chronic and debilitating psychological disorders (e.g., depression, manic-depressive and obsessive-compulsive disorders, schizophrenia)
Psychologist (clinical, counseling)	PhD, PsyD, or EdD	Grief, depression, psychosocial adjustment disorders, psychological disorders
Social worker	MSW	Mental health or environmental event that hinders life functioning
Counselor or marriage and family therapist	MS or MA	Depression, addiction, suicidal impulse, stress management, self-esteem
Sport psychologist (clinical, educational)	PhD, PsyD (MS or MA for some educational)	Motivation, relaxation, psychological obstacles in performance or healing
Academic counselor	MS, MA, or MEd	Career counseling, academic difficulties
Alcohol or drug abuse counselor	Varies	Substance misuse or abuse
Clergy	Varies	Spiritual guidance for adjustment issues

Adapted from Brewer, Petitpas, and Van Raalte 1999; Lemberger 2008.

situation arises requiring their expertise. This approach is essential for planning how to deal with the aftermath of catastrophic injuries or events but is also vital to one's ability to expeditiously consult on or refer patients dealing with less serious injuries. The proactive approach includes the following steps:

- Identifying potential professional mental health resources in the community
- Making initial contact with those resources and communicating with them regarding their comfort level in working with physically active people
- Defining the perceived areas of expertise of these resources
- Using these professionals for consultation and referral when needed

It may be beneficial for these professionals to have experience with the sport environment and an understanding of the unique pressures and challenges that participants within it face.

Making a Successful Psychosocial Referral

From a practical standpoint, once an athletic trainer has assessed that there might be some type of psychosocial dysfunction in a patient, the first step is to consult with a mental health care professional regarding an appropriate course of action (Brewer, Petitpas, and Van Raalte 1999). Without disclosing the identity of the patient, the athletic trainer can describe what he is witnessing in the patient and the reasons for concern. The mental health care professional can then offer advice as to a best course of action. Sometimes this will result in a recommendation for immediate referral; other times the mental health care professional may suggest an intervention that could be performed by the athletic training staff. If an intervention is suggested and is performed by the athletic trainer, the outcome of the intervention should always be discussed with the mental health professional to determine if further action is needed.

If referral is suggested (immediately or after the initial intervention), the athletic trainer can take the following steps to increase the likelihood that a patient will be receptive to the referral:

1. Gain the patient's trust and provide assurance that he has the patient's best interests in mind
2. Objectively describe the patient's behaviors that have caused concern

3. Express a desire to assist the patient, yet admit the limitations in his own scope of training and explain why he would not be the best provider of care in this situation

4. Assure the patient that another competent professional on the sports medicine team could provide better care

5. Offer to make an appointment with the other professional and accompany the patient to her first appointment.

Overcoming Resistance to Psychosocial Referral

Regardless of how the athletic trainer approaches the referral, he may encounter some hesitation on the part of the patient. Patients are often concerned with the perception that others (e.g., coaches, teammates, significant others) may have about seeking mental health assistance; therefore, it is essential to assure them that confidentiality will be strictly maintained throughout the process. Additionally, patients by nature are independent, self-sufficient people who find it difficult to seek help. Often there is a stigma within the athletic community that seeking mental health care is a sign of weakness. It is imperative that the athletic trainer attempt to minimize this stigma by normalizing mental health professionals as part of the sports medicine team and emphasizing that using their expertise is actually a sign of strength—the patient is taking control of health and healing by accessing the best-trained professionals to assist with the process. Just as the patient would not hesitate to seek additional medical assistance for physical aspects of her injury, she should use mental health consultations when struggling to cope with the psychological and

CASE STUDY

Case Study

Jill was excited about heading off to college and beginning her collegiate soccer career. She was expecting great things. However, 2 weeks into the school year, things are looking a little different. Jill was already anxious about having to take out the $8,000 in school loans to get her through the year, but her parents said they'd help her pay them off. She has just learned that her father has been laid off from his job due to slow economic times. Jill's mom doesn't currently hold a job because she stays home to care for her elderly mother, who lives with the family. To make matters worse, Jill's boyfriend of 3 years called last Friday to tell her that he wanted to break up with her, saying it was too difficult to maintain a long-distance relationship. Jill had already been struggling to keep up with her homework for classes (she never realized how hard she'd have to study in college), and now she finds concentrating even more difficult. She is having trouble sleeping because her mind keeps racing about everything that is going on, and she's experiencing headaches on almost a daily basis. Her sleep difficulty has left her feeling tired and fatigued during the day and is affecting her practices. Jill feels her play has fallen off dramatically since last year, and she is worried that she is letting down her coaches, who had recruited her heavily, and her teammates.

Think About It

1. What are some of the things in Jill's life that are stressful for her?

2. What might you observe about Jill that alerts you to the fact that she is feeling "stressed out"?

3. How might this stress be affecting her sport injury risk?

4. What are some things an athletic trainer could do to help reduce her stress levels?

emotional aspects. To further minimize the stigma of mental health consultation, it is a good idea, whenever possible, to introduce mental health professionals to the patients at the same time that other more traditional health care specialists (such as team doctors) on the sports medicine team are introduced.

Summary

To summarize, athletic trainers are expected to receive educational training and prepara-

tion to handle psychosocial aspects of sport injury. Despite these expectations, research has shown that athletic trainers sometimes feel unprepared to handle such situations (e.g., Stiller-Ostrowski and Ostrowski 2009). Even in these circumstances, athletic trainers can still serve several important functions. To fulfill these functions, they should know competent mental health professionals with whom they can consult; communicate with those professionals regarding a best course of action; and when necessary, make appropriate referrals.

Learning Aids

SUMMARY

It is no less important to consider the psychological aspects of sport injury than it is to consider the physical aspects. Psychological and sociocultural factors affect risk of sport injury and prevention efforts, recovery from sport injury, rehabilitation effectiveness, and return to play. A variety of interventions, such as imagery, goal setting, modeling, and patient education, provide psychological support and assistance to patients. Athletic trainers must be prepared to manage the psychological aspects of sport injury in the same ways they manage the physical aspects, through competent understanding of the scope and issues, effective proactive planning, consultation with other professionals, and the implementation of management plans. Evidence shows us that physical health is tied to psychological health, and patients are best served by a comprehensive athletic training approach that advantages both.

KEY CONCEPTS AND REVIEW

▸ **Outline the elements of the Sport Injury Risk Profile (SIRP).**

- Biological: internal physical and physiological characteristics of individual participants
- Psychological: internal mental characteristics of the individual participant
- Physical: external aspects of the physical environments surrounding participation
- Sociocultural: external aspects of the interpersonal, social, and cultural environment

▸ **Explain the relationship between stress and athletic injury.**

The more "stress" patients perceive, the more vulnerable they are to being injured, particularly if they do not have sufficient personal or social resources for buffering or coping with the stress.

▸ **Identify the psychological responses of patients to injury, including cognitions, affects, behaviors, and outcomes (CABO), using the model described in the chapter.**

- *Cognition:* The cognitions, or thoughts, of patients—immediately postinjury and dynamically throughout cycles of rehabilitation and recovery—involve mentally evaluating a variety of aspects of the sport injury. Patients appraise such things as meanings, losses, challenges, and perceptions.

- *Affect:* Emotions, feelings, or moods of patients during sport injury often arise from their thoughts, change throughout the injury and recovery process, and influence patient behaviors and recoveries. Some of the most commonly noted negative mood states following a sport injury are anxiety or tension, depression, and frustration; others include boredom, anger, and fatigue.

- *Behavior:* What patients do, their observable actions, have a great bearing on their recoveries. Examples of actions are adherence to or compliance with treatment regimens, use of mental skills and strategies, use of social networks, risk-taking behaviors, and the effort and intensity with which the patient pursues rehabilitation.

- *Outcome:* The results, effects, or consequences of patient cognition affect behavior over time, such as recovery progress, functional outcomes, or returning to training or competition.

▶ **Describe how characteristics of the sport injury socioculture affect participant health.**

Sport injury socioculture refers to the social and cultural structures, climates, processes, and interventions that influence sport injury risk and the participant's response to the injury, recovery, and return to play. The socioculture is one that encourages, rewards, and praises participants who risk injury and compete when injured and dismisses players who refuse to do so as weak or cowardly.

▶ **Explain the Integrated Rehabilitation Model (IRM) as presented in the text.**

The IRM provides a framework within which psychological interventions can be anchored so that they are relevant to the tissue healing process, psychological factors, and sport skills or return-to-play factors.

▶ **List and explain the psychological skills interventions that patients can use in sport injury situations.**

- Mental preparation: understanding the roles and responsibilities of being on the team, understanding expectations of teammates and coaches, and understanding what to expect after injury and during recovery and healing

- Relaxation: a physical and mental relaxation technique in which participants sense the tenseness of muscles and then progressively release the tension

- Imagery: visualizing the events, skills, or mechanics of both sport participation and the healing process

- Physical recovery confidence: the building of confidence and the dispelling of fear as achieved using stepwise progressions of skills or movements

- Rational emotive therapy: a therapy that focuses on overcoming negative thought patterns regarding sport participation or healing and recovery

- Goal setting: establishing measurable, performance-oriented, and realistic goals for sport participation and injury recovery and healing

- Patient education: helping patients gain knowledge of what rehabilitation involves and what the future holds

- Social support: the use of peers and groups to help the patient gain information and learn appropriate behaviors through talking to others who have coped successfully with a medical situation

▶ **Outline the things that would help athletic trainers recognize psychosocial distress in a patient.**

- Atypical behavior for the individual—the outgoing, energetic, boisterous individual becomes withdrawn and lethargic

- Changes in appearance—the individual appears tired or fatigued or shows decreased regard for physical appearance or hygiene

• Rehabilitation difficulties—the patient shows a lack of compliance with the rehabilitation program or a lack of effort during rehabilitation exercises

• Complaints of pain that seem incongruous with the amount of tissue damage the patient has suffered

• Psychophysiological complaints such as not sleeping or eating, tension headaches, or upset stomach

▶ **List the steps an athletic trainer should take to establish a psychosocial referral network before it is needed.**

• Identify potential professional mental health resources in the community

• Make initial contact with those resources and communicate with them regarding their comfort level in working with athletic patients

• Define the perceived areas of expertise of these resources

• Use these professionals for consultation and referral when needed

▶ **List the steps the athletic trainer could take to increase the likelihood that a patient will be receptive to psychosocial referral.**

• Gain the patient's trust and provide assurance that he has the patient's best interests in mind

• Objectively describe the patient's behaviors that have caused concern

• Express a desire to assist the patient, but admit the limitations in his own scope and explain why he would be not the best provider of care in this situation

• Assure the patient that another competent professional on the sports medicine team could provide better care

• Offer to make an appointment with that professional and accompany the patient to her first appointment

PRACTICE!

For hands-on practice in this area, go to the web resource and complete the following:

Level 3.3, Module N5: Rehabilitation Adherence and Motivation

Level 3.5, Module P3: Psychosocial Intervention

CRITICAL THINKING QUESTIONS

1. You are serving as the athletic trainer for the women's volleyball team. One of the senior members of the team has come to you in tears, saying that her mother has been diagnosed with cancer and has been given little hope for recovery. This is the same player who, earlier in the week, was telling teammates that her boyfriend of 3 years was cheating on her and that they had broken up. Do these factors raise any concern with you regarding her practice and sport participation? What might you watch for to ensure that she is staying focused on volleyball during practices and games?

2. One of the patients doing knee rehabilitation has appeared very lethargic and unmotivated in the last few sessions. How could you better understand what might be going on?

Evidence-Based Practice

Tamara C. Valovich McLeod, PhD, ATC, FNATA

OBJECTIVES

After reading this chapter, the student should be able to do the following:

- Define evidence-based practice (EBP).
- Describe the need for EBP in athletic training.
- Describe the five steps in the EBP process.
- Formulate an answerable clinical question using the PICO format.
- Describe the 5S approach to searching the medical literature.
- Understand the various criteria that are needed to appraise published research studies.
- Describe the process of integrating the evidence into clinical practice.
- Understand the usefulness of clinical decision rules and guidelines in patient care.
- Discuss the importance of measuring clinical outcomes in assessing the EBP process.
- Identify the questions you should ask during your self-evaluation of the EBP process.

This chapter provides an overview of evidence-based practice (EBP) for the athletic trainer. The concept of EBP is defined and the importance of EBP within the athletic training profession will be discussed. The chapter explores the five steps of the EBP process: defining a clinical question, searching for evidence, critically appraising the evidence, integrating the evidence, and evaluating the outcomes and one's performance of EBP. The last section of the chapter presents specific information about grading the levels of evidence and providing a strength of recommendation of the literature.

The Essence of Evidence–Based Practice

Evidence-based practice is formally defined as "the conscientious, explicit, and judicious use of the best evidence in making decisions about the care of individual patients" (Sackett et al. 1996, p.71). It is a process that incorporates a clinician's clinical expertise, the individual patient's values, and research regarding the **efficacy** and **effectiveness** of treatment or other findings into an integrated decision-making process (Sackett et al. 1996). The overarching goal of EBP is to improve clinical practice through improving a patient's outcomes.

Rather than providing a cookbook approach to health care, EBP uses a hierarchy of evidence to assist in answering clinical questions regarding individual patients (Guyatt et al. 2008). This evidence should be patient oriented and clinically relevant to the day-to-day care provided by athletic trainers (Steves and Hootman 2004). Patient-oriented evidence includes information from studies that evaluate outcomes deemed important by patients. These may include morbidity, symptom resolution, functional improvements, and quality of life (Hurwitz et al. 2000).

Furthermore, clinical decision making should take into account the experiences and expertise of the treating clinician, including the identification of each patient's unique

health status and weighing of the individual risks and benefits of the treatment for an individual patient (figure 23.1). The values of the patient and his family need to be accounted for as well as through an understanding of the unique preferences, concerns, and expectations of each patient. Lastly, the available health care resources play a role in the EBP clinical decision-making process. For example, it may be that a treatment modality with proven efficacy exists but that a secondary school athletic trainer does not have access to that particular modality in her setting.

The Importance of Evidence–Based Practice to Athletic Training

Evidence-based practice is essential for ensuring a scientific foundation for clinical athletic training practice (Sackett et al. 1996; Steves and Hootman 2004; Hertel 2005), as a central principle of EBP is to use the best research evidence to guide clinical decision making. Through the use of EBP, athletic trainers can apply tests and treatments supported by the evidence in their clinical practice in order to improve patient care.

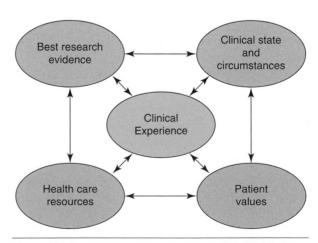

Figure 23.1 Evidence-based clinical decision making.

Based on Haynes, Devereaux, and Guyatt 2002; and DiCenso, Cullum, and Ciliska 1998.

The process of EBP also promotes critical thinking among clinicians. Clinicians must be open-minded about treatments and interventions that differ from what they have been taught but that are supported by evidence.

The inclusion of EBP in athletic training education is important, as the Institute of Medicine (2003) core competencies for health professions education promote the teaching and learning of EBP, and the PEW Health Professions Commission (1998) highlights that health care providers should provide evidence-based clinically competent care. Additionally, both agencies affirm the need for quality improvement in health professions education and clinical practice, which can be achieved through the evaluation of patient outcomes. Educators should provide students with the tools necessary to develop clinical questions, search for and appraise evidence, and model evidence-based practice in providing patient care.

Indirectly, the use of EBP in athletic training can further develop and advance the athletic training profession (Steves and Hootman 2004; Hertel 2005; Parsons et al. 2008). Promoting research on effective interventions and outcomes may enhance the reputation of the athletic training profession and increase opportunities for reimbursement.

The Steps of Evidence-Based Practice

Evidence-based practice is accomplished through a series of five interrelated steps that begins with identifying a clinical question regarding a specific patient and ends with evaluation of the patient's outcomes. The steps include (1) formulating an answerable clinical question, (2) searching the medical literature, (3) appraising published studies, (4) integrating the evidence into clinical practice, and (5) evaluating the EBP process and the patient's outcomes. The practice of EBP is a lifelong, self-directed learning process in which clinicians continually self-evaluate their abilities in order to improve the care they deliver to patients (Sackett and Rosenberg 1995).

Defining a Clinical Question

The first step in EBP is asking an answerable clinical question. Clinical questions are asked using the PICO format, in which the clinician identifies the patient population or clinical problem of interest (P), an intervention of interest (I), a treatment to which the intervention will be compared (C), and an outcome of interest (O). Ideally, the outcome of interest should be a patient-centered outcome that has the potential to change one's clinical practice (Hurwitz et al. 2000). The PICO format provides a standard template for asking answerable questions, ensures that clinicians are thoughtful in the formatting of questions, and aids in the later search for evidence that may answer the clinical question. Clinical questions are most often at the cutting edge of health care in the areas of therapy, diagnosis, or current theories regarding the pathology of injury or illness and can be directly applied to a specific patient or problem. PICO questions are categorized into diagnosis, therapy/prevention, harm/etiology, and prognosis, although they may include economic or decision analyses. Table 23.1 provides examples of clinical questions written in the PICO format.

Searching the Literature

Once a clinical question is formulated, the clinician needs to begin a search of the medical literature for relevant answers. The use of the answerable clinical question described earlier can allow clinicians to easily convert the PICO terms into keyword search terms. Search terms can then be linked using Boolean connectors (AND, OR, NOT) to broaden or focus the search. Using AND can broaden the search, and using OR can focus the search. The use of controlled vocabulary, such as Medical Subject Headings (MeSH), can ease the burden of the search by saving time and decreasing the

Table 23.1	Types of Clinical Questions	
	Definition	**Athletic training example**
Diagnosis	Studies that evaluate diagnostic tests, in order to exclude or confirm a diagnosis, based on their precision, accuracy, acceptability, safety, or expense	In active individuals (P), is the McMurray test (I) more accurate (O) in detecting meniscal lesions compared to the joint line tenderness test (C)?
Prognosis	Studies that estimate the patient's likely clinical course and any complications	Does massage (I) decrease healing time (O) in patients with hamstring strains (P) better than stretching (C)?
Therapy/Prevention/ Screening	Studies of treatments to offer patients that do more good than harm and that are worth the efforts and costs of using them Studies that investigate the chance of disease by identifying and modifying risk factors through early screening	In postsurgical patients (P), what is the effect of continuous passive motion (I) compared to immobilization (C) on acute range of motion gains (O)?
Etiology/Harm	Studies that identify risk factors or causes of disease	Are football players (P) with a history of multiple concussions (I) at greater risk for cognitive deficits (O) compared to those without a concussion history (C)?

chance of overlooking evidence that could answer the clinical question (Stillwell et al. 2010). Furthermore, the use of limits, including publication years, human subjects, and English language, can aid in streamlining the search.

With the abundance of published literature, a planned search strategy for information that is already summarized and appraised can greatly assist clinicians in finding answers to their clinical questions. The "5S" approach provides a strategy to search within an organized model of evidence-based information that is more relevant to point-of-care application (Haynes 2006). The 5S model depicted in figure 23.2 illustrates an approach in which clinicians begin their search for information that is already summarized and appraised to find a relevant answer to their clinical question efficiently; it also provides examples of databases that fit each level.

Systems refers to computerized decision support systems, ideally linked to a patient's electronic health record, that would automatically connect summarized evidence to the patient's clinical problem (Haynes 2001). The clinician would then have the latest evidence available at the time of the patient encounter to integrate with his clinical experience and the patient's preferences in order to make appropriate clinical decisions. At this time,

there are no systems that reach this level of sophistication in athletic training.

Summaries can include evidence-based electronic textbooks and abstracts that integrate evidence from the lower levels. Clinical topic summaries are advantageous because they tend to include information on multiple aspects of management for a given illness or condition, as opposed to the lower levels that often provide evidence for only one aspect of management (Haynes 2006).

Synopses are evidence-based journal abstracts that briefly describe **systematic reviews** and original research studies. These often provide clinicians with enough evidence to support a clinical decision, avoiding the need to search for and read the entire original paper (Haynes 2001).

Syntheses include systematic reviews and **meta-analyses** that are based on a clinical question of interest and follow a specific process for the identification, search, and selection of included investigations (Haynes 2001).

Studies include original journal articles accessed through Medline or similar databases. At this level, the clinician must not only search for the evidence but must also sort through numerous citations for relevance and critically appraise the evidence obtained. This level can include **randomized controlled trials**, **cohort studies**, **case-**

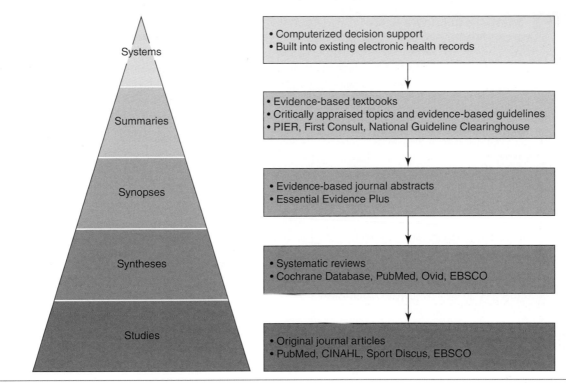

Figure 23.2 The 5S model of health care research evidence organization.

Adapted, by permission, from R.B. Haynes, 2006, "Of studies, syntheses, synopses, summaries, and systems: the "5S" evolution of information services for evidence-based health care decisions," *ACP Journal Club* 145(3): A8.

control studies, cross-sectional studies, case series, and case reports, among other study designs.

Appraising the Literature

The evidence obtained from searching at the studies or syntheses levels requires the clinician to evaluate or appraise the article before a decision can be made regarding its clinical usefulness. Not all published articles can be taken at face value, as there is the potential for bias in the reporting of study results. The rapid critical appraisal is advocated as a means to quickly evaluate an article for its validity, importance, and applicability to the clinical question and patient of interest (Guyatt et al. 2008). Table 23.2 provides examples of rapid critical appraisal questions asked for the various categories of studies. Additionally, critical appraisal checklists, specific to the study design, can be used to quantitatively evaluate the reporting of various elements within the article (table 23.3).

One can also appraise the evidence by evaluating the study design and assigning a **level of evidence** to a particular article. The study design hierarchy is important to understand as one means of interpreting the value of the results for clinical decision making. Studies can then be assigned a level of evidence based on the design as shown in figure 23.3. Levels of evidence are used with individual studies to help clinicians to determine the value of the results reported findings. One of the most widely used taxonomies, the Oxford Centre for Evidence-Based Medicine Levels of Evidence (2009), ranks studies from 1 through 5. Level 1 evidence is that gained from the most unbiased study designs: systematic reviews of randomized controlled trials or individual randomized controlled trials. The Strength of Recommendation Taxonomy (SORT) assigns levels of evidence initially based off the study outcome: disease-oriented evidence (DOE) or patient-oriented evidence (POE) (Ebell, 2004). Disease-oriented evidence includes physiological or surrogate outcomes such as blood pressure or blood sugar that may

Table 23.2 Questions to Ask in a Rapid Critical Appraisal

	Are the results valid?	What are the results?	How can I apply the results to patient care?
Diagnosis	Did participating patients present a diagnostic dilemma? Was there an appropriate, independent reference standard? Did investigators apply the same reference standard to all patients regardless of the results of the test under investigation?	What likelihood ratios were associated with the range of possible test results?	Will the reproducibility of the test result and its interpretation be satisfactory in my setting? Are the study results applicable to my patients? Will the test results change my management strategy? Will patients be better off as a result of the test?
Harm	Cohort: Were patients similar as to prognostic factors known to be associated with the outcome? Were the circumstances and methods for detecting outcome similar? Was the follow-up sufficiently complete? Case control: Were cases and controls similar with respect to the indication of circumstances that would lead to exposure? Were the circumstances and methods for determining exposure similar for cases and controls?	How strong is the association between exposure and outcome? How precise was the estimate of risk?	Were the study patients similar to my patient? Was follow-up sufficiently long? Was the exposure similar to what might occur in my patient? What was the magnitude of the risk? Are there any benefits known to be associated with the exposure?
Prognosis	Was the sample of patients representative? Were the patients sufficiently homogeneous with respect to prognostic risk? Was follow-up sufficiently complete? Were outcome criteria objective and unbiased?	How likely are the outcomes over time? How precise are the estimates of likelihood?	Were the study patients and their management similar to mine? Was the follow-up sufficiently long? Can I use the results in the management of my patients?
Therapy	Were patients randomized? Was randomization concealed? Were patients in the study groups similar with respect to known prognostic factors? To what extent was the study blinded? Was follow-up complete? Were patients analyzed in the groups to which they were randomized? Was the trial stopped early?	How large was the treatment effect? How precise was the estimate of the treatment effect?	Were the study patients similar to my patient? Were all patient-important outcomes considered? Are the likely treatment benefits worth the potential harm and costs?

Adapted from Guyatt et al. 2008.

Table 23.3 Critical Appraisal Checklists

Title	Use	Checklist
CONSORT: Consolidated standards of reporting trials	Evidence-based minimum set of recommendations for reporting the results of randomized controlled trials	25 items
STROBE: Strengthening the reporting of observational studies in epidemiology	Checklist of items to include in articles reporting observational studies including cohort, case control, and cross-sectional	22 items
STARD: Standards for the reporting of diagnostic accuracy studies	Evaluation of studies of diagnostic accuracy to assess the potential for bias and to evaluate generalizability	25 items
PRISMA: Preferred reporting items for systematic reviews and meta-analyses	Evidence-based minimum set of standards for reporting systematic reviews and meta-analyses	27 items
MOOSE: Meta-analysis of observational studies in epidemiology	Guidelines to evaluate the reporting of observational meta-analyses	35 items

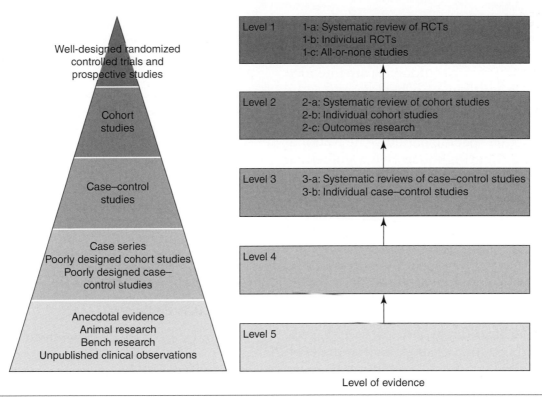

Figure 23.3 Evidence hierarchy with study design.

Reprinted, by permission, from J.M. Medina, P.O. McKeon, J. Hertel, 2006, "Rating the levels of evidence in sports-medicine research," *Athletic Therapy Today* 11(5): 42-45.

not reflect that a patient's outcomes have improved, while POE includes outcomes that matter to patients, including mortality, morbidity, and a reduction of symptoms (Ebell, 2004). All studies of DOE are assigned a Level 3, and POE studies are assigned Level 1 for higher quality study design and Level 2 for lower quality study design.

Systematic reviews or detailed searches of a body of literature may also be assigned a **strength of recommendation** (SOR), which provides a mechanism for clinicians to evaluate the evidence for its applicability and use in clinical practice. The SOR is usually assigned an A, B, C, D, or I depending on the quality, quantity, and consistency of the included studies. For example, a grade of A may be given when a body of evidence consists of numerous Level 1 studies with similar findings or consistent results; a grade of B represents consistent Level 2 or 3 studies; a grade of C denotes conflicting evidence or evidence from Level 4 studies; a grade of D or I indicates insufficient evidence available

to make a clinical recommendation (Medina et al. 2006).

Integrating the Literature Into Practice

Once the evidence has been appraised, clinicians need to find a way to integrate the valid, important, and applicable evidence into their clinical decision making along with their experiences and the patient's values. This may be the most difficult aspect of EBP for some clinicians, as the best available evidence may not fit with their individual clinical expertise or the patient's preference. It is important to note that the evidence cannot be used in isolation from the other aspects needed for clinical decision making.

For some conditions, evidence-based clinical guidelines or prediction rules may be a useful way of integrating the evidence with specific findings for a particular patient. **Clinical practice guidelines**, which are systematically developed statements regarding specific illnesses, conditions, or circumstances, can assist clinicians and patients in making health care decisions (Field and Lohr 1990). Practice guidelines are intended to provide guidance on best practices by defining how to use clinical findings to make decisions about what course of action to take with a specific patient. The National Guideline Clearinghouse (www.guideline.gov) provides a searchable database of published practice guidelines. **Clinical prediction rules** are more specific than guidelines and are typically used to aid the clinician in making decisions regarding the evaluation and diagnosis of particular conditions. Prediction rules provide guidance on a course of action based on three or more variables obtained from the patient's history, physical examination, or diagnostic test results, such as the Ottawa Ankle Rules (Bachmann et al. 2003) or Wells' Clinical Prediction Rule for Deep Vein Thrombosis (Wells et al. 1995).

Evaluating the Outcomes

The clinician must evaluate the patient's outcome following the integration of the evidence into the patient's assessment or treatment. It is important to note whether the treatment improved the patient's symptom reports, function, or disability and whether the treatment effects lasted over longer periods of time. Outcomes should be evaluated on an individual or patient level and also within the context of research to determine the efficacy of athletic training interventions. It is best to include both clinician-report (e.g., strength, range of motion) and patient-report (e.g., pain scale, quality of life instrument) outcomes measures to determine how the integration of evidence affected the entire continuum of the disablement spectrum (Snyder et al. 2008; Valovich McLeod et al. 2008).

Evaluating the Evidence-Based Practice Process

The final step of EBP allows the clinician to reflect on the entire EBP process and self-evaluate her ability to ask questions, search, appraise, integrate, and measure outcomes. Since EBP is a self-directed process of life-long learning (Sackett and Rosenberg 1995), there is a continued need for reflection and improvement in all aspects of EBP. The self-evaluation requires careful consideration and critical thinking about each of the EBP steps, and it takes time and practice to improve individual skills in EBP.

Learning Aids

SUMMARY

Evidence-based practice is a systematic process of improving patient outcomes through the inclusion of the best research evidence with clinical expertise and patient preferences. In athletic training, EBP can be used to help select the most accurate diagnostic tests during an evaluation to determine the most effective treatment for athletic injuries and illnesses. Evidence-based practice promotes critical thinking and is an important means of professional development.

KEY CONCEPTS AND REVIEW

▸ **Define evidence-based practice (EBP).**

The integration of the best research evidence, clinical experience, and patient preferences and values

▸ **Describe the need for EBP in athletic training.**

Evidence-based practice ensures a scientific foundation for athletic training practice. It improves critical thinking in the clinical setting, may increase our standing in the medical community, and can lead to the development of best practice guidelines.

▶ **Describe the five steps in the EBP process.**

Define the clinical question, search for evidence, appraise evidence, integrate evidence with clinical expertise and patient preference, evaluate outcomes, and perform self-evaluation of the EBP process

▶ **Formulate an answerable clinical question using the PICO format.**

An answerable question has the following components: P, patient; I, intervention of interest; C, comparison; O, outcome of interest.

▶ **Describe the 5S approach to searching the medical literature.**

Ideally, start with systems, which are integrated patient medical records with point-of-care evidence and information. If this is not available, move down the pyramid, to summaries, synopses, and syntheses and eventually to searching for individual studies through databases such as PubMed or CINAHL.

▶ **Understand the various criteria that are needed to appraise published research studies.**

The rapid critical appraisal evaluates all research on the following three main questions: (1) Is the evidence valid? (2) Is the valid evidence important? and (3) Is the valid, important evidence applicable to my patient? Additionally, numerous checklists have been developed for various study designs that can be used to appraise the literature; these include CONSORT, STROBE, STARD, PRISMA, and MOOSE.

▶ **Describe the process of integrating the evidence into clinical practice.**

Clinicians must learn to integrate the valid, important, and applicable evidence into their clinical practice, taking into account their own clinical expertise and the preferences and values of their patient. Integration may be a slow process and should evolve over time.

▶ **Understand the usefulness of clinical decision rules and guidelines in patient care.**

Decision rules and practice guidelines are intended to provide guidance for best practices in patient care. However, clinicians must take into account their own experiences and the values of their patient in determining the best course of diagnosis or treatment.

▶ **Discuss the importance of measuring clinical outcomes in assessing the EBP process.**

To determine whether the integration of the best evidence with one's clinical expertise and the patient's values made a difference in outcome for the patient, one must assess patient-report clinical outcomes. Numerous outcomes scales are available, including generic and specific scales.

▶ **Identify the questions you should ask during your self-evaluation of the EBP process.**

Clinicians need to evaluate their own performance at each of the five steps of the EBP process. This self-evaluation is critical in improving one's use of EBP.

PRACTICE!

For hands-on practice in this area, go to the web resource and complete the following:

Level 1.2, Module A2: Becoming a Critically Thinking Clinician

CRITICAL THINKING QUESTIONS

1. Define EBP within the context of athletic training.

2. Describe the need for critical thinking in athletic training and explain why appraising the evidence is an important aspect of EBP.

3. Discuss how and when athletic trainers can develop clinical questions to facilitate EBP.

Glossary

asthma—A chronic lung disorder in which air becomes trapped in the small alveoli and the patient has difficulty expelling air and consequently difficulty inhaling a full breath. Asthma can be induced by exercise (exercise-induced asthma or EIA) rather than occurring as the inflammatory reaction associated with typical asthma. Both types are usually easily controlled with inhaled medication. Asthma attacks can be life threatening if not understood and treated appropriately.

abandonment—The desertion of a patient–practitioner relationship by the health care provider without the consent of the patient.

acclimatization (acclimation)—The process of adjusting to differences in environment, whether these are day-to-day differences or a difference due to a change in geographical location.

accommodating resistance—Resistance provided to a muscle that changes as the muscle moves through its range of motion.

active stretching—The patient's active muscle contraction of the antagonistic muscle controls and provides the stretching of the agonist muscle.

actual cause—The degree to which a health care practitioner's actions are associated with the adverse outcomes of a patient's care.

acute (inflammatory) phase—The phase following injury occurrence that is characterized by such reactions as pain, inflammation, bleeding, or loss of function.

adipose tissue—Body fat.

AED—Automatic external defibrillator; a portable electronic device that automatically diagnoses heart rate and rhythm disturbances and is able to treat the condition.

aerobic—"With air" or requiring air, where air is oxygen. Usually this adjective is coupled with "exercise," where the exercise is one that requires air or uses air.

affective responses—Emotions, feelings, and moods such as anxiety, anger, sadness, or energy that occur in response to sport injury situations.

agility—The ability to control the direction of a body or its parts during rapid movement.

agonist[1]—In exercise, a muscle that acts with another muscle to produce a movement.

agonist[2]—An agent that works in concert with another agent. Two systems working agonistically are often able to produce a greater effect.

agonistic muscle pattern—Pattern in which a muscle acts as prime mover to produce a motion.

alimentary—Relating to the digestive tract.

allopathic—Referring to a branch of the medical profession leading to the designation MD (Medical Doctor).

ALS—Advanced Life Support; a portion of the training of paramedics that gives them skills in administration of intravenous (IV) therapy, advanced pharmacology, cardiac monitoring, defibrillation, advanced airway maintenance, and intubation as well as other advanced assessment and treatment skills.

alveoli—Anatomical pouches or hollow cavities located in the end of the respiratory tree; the point in the bronchial tree at which gas exchange occurs.

AMA—The American Medical Association; the governing body for the medical profession.

ambulatory—Related to the ability to walk.

amortization—The second phase of a plyometric activity; a rapid transition from eccentric to concentric motion.

amplification—The act or result of increasing magnitude.

anaerobic—"Without air" or not requiring air (oxygen). Usually this adjective is coupled with "exercise," where the exercise is one that does not require air. An example is a short sprint in which breathing is suspended until the end of the sprint. Swimming underwater is an easy example to understand.

analgesic—A drug used to reduce pain.

anaphylaxis—A severe, whole-body allergic reaction. Once the patient is exposed to a particular drug, chemical, or other substance, the body becomes sensitized, and future exposures to that offensive substance result in the allergic response.

anchor strip—A tape layer used to secure tape applied subsequently.

anecdotal—Referring to a report based on the experience or observations of an individual, not necessarily with any scientific support.

anesthesia—A reversible loss of sensation (local anesthesia) or loss of consciousness (general anesthesia). A drug used to create anesthesia is called an anesthetic.

angioedema—Swelling similar to hives but under the skin surface rather than on top.

antagonist[1]—In exercise, a muscle whose action is opposite the action of the agonist muscle. An example is the triceps (antagonist to elbow flexion), which opposes the action of the biceps brachii (agonist for elbow flexion).

antagonist[2]—An agent that works against another agent. In medicinal therapy, a drug that could counteract the effect of another drug is an antagonist.

antagonistic muscle pattern—Pattern in which a muscle opposes the motion of another muscle.

anthropometry—The study of the human form; in exercise medicine, it includes physical attributes such as circumferences of body parts and thickness of a fold of skin.

anticoagulation—Against clotting (coagulation); an anticoagulant drug thins the blood.

antihistamines—Literally, against a histamine. The histamine is the factor that causes the symptom of allergies, so the antihistamine reduces the symptoms of allergy.

antihypertensive—Drug designed to reduce high blood pressure.

antipyretic—A drug that reduces fever. *Pyretic* means "fire," so *antipyretic* means "against the fire."

antitussive—A drug that works against or controls a cough. *Tussive* means "of or pertaining to a cough."

aplastic anemia—A blood disorder in which the bone marrow fails to produce enough new blood cells.

arrhythmia—Rhythm disturbance of the heart.

articular cartilage—Cartilage located at the ends of long bones that come together to form joints.

articulation—A union (joint) between two bones.

ASTM—The American Society for Testing and Materials, one of the largest voluntary standards development organizations in the world.

atherosclerosis—A condition in which an artery wall thickens with a buildup of fats like cholesterol; often referred to as hardening of the arteries.

autoclave—A device used to sterilize equipment by subjecting it to high-pressure saturated steam (121° F) for 10 to 15 min.

avulsion fracture—Injury in which a violent contraction or excessive stretch causes traction forces through the muscular tendon to such a degree that a bony fracture occurs at the attachment site.

axial loading—A force that is applied along the long axis of a structure.

axilla—The armpit; the anatomical location of the axillary artery and the brachial plexus of nerves.

balance—The body's ability to maintain its equilibrium by controlling the center of gravity over the base of support.

ballistic stretching—An active or passive stretching that includes bouncing at the end of the range of available motion.

baroreceptor—A nerve ending in the wall of an artery that senses a change in pressure (blood pressure).

behavioral responses—Efforts, actions, or activities carried out in response to sport injury situations.

biceps brachii—A two-headed muscle of the arm—a flexor of the shoulder and the elbow and a strong supinator of the forearm.

bile—A green-brown fluid produced by the liver. It is used in the small intestine to break down fats.

bioelectrical impedance—A method of estimating a person's body fat percentage using the speed of electrical conduction through the body. Fat is a poor conductor of electrical current, while lean muscle transmits the electrical current; thus the fat percentage can be calculated. Often this method is wrought with error if factors are not controlled.

biomechanical—Referring to the application of mechanical principles to living organisms; in exercise medicine, the mechanical properties of muscles and joints.

biomechanics—The study of the mechanics of living; in the case of the athletic trainer, the mechanics of human movement and the way in which joints move.

blocker's exostosis—Also known as tackler's exostosis or blocker's spur; excessive bone formation or a palpable spur due to repetitive insult or irritation of the upper or lateral humerus.

bloodborne pathogen—Contaminants that are carried in the bloodstream.

boxer's fracture—Fracture of the neck of the fifth metacarpal.

brachial artery—The major artery of the arm—a continuation of the axillary artery from the shoulder region that changes into the radial and ulnar arteries at the elbow.

bradycardia—A very slow heart rate; occurs naturally with heavy endurance training. A sudden slowdown of the heart rate may indicate a heart (pacemaker) problem or internal bleeding.

brain stem—The lower end of the brain, connecting the brain to the spinal cord.

breach of contract—An unexcused failure to perform the services specified in a contract, either formal or informal.

bronchioles—The first part of the bronchial tree that does not contain cartilage and the last segment before the terminal alveolar sacs.

bronchitis—Inflammation of the mucous membranes of the bronchi, the part of the bronchial tree between the trachea and the lungs.

bronchodilator—A drug that dilates, or opens up, the brochioles, thus allowing the patient to breathe more freely.

bronchospasm—Constriction of the muscular walls of the brochioles, causing difficulty breathing. *See also* brochodilator.

budget—A type of operational plan for the coordination of resources and expenditures.

buoyant—Related to the ability to float.

bursitis—An inflammatory condition of fluid accumulation within a bursa.

CAAHEP—The Commission on Accreditation of Allied Health Higher Education Programs; the accrediting agency for college allied health programs.

CAATE—The agency responsible for the accreditation of entry-level athletic training educational programs. The American Academy of Family Physicians (AAFP), the American Academy of Pediatrics (AAP), the American Orthopedic Society for Sports Medicine (AOSSM), and the

National Athletic Trainers' Association (NATA) collaborate in developing the Standards for Entry-Level Athletic Training Educational Programs.

CAHEA—The Committee on Allied Health Education and Accreditation, a program of the American Medical Association.

calcaneal exostosis—Also known as a "pump bump"; chronic irritation at the Achilles tendon attachment to the calcaneus, characterized by localized pain, swelling, and possible enlargement of the calcaneal apophysis.

capitation—A system whereby medical vendors receive a fixed amount per patient.

carbohydrate—An organic compound that consists of only carbon, hydrogen, and oxygen. In biochemistry, a carbohydrate is a saccharide that can be divided into four chemical groups: monosaccharides, disaccharides, iliogosaccharides, and polysaccharides. The first two of these are sugars.

cardiac output—The amount (volume) of blood being pumped by the heart.

cardiopulmonary—Relating to the heart and lungs.

cardiorespiratory—Relating to the structure and function of the heart and lungs.

cardiovascular collapse—A failure of the cardiac circulation; often caused by shock or trauma from injury or surgery.

carotid sinus—A localized dilation of the internal carotid artery at its origin from the common carotid bifurcation.

case report—A retrospective report of one patient's unique clinical presentation or outcome.

case series—A report of several clinical observation cases with a common outcome or course.

case-control study—Retrospective study that compares two groups, one with the condition of interest and one without.

central nervous system—The brain and spinal cord.

certification[1]—A nongovernmental process by which standards are measured and verified; the Board of Certification uses certification to credential athletic trainers nationally.

certification[2]—A form of title protection, established by state law or sponsored by professional associations, designed to ensure that practitioners have essential knowledge and skills sufficient to protect the public.

cervical whiplash—An injury mechanism whereby the cervical spine is suddenly forced into extension followed by sudden forced flexion.

chancre—A sore or ulcer.

charting by exception—A type of medical record that notes only those patient responses that vary from predefined norms.

check reign—A material or fabric used to restrict the excursion of an opening or a hinge-like structure (joint).

chemotaxis—Cellular movement based on chemical signals.

cholesterol—A wax-like steroid found in cell membranes of mammals. Cholesterol is important and necessary, but high levels of cholesterol in the blood may be a warning sign of heart disease.

chondrocytes—Cells found in cartilage.

chronic inflammation—An inflammatory process that lasts longer than expected or does not resolve in a normal amount of time.

chronic instability—Subluxation of a joint that is chronic, repetitive, or both.

clinical practice guidelines—Systematically developed statements that contain recommendations based on evidence, intended to assist clinicians and patients in making specific health care decisions.

clinical prediction rule—Studies in which the best combination of signs, symptoms, physical findings, and diagnostics are used to predict the probability of a diagnosis or outcome following treatment.

clonic—Referring to a rapid contraction and relaxation of a muscle or muscle group.

closed kinetic chain (CKC)—Characterizes a motion in which the distal segment of an extremity is weight bearing and the body moves over the hand or foot.

code of ethics—A set of rules adopted by an organization to assist with decisions regarding the professional conduct of its members.

cognitive appraisal—Personal interpretations, appraisals, or beliefs concerning the meaning, threat, or challenge of sport injury situations and the coping resources available for managing them.

cognitive—A scientific term that refers to processes of the mind.

coherence—A property of laser light; all discharged photons are in sync with each other and travel in parallel.

cohort study—Study in which patients with a certain condition are followed prospectively and compared to patients without the condition on an outcome of interest.

cold urticaria—An allergic reaction to cold exposure.

collimation—A property of laser light; the light travels in one direction without diverging. Once a medium change is encountered, there is a possibility for reflection, refraction, and absorption of the light.

commission—An act of committing something that is unhelpful or harmful to one's patient.

common fibular nerve—A branch of the sciatic nerve; the lateral-lying nerve that supplies the lateral (superficial fibular nerve) and the anterior (deep fibular nerve) compartments of the leg.

compartment syndrome—Pressure buildup in a muscle compartment from either a chronic or acute etiology. In severe cases, the pressure leads to neurovascular compromise and associated pathologies.

complete blood count (CBC)—A combination of tests of the patient's blood. The CBC as used in the United States evaluates the white cell count (WBC), hemoglobin (Hb), hematocrit (Hct), and platelets (Plt).

concentric—Referring to a dynamic activity in which the muscle shortens.

concussion—Transient alteration in brain function with or without structural damage.

conduction—The transfer of heat from a warmer area to a cooler area. The two areas must be in physical contact with each other.

conformability—The ease with which a fabric or material molds to the part being covered.

constriction—A narrowing of a passageway.

contamination—The presence of an unwanted substance in a wound; a bacterium or other foreign element.

continuous passive motion (CPM)—Process in which a joint is slowly moved through its available range of motion; typically occurs with use of an external device.

contract–relax technique—Proprioceptive neuromuscular facilitation technique used with patients who have limited range of motion. Involves a contraction of antagonist muscle followed by stretch of antagonist muscle.

contracture—Shortening or shrinking of a structure, such as scar tissue or muscle. In a muscle contracture, the muscle is in a semi-rigid, shortened state, making it difficult to stretch.

controlled substances—Substances covered by the Controlled Substances Act, a Congress-controlled law which regulates the distribution and use of drugs that are considered to have a potential for abuse.

contusion—A bruise.

convection—The transfer of heat into cooler circulating air or fluid.

coordination—The ability of muscles and muscle groups to perform complicated movements.

COPD—Chronic obstructive pulmonary disease; a co-occurrence of chronic bronchitis and emphysema, both of which cause narrowed airways. It is seldom reversible.

coping resources—Personal capabilities and social network sources of assistance available to individuals that are helpful for adapting to stressful situations such as sport injury.

corticosteroids—A class of medicine used for combating inflammation.

costochondritis—Chronic irritation and inflammation of the costochondral junction.

creep—Property of a connective tissue, based on its components, that results in a gradual change in tissue length with a sustained stress.

crepitus—A crackling, grating, or grinding sensation caused by abnormal movement between two structures.

cross-sectional study—Study in which specific populations are evaluated at the same point in time to determine the prevalence of a condition or outcome.

cross-training—Exercise of the contralateral body part in an effort to improve strength in an injured body segment.

DAPRE—Daily Adjustable Progressive Resistive Exercise.

debridement—The removal of dead or infected tissue to improve healing.

deconditioned—Referring to a low level of fitness or condition as a result of decreased physical activity, prescribed bed rest, or illness.

defendant—In law, the person or persons against whom an action (suit) is brought.

deformation—The act or process of changing shape or distorting.

denervated—Referring to muscle that has lost innervations due to injury to the low (alpha) motor neuron.

diabetes (diabetes mellitus)—A disease of the metabolic system in which the person has high blood sugar either because the body does not produce sufficient insulin or because the insulin produced is not effective in breaking down sugar.

diarrhea—Loose or liquid bowel movement (stool).

diastolic—Relating to the period of time in which the heart chambers are filling or

to the lower number listed in recording blood pressure.

dislocation—Discongruity of a joint with obvious deformity as the joint surfaces do not reduce or return to anatomical position.

distal—Away from the center of the body.

dynamic activity—Activity in which movement occurs.

dysphagia—Pain with swallowing.

dyspnea—Difficulty with breathing.

dyssynchrony—A misfiring or mistiming of a muscle contraction.

eccentric—Referring to dynamic activity in which muscle lengthens.

effectiveness—The extent to which a treatment or intervention works in clinical practice or real-world situations.

efficacy—The extent to which a treatment or intervention works in clinical trials or laboratory studies.

effleurage—Stroking massage.

elastin—Primary component of connective tissue; a protein that helps tissues regain their shape after being stretched or contracted.

electrode—As used in sports medicine, the electrode is a small, often rubber or gel pad that is connected to a wire. The wire is connected to a machine or device that delivers or receives electrical impulses to or from the electrode.

electromyographic (EMG)—Referring to a measure of the electrical activity in muscle.

emergency action plan (EAP)—A blueprint for handling emergencies that helps establish accountability for their management.

emesis—Vomiting. An agent used to reduce the occurrence of vomiting is an antiemetic.

EMS—Emergency Medical Services; "activate EMS" indicates that a call should be placed to 911 or other designated numbers from which emergency help will be dispatched.

EMT—Emergency medical technician, a health care professional dealing with accidents and sudden illnesses. Procedures performed are regulated by jurisdiction, but usually include cardiopulmonary care and resuscitation, defibrillation, control of bleeding, shock prevention, and care and immobilization of bones and joints.

EMT-P—Paramedic; an emergency medical technician who has undergone advanced-level training. A paramedic is allowed to administer medications through injection and has advanced life support training.

end feel—The quality of the feel or sensation experienced by the examiner when applying pressure to the joint at the end of the range of motion.

endogenous—Having an internal cause or origin. An endogenous chemical is one produced within the body.

endorphin—A member of a group of hormones secreted by the brain and nervous system. These are natural chemicals that cause an analgesic (pain reducing) effect.

enkephalin—A family of five-peptide chain transmitter substances that inhibit synaptic transmission in nociceptive pathways.

ENT—Abbreviation for the medical specialty concerned with the evaluation and treatment of conditions of the ear, nose, and throat.

enteral—Passing through the digestive tract, usually through the mouth, but the route of administration can also begin at the rectal end of the digestive tract.

ephedrine—A drug that is used as an appetite suppressant but that may also be included in drugs to treat congestion or hypotension associated with anesthesia.

epicondyle—The area of bone just above the articular (joint) surface. In the elbow, it is the point of muscle attachment.

epinephrine—A type of adrenaline; a hormone and a neurotransmitter.

epiphyseal plate—"Growth plate"; location at ends of bone where growth occurs during childhood and adolescence.

epistaxis—"Nosebleed."

ergonomic—Referring to a design intended to provide optimum comfort and to avoid stress or injury.

erythema—Redness of the skin, often only superficial and splotchy in appearance.

essential amino acid—An amino acid that cannot be produced by the body and must be supplied in the diet; amino acids are the building blocks of proteins.

evaporation—The change of a liquid into a gas. In the text, refers to the change of sweat or of the water in exhaled air into gas, which provides a superficial cooling effect.

evolutionary—Referring to the changing of a process or object over a period of time. Often the evolution includes improvements in design or function.

exclusive provider organization (EPO)—A type of preferred provider organization (PPO) in which medical services are reimbursed only if the patient uses contracted providers.

exemption—A legislative mechanism used to release members of one profession from the liability of violating another profession's practice act.

exercise-induced asthma (EIA)—Asthmatic condition with no trigger other than exercise; patients do not experience asthma under any other circumstances.

expectorant—A cough medication that helps to loosen phlegm associated with an upper respiratory irritation.

extraction collar—A specially designed device that fills the space between a patient's shoulders and base of the skull to immobilize the cervical spine and allow her to be transported to a medical facility.

fabrication—The process of making or constructing something.

fee-for-service plan—Known as an indemnity plan; a type of traditional medical insurance plan in which patients are free to seek medical services from any provider. The plan covers a portion of the cost of covered procedures, and the patient is responsible for the balance.

FERPA (Family Educational Rights and Privacy Act)—Sometimes referred to as the Buckley Amendment. A 1974 federal law requiring student authorization to release educational records to a third party and ensuring access for students to their records.

fibroadenomas—Benign tumors that occur most frequently in women between the ages of 18 and 35; characterized by solid lumps of fibrous and glandular tissue.

fibroblastic (proliferative) phase—Phase of injury rehabilitation in which tissue breaks down and builds up.

fibrocartilage—Tough and strong tissue made up of collagen bundles; has strong shock-absorbing properties.

fibrocystic changes—Changes that do not represent a disease state but rather a benign development of multiple fibrous lumps or small cysts.

fibular head—The proximal or top end of the fibula.

first responder—A person who is trained in emergency care but has less training than those on the ambulance; the first responder helps with the patient prior to the arrival of emergency trained medical professionals.

flexibility—The ability of muscles and other soft tissue to sufficiently elongate to achieve a full, unrestricted range of motion.

flushing—A reddening of the skin of the face and other areas of the body.

focus charting—A medical record that registers a patient's complaint data, the health care practitioner's actions, and the patient's response.

force—Stress × area.

foreseeability—The ability to project the likely outcome of an act.

friction—Resistance to movement between two surfaces.

functional activities—Activities that mimic the stresses, demands, and skills of an activity, sport, or movement.

functional and activity-specific exercises—Functional exercises are activities that precede sport-specific or activity-specific exercises in a rehabilitation program. They commonly involve multiplanar movements and provide greater stresses and demands than strength exercises. Sport-specific or activity-specific exercises include drills involving a specific sport or work performance.

functional evaluation—Assessment of the patient's ability to perform an exercise or skill.

gamekeeper's thumb—Injury that involves the ulnar collateral ligament of the metacarpophalengeal joint of the thumb. Injury results from forced abduction and hyperextension of the thumb.

glucocorticoid—A member of a group of steroids that act on the glucose molecule. They are important in reducing inflammation.

glycemic index—A measure of the effects of carbohydrates on blood sugar. Carbohydrates that break down quickly and release glucose into the bloodstream rapidly have a high glycemic index (GI); carbohydrates that release glucose more gradually have a low GI.

golfer's elbow—Medial epicondylitis, an inflammatory condition of the wrist flexor and pronator muscles at their common attachment site at the lateral epicondyle of the humerus.

Golgi tendon organ (GTO)—A part of the tendon that provides sensory information and assists in tendon reflexes.

goniometer—Tool used to measure joint range of motion.

gout—A form of arthritis caused by high levels of uric acid in the blood. The uric acid can be deposited in joints, causing them to become tender, red, hot, and swollen. Gout most often affects the metatarsophalangeal joint of the great toe.

half-life—The period of time it takes for the concentration of a substance or chemical in the body to decrease by half.

health insurance—A type of policy designed to reimburse the cost of preventive as well as corrective medical care.

health maintenance organization (HMO)—A health insurance plan that requires policyholders to use only those medical vendors approved by the company. A primary care physician, who acts as a gatekeeper to specialty services, coordinates all medical services.

heat exhaustion—A form of heat illness that occurs due to low body fluids and high body temperatures. The body sweating causes dehydration, and the individual may experience headache, dizziness, nausea, or rapid breathing. Other signs are heavy sweating, paleness, and fainting.

heat index—An index that combines air temperature and relative humidity in an attempt to determine the human response to temperature.

heatstroke—The most severe heat illness, marked by the body's inability to dissipate heat; sweating and temperature control are inadequate. This is a medical emergency. Signs of heatstroke are high body temperature (usually higher than 104° F), changes in mental status (irritability, confusion, unconsciousness), rapid heart rate, dry and hot skin, and rapid breathing.

helmetry—The athletic term used to describe the science behind the study of protective helmets.

hematocrit (Hct)—The volume or proportion of red blood cells in whole blood. Normally the Hct is about 48% for males and 38% for females.

hematoma—A localized mass or "blood [hema] tumor [toma]" caused by an accumulation of blood in a confined area of a tissue or space.

hematuria—Blood in the urine.

hemoglobin (Hb)—The oxygen-carrying part of the red blood cell, with a high content of iron. High hemoglobin levels may result from training at high altitudes, smoking, or dehydration; low hemoglobin levels may indicate blood loss, nutrition deficiencies, kidney disease, and abnormal hemoglobin due to sickle cell disease.

hemorrhage—Bleeding.

hemothorax—Condition that occurs when blood enters the pleural cavity located between the lung and chest wall, thus reducing the volume of the lung.

hernia—Pathology characterized by the protrusion of abdominal or pelvic contents through a weakened area of the anterior abdominal wall.

herringbone—A pattern of weave consisting of columns of short parallel lines, with all the lines in one column sloping one way and all the lines in the next column sloping the other way so as to resemble the bones in a fish.

high-density lipoprotein (HDL) cholesterol—One of the five main groups of lipoproteins. HDL particles containing cholesterol can remove cholesterol from arteries and move it to the liver. Often called "good cholesterol" due to its ability to rid the bloodstream of cholesterol.

hip pointer—Contusion of the iliac crest.

HIPAA—The Health Insurance Portability and Accountability Act of 1996; helps employees transfer their health insurance when they switch employers, ensures that their health information will remain private, and gives people more access to their own health care information.

hold–relax technique—Proprioceptive neuromuscular facilitation technique consisting of a maximal isometric contraction of the antagonist at the end range of the agonist. The antagonist is then relaxed, and the agonist is used actively without resistance to increase motion of the antagonist. This technique is used to relax muscle spasm.

humeral head—The proximal (shoulder) end of the long bone of the arm.

hyaline cartilage—Most abundant cartilage; forms supportive tissue in the nose, ears, trachea, and articular (joint) surfaces of bones.

hyperextension—Extension of a joint beyond the normal range.

hypertension—Elevated blood pressure.

hyperthermia—A condition in which the core temperature rises above normal levels (usually 98° to 100° F). Signs of hyperthermia are profuse sweating, red and hot skin; as hyperthermia continues, the body may run out of water and the sweating diminishes, signaling a medical emergency.

hypertrichosis—Abnormal growth of body hair.

hypertrophy—The increase in the size (volume) of an organ or tissue due to enlargement of its individual cells. In exercise medicine, hypertrophy is the enlargement of skeletal muscle as a result of strength training.

hyphema—An accumulation of blood in the anterior chamber of the eye.

hypotension—Abnormally low blood pressure.

hypothermia—A condition in which core temperature drops below normal levels (usually 98-100° F). Signs of hypothermia are shivering, mental confusion, and blueness (cyanosis) of lips, ears, and digits.

hypoxia—A condition in which the body or specific tissues do not have a sufficient oxygen supply.

hysteresis—A phenomenon that occurs with repeated stress to a material; the term comes from the Greek for "lagging behind." A new stress is placed on the material during the recovery or stress-relaxation, and the new strain or change in length is compounded because the tissues take longer to respond.

iatrogenic—Caused by the treatment; for example, an incision to remove a cyst cuts through a muscle, causing an iatrogenic injury to that muscle.

iliotibial band friction syndrome—Condition caused by excessive friction between the iliotibial (IT) band and the lateral femoral epicondyle.

illumination—Light or lighting in a room or space.

impervious—Not able to be penetrated, for example by water or light.

individual practice association (IPA)—A managed care model whereby an HMO provides health care services through a network of individual medical practitioners. Care is provided in a physician's office as opposed to a large, multifunctional medical center.

inhaler—A medical device for delivering medicine into the body via the lungs.

instability—Abnormal joint movement caused by disruption of ligament or capsular integrity.

intercostal muscles—Small muscles between the ribs.

internship—A paid or nonpaid position that offers on-the-job training much like an apprenticeship.

intracranial hemorrhage—Condition characterized by tissue edema or bleeding within the intracranial space.

intracranial—Within the skull.

iontophoresis—Use of an electrical current to drive medications into the tissues.

irritability—A characteristic of an injury that is classified as mild, moderate, or severe based on the intensity of pain, the amount of time the pain has been present, and how much the pain interferes with activity and sleep. Irritability relates to the stage of the injury, its extent, the structures injured, and the patient's level of pain tolerance.

ischemia—Tissue anemia caused by lack of blood flow to an area.

ISO—the universal short form for the International Organization for Standardization, an organization that develops rules (standards) for many of the products we use on a daily basis. Subcommittees exist that concentrate on standards for athletic equipment and sport surfaces.

isokinetics—A movement pattern in which the velocity of the movement remains constant but the force generated may vary.

This is achieved on specialized testing or exercise machines.

isometric—Referring to a muscle contraction that does not produce movement.

isotonic—Referring to a movement pattern in which the tension in the muscle remains constant.

jersey finger—Rupture or avulsion of the flexor digitorum profundus tendon at the distal phalanx resulting in lost ability to flex the distal portion of the finger.

job description—A written description of the specific responsibilities a position holder will be accountable for in an organization.

job specification—A written description of the requirements or qualifications a person should have to fill a particular role in an organization.

joint mobilization—Passive joint movement for increasing joint mobility or reducing pain.

Jones fracture—Fracture that occurs at the base of the fifth metatarsal of the foot. Should not be confused with a styloid process fracture of the same bone.

ketoacidosis—A chronic condition of high concentrations of ketones in the bloodstream. Ketones are formed by the breakdown of fats and proteins. Ketoacidosis is often detected by the smell on a person's breath, which is similar to that of fruit or nail polish. Ketoacidosis is common in untreated type 1 diabetes.

kilocalorie (calorie)—A unit of energy; the approximate energy needed to increase the temperature of 1 g of water by 1° C.

kinesiology—The study of human movement and how muscles move the body.

laceration—A jagged tear of the skin.

laminectomy—Surgery to remove the posterior arch of a vertebra.

laryngeal edema—Swelling in and around the larynx (voice box).

lateral stays—As used in braces, plastic strips of material inserted into the sides of a brace to increase the stability of the brace material.

laxity—Hypermobility or increased joint movement.

legislation—A law that has been issued by a legislature or other governing body.

level of evidence—The validity of an individual study based on the assessment of study design .

liability—Indication of responsibility.

licensure—A form of state credentialing, established by statute and intended to protect the public, that regulates the practice of a trade or profession by specifying who may practice and what duties they may perform.

lipids—A large group of molecules with a main function of energy storage. The term is used to denote fats, yet fats are a subgroup of lipids called triglycerides. Lipids include fatty acids and cholesterol.

Lisfranc fracture—With reference to the Lisfranc joint, a fracture that occurs between the midfoot and forefoot in the area of the first and second cuneiform and the base of the first and second metatarsals.

little league elbow—Apophyseal (growth) plate injury of the medial elbow in adolescents, particularly those involved in throwing sports.

little league shoulder—Epiphyseal fracture of the proximal humeral growth plate.

long sitting—Sitting erect with hips flexed to 90° and knees straight.

long-term goal—The final or desired outcome.

low-density lipoprotein (LDL) cholesterol—One of the five major groups of lipoproteins; helps with the transport of lipids (cholesterol and triglycerides) through the bloodstream. High LDL levels are associated with higher risks of atherosclerosis.

macrophages—Cells that fight infections or foreign substances.

macrotrauma—Injury occurring from impact trauma or sudden overload.

major life events—Major events or changes in an individual's status or circumstances that are often perceived as stressful.

malaise—A vague, general feeling of illness and fatigue.

mallet finger—Rupture or avulsion of the extensor digitorum tendon at the distal phalanx resulting in lost ability to extend the distal portion of the finger.

malpractice—Liability-generating conduct associated with an adverse outcome of patient treatment (Scott 1990, p. 6).

manipulation—Passive joint movement used to increase joint mobility.

manual resistance exercise—The use of hands-on techniques to create resistance for a patient.

manual therapy—The use of hands-on techniques for evaluating, treating, and improving the status of neuromusculoskeletal conditions.

massage—Manual manipulation used to change characteristics of soft tissue.

maturation (remodeling) phase—A sport-specific or functional phase of injury rehabilitation.

medial tibial stress syndrome (MTSS)—Commonly called "shin splints"; an inflammation of the periosteum along the posterior medial tibial border at or near the insertion of the long toe or ankle flexors.

medical insurance—A contract between a policyholder and an insurance company to reimburse a percentage of the cost of the policyholder's medical bills.

medical practice act—A state law regulating the practice of medicine, usually by specifying who may practice and under what circumstances.

medical records—The physical file folder or digital file containing a single patient's medical reports and information, as well as the information that makes up the patient's health history. The medical record is a personal and private record and cannot be viewed by a third party (a person other than the patient and provider) without explicit, written permission from the patient (*see* HIPAA).

menarche—Initiation of the menstrual cycle.

meta-analysis—A systematic review in which the data from the included studies are pooled for additional analyses and a summary estimate of effect.

metabolic disorders—A large class of genetic diseases related to disorders of metabolism. Most metabolic disorders cause an accumulation of substances that cannot be broken down by the faulty metabolic system.

metabolism—The chemical reactions that occur in the body to sustain life.

methodology—A system of methods used in a particular area of study or activity.

microtrauma—Small injuries caused by repetitive overuse without adequate recovery; cumulative microtrauma can eventually lead to major injury if left untreated.

mineralocorticoid—A steroid that works to maintain the salt balance in the body.

mission statement—A written expression of an organization's philosophy, purposes, and characteristics.

modeling—A process in which knowledge and support are gained from observing others; actions and attitudes are learned through observation.

monochromaticity—The quality or state of having only one color.

mucolytic—A chemical that reduces thick mucus to help thin it for expectoration (coughing out or expelling). *See also* expectorant.

muscle endurance—The ability of a muscle or group of muscles to perform a movement or movement pattern repetitively for a sustained period of time.

muscle energy—Manual therapy technique used to correct alignment and improve function.

muscle power—The ability to lift a weight through a large range of motion in a short period of time; work produced over time.

muscle strength—The maximal force a muscle can generate in a specific movement pattern at a specific velocity; a muscle's relative ability to resist or produce a force.

muscle strength imbalance—Nonequal or noncompatible muscle strength between agonist and antagonist muscles leading to overpowering and increasing risk of injury.

musculotendinous junction—Point where muscle tissue fibers change into tendon tissue.

musculotendinous unit—The structure comprising both the muscle and tendon.

myofascial pain syndrome—Persistent pain of soft tissue; origins are characterized by taut fibrous bands and focal areas of hypersensitivity called trigger points.

myofascial release—Hands-on technique similar to massage with the purpose of reducing adhesions in myofascial tissue.

myofibroblasts—Cells that have contractile properties.

myositis ossificans—Calcium formation within muscle tissue following unresolved hematoma.

narrative charting—A method of recording the details of a patient's assessments and treatments using a detailed, prose-based format.

NATA—The National Athletic Trainers' Association; the governing body for the athletic training profession.

nature—A characteristic of an injury that is classified according to the type of injury and the structure involved. A sprain or dislocation is an injury of a ligament or capsule; a strain is an injury of a muscle or tendon; a fracture is an injury of a bone; and an open wound is an injury of the skin and possibly other structures.

negligence—In law, failure to exercise the degree of care considered reasonable under the circumstances, resulting in an unintended injury to another party.

neurogenic—Originating in or controlled by the nervous system.

neuroimaging—Varied techniques for imaging the structure and function of the brain.

neuropsychological—Referring to the structure and function of the brain, related to specific psychological processes and behaviors.

neuropsychologists—Medical specialists who focus on the function of the brain.

NOCSAE—The National Operating Committee on Standards for Athletic Equipment; a standards group that focuses on safety properties of athletic equipment.

nonproprietary—Not registered or restricted, usually freely available on the market.

nonsteroidal—Not of the steroid family; nonsteroidal drugs are often used to reduce inflammation. It is thought that when a medication contains no steroid, the side effects are fewer.

normative culture—Customary beliefs, attitudes, and behaviors expected within a certain social structure or group such as a sport or sport team.

noxious—Harmful, very unpleasant, pain provoking.

NSAIDs—Nonsteroidal anti-inflammatory drugs.

omission—A failure to act when there was a legal duty to do so.

open kinetic chain (OKC)—Characterizes a motion in which the distal segment of an extremity moves freely in space.

operational plan—A type of plan that defines organizational activities in the short term, usually no longer than 2 years.

orthopedic—Relating to a medical specialization that deals with disorders of bones and joints.

orthostatic hypotension—Reduced blood pressure upon standing; usually a drop of 20/10 mmHg.

OSHA—Occupational Safety and Health Administration; an agency of the federal government that regulates workplace safety and health.

ossification—Process of bone formation.

osteoarthritis—A type of arthritis that affects the joint surfaces. This disease process can be inherited or may develop in a joint following trauma or injury.

outcomes—Results, effects, or consequences associated with sport injury situations.

overload principle—Principle stating that a muscle must be overloaded beyond its accustomed level if it is going to gain strength.

palmar—On the palm side of the hand.

palpable—Detectable by touch or feel.

palpation—Examination by the use of touch.

paramedic—Also designated as EMT-P, the paramedic has advanced training in emergency and advanced life support (ALS). United States law restricts the use of the title "paramedic," and the person must hold a valid registration with a governing agency.

parenteral—Referring to administration of drugs via routes other than the digestive tract.

passive stretching—Acted upon by an external agent; in therapy and stretching, a procedure is passive when a patient is moved either through a range of motion or in a stretch; the patient does not cause the movement or aid in the stretching.

patellofemoral pain syndrome (PFPS)—Vague and general anterior knee pain; also known as miserable malalignment syndrome or patellofemoral stress syndrome (PFSS).

pathophysiology—The study of an alteration in normal mechanical, physical, or biochemical functions that may result from disease or damage to tissues.

pectoralis major—A large muscle of the chest area; the major muscle used in bench press.

periodization—An exercise prescription designed to gradually change the type, intensity, and amount of training to allow the individual to achieve optimal gains in strength and power.

periorbital hematoma—"Black eye."

periosteum—Membrane that covers the outside of many long bones.

peripheral—Away from the body center.

petrissage—Compression or kneading type of massage.

pharmacodynamics—Study of the effects of drugs and their mechanism of action.

pharmacokinetics—Study of the movement of drugs in the body.

pharmacology—The branch of medicine that deals with the uses, effects, and actions of drugs.

pharmacotherapeutics—Study of the effects of drugs on the body.

photon—A measurement of electromagnetic energy that lacks mass, lacks an electrical charge, and has an indefinite lifetime. Photons contain a specific amount of energy depending on their wavelength.

physical agents—Treatments that cause some change to the body.

physician's assistant—A medical professional who works under a licensed physician, extending that physician's care.

physiology—The study of the function of human systems and the interaction of the systems.

plaintiff—The person or persons who institute a suit in a court of law.

plastic deformation—Deformation that exceeds the plastic limit, causing a structure to deform and remain deformed.

plyometrics—A type of exercise that uses fast, powerful movements to improve the function of the neuromuscular system. Plyometrics usually involve rapid loading and unloading of muscles with an element of stretch imposed prior to a contraction.

pneumatic—Using pressurized gas (air).

pneumothorax—Condition that occurs when air enters the pleural cavity located between the lung and chest wall, thus reducing the volume of the lung.

point-of-service plans (POS)—Managed care plans that are similar to preferred provider organizations (PPOs) except that primary care physicians are assigned to patients to coordinate their care.

policy[1]—A type of plan that expresses an organization's intended behavior relative to a specific program subfunction.

policy[2]—A contract between an insurance company and an individual or organization.

porous—Referring to a material that has small spaces or holes through which liquid or air may pass.

position description—A formal document that describes the qualifications, work content, accountability, and scope of a job.

potency—A measure of the strength of the effect produced by an agent.

practice—The action that takes place in response to administrative problems.

preferred provider organization (PPO)—A health insurance plan that provides financial incentives to encourage policyholders to use medical vendors approved by the company.

preparticipation physical examination (PPE)—The medical physical exam that must be completed before an individual is allowed to participate in the chosen sport.

primary coverage—A type of health, medical, or accident insurance that begins to pay for covered expenses immediately after a deductible has been paid.

primary intention—A healing process that occurs throughout a bridge of tissue when the wound edge separation is small.

proactive approach—Approach in which one takes the initiative to be prepared in advance for a situation or event such as a mental health referral, anticipating what will be needed before things happen.

procedure—A type of operational plan that provides specific directions for members of an organization to follow.

process—A collection of incremental and mutually dependent steps designed to direct the most important tasks of an organization.

prodrug—A chemical that remains inactive until it is metabolized, thus exerting its effect only when it reaches a place where it can be distributed.

progressive overload—Exercise progression in which increasing loads are imposed to muscle for the purpose of developing strength.

proliferation phase—Stage of healing process that is characterized by disposal of dead tissue, early scar formation, and restoration of circulation.

pronator teres syndrome—A condition caused by compression of the median nerve between the two heads of the pronator teres or fibrous tissue at the elbow.

prone—Position in which patient lies on the stomach, facedown.

proprioception—The body's ability to transmit afferent information regarding position sense, to interpret the information, and to respond consciously or unconsciously to stimulation through posture or movement.

proprioceptive neuromuscular facilitation (PNF)—In exercise medicine, a specialized manual therapy technique to help train the interplay between the nervous and muscular systems. The technique involves a stretch to stimulate the muscle spindle, resistance to stimulate muscular strength, and specific movement patterns.

proprioceptors—Receptors that provide feedback on position sense.

proteoglycan—A constituent of the connective tissue ground substance; a protein core with a glycosaminoglycan (GAG) chain covalently attached to form a gel-like substance.

protocol—A guideline.

proximal—Closer to the center of the body.

proximate (legal) cause—The degree to which the harm caused by a health care practitioner was foreseeable.

pruritus—A sensation that causes the desire to scratch.

psychological skills interventions—Intentional actions used to improve the sport injury situation for the better; strategies employed to achieve better psychological and physical cycles of responses and outcomes.

psychology—The study of mental functions and human behavior.

psychomotor—Relating to the origination of movement in conscious mental activity.

pursed-lip breathing—A special technique of exhalation used by asthmatic patients.

radicular—Following the course of a peripheral nerve.

radiograph—An X ray.

radiology—The specialty area of imaging the body by radiation (X rays).

radiolucent—Relating to a material that allows the radiation of X rays to pass through. The material shows up an opaque white on the radiograph.

randomized controlled trial—Study in which patients are randomly assigned to an experimental or control group and then prospectively followed to determine the effect of the intervention on the outcome of interest.

range of motion—The amount of mobility at a joint; affected by the structure of the joint and the flexibility of the muscles that act upon it.

registration—A type of state credentialing that requires qualified members of a profession to register with the state in order to practice.

rehabilitation—Returning an individual to a previous physical and psychological condition.

reliability—A statistical statement of the consistency of measurement.

remodeling phase—Stage of healing process that is characterized by scar maturation and increases in tissue tensile strength.

respiratory rate—The number of breaths taken per minute. Respiratory rate is one of the vital signs.

rickets—A vitamin D deficiency disease that causes softening of the bones. Lack of calcium in the diet can also cause rickets.

risk management—A process designed to prevent losses of all kinds for everyone associated with an organization, including its directors, administrators, employees, and clients.

rotary—Revolving around an axis.

sciatica—Nerve pain referred along the course of the sciatic nerve.

scurvy—A vitamin C deficiency disease that causes bleeding of the mucous membranes (mouth, nose) and softening of the gums. Patients look pale and feel depressed, and they often lose teeth due to gum softening.

secondary coverage—A type of health, medical, or accident insurance that begins to pay for covered expenses only after all other sources of insurance coverage have been exhausted. Also known as excess insurance.

secondary intention—A healing process in which new tissue fills in the wound from the sides and bottom; occurs when the wound edge separation is large.

secondary school—The school years after elementary school and prior to college; usually called junior high and high school but also includes middle school.

secondary survey—In emergency medicine, evaluation of the patient after cardiopulmonary function has been established.

second-impact syndrome—Condition characterized by an autoregulatory dysfunction that causes rapid and fatal brain swelling.

severity—A characteristic of an injury that determines whether or not to refer the patient to a physician or other medical specialist. Severity, categorized as mild, moderate, or severe, is identified by the magnitude of the signs and symptoms: The more intense the signs and symptoms, the more severe the injury.

shock—A life-threatening medical condition that happens when not enough blood is present in circulation to sustain cellular activity.

short sitting—Sitting erect with hips and knees flexed to 90°, as in sitting on the edge of a table.

short-term goals—Intermediate goals that should be reached as steps toward obtaining a long-term or end goal.

sickle cell anemia—A genetic blood disorder in which some of the red blood cells become abnormal, rigid, and shaped like a sickle. Persons with sickle cell disease often have intense, painful crises that result when the sickled cell clogs an artery and causes decreased blood flow to that area.

sickle cell trait—A genetic blood disorder in which one of the genes for hemoglobin is normal and one is for the sickling trait. Individuals with this disorder are less prone to the severe symptoms of the sickle cell disease, in which the patient carries both genes for sickling. Those with the trait may have difficulty with anaerobic exercise, especially if dehydrated and exercising in a hot environment.

sign—A finding that is observable or that can easily be measured.

sling psychrometer—A simple device for measuring relative humidity (hydrometer). The psychrometer has two thermometers, one dry bulb and one wet bulb; and a formula using the two temperatures determines relative humidity. Electronic psychrometers are available to reduce the time and effort needed to obtain the values.

slow reversal-hold-relax technique—Concentric contraction of the agonist into the range-limited motion of the antagonist followed by an isometric contraction of the antagonist. This is followed by relaxation of the antagonist, then concentric movement by the agonist.

Snellen eye chart—A chart showing letters in successively decreasing size, used to evaluate visual acuity. The chart was developed in 1862 by a Dutch ophthalmologist. Variations of the chart are in common use today.

social support—Help, comfort, and assistance from other people in challenging life situations such as sport injury.

spasm—A reflex muscular contraction produced to minimize and protect a body part; involves tonic muscle activity and can be painful.

spending-ceiling model—A type of expenditure budgeting that requires justification only for those expenses that exceed those of the previous budget cycle. Also known as the incremental model.

spending-reduction model—A type of budgeting used during periods of financial retrenchment that require reallocation of institutional funds, resulting in reduced spending levels for some programs.

sphygmomanometer—A blood pressure meter.

spinal stenosis—Condition characterized by developmental or congenital narrowing of the spinal canal, increasing the risk of spinal cord compression and injury.

spine board—A stiff plastic or wooden board used to stabilize a patient's spine for transport.

splanchnic nerves—A special set of thoracic and abdominal nerves that carry autonomic nervous system information, especially sympathetic.

spondylitis—Inflammation of the facet joint and surrounding capsule between adjacent vertebrae.

spondylolisthesis—Fracture of the pars interarticularis with forward subluxation of vertebrae; condition in which the fracture in spondylolysis becomes unstable and forward subluxation of the involved vertebrae occurs.

spondylolysis—Condition involving a stress fracture or congenital weakening of the pars interarticularis portion of the lumbar vertebrae.

spontaneous emission—Random discharge of a light wave that occurs naturally. An atom absorbs energy to raise its valence level, and the same amount of energy is emitted spontaneously when the atom releases a photon.

sport injury psychology—Psychological thoughts (cognitions), feelings (affect), actions (behaviors), and interventions that affect the sport injury risk, response, recovery, and return of participants.

sport injury socioculture—Social and cultural structures, climates, processes, and interventions that influence the sport injury risk, response, recovery, and return of participants.

sport-specific activities—Activities that mimic the demands and requirements of a specific sport or position.

staff selection—The procedures used as the basis for any employment decision, including recruitment, hiring, promotion, demotion, retention, and performance evaluation.

standard of care—The legal duty to provide health care services consistent with what other health care practitioners of the same training, education, and credentialing would provide under the circumstances.

standards of practice—Widely accepted principles intended to guide the professional activities of a health care practitioner.

static activity—An isometric activity in which no movement occurs.

statute—A formal written decree issued by a legislative authority that governs a state, city, or country.

stenosis—An abnormal narrowing of a blood vessel or other tubular organ or anatomical structure.

stethoscope—An acoustic device that magnifies the sound of the heart or lungs; the hearing device used to measure blood pressure with a sphygmomanometer.

strength of recommendation—Grading the strength of a body of evidence for clinical practice decisions. Assigning a strength of recommendation is a way to grade the evidence for use in clinical decision making.

stress—Force / area.

stress response—Cognitive and physiologic changes such as narrowed attention, increased heart rate, rapid breathing, and perspiring; occur in situations such as sport injury that are perceived as threatening.

stress testing—Method of applying tension to a joint to evaluate the integrity of a ligament.

stress-relaxation—A tissue's ability to relax or reduce tension in response to a constant deformation.

subcutaneous—Beneath the skin.

subluxation—Discongruity of a joint with immediate or spontaneous reduction. Upon examination, joint surfaces are in or close to their anatomical position.

submerge—To put under water.

supine—Lying position in which patient is on the back, face up.

symptom—A subjective complaint or an abnormal sensation that the patient describes but that cannot be directly observed.

syncope—A loss of consciousness (fainting) caused by insufficient blood flow to the brain.

systematic review—A critical review of existing evidence, performed in a systematic manner to answer a focused clinical question.

systemic—Affecting the entire body.

systolic—Referring to the contraction phase of the heart.

tachycardia—A heart rate that exceeds normal.

tennis elbow—Lateral epicondylitis, which is an inflammatory condition of the wrist extensor and supinator muscles at their common attachment site at the lateral epicondyle of the humerus.

tensiometry—Measurement of the amount of tension generated during muscle contraction.

theater sign—Poorly localized anterior knee pain that is exacerbated by prolonged sitting as required for watching a movie.

therapeutic modality—A device or apparatus having curative powers.

thermal radiation—Electromagnetic waves produced by a heat source and transferred into the environment. The radiant heat produced by a space heater is an example. On a very cold day you may be able to see heat waves rising from the scalp of an exercising individual. She is radiating heat into the environment.

thermistor—A small plastic (polymer) device that detects temperature.

third party—A medical vendor with no binding interest in a particular insurance contract.

third-party reimbursement—The process by which medical vendors receive reimbursement from insurance companies for services provided to policyholders.

thoracic outlet syndrome (TOS)—A vascular condition in the cervical region due to compression of the subclavian artery as it passes through the thoracic outlet marked by the scalene muscles and the first rib.

Tinel's sign—Radiating pain or paresthesia caused by light tapping or percussion over an inflamed nerve.

tinnitus—Ringing in the ears.

tonic—Referring to a sustained contraction of a muscle or muscle group.

tornado—A violent, rotating column of air, with the narrow end touching the earth.

tort—Damage, injury, or a wrongful act done willfully, negligently, or in circumstances involving strict liability but not involving breach of contract, for which a civil suit can be brought; a remedy normally will be provided, usually in the form of monetary damages.

tourniquet—A constricting device used to control serious bleeding. The pressure is applied circumferentially around the limb.

toxicology—Study of the nature and effects of poisons and harmful drugs and chemicals.

transcutaneous electrical nerve stimulation (TENS)—The use of a therapeutic device that stimulates peripheral nerves by passing an electrical current through the skin.

transdermal—Across the skin; transdermal application is used in pharmacology to transmit a drug across the dermis (skin).

transient neuropraxia—Condition in which neuropraxic and nerve symptoms such as sensory and motor changes usually subside within a few minutes to a few days.

traumatic brain injury—Damage to the brain from impact or acceleration.

triglyceride—A chemical compound made by the combination of glycerol and three fatty acids. It is the main component of vegetable oil and animal fats.

tropocollagen—A molecule that composes collagen in a triple helix strand. Tropocollagen is made of three intertwining polypeptide strands held together by hydrogen bonds.

turf toc—A sprain of the first metatarsophalangeal typically caused by excessive extension or dorsiflexion.

type I collagen—The strongest, most abundant collagen in the human body; composes ligaments, tendons, and muscles as well as mature scar tissue following the inflammatory process.

type II collagen—The collagen present in hyaline cartilage among other types of tissues; has specialized functions.

type III collagen—The major component of granulation tissue, produced by fibroblasts. It is less able to resist stress than the other types of collagen, and damage results if forces exceed its tensile strength.

ulnar—On the little-finger side of the hand, wrist, or forearm.

ultrasound—High-frequency acoustic energy.

unconscious—Relating to a mental state that renders the patient unresponsive.

undescended testicle—A birth defect, also called cryptorchidism, in which the testicle fails to migrate out of the abdominopelvic area through the inguinal canal to enter the scrotum. Usually the testicle descends within the first year of life.

Universal Precautions—A technique used to protect the clinician from exposure to bloodborne pathogens.

urinalysis (UA)—A series of tests performed on a specimen of urine; a routine test that is commonly a part of both athletic physicals and general, well-person physicals.

valgus stress—Joint stress that occurs in the frontal plane toward the midline.

validity—In statistics, the extent to which a measurement is within an acceptable range.

valsalva maneuver—Holding of the breath to increase intrathoracic pressure.

varus stress—Joint stress that occurs in the frontal plane away from the midline.

vasoconstriction—Constriction of blood vessels, effectively decreasing blood flow through them.

vasodilation—Dilation of blood vessels, effectively increasing blood flow through them.

ventilator—A machine that mechanically moves air into and out of the lungs.

vision statement—A concise statement that describes the ideal state to which an organization aspires.

wheal—A reaction of the skin surface characterized by an elevated patch of skin that appears smooth and red.

wheeled transporter—Any device with wheels that makes moving an individual easier; may be machine powered or moved by human power.

windchill—The effect of wind on the feeling of low air temperature on the skin.

Young's modulus of elasticity—Graph to explain the change in length of a material in relation to the stress applied. The slope of the line is the stiffness of the material, while the inverse of the slope is the compliance of the tissue.

References

Part Openers

NATA-BOC, 2011, "Athletic Training Education Competencies", 5th Edition, NATA, pp. 1-31

Introduction

Laster-Bradley, M., and B.A. Berger. 1991. Evaluation of drug distribution systems in university athletic programs: Development of a model of "optimal" distribution system for athletic programs. Unpublished report. Auburn University, Alabama.

Chapter 1

American Heart Association. 2007. Recommendations and considerations related to pre-participation screening for cardiovascular abnormalities in competitive athletics: 2007 update. *Circulation* 115(March):1643-1655.

Maron, B.J., and D.P. Zipes. 2005. Introduction: Eligibility recommendations for competitive athletes with cardiovascular abnormalities-general considerations. 36th Bethesda Conference. *Journal of the American College of Cardiology* 45:1318-1321.

National Collegiate Athletic Association. 2010. *2010-2011 NCAA sports medicine handbook.* Indianapolis: National Collegiate Athletic Association. Retrieved June 10, 2011 from www.ncaapublications.com/p-4203-2010-2011-sports-medicine-handbook.aspx.

Rice, S.G. and the American Academy of Pediatrics' Council on Sports Medicine and Fitness. 2008. Medical conditions affecting sports participation. *Pediatrics* 121(4, April):841-848.

Chapter 2

Fleck, S.J., and W.J. Kraemer. 2004. *Designing resistance training programs,* 3rd ed. Champaign, IL: Human Kinetics.

Hettinger, R. 1961. Effect of isometric training on the elbow flexion force torque of grade five boys. *Research Quarterly for Exercise and Sport* 47:41-47.

Shultz, S.A., P.A. Houglum, and D.H. Perrin. 2010. *Examination of musculoskeletal injuries,* 3rd ed. Champaign, IL: Human Kinetics.

Chapter 3

Boden, B., D.C. Osbahr, and C. Jimenez. 2001. Low-risk stress fractures. *American Journal of Sports Medicine* 29(1): 100-111.

Centers for Disease Control and Prevention. 1998. Hyperthermia and dehydration-related deaths associated with intentional rapid weight loss in three collegiate wrestlers—North Carolina, Wisconsin, and Michigan November-December, 1997. *Morbidity and Mortality Weekly Report* 47(6):105-108.

Chapter 4

Binkley, H.M., J. Beckett, D.J. Casa, D.M. Kleiner, et al. 2002. National Athletic Trainers' Association position statement: Exertional heat illnesses. *Journal of Athletic Training* 37(3):329-343.

Casa, D.J., L.E. Armstrong, S.K. Hillman, et al. 2000. National Athletic Trainers' Association position statement: Fluid replacement for athletes. *Journal of Athletic Training* 35(2):212-224.

Chapter 5

Appenzeller, H. 1985. *Sports and law: Contemporary issues.* Charlottesville, VA: Michie.

Austria v. Bike Athletic Co. 810 P. 2d 1312 (1991).

Brahatcek v. Millard School District. 273 N.W. 2d 680, 202 Neb. 86 (1979).

Centers for Disease Control and Prevention. 2008. Potential exposure to lead in artificial turf: Public health issues, actions and recommendations. Official CDC Health Advisory, distributed via Health Alert Network, June 18, 2008.

Mitten, M.J. 2002. Emerging legal issues in sports medicine: A synthesis, summary and analysis, *St. John's Law Review* 76(1):1-21.

Monaco v. Raymond (superintendent of Yonkers City School District), 122 Misc.2d 370 (1984).

Rawlings Sporting Goods Co., Inc. v. Daniels. 619 S.W. 2d 435 (Tex. Civ. App. 1981).

Chapter 6

Beam, J.W. 2006. *Orthopedic taping, wrapping, bracing, and padding.* Philadelphia: Davis.

Hillman, S.K. 2005. *Introduction to athletic training.* Champaign, IL: Human Kinetics.

Perrin, D. 2012. *Athletic taping and bracing,* 3rd ed. Champaign, IL: Human Kinetics.

Chapter 7

Bonfiglio, R., L.A. Cone, and F.P. Lagattuta. 1998. Pathophysiology of soft tissue injuries. In R.E. Windsor and D. Lox (eds.), *Soft tissue injuries: Diagnosis and treatment.* Philadelphia: Hanley & Belfus.

Harris, R.B. 1983. *Textbook of disorders and injuries of the musculoskeletal system,* 2nd ed. Baltimore: Williams & Wilkins.

Moore, K.L., A.F. Dalley, and A. Aqur. 2009. *Clinically oriented anatomy,* 6th ed. Baltimore: Lippincott, Williams & Wilkins.

Chapter 8

Maitland, D.G. 1991. *Peripheral manipulation.* Boston: Butterworth-Heinemann.

Ray, R., and J. Konin. 2011. *Management strategies in athletic training,* 4th ed. Champaign, IL: Human Kinetics.

Shultz, S.J., P.A. Houglum, and D.H. Perrin. 2010. *Examination of musculoskeletal injuries,* 3rd ed. Champaign, IL: Human Kinetics.

Chapter 9

Andrews, J.R., and J.A. Whiteside. 1993. Common elbow problems in the athlete. *Journal of Orthopedic and Sports Physical Therapy* 17(6):289-295.

Shultz, S.J., P.A. Houglum, and D.H. Perrin, 2010. *Examination of musculoskeletal injuries,* 3rd ed. Champaign, IL: Human Kinetics.

Chapter 10

Shultz, S.J., P.A. Houglum, and D.H. Perrin. 2010. *Examination of musculoskeletal injuries,* 3rd ed. Champaign, IL: Human Kinetics.

Chapter 11

Cantu, R.C. 2001. Posttraumatic retrograde and anterograde amnesia: Pathophysiology and implications in grading and safe return to play. *Journal of Athletic Training* 36(3):244-248.

Cantu, R.C., and R. Voy. 1995. Second-impact syndrome. *Physician and Sportsmedicine* 23: 27-34.

Moore, K.L. 1992. *Clinically oriented anatomy,* 3rd ed. Baltimore: Williams & Wilkins.

Shultz, S.J., P.A. Houglum, and D.H. Perrin. 2010. *Examination of musculoskeletal injuries,* 3rd ed. Champaign, IL: Human Kinetics.

Torg, J.S., R.J. Naranja, H. Palov, B.J. Galinat, R. Warren, and R.A. Stine. 1996. The relationship of developmental narrowing of the cervical spinal canal to reversible and irreversible injury of the cervical spinal cord in football players. *Journal of Bone and Joint Surgery* 78A:1308-1314.

Chapter 12

American Heart Association. 2003. Atherosclerosis. Retrieved November 2, 2004, from www.americanheart.org/presenter.jhtml?identifer=4440.

Venes, D., ed. 2010. *Taber's cyclopedic medical dictionary,* 21st ed. Philadelphia: Davis.

Chapter 13

Boissy, P., I. Shrier, S. Briere, J. Mellete, L. Fecteau, G.O. Matheson, D. Garza, W.H. Meeuwisse, E. Segal, J Boulay, and R.J. Steele. 2011. Effectiveness of cervical spine stabilization techniques. *Clinical Journal of Sport Medicine* 21(2):80-88.

Centers for Disease Control and Prevention. 2010 update. Bloodborne infectious diseases: HIV/ AIDS, hepatitis B, hepatitis C. Retrieved June 21, 2001, from www.cdc.gov/niosh/topics/bbp/.

Domeier, R.M. 1999, March. Indications for prehospital spinal immobilization. Position paper, National Association of EMS Physicians. Retreived July 6, 2011 from www.naemsp.org/pdf/spinal.pdf.

Huynh, P.N., E.K. Hu, J.F. Linzer, L Scott, and S. Thobani. 2011, March 29 update. Exercise-induced anaphylaxis. Retrieved June 21, 2001, from http://emedicine.medscape.com/article/886641.

McCrory, P., W. Meeuwisse, K. Johnston, J. Dvorak, M. Aubry, M. Molloy, and R. Cantu. 2009, May. Consensus Statement on Concussion in Sport – the 3rd International Conference on Concussion in Sport, held in Zurich, November 2008. *Clinical Journal of Sport Medicine* 19(3):185-195.

The Section on Disorders of the Spine and Peripheral Nerves of the American Association of Neurological Surgeons and the Congress of Neurological Surgeons. 2001, September. Pre-hospital spinal immobilization following trauma. Retrieved July 6, 2011 from http://static.spineuniverse.com/pdf/traumaguide/1.pdf.

Chapter 14

Ray, R. and J.G. Konin, 2011. *Management strategies in athletic training,* 4th ed. Champaign, IL: Human Kinetics.

Chapter 15

Hildebrand, K.A., C.L. Gallang-Behm, A.S. Kydd, and D.A. Hart. 2005. The basics of soft tissue healing and general factors that influence such healing. *Sports Medicine and Arthroscopy Review* 11(3):136-144.

Kubler-Ross, E. 1969. *On death and dying.* New York: Macmillan.

Peterson, P. 1986. The grief response and injury. *Athletic Training* 21:312-314.

Rotella, R.J. 1985. The psychological care of the patient. In *Sports psychology: Psychological consideration in maximizing sport performance.* Ann Arbor, MI: McNaughton and Gun.

Chapter 16

Bjordal, J.M., R.A. Lopes-Martins, J. Joensen, C. Couppe, A.E. Ljunggren, A. Stergioulas, and M.I. Johnson. 2008, May. A systematic review with procedural assessments and meta-analysis of low level laser therapy in lateral elbow tendinopathy (tennis elbow). *BMC Musculoskeletal Disorders* 9:75.

Denegar, C.R., E. Saliba, and S. Saliba. 2010. *Therapeutic modalities for musculoskeletal injuries,* 3rd ed. Champaign, IL: Human Kinetics, 206.

Draper D.O., J.C. Castel, and D. Castel. 1995. Rates of temperature increase in human muscle during 1 MHz and 3 MHz continuous ultrasound. *Journal of Orthopaedic and Sports Physical Therapy* 22:142-150.

Enwemeka, C.S., J. Parker, D. Dowdy, E. Harkness, L.E. Sanford, and L.D. Woodruff. 2004. The effects of laser therapy on tissue repair and pain control. A meta analysis of the literature. *Photomedicine and Laser Surgery* 22(4):323-329.

Fond, D., and B. Hecox. 1994. Intermittent pneumatic compression. In B. Hecox, T.A. Mehreteab, and J. Weisberg, eds., *Physical agents.* Norwalk, CT: Appleton & Lange, 419-428.

Fritz, J.M., W. Lindsay, J.W. Matheson, G.P. Brennan, S.J. Hunter, S.D. Moffit, A. Swalberg, and B. Rodriquez, 2007. Is there a subpopulation of patients with low back pain likely to benefit from mechanical traction? Results of a randomized clinical trial and subgrouping analysis. *Spine* 32:E793-800.

Gersten, J. 1958. Effect of metallic objects on temperature rises produced in tissue by ultrasound. *American Journal of Physical Medicine* 37:75-82.

Hernandez., L.C., P. Santisteban, and M.E. del Valle-Soto. 1989. Changes in mRNA of thyroglobin, cytoskeleton of thyroid cell and thyroid hormone levels induced by IR-laser radiation. *Laser Therapy* 1(4):203-208.

Hooker, D. 1998. Intermittent compression devices. In W.E. Prentice, ed., *Therapeutic modalities for allied health professionals.* New York: McGraw-Hill, 392-403.

Hopkins, J.T., T.A. McLoda, J.G. Seegmiller, and G.D. Baxter. 2004, September. Low-level laser therapy facilitates superficial wound healing in humans: A triple-blind, sham-controlled study. *Journal of Athletic Training* 39(3):223-229.

Johns, L.D., S.J. Straub, and S.M. Howard. 2007a. Analysis of effective radiating area, power, intensity, and field characteristics of ultrasound transducers. *Archives of Physical Medicine and Rehabilitation* 88:124-129.

Johns, L.D., S.J. Straub, and S.M. Howard. 2007b. Variability in effective radiating area and output power of new ultrasound transducers at 3 MHz. *Journal of Athletic Training* 42:22-28.

Lehmann, J.F., B. Delateur, and D.R. Silverman. 1966. Selective heating effects of ultrasound in human beings. *Archives of Physical Medicine and Rehabilitation* 47:331-338.

Seiger, C., and D.O. Draper. 2010, September. Use of pulsed shortwave diathermy and joint mobilization to increase ankle range of motion in the presence of surgical implanted metal: A case series. *Journal of Orthopaedic and Sports Physical Therapy* 36(9):669-677.

Shooshtari, S.M., V. Badiee, S.H. Taghizadeh, A.H. Nematollahi, A.H. Amanollahi, and M.T. Grami. 2008, June-July. The effects of low level laser in clinical outcome and neurophysiological results of carpal tunnel syndrome. *Electromyography and Clinical Neurophysiology* 48(5):229-231.

Sicard-Rosenbaum, L., D. Lord, J.V. Danoff, A.K. Thom, and M.A. Eckhaus. 1995. Effects of continuous therapeutic ultrasound on growth and metastasis of subcutaneous murine tumors. *Physical Therapy* 75:3-11.

Stergioulas, A., M. Stergioula, R. Aarskog, R.A. Lopes-Martins, and J.M. Bjordal. 2008, May. Effects of low-level laser therapy and eccentric exercises in the treatment of recreational athletes with chronic achilles tendinopathy. *American Journal of Sports Medicine* 36(5):881-887.

Straub, S.J., L.D. Johns, and S.M. Howard. 2008. Variability in effective radiating area at 1 MHz affects ultrasound treatment intensity. *Physical Therapy* 88(1):50-57.

Travel, J.G., and D.G. Simons. 1983. *Myofascial pain and dysfunction: The trigger point manual.* Baltimore: Williams & Wilkins.

Tsang, K.K.W., J.H. Hertel, C.R. Denegar, and W.E. Buckley. 2001. The effects of elevation and intermittent compression on the volume of injured ankles (Abstract). *Journal of Athletic Training* 36:S-50.

Tume, K.G., and S. Tume. 1994. *A practitioner's guide to laser therapy and musculoskeletal injuries.* Port Noarlunga, South Australia: Southern Pain Control Centre, 16.

Tuner, J., and L. Hode. 2002. *Laser therapy: Clinical practice and scientific background.* Tallinn, Estonia, 103.

U.S. Department of Health and Human Services Food and Drug Administration, Washington, DC (03/23/04) Final 510(K) Summary of Application #K032816. Retrieved 02/28/2011.

U.S. Department of Health and Human Services Food and Drug Administration, Washington, DC (07/29/02) Acculaser, Inc. Summary of 510(k) Premarket Notification KO20657. Retrieved 02/28/2011.

Walker, N.A., C.R. Denegar, and J. Preische. 2007. Systematic review of LIPUS and PEMF in treatment of tibial fractures. *Journal of Athletic Training* 42:530-535.

Wohlgemuth, W.A., G. Warner, T. Reiss, T. Wagner, and K. Bohndorf. 2001. In vivo laser-induced interstitial thermotherapy of pig liver with a temperature-controlled diode laser and MRI correlation. *Lasers in Surgery and Medicine* 29(4):374-378.

Woodruff, L.D., J.M. Bounkeo, W.M. Brannon, K.S. Dawes Jr., C.D. Barham, D.L. Waddell, and C.S. Enwemeka. 2004. The efficacy of laser therapy in the treatment of wounds: A meta-analysis of the literature. *Photomedicine and Laser Surgery* 22(3):241-247.

Chapter 17

Cyriax, J.H. 1977. *Textbook of orthopedic medicine.* Vol. 2, *Treatment by manipulation, massage and injection.* Baltimore: Williams & Wilkins.

Houglum, P.A. 2010. *Therapeutic exercise for musculoskeletal injuries,* 3rd ed. Champaign, IL: Human Kinetics.

Kaltenborn, F.M. 2002. *Mobilization of the extremity joints,* 5th ed. Vol. 1, *The extremities.* Minneapolis: OTPT.

Knight, K.L. 1985. Guidelines for rehabilitation of sports injuries. *Clinics in Sports Medicine* 4:405-416.

Maitland, G.D. 1991. *Peripheral manipulation.* London: Butterworth-Heinemann.

Mennell, J.M. 1964. *Joint pain: Diagnosis and treatment using manipulative techniques.* Boston, MA: Little, Brown & Co.

Paris, S.V., and C. Patla. 1988. *E1 course notes: Extremity dysfunction and manipulation.* St. Augustine, FL: Patris.

Saal, J.S. 1987. Flexibility training. In J.A. Saal, ed., *Rehabilitation of sport injuries.* Philadelphia: Hanley & Belfus.

Chapter 18

Denegar, C.R., E. Saliba, and S. Saliba. 2010. *Therapeutic modalities for musculoskeletal injuries,* 3rd ed. Champaign, IL: Human Kinetics.

Houglum, P.A. 2010. *Therapeutic exercise for musculoskeletal injuries,* 3rd ed. Champaign, IL: Human Kinetics.

Mycek, M.K, R.A. Harvey, and P.C. Champe. 2000. *Pharmacology: Lippincott's illustrated reviews.* Baltimore: Lippincott, Williams & Wilkins.

Ray, R., and J. Konin. 2011. *Management strategies in athletic training,* 4th ed. Champaign, IL: Human Kinetics.

Smith SM, Schroeder K, Fahey T. Over-the-counter medications for acute cough in children and adults in ambulatory settings. Cochrane Database of Systematic Reviews 2008. Issue 1. Art No:CD001831. DOI 10.1002/14651858. CD001831.pub3

Chapter 19

Block, P. 1987. *The empowered manager: Positive political skills at work.* San Francisco: Jossey-Bass.

Bruce, S.D. 1986. *Prewritten job descriptions.* Madison, CT: Business and Legal Reports.

Castetter, W.B. 1992. *The personnel function in educational administration,* 5th ed. New York: Macmillan.

Equal Employment Opportunity Commission. 1978. *Uniform guidelines on employee selection procedures.* Washington, DC: Bureau of National Affairs.

Fowler, A.R., and S.C. Bushardt. 1986. T.O.P.E.S.: Developing a task oriented performance evaluation system. *Advanced Management Journal* 51(4):4-8.

Gabriel, A.J. 1981. Medical communications: Records for the professional athletic trainer. *Athletic Training* 16(l):68-69.

Garofalo, M.J. 1989. How strategies can get lost in the translation. *Business Month* 134(10):82-83.

Gibson, C.K., D.J. Newton, and D.S. Cochran. 1990. An empirical investigation of the nature of hospital mission statements. *Health Care Management Review* 15(3):35-45.

Haddad, S.A. 1985. Compensation and benefits. In W. Tracey, ed., *Human resources management and development handbook.* New York: AMACOM, 638-660.

Hawkins, J.D. 1989. Sports medicine record keeping: The key to effective communication and documentation. *Sports Medicine Standards and Malpractice Reporter* 1(2):31-35.

Horine, L. 1991. *Administration of physical education and sport programs,* 2nd ed. Dubuque, IA: Brown.

Jones, R.L., and H.G. Trentin. 1971. *Budgeting: Key to planning and control,* 2nd ed. New York: American Management Association.

Kettenbach, G. 1995. *Writing S.O.A.P. notes,* 2nd ed. Philadelphia: Davis.

Kettenbach, G. 2009. *Writing patient/client notes,* 4th ed. Philadelphia: Davis.

Mayo, H.B. 1978. *Basic finance.* Philadelphia: Saunders.

Miles, B.J. 1987. Injuries on the road: Good information reduces problems. *Athletic Training* 22(2):127.

Nelson, S., E. Altman, and D. Mayo. 2000. *Managing for results.* Chicago: American Library Association.

Pearce, J.A. 1982. The company mission as a strategic tool. *Sloan Management Review* 23(2):15-23.

Ray, R.R. 1990. An injury-free budget. *College Athletic Management* 2(l):42-45.

Spallina, J.M. 2004. Strategic planning—getting started: Mission, vision and values. *Journal of Oncology Management* 13(1):10-11.

U.S. Small Business Administration. 1980. *Job analysis, job specifications, and job descriptions.* Washington, DC: U.S. Government Printing Office.

Wildavsky, A. 1975. *Budgeting: A comparative theory of budgetary processes.* Boston: Little, Brown.

Yate, M. 2002. *Knock 'em dead.* Avon, MA: Adams.

Young, I. P. 2007. *Human resource function in the educational administration,* 8th ed. Upper Saddle River, NJ: Prentice Hall.

Chapter 20

Albohm, M.J., and G.B. Wilkerson. 1999. An outcomes assessment of care provided by certified athletic trainers. *Journal of Rehabilitation Outcomes Measurement* 3(3):51-56.

Andersen, J.C., R.W. Courson, D.M. Kleiner, and T.A. McLoda. 2002. National Athletic Trainers' Association position statement: Emergency planning in athletics. *Journal of Athletic Training* 37:99-104.

Binkley, H. M., Beckett, J., Casa, D. J., Kleiner, D. M. and Plummer, P. E., National athletic trainers association position statement; exertional heat illness. *Journal of Athletic Training* 37(3):329-343.

Board of Certification (2010). The 2009 Athletic Trainer Role delineation study, Omaha, NE: Stephen B. Johnson Retrieved from: http://www.bocatc.org/index.php?option= com_content&view=article&id=109:role-delineation-study&catid=14:resources.

Chambers, R.L., N.V. Ross, and J. Kozubowski. 1986. Insurance types and coverages: Knowledge to plan for the future (with a focus on motor skill activities and athletics). *Physical Educator* 44(l):233-240.

Ciccolella, M. 1991. Caught in court. *College Athletic Management* 3(4):10-13.

Consensus statement on concussion in sport: The 3rd international conference on concussion in sport held in Zurich, 2008. 2009. *Clinical Journal of Sport Medicine* 19(3):185-200.

Culp, B., N.D. Goemaere, and E. Miller. 1985. Risk management: An integral part of quality assurance. In C.G. Meisenheimer, ed., *Quality assurance: A complete guide to effective programs.* Rockville, MD: Aspen, 169-192.

Danzon, P.M. 1985. *Medical malpractice.* Cambridge, MA: Harvard University Press.

DeCarlo, M.S. 1997. Reimbursement for health care services. In J.G. Konin, ed., *Clinical athletic training.* Thorofare, NJ: Slack, 89-104.

Drowatzky, J.N. 1985. Legal duties and liability in athletic training. *Athletic Training* 20(l):10-13.

Gieck, J., J. Lowe, and K. Kenna. 1984. Trainer malpractice: A sleeping giant. *Athletic Training* 19(l):41-46.

Godek, J.J. 1992. Sports rehabilitation in the '90s: Who's who? *Journal of Sport Rehabilitation* 1:87-94.

Gorse, K., R. Blanc, F. Feld, and M. Radelet. 2010. *Emergency care in athletic training.* Philadelphia: Davis.

Graham, L.S. 1985. Ten ways to dodge the malpractice bullet. *Athletic Training* 20(2):117-119.

Hart, P.M., and S.L. Cole. 1992. Subtracting insult from injury. *Athletic Business* 16(5):39-42.

Herbert, D.L. 1990. *Legal aspects of sports medicine.* Canton, OH: Professional Reports Corporation.

Horsley, J.E., and J. Carlova. 1983. *Testifying in court.* Oradell, NJ: Medical Economics.

Inter-Association Task Force on Exertional Heat Illnesses Consensus Statement. 2003. Retrieved from http://www.nata.org/sites/default/files/inter-association-task-force-exertional-heat-illness.pdf.

Lehr, C. 1992. Status of medical insurance provided to student-athletes at NCAA schools. *Journal of Legal Aspects of Sport* 2(l):12-22.

Leiske, A.M. 1985. Standards: The basis of a quality assurance program. In C.G. Meisenheimer, ed., *Quality assurance: A complete guide to effective programs.* Rockville, MD: Aspen, 45-72.

Leverenz, L.J., and L.B. Helms. 1990a. Suing athletic trainers: Part I. *Athletic Training* 25(3):212-216.

Leverenz, L.J., and L.B. Helms. 1990b. Suing athletic trainers: Part II. *Athletic Training* 25(3):219-226.

May, C.A., C. Schraeder, and T. Britt. 1996. *Managed care and case management: Roles for professional nursing.* Washington, DC: American Nurses.

National Collegiate Athletic Association. 2010. *2010-2011 NCAA sports medicine handbook.* Indianapolis: National Collegiate Athletic Association.

O'Leary, M.R. 1994. *Lexicon.* Oakbrook Terrace, IL: Joint Commission on Accreditation of Healthcare Organizations.

Rankin, J.M., and C. Ingersoll. 2000. *Athletic training management: Concepts and applications,* 2nd ed. New York: McGraw-Hill.

Rehberg, R.S. 2007. *Sports emergency care: A team approach.* Thorofare, NJ: Slack.

Rowell, J.C. 1989. *Understanding medical insurance reimbursement: A step-by-step guide.* Oradell, NJ: Medical Economics.

Scott, R.W. 1990. *Health care malpractice.* Thorofare, NJ: Slack.

Sideline preparedness for the team physician: A consensus statement. 2000. Retrieved from: www.amssm.org/MemberFiles/SidelinePrepare.pdf. Publication by six sports medicine organizations: AAFP, AAOS, ACSM, AMSSM, AOSSM, and AOASM.

van der Smissen, B. 2001. Tort liability and risk management. In B.L. Parkhouse, ed., *The management of sport: Its foundation and application.* New York: McGraw-Hill, 177-198.

Wadlington, W., J.R. Waltz, and R.B. Dworkin. 1980. *Law and medicine.* Mineola, NY: Foundation Press.

Walsh, K.M., B. Bennett, M. Cooper, R.L. Holle, R. Kithill, and R.E. Lopez. 2000. National Athletic Trainers' Association position statement: Lightning safety for athletics and recreation. *Journal of Athletic Training* 35:471-477.

Chapter 21

Chandrashekar, N., J. Hashemi, J. Slauterbeck, and B.D. Beynnon. 2008. Low-load behaviour of the patellar tendon graft and its relevance to the biomechanics of the reconstructed knee. *Clinical Biomechanics (Bristol, Avon)* 23:918-925.

Denegar, C.R, E. Saliba, and S. Saliba. 2010. *Therapeutic modalities for musculoskeletal injuries,* 3rd ed. Champaign, IL: Human Kinetics.

Egan, J.M. 1987. A constitutive model for the mechanical behaviour of soft connective tissues. *Journal of Biomechanics* 20:681-692.

Houglum, P.A. 2010. *Therapeutic exercise for musculoskeletal injuries,* 3rd ed. Champaign, IL: Human Kinetics.

Magnusson, S.P., P. Aagaard, E.B. Simonsen, and F. Bojsen-Moller. 2000. Passive tensile stress and energy of the human hamstring muscles in vivo. *Scandinavian Journal of Medicine and Science in Sports* 10:351-359.

Moger, C.J., K.P. Arkill, R. Barrett, P. Bleuet, R.E. Ellis, E.M. Green, and C.P. Winlove. 2009. Cartilage collagen matrix reorientation and displacement in response to surface loading. *Journal of Biomechanical Engineering* 131:031008.

Pietrosimone, B.G., J.M. Hart, S.A. Saliba, J. Hertel, and C.D. Ingersoll. 2009. Immediate effects of transcutaneous electrical nerve stimulation and focal knee joint cooling on quadriceps activation. *Medicine and Science in Sports and Exercise* 41:1175-1181.

Rees, J.D., N. Maffulli, and J. Cook. 2009. Management of tendinopathy. *American Journal of Sports Medicine* 37:1855-1867.

Sharma, P., and N. Maffulli. 2005. Tendon injury and tendinopathy: Healing and repair. *Journal of Bone and Joint Surgery, American* 87:187-202.

Sharma, P., and N. Maffulli. 2006. Biology of tendon injury: Healing, modeling and remodeling. *Journal of Musculoskeletal and Neuronal Interactions* 6:181-190.

Shultz, S.J., P.A. Houglum, and D.H. Perrin. 2010. *Examination of musculoskeletal injuries,* 3rd ed. Champaign, IL: Human Kinetics.

Viidik, A. 1973. Functional properties of collagenous tissues. *International Review of Connective Tissue Research* 6:127-215.

Chapter 22

Andersen, M.B., and J.M. Williams. 1988. A model of stress and athletic injury: Prediction and prevention. *Journal of Sport and Exercise Psychology* 10:294-306.

Board of Certification. 2010. *The 2009 athletic trainer role delineation study.* Omaha: Stephen B. Johnson.

Brewer, B.W., A.J. Petitpas, and J.L. Van Raalte. 1999. Referral of injured athletes for counseling and psychotherapy. In R. Ray and D.M. Wiese-Bjornstal, eds., *Counseling in sports medicine.* Champaign, IL: Human Kinetics, 127-141.

Flint, F.A. 1991. The psychological effects of modeling in athletic injury rehabilitation. Unpublished doctoral dissertation, University of Oregon, Eugene. Microform Publications No. BF 357.

Flint, F.A. 1998a, January. Sport psychology and rehabilitation. Paper presented at the annual conference of the Eastern Athletic Trainers' Association, Buffalo, NY.

Flint, F.A. 1998b. *Psychology of sport injury*. Champaign, IL: Human Kinetics.

Flint, F.A. 2007a. Modeling in injury rehabilitation. In D. Pargman, ed., *Psychological bases of sport injury*, 3rd ed. Morgantown, WV: Fitness Information Technology, 95-107.

Flint, F.A. 2007b. Matching psychological strategies with physical rehabilitation. In D. Pargman, ed., *Psychological bases of sport injury*, 3rd ed. Morgantown, WV: Fitness Information Technology, 319-334.

Kulik, J. A. and Mahler, H. I. 1987. Effects of pre-operative roommate assignment on postoperative anxiety and recovery from coronary-bypass surgery. *Health Psychology* 6:525-543.

Lemberger, M.E. 2008. Systematic referrals: Issues and processes related to psychosocial referrals for athletic trainers. In J.M. Mensch and G.M. Miller, eds., *The athletic trainers' guide to psychosocial intervention and referral*. Thorofare, NJ: Slack, 65-99.

National Athletic Trainers' Association. 2005. *NATA code of ethics*. Retrieved February 2, 2009, from http://www.nata.org/codeofethics.

National Athletic Trainers' Association. 2011. *Athletic training educational competencies*, 5th ed. Retrieved March 28, 2011, from www.nata.org/education/competencies.

Stiller-Ostrowski, J.L., and J.A. Ostrowski. 2009. Recently certified athletic trainers' undergraduate educational preparation in psychosocial intervention and referral. *Journal of Athletic Training* 44(1):67-75.

Wiese-Bjornstal, D.M. 2009. Sport injury and college athlete health across the lifespan. *Journal of Intercollegiate Sports* 2:64-80.

Wiese-Bjornstal, D.M. 2010. Psychology and socioculture affect injury risk, response, and recovery in high-intensity athletes: A consensus statement. *Scandinavian Journal of Medicine and Science in Sport* 20 (Suppl 2):108-116.

Chapter 23

Bachmann, L.M., E. Kolb, M.T. Koller, J. Steurer, G. ter Riet. 2003. Accuracy of Ottawa ankle rules to exclude fractures of the ankle and midfoot: Systematic review. *British Medical Journal* 326(7386):417.

Ebell, M.H., J. Siwek, B.D. Weiss, S.H. Woolf, J. Susman, B. Ewigman, M. Bowman. 2004. Strength of recommendation taxonomy (SORT): a patient-centered approach to grading evidence in the medical literature. *Journal of the American Board of Family Practice*, 17(1):59-67.

Field, M.J., and K.N. Lohr 1990. *Clinical practice guidelines: Directions of a new program*. Washington, DC: National Academy Press.

Guyatt, G., R. Drummond, M. Meade, D. Cook. 2008. *Users' guides to the medical literature: A manual for evidence-based clinical practice*, 2nd ed. New York: McGraw-Hill Medical.

Haynes, R.B. 2001. Of studies, summaries, synopses, and systems: The "4S" evolution of services for finding current best evidence. *Evidence-Based Mental Health* 4(2):37-39.

Haynes, R.B. 2006. Of studies, syntheses, synopses, summaries, and systems: The "5S" evolution of information services for evidence-based health care decisions. *ACP Journal Club* 145(3):A8.

Hertel, J. 2005. Research training for clinicians: The crucial link between evidence-based practice and third-party reimbursement. *Journal of Athletic Training* 40(2):69-70.

Hurwitz, S.R., D. Slawson, A. Shaughnessy. 2000. Orthopaedic information mastery: Applying evidence-based information tools to improve patient outcomes while saving orthopaedists' time. *Journal of Bone and Joint Surgery, American* 82(6):888-894.

Institute of Medicine. 2003. *Health professions education: A bridge to quality*. Washington, DC: Institute of Medicine.

Medina, J.M., P.O. McKeon, J. Hertel. 2006. Rating the levels of evidence in sports-medicine research. *Athletic Therapy Today* 11(5):42-45.

Oxford Centre for Evidence-Based Medicine. (2009). Levels of Evidence. http://www.cebm.net/?o=1025.

Parsons, J.T., T.C. Valovich McLeod, A.R. Snyder, E.L. Sauers. 2008. Change is hard: Adopting a disablement model for athletic training. *Journal of Athletic Training* 43(4):446-448.

Pew Health Professions Commission. 1998, December. *Recreating health professional practice for a new century: The fourth report of the Pew Health Professions Commission*.

Sackett, D.L., and W.M. Rosenberg. 1995. The need for evidence-based medicine. *Journal of the Royal Society of Medicine* 88(11):620-624.

Sackett, D.L., W.M. Rosenberg, J.A. Gray, R.B. Haynes, W.S. Richardson. 1996. Evidence based medicine: What it is and what it isn't. *British Medical Journal* 312(7023):71-72.

Snyder, A.R., J.T. Parsons, T.C. Valovich McLeod, R.C. Bay, L.A. Michener, E.L. Sauers. 2008. Utilizing disablement models and clinical outcomes assessment to enable evidence-based athletic training practice: Part I - disablement models. *Journal of Athletic Training* 43(4):428-436.

Steves, R., and J.M. Hootman. 2004. Evidence-based medicine: What is it and how does it apply to athletic training? *Journal of Athletic Training* 39(1):83-87.

Stillwell, S.B., E. Fineout-Overholt, B.M. Melnyk, K.M. Williamson. 2010. Evidence-based practice, step by step: Searching for the evidence. *American Journal of Nursing* 110(5):41-47.

Valovich McLeod, T.C., A.R. Snyder, J.T. Parsons, R.C. Bay, L.A. Michener, E.L. Sauers. 2008. Utilizing disablement models and clinical outcomes assessment to enable evidence-based athletic training practice: Part II - clinical outcomes assessment. *Journal of Athletic Training* 43(4):437-445.

Wells, P.S., J. Hirsh, D.R. Anderson, A.W. Lensing, G. Foster, C. Kearon, J Weitz, R. D'Ovidio, A. Cogo, P. Prandoni.1995. Accuracy of clinical assessment of deep-vein thrombosis. *Lancet* 345(8961):1326-1330.

Index

Note: The letters *f* and *t* after page numbers indicate figures and tables, respectively.